FORENSIC NURSING

Evidence-Based Principles and Practice

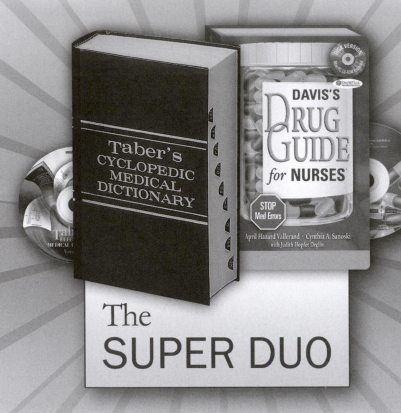
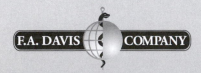

FORENSIC NURSING

Evidence-Based Principles and Practice

Rose E. Constantino, PhD, JD, RN, FAAN, FACFE
Associate Professor
Department of Health & Community Systems
University of Pittsburgh School of Nursing
Pittsburgh, Pennsylvania

Patricia A. Crane, PhD, MSN, RNC, WHNP
Assistant Professor, School of Nursing
University of Texas Medical Branch Galveston
Galveston, Texas

Susan E. Young, PhD Candidate, RN
Doctoral Candidate
School of Nursing
University of North Carolina at Chapel Hill
Chapel Hill, North Carolina

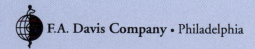

F.A. Davis Company • Philadelphia

F. A. Davis Company
1915 Arch Street
Philadelphia, PA 19103
www.fadavis.com

Printed in the United States of America

Last digit indicates print number: 10 9 8 7 6 5 4 3 2 1

Sr. Acquisitions Editor: Thomas Ciavarella
Director of Content Development: Darlene D. Pedersen
Manager of Art and Design: Carolyn O'Brien
Project Editor: Elizabeth Hart
Electronic Project Editor: Sandra Glennie

As new scientific information becomes available through basic and clinical research, recommended treatments and drug therapies undergo changes. The author(s) and publisher have done everything possible to make this book accurate, up to date, and in accord with accepted standards at the time of publication. The author(s), editors, and publisher are not responsible for errors or omissions or for consequences from application of the book, and make no warranty, expressed or implied, in regard to the contents of the book. Any practice described in this book should be applied by the reader in accordance with professional standards of care used in regard to the unique circumstances that may apply in each situation. The reader is advised always to check product information (package inserts) for changes and new information regarding dose and contraindications before administering any drug. Caution is especially urged when using new or infrequently ordered drugs.

Library of Congress Cataloging-in-Publication Data

Constantino, Rose Eva Bana.
  Forensic nursing : evidence-based principles and practice / Rose E. Constantino, Patricia A. Crane, Susan E. Young.
     p. ; cm.
  Includes bibliographical references.
  ISBN 978-0-8036-2185-5 (pbk. : alk. paper)
  I. Crane, Patricia A. II. Young, Susan E. III. Title.
  [DNLM: 1. Forensic Nursing—methods. 2. Evidence-Based Nursing—methods. WY 170]

614.15—dc23

2012010880

To Virginia Lynch, forensic nurse pioneer, scientist, and practitioner and all of the forensic clinicians whom she has inspired who continue the global development of forensic nursing practice, research, and education.

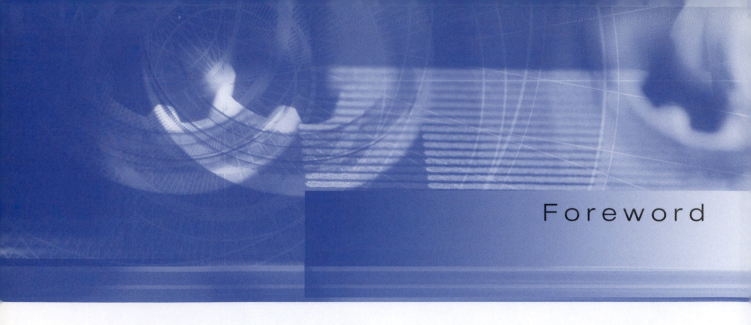

Foreword

It is a privilege to have been invited to write the foreword for this exceptionally relevant, timely, and invaluable resource for the practice of forensic nursing. The knowledge, skills, and advanced practice guidelines are consistent with evidence-based practice in the 21st century. Nursing roles within a collaborative practice model enhance assessment and broaden the scope of practice not only in nursing but in other disciplines as well. The art and science of nursing are reflected throughout the text as is the framework that grounds nursing practice from an ethical, legal, and culturally relevant perspective.

The integration of the foundations of nursing practice is evidenced by the comprehensive in-depth descriptions and competencies described throughout the text. The outcomes in nursing in general and forensic nursing in particular will benefit the patient both in the short term and in the future. As well, the challenges of global issues and considerations for practice are well addressed and thought-provoking.

Best practices are reflected throughout the text and guide forensic nursing practice and research. The challenges posed by a forensic focus could result in a dehumanizing experience for the patient, and this is thoughtfully addressed. As advanced practice becomes even more complex, this text will serve as a guide for meeting these challenges. This text will benefit both the experienced practitioner and the novice and serve as a reference for practitioners in novel settings such as long-term care and correctional facilities. Forensic nursing practice is on the cutting edge of current trends and advancements in a unique and specialized area of nursing practice.

Barbara A. Moynihan, PhD, APRN, BC, AFN
Faculty, Quinnipiac University

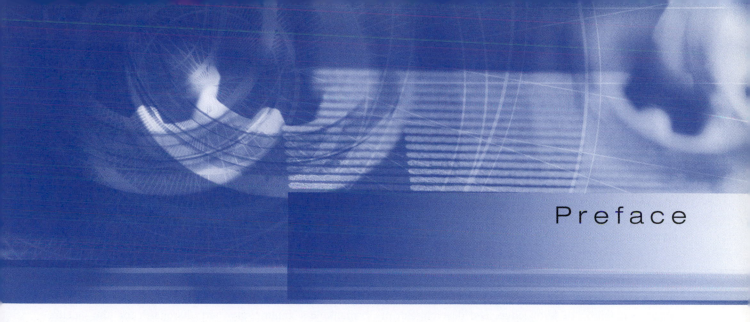

Forensic nursing is defined as the application of forensic science, biopsychosocial knowledge, and clinical nursing skills in the scientific investigation, collection, preservation, analysis, and examination of evidence. Forensic nursing is formally organized and is represented by a nursing specialty association—the International Association of Forensic Nurses (IAFN).

In the late 1990s, a textbook that comprehensively covered the principles and practice of forensic nursing could not be found. Fortunately, the IAFN and the American Nurses Association (ANA) published the scope and standards of forensic nursing practice in 1997. This publication guided educators in course development in forensic nursing at some schools of nursing in the United States. Then in 2006, Virginia Lynch's *Forensic Nursing,* which covered the breadth and depth of forensic nursing, was published. However, students and teachers alike sought a textbook to give them not only background but also foreground information accompanied by evidence-based nursing interventions that are translatable into forensic nursing practice. The inclusion of evidence-based data and its conceptual inductive organization sets this book apart from others.

Our systems of laws, health care, research, and education are based on credible evidence. Evidence-based practice in forensic nursing is an important guide for nursing students, educators, researchers, and administrators. It provides a clear and succinct summary of current, relevant nursing and related multidisciplinary research. Forensic nursing in the 21st century is replete with challenges and opportunities as nurses continue to be thoughtful and deliberate in heeding and interfacing with laws, policies, and regulations laid before them as roadmaps in forensic nursing practice, education, research, and administration. Challenges are met as nurses embrace technology in transforming and translating forensic nursing science and research into evidence-based practice. No forensic nurse stands alone because forensic nursing is an open system connected to other systems in interactive complexity and synergy with larger systems as presented in Unit 1, Chapters 1 through 6. As an open system, forensic nursing is dynamic, permeable, and constantly evolving. Our goal is to provide a roadmap to forensic nurses nationally and globally as they continue to make a difference in their specific area of practice.

We invite the more than three million nurses in the United States, who represent the largest group of health professions and nurses all over the world, to examine this book. In their capacity as clinicians, researchers, administrators, or educators, they come in contact not only with patients and their families but also with precious physical and nonphysical evidence that, if left uncollected, unrecorded, or unpreserved, can be detrimental to the assessment, treatment, evaluation, investigation, and disposition of the case or to comprehensive nursing care. This book provides a roadmap for nurses who are already forensic nurses or who are looking forward to a role in forensic nursing. There is a compelling need to develop a book such as this as nurses search for additional knowledge and skills in an area of practice where evidenced-based research and studies are few, far between, and do not proximately address their impact on the role of the forensic nurse.

Unit One, Introduction to Forensic Nursing Practice, provides an overview of the process by which nursing knowledge and skills and forensic science are integrated into forensic nursing. It provides introductory information to areas of nursing in general and specifically to forensic nursing education, research, and practice (Chapters 1, 5, and 6). Areas of the law, the anatomy and physiology of a lawsuit, and ethical, legal, and social issues (ELSI) related to forensic nursing are discussed in Chapters 3 and 4. Principles and practice of forensic nursing are presented in Chapter 2 in conjunction with the theoretical and conceptual frameworks and models for understanding forensic nursing.

Unit Two, Forensic Nursing in Interpersonal Violence, provides specific learning principles that focus on the development of investigative techniques in forensic nursing examination. In Chapters 7 through 12, emphasis is placed on the application of nursing skills and knowledge to questions of law and health in examinations, investigations, and other forensic issues. Case studies on the typology of violence; intimate partner, child, and elder abuse; sexual assault, and evidence collection allow for critique, acquisition of knowledge, and development of skills relevant to the various roles in forensic nursing practice. Principles and practice and role responsibilities inherent to forensic nursing are presented with an overview of roles throughout the life span for breadth and depth, the preservation and examination of databases in cold cases, self-directed violence, and death investigation. Techniques of forensic assessment and physical examination, evidence collection, chain of custody, and forensic documentation that withstands courtroom scrutiny and legal challenges are discussed.

Unit Three, Forensic Nursing in Special Areas of Practice, includes the forensic nurse as a psychiatric mental health nurse, correctional nurse, legal nurse consultant, and emergency and acute care nurse. Screening cases, analyzing professional malpractice cases, performing hospital/medical records review and examination, performing quality assurance and risk management, and preparing effective written and verbal reports and abstracts are discussed in Chapters 13 through 17. Unit Three invites the registered nurse in any practice setting to combine nursing knowledge with forensic science and nursing research in scientific investigation, evidence collection and preservation, analysis, and legal documentation or in providing sound evidence-based nursing care.

Unit Four, Forensic Nursing in Collective Violence, provides an overview of forensic nursing in collective violence. As forensic nurses participate in the globalization of nursing, Chapters 18 through 20 introduce the nurse to an understanding of violence and disasters in a shrinking and aging world, including violation of human rights through trafficking, exploitation, torture, genocide, wars, and natural disasters. The history of mankind's inhumanity and disregard for the health, safety, and life of vulnerable groups is described. Disasters are classified as either natural or technological in which the nurse can be a vital team member or leader. Natural disasters are environmental events, such as volcanic eruptions, earthquakes, floods, cyclones, or more long-term epidemics, drought, or famine (catastrophic food shortage). Technological disasters are primarily caused by hardware failure and human error, resulting in toxic emissions, explosions, and transport accidents that may cause a chemical spill; insidious air, water, and soil pollution; or food contamination. The roles of the forensic nurse are discussed in detail throughout Unit Four.

An important part of every chapter is the inclusion of a useful quotation that is well worth reading. Each chapter also includes competencies, evidence-based practice, review questions, and references.

Rose Constantino, Patricia Crane, and *Susan Young*

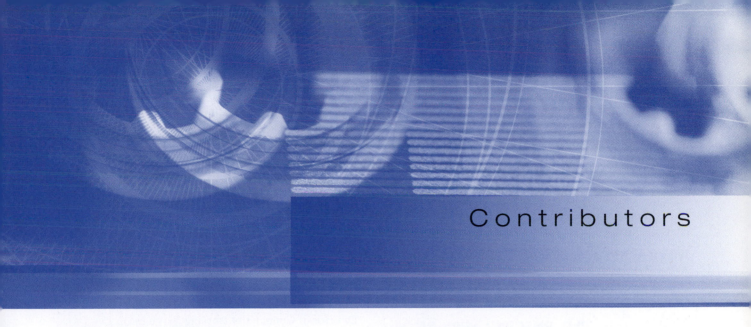

Contributors

Jocelyn Anderson, MSN, RN
PhD Student
Johns Hopkins University School of Nursing
Baltimore, Maryland

**Christine Cassesse, MSN, FNP-BC,
  FPMHNP-BC**
Nurse Practitioner, Integrated Pediatric/Behavioral
   Health Practice
Children's Community Pediatrics, Armstrong
Kittanning, Pennsylvania

Alison Cole, PhD
Clinical Psychologist
Binghamton University
Oneonta, New York

**Diana K. Faugno, MSN, RN, CPN, SANE-A,
  SANE-P, FAAFS, DF-IAFN**
Forensic Nurse Consultant
Eisenhower Medical Center
Palm Desert, California

Allyson Havill, PhD, RN, PMHCNS-BC
Clinical Nurse Specialist
VA Pittsburgh Healthcare System
Pittsburgh, Pennsylvania

Anita Hufft, PhD, RN
Dean and Professor of Nursing
Valdosta State University
Valdosta, Georgia

Nursine Shuman Jackson, MSN, RN
Legal Nurse Consultant/Cardiovascular Clinical Nurse
   Specialist
Adjunct Faculty
University of Pittsburgh
New York, New York

Irene Kane, PhD, RN, HFS, CNAA
Assistant Professor of Nursing
RN Options Coordinator
University of Pittsburgh School of Nursing
Pittsburgh, Pennsylvania

Diane Kjervik, JD, MSN, RN, FAAN
Professor Emeritus
University of North Carolina at Chapel Hill
   School of Nursing
Chapel Hill, North Carolina

Elizabeth LaRue, PhD, MLS
Assistant Professor
University of Pittsburgh
Pittsburgh, Pennsylvania

Louanne Lawson, PhD, RN
Associate Professor
UAMS College of Nursing
Little Rock, Arkansas

Cheyenne Martin, PhD, RN
Rebecca and Edwin Gale Professor of Ethics
University of Texas Medical Branch (UTMB)
Graduate School of Biomedical Sciences and School
   of Nursing
Galveston, Texas

Nancy Martin, EdD, MSN, RN, FCNS
Forensic Nurse Educator
Forensic Nursing Health Science Services
Lexington, Ohio

Patricia R. Messmer, PhD, RN-BC, FAAN
Consultant Nursing Education and Research
Miami Dade College
Miami, Florida

Ann M. Mitchell, PhD, RN, FAAN
Associate Professor of Nursing and Psychiatry
University of Pittsburgh School of Nursing
Pittsburgh, Pennsylvania

Stacey A. Mitchell, DNP, MBA, RN, SANE-A, SANE-P
Director, Forensic Nursing Services
Harris County Hospital District
Houston, Texas

Karen A. Monsen, PhD, RN, FAAN
Assistant Professor
University of Minnesota School of Nursing
Minneapolis, Minnesota

Mary Muscari, PhD, RN, CPNP, APRN-BC
Associate Professor of Nursing
Binghamton University
Affiliate Faculty Criminology
Regis University
Binghamton, New York

Elaine Pagliaro, MS, JD
Grants and Research Coordinator
Henry C. Lee Institute of Forensic Science
Grants and Research Coordinator
University of New Haven
West Haven, Connecticut

Angela Primeau, MSN, RN, CNS-BC, SANE-A, FNE-A
Nurse Coordinator
Stanford Hospital and Clinics
Stanford, Connecticut

Sara Rowe, PhD, RN
Clinical Assistant Professor
University of Arkansas for Medical Science
College of Nursing
Little Rock, Arkansas

Daniel J. Sheridan, PhD, RN, FAAN
Associate Professor
Johns Hopkins University
Baltimore, Maryland

Catherine J. Carter-Snell, RN, PhD, SANE-A, ENC-C
Associate Professor, Forensic Studies
Mount Royal University
Calgary, Alberta, Canada

Patricia M. Speck, DNSc, APN, FNP-BC, DF-IAFN, FAAFS, FAAN
Associate Professor and Public Health Nursing Option Coordinator
University of Tennessee Health Science Center College of Nursing
Memphis, Tennessee

Kathleen Thimsen, RN, MSN, WOCN, FNS
Director of Community Nursing Services
Southern Illinois University at Edwardsville
East St. Louis, Illinois

Tasha Venters, MS
Victims Advocate Program Manager
Woodbridge, Virginia

Daniele Wilcox, RN
Forensic Health Student
Binghamton University, 2007
Binghamton, New York

David Williams, DDS, MS, MPH, FACD
Assistant Clinical Professor
University of Maryland School of Dentistry
Baltimore, Maryland

Joyce P. Williams, DNP, RN
Assistant Professor
University of Tennessee, Memphis
Memphis, Tennesee

Margarete L. Zalon, PhD, RN, ACNS-BC, FAAN
Professor
University of Scranton
Dept. of Nursing
Scranton, Pennsylvania

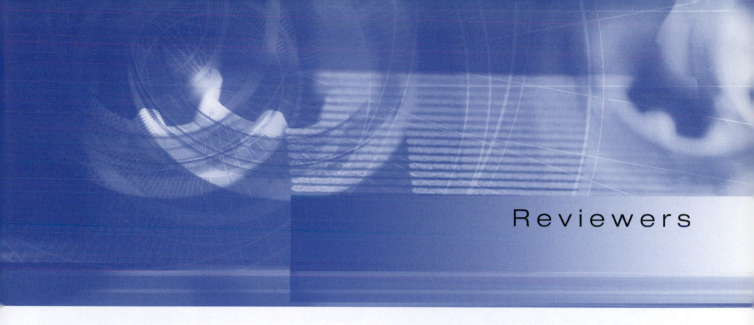

Reviewers

Lynda D. Benak MSN, BS, RN
Clinical Risk Manager
Central Maine Healthcare
Auburn, Maine

Tatayana Bogopolskiy ARNP, MSN
Clincal Assistant Professor
Florida International Professor
North Miami, Florida

Venive Cuningkin BSN, RN
Faculty
Baptist Health School of Nursing
Little Rock, Arkansas

**Renae Diegel RN, BBL, CEN, CFN, D-ABMDI,
SANE-A, CMI-III, CFC**
Medicolegal Death Investigator
Macomb County Medical Examiner's Office
Mt. Clemens, Michigan

Ann Ersland RN, MSN, CNM, ARNP
Associate Professor
Iowa Valley Community College
Iowa Falls, Iowa

Brenda M. Ewen MSN
Forensic Nurse Consultant/Adjunct Faculty
University of Delaware
Wilmington, Delaware

Cris Finn PhD, RN
Assistant Professor
Regis University
Denver, Colorado

Jim W. Flahive MSN, RN
Instructor
University of Texas at El Paso
El Paso, Texas

**Jodie A. Flynn MSN, RN, SANE-A, SANE-P,
D-ABMDI**
Instructor
MedCentral Health System
Forensic Nurse Investigator
Richland County Coroner Office
Mansfield, Ohio

Pauline Freedberg MSN, RN
Professor of Nursing
Westmoreland County Community College
Youngwood, Pennsylvania

Barbara A. Gilbert RN, MSN, FN
BSN Nursing Faculty
Excelsior College
Albany, New York

Terry L. Kerns RN, MSN
Supervisory Special Agent
Quantico, Virginia

Valerie Kuenkele RN, MSN, CNP
Assistant Professor
MedCentral College of Nursing
Mansfield, Ohio

Kathleen A. LuPone
Clinical Assistant Professor
Arizona State University
Phoenix, Arizona

Carl Mangum RN, MSN, PhD(c), CHS
Assistant Professor
Emergency Preparedness and Response
  Specialist
University of Mississippi

Nancy Martin RN, MSN, FCNS
Forensic Clinical Nurse Specialist
Sole Proprietor of Forensic Nursing and Health Science
    Services
International Association of Forensic Nurses
Lexington, Ohio

Elaine Mordoch RN, BN, MN, PhD
Assistant Professor
University of Manitoba
Winnipeg, Manitoba, Canada

Mary Muscari PhD, CPNC, APRN-BC, FCNS
Pediatric Nurse Practitioner
Psychiatric Clinical Nurse Specialist
Forensic Clinical Nurse Specialist
Professor/Director of Forensic Health
University of Scranton
Scranton, Pennsylvania

Christie Obritsch MSN, RN
Assistant Professor
University of Mary
Bismarck, North Dakota

Jennifer Pfeiffer DNP, MPH, PHN, CIC
Clinical Assistant Professor
University of Minnesota
Minneapolis, Minnesota

Paula Pillone MS, NP-P
Assistant Professor of Clinical Nursing
Columbia University
Nurse Practitioner
St. Luke's Roosevelt Hospital Center
New York, New York

Norma Poirier PhD, MN, MaEd
Nursing Professor
Université de Moncton
Moncton, New Brunswick, Canada

Tony Ramsey AAS, BBA
Director of Health, Wellness and PSS
Davidson County Community College
Lexington, North Carolina

Russell R. Rooms MSN, APRN-BC
Assistant Professor
University of Rochester
President and CEO
National Forensic Nursing Institute
Oklahoma City, Oklahoma

LeAnn E. Schlamb RN-BC, MSN, CFN
Coordinator of Allied Health Education and Consultative
    Education Services
Butler Technology and Career Development School
Fairfield Township, Ohio

Donna Thompson MS, APRN, FNE, CFC
Nursing Faculty/Forensic Nursing Examiner
Salt Lake Community College
West Jordan, Utah

Karen Ursel RN, BN, MHSA
Senior Nursing Instructor
University of New Brunswick
Moncton, New Brunswick, Canada

Sharon Weidner MSN/CNS, RN
Instructor
St. Luke's School of Nursing
Bethlehem, Pennsylvania

Cathy H. Williams DNP, MSN, RN
Associate Professor/BSN Coordinator
Albany State University
Tifton, Georgia

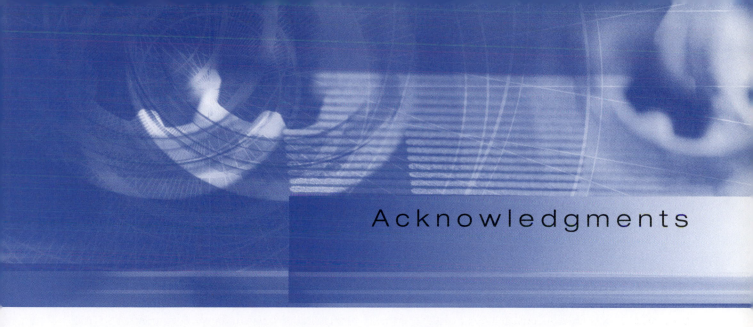

Acknowledgments

In order to present the work in a publication of this type, we must acknowledge the many people who have influenced forensic nursing since its inception and its recognition as a nursing specialty. All the leaders, experts, instructors/ faculty/professors, mentors, and researchers have in some way contributed to the advancement of forensic nursing knowledge. With the development of knowledge, sharing of resources, and mentorship, professionals are able to push the refined knowledge like fruit through a sieve, out into practices and global settings where forensic knowledge is limited, and share it with other professionals.

Our application of forensic knowledge to nursing practice started with a thirst and passion. The global health-care experiences of our patients who suffer from mental and psychological trauma, violence, torture, and human rights abuses challenged existing knowledge. To improve forensic patient outcomes, we had to find new answers, acquire new skills, attempt new management strategies, write new protocols, and collaborate in a meaningful way with many other professionals to adapt our practice of nursing to meet the needs of our patients. Change agents in nursing continue to share knowledge in many ways around the globe with education, training, support, and mentorship.

Our inspiration was ignited by Virginia Lynch, Ann Burgess, Linda Ledray, and many other science professionals, pioneers, and organizations. The seeds they planted keep the science of forensic nursing growing.

All the experts and leaders in forensic nursing cannot be named or recognized in one book. We have recognized so few here, but we all have our own inspirational leaders and those who supported and drove us forward. I think none would deny this: the most powerful driving force, the greatest inspiration, the most significant inspiration to acknowledge for each of us in forensic nursing practice are the men, women, and children who experienced trauma, tragedy, torture, violence, and abuse and came to us for care. They trusted us to tell their story. They told us of their terror. Young ones opened their hearts to us and revealed family secrets of years of abuse. Their voices should continue to be our inspiration. We acknowledge them all for their bravery in speaking out and bringing light to their experiences—because their experiences changed the way we practice nursing.

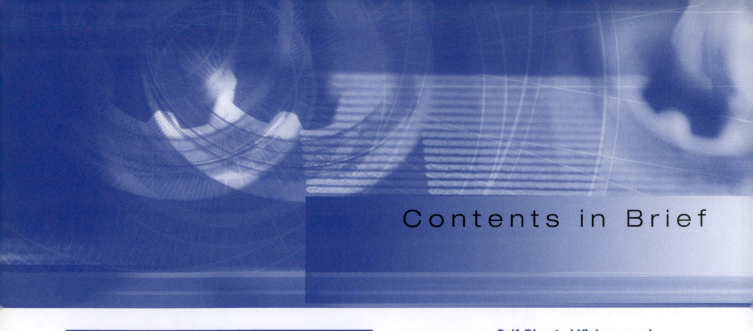

Contents in Brief

Table of Contents

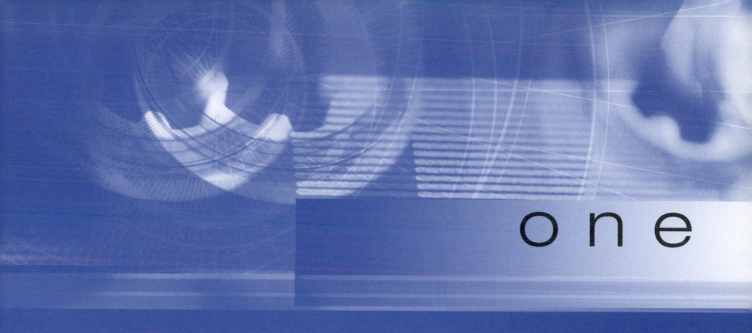

one

INTRODUCTION TO FORENSIC NURSING PRACTICE

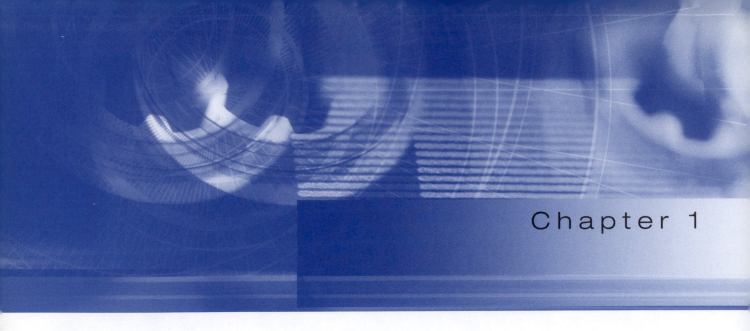

Chapter 1

FUNDAMENTALS OF CONTEMPORARY FORENSIC NURSING PRACTICE, EDUCATION, AND RESEARCH

Margarete L. Zalon, Rose E. Constantino, and Patricia A. Crane

"Never underestimate the power of a small group of individuals to change the world. Indeed it is the only thing that ever has."

Margaret Mead

Competencies

1. Understanding the definition and scope of practice of forensic nursing.
2. Analyzing the historical development of forensic nursing practice in relation to contemporary practice issues.
3. Describing the standards of forensic nursing practice.
4. Assessing avenues for obtaining education in forensic nursing.
5. Investigating resources for evidence-based forensic nursing practice and education.

Key Terms

Evidence-based practice
Evidence-based nursing practice
Forensic
Forensic nursing
Sexual Assault Nurse Examiner (SANE)
Standards
Therapeutic jurisprudence
Translation science

INTRODUCTION

This chapter introduces the topics of the scope of practice and standards of care in forensic nursing, education for forensic nursing, and the use of research evidence for the practice of forensic nursing. Forensic nurses seek the truth about when, what, where, how, and who was involved in a traumatic or catastrophic event. Forensic nurses seek to improve acute and long-term health outcomes that stem from intentional violence and trauma. Nurses in many different settings encounter patients who have experienced violence, intentional injuries, or trauma who could be categorized as forensic patients, those patients whose condition, safety, and future health involve a health-care issue that intersects with the law. Forensic nursing actions require that health-care professionals and the public, through various agencies, take direct action to address the consequences and prevent the recurrence of intentional violence and trauma. Such action requires collaboration among professionals in health care, law enforcement, social services, and various other community and governmental agencies.

Violence as a Public Health Problem

Violence is a public health problem. Each year, 1.6 million people die due to violence, and many more are injured and have physical, sexual, reproductive, and mental health problems. Among people age 15 to 44 years, violence is among the leading causes of death, accounting for 14% of deaths among males and 7% of deaths among females. In the United States, according to the National Crime Victimization Survey, 5.2 million people were victims of violent crime in 2007, with one rape or assault occurring for every 1000 persons and one murder occurring for every 100,000 persons. In 2006, there were 27.7 million visits to emergency departments for unintentional injuries and 2.5 million visits for intentional injuries. In addition, the United States has one of the largest per capita prison populations in the world, with over 2.3 million persons incarcerated in federal, state, and local prisons. It has been estimated that the number of Americans age 65 and over who have been injured, exploited, or otherwise mistreated by someone on whom they depend for care or protection is between one and two million. Thus, it is highly likely that nurses will encounter individuals whose lives have been altered due to violence, injury, and trauma. Nurses have the opportunity to prevent violence and reduce its sequelae as both victims and perpetrators of violence enter the health-care system for care.

The Forensic Nurse

Forensic nursing helps to collect evidence in settings such as the emergency room, intensive care unit, critical care unit, labor and delivery unit, pediatric unit, as well as the general medical, surgical, psychiatric units, and extended care settings. Forensic nursing can be performed in settings wherever nurses practice, including schools, prisons, and the community. Forensic nurses provide care to patients in an objective and impartial manner, seeking the truth and supporting the provision of care that is sensitive and respectful and that also incorporates scientific knowledge and evidence-based practice. Because nurses are frequently the first professionals to see a patient in a health-care setting and may have 24-hour responsibility for the provision of nursing care, trained and experienced forensic nurses are vital in the clinical setting. In this capacity, the nurse comes in contact with various types of patients and their families and must also address issues related to critical physical and nonphysical evidence. Initial and long-term contact offer opportunities for the forensic nurse to address documentation, collection, protection, and storage of evidence that is critical to assessment, treatment, evaluation, investigation, and disposition of the patients' health care and the legal outcome of a case.

Definitions of Forensic and Forensic Nursing Practice

"Forensic" refers to the application of scientific knowledge to legal problems, and it can be used to describe medicine, psychology, and nursing. *Forensic* is derived from the Latin *forensis,* which refers to public debate or discussion; hence, the legal system is the location for the public discussion and debate. According to the American Academy of Forensic Sciences (AAFS, n.d), forensic science is used in public and in the justice system; any science that is used for the purposes of the law is a forensic science. Whereas the general public may associate forensic science with criminal or death investigations, it is in fact much broader, including an investigation of trauma and violence in the living and care for the offenders who caused the injuries. Forensic science includes such specialties as criminalistics, digital and multimedia sciences, toxicology, odontology, engineering, pathology and biology, anthropology and physical sciences, and psychiatry and behavioral sciences. Clinical forensic practice is the application of medical and nursing sciences to the care of living patients who may be involved in some way in a criminal or liability-related incident (Lynch, 2013).

Forensic nursing practice demonstrates the scientific and forensic base in health care. Forensic nursing has its roots in forensic medicine, and it has advanced its own specialization within nursing, including the development of scope and standards of forensic nursing practice statements. The science of forensic nursing is the appraisal, analysis, and synthesis of methods and outcomes and translation of best-evidence outcomes to the practice setting and population. Patient or client preferences and choices are incorporated into forensic nursing care. Forensic nurses work with abused children, adolescents, adults, substance and person abusers, convicted criminals, families of patients who are donating organs for transplant, the criminally insane, and with the judicial and law enforcement system. Forensic nurses are also committed to minimum standards of assessment, evidence collection, and crime reporting. Forensic nursing includes a blend of overlapping responsibilities in practice that is unique and complex, with synergy and general systems concepts forming its foundation.

The International Association of Forensic Nurses (IAFN, 2008) adopted the following definition: "Forensic nursing is the practice of nursing globally when health and legal systems intersect." Forensic nursing is a nursing specialty and has been recognized as such by the American Nurses Association (ANA) since 1995. Forensic nursing integrates and accommodates nursing, forensic science, and technology. Accommodation is at the cutting edge of forensic nursing, addressing all areas of interface between law and nursing. Forensic nurses address such wide-ranging issues as deviations in standards of care in health-care settings; primary, emergency, and critical care examination; toxicology report interpretations; evaluation of professional negligence and other professional wrongdoing; evaluation of survivors of persecution and torture who are seeking asylum; sexual violence; human-caused or natural disasters; domestic violence; child neglect; and child and elder abuse. Nurses can practice forensic nursing in as many specialties as there are for nursing. Like other specialties, there is a distinct body of knowledge for forensic nursing. According to the ANA and the IAFN, forensic nursing "focuses on the identification, management, and prevention of intentional and unintentional injuries in a global community. Forensic nurses collaborate with agents in healthcare, social, and legal systems to investigate and interpret clinical presentations and pathologies by evaluating physical and psychological injury, whether intentional or unintentional; describing the scientific relationships of the injury and evidence; and interpreting the associated influencing factors." Furthermore, the role of forensic nurses is to "integrate forensic and nursing sciences in their assessment and care of victims and perpetrators of physical, psychological, or social trauma."

The Forensic Nurse's Responsibilities to the Public

Because truth is the guiding principle of forensic nursing, it is important that nurses understand that advocacy is best accomplished in an impartial manner. The nurse's obligation to patients is not based on what the patients did, their lifestyle, or personal characteristics, but rather on their need for nursing care. For many years, nurses have earned the reputation as being the most trusted profession as indicated in the annual Gallup poll of the public's ratings of honesty and ethical standards of various professions. In the United States, 84% believe that nurses' honesty and ethical standards are "high" or "very high." Trust implies impartiality.

The application of trust to forensic nursing is illustrated when a nurse is asked to testify in court. If the nurse's support for the victim is obvious, then it is less likely that critical testimony will be perceived as accurate and impartial. That, in turn, creates doubts in the minds of jurors, who may find it difficult to render a guilty verdict. Canaff (2009), a prosecutor, describes three important intersecting roles of the **Sexual Assault Nurse Examiner (SANE)**—comfort and care of patients reporting sexual assault, competent and consistent evidence collection, and expert testimony on anatomy and tissue—emphasizing that SANEs will do more for victims, legal advocacy, and the elimination of sexual violence through their objectivity. Williams (2008) explores this question from the perspective of the ethical principle of utilitarianism in that the forensic nurse, when providing testimony, very often is doing so from the perspective of the community's interest. Similarly, in providing care to perpetrators in the criminal justice system, forensic nurses have an obligation to be nonjudgmental. Very often these perpetrators may be stigmatized, marginalized, and subject to discrimination. Indeed, the *Code of Ethics for Nurses* focuses on the nurse's obligations to the patient regardless of the patient's personal characteristics and also mandates that nurses fulfill their responsibilities to society as a whole in promoting the public's health.

Contemporary consumers are no longer satisfied with the delivery of forensic nursing care in an ordinary way. In a world of increasingly expensive forensic technology, consumers no longer accept the ordinary, ineffective, or unsuccessful procedures. The public anticipates effective, efficient, and authentic technology that produces accurate results that are consistent, honest, reliable, transparent, and trustworthy. Health-care consumers develop loyalty to a service provider or setting based on their total overall experience. Health-care organizations will have a competitive edge if they can provide their patients with a standardized experience that is responsive to patients' needs. The most mundane patient contact or an extended hospital stay can be transformed into an opportunity to engage patients and families in a health-enhancing way. The winning performance is an operational model that ramps up performance to create exceptional experiences for health consumers.

Forensic nursing in the 21st century is replete with opportunities as nurses continue to be thoughtful and deliberate in heeding and interfacing with the laws, policies, and regulations that serve as roadmaps in forensic nursing practice, education, research, and administration. Challenges are met as they embrace technology in transforming and translating forensic nursing science and research into evidence-based practice. No forensic nurse stands alone because forensic nursing is an open system connected to other systems in interactive complexity with even larger systems. As an open system, forensic nursing is dynamic, permeable, and constantly expanding.

THE DEVELOPMENT OF FORENSIC NURSING

Forensic nursing is interconnected with the criminal justice system. The term *forensic nursing* was first used by Virginia Lynch in her master's thesis at the University of Texas at Arlington. Lynch (1993) defined forensic nursing as "the application of nursing process to public or legal proceedings, and the application of forensic health care in the scientific investigation of trauma and/or death related to abuse, violence, criminal activity liability, and accidents." In her pioneering research, Lynch identified forensic role behaviors and clarified expectations for nurses working with trauma patients in emergency departments. She was the first to propose forensic nursing as a specialty.

THE SEXUAL ASSAULT NURSE EXAMINER ROLE

During the 1970s, SANE programs were developing in different parts of the United States and Canada. The nurses with this specialized training brought the highest standards of care to their patients with sensitivity, skilled and uncompromised evidence collection, and reliable courtroom testimony. Around the same time, Ann Wolbert

Burgess, DNS, RN, FAAN, began her groundbreaking work in the treatment of victims of trauma and abuse, cofounding the first hospital-based crisis counseling programs at Boston City Hospital. She subsequently demonstrated the value of the nursing perspective in her work with the FBI in examining the relationships between child abuse, juvenile delinquency, and subsequent criminal activity.

The International Association of Forensic Nurses

In 1992, a group of 72 nurses, primarily from 31 SANE programs in the United States and Canada, led by Linda Ledray, PhD, RN, SANE-A, FAAN, met in Minneapolis, Minnesota. The meeting resulted in the formation of the IAFN, which was incorporated the following year. Active leadership of the board of directors of IAFN has been critical, so that, with the professional and global transition and dynamic growth of forensic nursing practice, the organization is vital; it maintains the currency of its mission, goals, policies, and bylaws and has published the recently updated *Scope and Standards of Forensic Nursing Practice*. Most important, at all stages of growth and development, the inclusion of nurses practicing in all forensic nursing roles and specialties internationally ensures contemporary representation of the diverse membership and practice roles (ANA & IAFN, 2009).

The current mission of the IAFN is to provide leadership in forensic nursing practice by developing, promoting, and disseminating information globally about forensic nursing science. The goals of the IAFN are to promote violence-prevention strategies, improve standards of evidence-based forensic nursing, exchange ideas and develop knowledge, and establish standards of ethical conduct for forensic nurses.

Since the incorporation of the IAFN, the organization has grown to over 3000 members and holds well-attended annual international scientific assemblies and regional training events. The IAFN publication *On the Edge* was initiated in the mid-1990s, but a more formal scientific journal was a long-time goal, leading to the launch of *Journal of Forensic Nursing* in 2005. A history of key events in the development of forensic nursing are listed in Table 1.1.

Growth of Forensic Nursing

Early programs in forensic nursing focused on training of nurses to conduct sexual assault examinations. A nurse who completed these programs was called a Sexual Assault Nurse Clinician (SANC) or a SANE. Other terms used

TABLE 1.1 **Key Events**

Date	Event
1948	United Nations Universal Declaration of Human Rights declares that no one should be subjected to torture or to cruel or unusual punishment.
1984	Violence identified as a public health issue by the U.S. Surgeon General (Koop, 1986).
1990	Virginia Lynch analyzes the role of the forensic nurse in her master's thesis (Lynch, 1990).
1991	American Association of Colleges of Nursing position paper states that violence against women is a nursing practice problem (AACN, 1991).
1991	American Academy of Forensic Sciences recognizes forensic nursing.
1992	The International Association of Forensic Nurses (IAFN) is established.
1994	Violence Against Women Act (VAWA) signed into law.
1995	American Nurses Association (ANA) recognizes forensic nursing as a specialty.
1996	IAFN adopts the term *Sexual Assault Nurse Examiner (SANE)* and SANE standards of nursing practice.
1997	ANA and IAFN publish the first *Scope and Standards for Forensic Nursing Practice*.
2002	IAFN offers the Sexual Assault Nurse Examiner certification examination for adult/adolescent (SANE-A).
2005	IAFN creates the Forensic Nursing Certification Board.
2006	IAFN offers the Sexual Assault Nurse Examiner certification examination for pediatric/adolescent (SANE-P).
2008	IAFN Certification Board becomes sole owner of title of "SANE" to used after passing certification examination.
2009	ANA and IAFN revised the *Scope and Standards for Forensic Nursing Practice*.

include Sexual Assault/Forensic Nurse Examiners (SAFE) or forensic nurse examiners. However, the IAFN adopted the term Sexual Assault Nurse Examiner-Adult/Adolescent (SANE-A) and Sexual Assault Nurse Examiner-Pediatrics/Adolescent (SANE-P). Since then, certificate programs in forensic nursing have grown extensively, with over 535 programs in the United States, Canada, and Australia listed on the IAFN Web site. The first master's degree program with a specialization in forensic nursing was established at the University of Texas at Arlington in 1986. Since then, many universities in the United States and around the world offer formal courses, forensic nursing continuing education, and specialty tracks of study at the baccalaureate, graduate, and doctoral levels (see Chapter 6 for more information).

The growth, expansion, and formalization of forensic nursing as a subspecialty is a response to nursing interest and market demand. Solid educational resources are critical in the face of a developing subspecialty. More important, however, educational opportunities meet a variety of policy requirements and guidelines for health-care organizations and institutions, nursing organizations, and other health-care providers. Forensic nursing expert educators and clinicians must be knowledgeable so that the educational opportunities are adequate and allow for safe and ethical nursing practice in all settings and with diverse populations. Forensic nursing competencies are often a minimal part of the nursing education formal curriculum. Strategic growth of forensic nursing knowledge is required by the organizational structure and culture because it is demanded by societal needs and legal and ethical trends in health care. Health-care policy derived from legislation strongly influences nursing practice, education, and regulatory issues. Currently, there are many legislative bodies and policy-developing organizations that aim to fund and require nursing educational preparation to meet the needs of forensic patients.

Forensic medicine has not experienced the same growth as forensic nursing in the United States. Whereas pathology as a medical specialty has been well established, forensic medicine, associated with care for the living, is only recently receiving attention. Consequently, this means that very often the forensic nurse may be the only health-care professional with specific training in the care of victims, offenders, and the collection and preservation of evidence. Hence, the collaborative role of the forensic nurse is critical to the outcomes of care for these vulnerable populations. There is considerable evidence for the effectiveness of SANE or other sexual assault/domestic violence programs. Plichta, Clements, and Houseman (2007) examined SANE delivery models in emergency departments (EDs) in Virginia; the results indicate that systems that called in off-site SANEs and full coverage of services by ED SANEs provided a higher quality of care. Similar findings are reported by pediatric emergency departments (Bechtel, Ryan & Gallagher, 2008; Sampsel, et al., 2009) and in Ontario, Canada. However, interdisciplinary collaboration is important for all forensic nursing roles. Mason and Carton (2002) identified 13 common areas with approximately 250 content items suitable for interdisciplinary forensic education. Several large academic centers have established interdisciplinary teams to provide clinical forensic consultation, with forensic nurses playing an integral role in the provision of care, consultation, and education of health-care providers.

SCOPE OF FORENSIC NURSING PRACTICE

Forensic nursing is a complex specialty that has experienced tremendous growth. There are as many areas in which forensic nursing can be practiced as there are specializations in nursing. This growth indicates that the original pioneers of forensic nursing, Lynch and others, were accurate in their futuristic thinking. The application of forensic science to the nursing care of diverse populations of children, adults, the elderly, vulnerable groups, and incarcerated individuals was a necessary and innovative revitalization of specialty nursing practice and can affect not only health outcomes but also legal outcomes. Envisioning the need for specialty education for nurses, Lynch developed an integrated practice model for forensic nursing that includes the theoretical foundation for forensic nursing: field of expertise, the health-care system, and societal impact. The fields of expertise include nursing science, forensic science, and criminal justice. The health-care system includes interactions of nurses with victims and offenders within the health-care system. The societal impact includes human behavior; social sanctions, including the law; and crime and violence. This model reflects the integration of multiple aspects of forensic nursing and is illustrated in Figure 1.1.

Foundation for Forensic Nursing

The scope and standards of forensic nursing practice are derived from nursing's seminal documents: *Nursing's Social Policy Statement,* the *Code of Ethics for Nurses,* and *ANA Nursing: Scope and Standards of Practice. Nursing's Social Policy Statement* defines nursing's obligations to society and includes six critical elements of nursing: provision of a caring relationship, attention to human experiences and responses to health and illness, integration of objective data with the patient's subjective experience, application of scientific knowledge, advancement of professional knowledge, and the promotion of social justice. For forensic nursing, this means the provision of sensitive care by nurses who are knowledgeable about evidence-based forensic nursing practice and health-care advocacy for forensic patients. The ANA's *Nursing: Scope and Standards of Practice* provides the framework for nursing practice and serves as the template for the development of

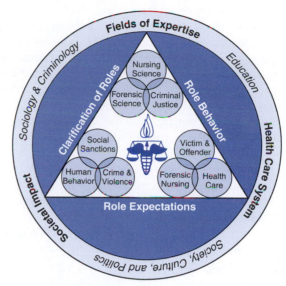

■ FIGURE 1.1 Integrated practice model for forensic nursing science. (Reprinted with permission from Lynch, V.A. & Duvall, J.B. [2011]. *Forensic nursing science.* [2nd ed.]. St. Louis: Elsevier Mosby.)

specialty scopes and standards. **Standards** are authoritative statements put forth by the profession by which the quality of practice, service, and education can be judged. In addition to *ANA Nursing: Scope and Standards of Practice,* numerous specialty standards documents are also critical resource documents for blended forensic nursing practices. The documents that may be of particular interest to forensic nurses in specialty practice include *Corrections Nursing: Scope and Standards of Practice, Legal Nurse Consulting: Scope and Standards of Practice,* and *Transplant Nursing: Scope and Standards of Practice.*

The Forensic Nurse Role

Forensic nursing can be practiced with individuals, families, and communities whose care is influenced or affected by the legal system or forensic issues. For example, a nurse in an emergency room prepared as a SANE-A can care for the victim of a sexual assault. In addition, the nurse may be required to collect evidence from an accused perpetrator who is hospitalized or incarcerated. A family nurse practitioner may be required to assess a child experiencing abuse as well as the child's family. Public health nurses need to assess community health resources, safety issues, and care for vulnerable persons who have been displaced by natural disasters. Forensic nursing practice is concerned with patients who are victims, accused perpetrators, and convicted felons who are involved with traumatic events, as well as with their families, communities, and the systems that respond to them. Trauma may be inclusive of interpersonal violence such as child abuse, intimate partner abuse, and assault, rape, and gang violence. However, human-caused catastrophes and natural causes of trauma and population evacuation are also health-care events with legal applications governing the health care provided. Environmental health hazards that may affect thousands within a town or community require much interaction between nursing and the legal authorities to ensure safety and the meeting of health needs for the populations at risk.

Nurses apply forensic science and must be cognizant of related laws when working with institutions and families for the procurement and transfer of organs and other body parts from the deceased or the living for medical uses. Integral to forensic nursing practice is collaboration with members of the health-care team, law enforcement and the criminal justice system, public health departments, and social service agencies. All professionals may be equal partners and have equal interest in private and public health issues, and all will benefit from all parties being respected and present at the management and decision-making table. Forensic nurses are also involved with investigation and interpretation of clinical presentations and pathological evaluations of physical and psychological injury. Great depth of understanding is required to hypothesize and describe the relationships between persons, intentional or unintentional injury, scientific evidence, and interpretation of factors that might influence the injury and evidence. It is unlikely that any individual has all the knowledge needed to perform the aforementioned tasks and roles at the expert level. The

sign of the true expert, however, is one who knows the best resources to consult in order to find the truth.

The distinctive feature of forensic nursing practice is the nurses' knowledge of how legal and social systems intersect with the health-care system. Forensic nurses have integral roles in health-care settings that are responsible for provision of health care for individuals who have experienced personal trauma and injury intentionally at the hand of another. Forensic nurses may provide for safety of workers and provide care in correctional and secure environment settings. They may work in health-care organizations as risk managers and in medical examiner or coroner's offices as death investigators. However, Lynch points out that the role of a forensic nurse in any setting is that of a clinical investigator rather than a criminal investigator. Forensic nursing roles allow for the application of skilled communication with balanced sensitivity to collect subjective and objective data and come to a conclusion or diagnosis for ongoing treatment and evaluation of an investigation.

The process, known as the nursing process, plays an important part and may also inform a legal investigation of any kind, for either the living or the deceased (see Table 1.2).

Additional forensic nursing responsibilities may include documentation of violence risk factors for medical issues to plan community interventions. Forensic nurses investigate the causes and epidemiology of trauma, abuse, and toxic events in hospitals and community settings such as home health agencies, group homes for wards of the state, and public health departments. The growth of

TABLE 1.2 **Nursing Process Applied to an Elderly Emergency Room Patient Potentially Experiencing Mistreatment/Abuse**

Nursing Process	General Guidelines	Specific components for elderly patient potentially experiencing mistreatment/abuse.
Assessment	Collection of data from subjective health history (what the patient says); Objective data (observations by nurse on physical and behavioral patient responses, physical examination) that are documented. This includes laboratory work, past procedures, and history and recording the data to help direct critical thinking toward a diagnosis.	Emotional abuse: fear, withdrawal, anger, denial, depression, helplessness. Assess for cognitive change, delirium and willingness to talk about living conditions. Physical signs of abuse: absence of scalp hair, bruises or evidence of trauma, underweight, bite or cigarette marks, lacerations, burns, welts, imprint or rope marks. Indicators of neglect: poor hygiene, smell of urine or feces, poorly clothed, dehydrated, pressure ulcers, untreated medical conditions, failure to adhere to medication regime. Financial abuse. Sexual abuse: vaginal or anal bleeding, sexually transmitted diseases. Review low or high serum levels of medications, serum sodium, serum protein, hematocrit. Assess caregiver stress.

Nursing Process	General Guidelines	Specific components for elderly patient potentially experiencing mistreatment/abuse.
Diagnosis	Identify nursing problems and characteristics and the potential problems in order to develop further analysis of data, strengths, and resources.	Potential nursing diagnoses specific to elder mistreatment/abuse may include risk for injury; violence, risk for other-directed; anxiety; caregiver role strain; risk for caregiver role strain; fear; fluid volume deficient; health maintenance; ineffective; powerlessness; nutrition, imbalanced, less than body requirements; rape-trauma syndrome; social isolation; thought process, disturbed; neglect, unilateral.
Outcomes	Describe measurable outcomes.	Patient is protected from harm and removed from unsafe situation if necessary. Decrease in risk for elder mistreatment/abuse. Decrease in caregiver strain.
Planning	Based on measurable outcomes; assign priorities to diagnoses and to interventions and therapies; collaborate with interdisciplinary team members. Initiate appropriate referrals.	Develop plan for safety that includes reporting to the appropriate agency and providing a safe placement either in home or hospital. Coordinate services with social work and other members of the health-care team.
Interventions	The nursing plan is put into action; responsibilities of family and other providers and referral resources involved in patient care are coordinated.	Implement safety plan (hospital admission) depending on the risk for injury. Treat any injuries. Mandatory report to appropriate agency. Document assessment findings, which may include photographic evidence, before treatment is instituted. Collect and preserve physical evidence. Depending on risk for injury, initiate safety plan such as hospital admission. Provide education to patient that mistreatment or abuse tends to escalate over time. Obtain assistive devices such as eyeglasses or hearing aids. Teach family members strategies to reduce caregiver strain.
Evaluation	Compare outcomes with what was intended; determine if the outcome is acceptable, or if the problem resolved; involve family and other disciplines; alterations in patient status resulting from plan and implementation are documented at this time.	Determine whether patient has been safe. Reassess patient for reduction of risk factors and healing of physical injuries. Assess for recurring problems related to elder mistreatment/abuse. Assess for new onset of emotional problems.

forensic nursing is due to nurses' application of forensic science to their individual practices in critical care, neonatal and burn units in health-care institutions, health care with trafficking and disaster assistance programs, and research teams. Rapidly expanding opportunities for nurses develop when nurses are exposed to forensic science and grasp the value of forensic education for improving or expanding their role to provide more holistic care. The IAFN has identified areas of forensic nursing practice, which are listed in Box 1.1.

In addition, nurses in various settings may seek additional education to ensure competency in specialty area practice that may overlap with the IAFN-identified roles. For example, a pediatric nurse practitioner in primary care may be certified as a SANE-P, but work with risk management and patient safety in the hospital to investigate, track, and prevent abuse of patients. A nurse's forensic practice, and the knowledge and education that are the foundation for that practice, informs additional practice roles.

Practice Settings

Forensic nurses deal with vulnerable populations, those who are exposed to being attacked or harmed. Vulnerable patients need appropriate health-care services as well as advocacy support in negotiating the complex health, legal, and social systems that are involved when forensic health-care services must be provided. The forensic nurse is directly involved and may be instrumental in ensuring that the forensic patient's health-care needs are met in a respectful

Box 1.1   Areas of Forensic Nursing Practice

Interpersonal violence
Domestic violence/sexual assault
Child and elder abuse and neglect
Physiological/psychological abuse
Occult/religious
Human trafficking
Forensic mental health nursing
Corrections nursing
Legal nurse consulting
Emergency/trauma services
   Accidents
   Traumatic injuries
   Work-related injuries
   Suicide attempts
   Disasters
Patient care/facility issues
   Accidents/injuries/neglect
   Inappropriate treatment/medication
Public health and safety
   Environmental hazards
   Drug/alcohol abuse
   Food and drug tampering
   Epidemiological issues
   Tissue/organ donation
Death investigation
   Homicides/suicides
   Suspicious deaths
   Mass disasters

Adapted from the International Association of Forensic Nurses. (2006). *What is forensic Nursing?* Retrieved August 17, 2009 from http://www.iafn.org

and humane manner. In this capacity, the nurse must have good communication with the patient and family and other team members, such as other health-care, social, and mental health–care workers. The forensic nurse may also have a responsibility to separate all people involved so they are not all in one room or one area of the clinical setting. Each person involved needs his or her own separate interview and no contact with others involved. Limiting the people who come in contact with biological evidence, so as to preserve its integrity, may be an initial responsibility of the forensic nurse. Documentation of evidence collected to maintain chain of custody and documentation of statements made by witnesses are essential responsibilities. Lack of forensic knowledge and an inability to multitask can lead to the nurse being unable to conduct the interview, evidence collection, and storage procedures appropriately, which could be detrimental to

the assessment of treatment and evaluation, investigation, and disposition of a case.

A traditional role in which forensic nurses have made a significant impact is that of the SANE. Nurses prepared as a SANE-A or SANE-P are specially qualified to deal with persons who have been sexually assaulted and who are at a vulnerable time in their lives. The SANE is able to collect appropriate data and evidence and intervene while preserving the dignity of the victim in an effort to deal with the effects of sexual violence. Programs preparing SANE nurses are designed to meet the needs of sexual assault victims by providing immediate, compassionate, culturally sensitive, and comprehensive forensic evaluation and treatment by trained, professional nurse experts (see Chapter 9 for more information).

As a nurse death investigator, forensic nurses investigate suspicious deaths or deaths suspected to be from homicide, suicide, or natural disaster. Also, nurses investigate accidents, injuries, and environmental hazards. In a death investigation, the forensic nurse brings knowledge of forensic science blended with the preservation of dignity for the deceased and an understanding of how to address the emotional needs of families and loved ones. Many areas of nursing knowledge are used, from basic communications skills and anatomy and physiology to knowledge of pharmacology and pathophysiology, mathematics and physics, psychiatric health, and education. The forensic nurse serves as an impartial observer striving to protect the rights of the deceased and others who may be involved. As an investigator, the forensic nurse brings knowledge of the following: standards for screening, indicators of criminal activity and/or abuse, risk for injury, intentional or unintentional injury determination, and analysis and preservation of evidence. In the investigation of environmental hazards, the forensic nurse brings knowledge of public health levels of prevention, situational analysis, science, and psychological behavior that commonly follows a mass event. Nurses may be the only professionals involved in a disaster scene who have the insight to apply appropriate safeguards for the protection of individuals and their families, communities, and broader populations from physical, environmental, and psychological harm. The holistic outlook is an invaluable asset often found only with the involvement of the nurse professional.

Nurse provision of psychiatric care is another role in which the application of holistic concepts enhances the nursing assessment process. Functions of the psychiatric forensic nurse include legal sanity evaluation, safety and security evaluations, competency evaluation, assessment of capacity for intent, assessment of violence potential, prediction of dangerousness, parole and probation considerations, consultation on violence management, assessment of racial and cultural factors in crime, jury selection assistance, investigation of criminal history, assessment of personality disorders, sexual predator screening, and consultation in legal proceedings. The majority of the forensic nurse's responsibilities might be caring for the living. However, after a person dies, the forensic psychological evaluation of an individual and his or her behavior around the time of death, often called the psychological autopsy, may be crucial in determining the cause and manner of death.

The development of forensic nursing and what constitutes forensic nursing may vary by country due to the distinctive history and development of health care, nursing, and the particular practice specialty. Differences in history, economic and political development, cultural influences, and types of services available in different countries all influence the prevalence and practice role of forensic nursing. For example, nurses working in correctional settings in the United Kingdom are commonly referred to as forensic mental health nurses, although this has been expanded to include nurses working with individuals who have histories of offending regardless of the setting in which they are found (Kettles, et al., 2011). Coram points out that forensic nursing is not determined by the location of the patient but rather by the nurse-patient relationship and the role and functions performed.

STANDARDS OF FORENSIC NURSING PRACTICE

Sources of Standards

Nurses are held to standards from a variety of sources that include but are not limited to the nursing practice act and the laws and regulations of the jurisdiction where a nurse practices; the *Code of Ethics for Nurses*, the *Scope and Standards of Nursing Practice*, the *Scope and Standards of Forensic Nursing Practice* accrediting organization standards; and institutional policies. In contemporary health, it is an expectation that best practice standards derived from research or evidence-based literature guide nursing actions. Additional standards may be derived from case law; common law; state and federal regulations governing healthcare facilities, correctional institutions or other settings where nursing is practiced; and institutional policies.

Forensic nurses, like all health-care professionals, are expected to have the competencies set forth by the Institute of Medicine for health professions education

(Greiner & Knebel, 2003). This includes patient-centered care delivered as part of an interdisciplinary team, with an emphasis on an evidence-based practice and quality improvement approach, as well as the use of informatics.

Ethics

The *Code of Ethics for Nurses* is the nonnegotiable standard every nurse entering the profession must follow. It is in essence what one agrees to when becoming a nurse. The International Council of Nurses (ICN) has an *International Code of Ethics for Nurses* (2006). These codes provide a guide for practice and address nurses' obligations to the people to whom they provide care. They also describe nurses' responsibilities for collaboration with other health-care professionals, advocacy, and advancement of the profession. The need to articulate the importance of fairness, objectivity, and impartiality in forensic nursing was recognized by forensic nursing leaders when the IAFN adopted a vision for ethical practice in 2008. The IAFN vision paper indicates that nurses should practice within an ethical framework for decision making that is guided by the ethical principles of autonomy, beneficence, justice, and non-maleficence. The IAFN vision provides guidelines for the context of ethical forensic nursing practice by fidelity to patients and clients, obligation to the public, obligation to science and its advancement, and dedication to colleagues. The concept of fidelity to patients and clients recognizes, along with the ICN and ANA codes, that forensic nurses are obligated to their patients and that confidentiality must be respected. The limits of confidentiality are disclosed to patients and clients. Forensic nurses are obligated as promoters of public health within the global community to understand societal factors related to violence and their responsibilities for violence prevention. Forensic nurses are also responsible for translating scientific evidence into nursing best practices to enhance the patient outcomes. The forensic nurse must be precise when making public comments on scientific matters and make sure that their statements are substantiated. Furthermore, the vision addresses the forensic nurse's responsibilities for collegiality and the mentorship of students. Professional behaviors related to scholarship are critical for the advancement and dissemination of forensic nursing science and related interdisciplinary scientific work.

Scope and Standards of Practice

Forensic Nursing: Scope and Standards of Practice includes standards of practice that build upon the nursing process components of assessment, diagnosis, outcomes identification, planning, implementation, and evaluation. Measurement criteria are identified for the forensic nurse and the forensic advanced practice nurse as well as the forensic nurse in a nursing role specialty. An illustration of how standards for nursing practice and selected measurement criteria can be applied in forensic nursing appears in Table 1.3.

The forensic nursing practice standards also include professional performance standards for the forensic nurse, the forensic advanced practice nurse, and the forensic nurse in a nursing role specialty. Regardless of the practice setting, educational preparation, or role, forensic nurses have a responsibility to foster high standards

through quality of practice, education, professional practice evaluation, collegiality, collaboration, ethics, research, resource utilization, and leadership. High-quality practice is accomplished by participation in quality improvement activities to improve forensic nursing practice and to achieve recognition of expertise by seeking appropriate certification. Forensic nurses are expected to pursue ongoing educational activities to attain knowledge, maintain competency, and engage in appropriate activities for the evaluation of forensic nursing practice. The dynamic growth and development of the specialty, its influence over other nursing practice settings and specialties, and the impact of forensic health issues within the context of

TABLE 1.3   Application of Forensic Nursing Practice Standards

Element	Measurement Criterion Example	Practical Application From the Literature
Assessment	Collect data with focus on medical-legal implications	The purpose of the forensic examination by a Sexual Assault Nurse Examiner (SANE) is to provide health care and to collect evidence. Sommers' (2007) review of medical records for genital injury variables indicates a need for refined measurement strategies for injury severity and skin color to fully describe the nature of genital trauma. The forensic nurse is familiar with standards for accurate and complete data collection in cases of sexual assault.
Diagnosis	Uses complex data and information and review of medical-legal evidentiary documents in identifying diagnoses	A variety of tools are available for the assessment of intimate partner violence. McFarlane and colleagues (2001) developed a valid and reliable three-question tool, the Abuse Assessment Screen, which can be used in clinical settings. More recently, the tool as been adapted for use with individuals who depend on others for care. Campbell and colleagues (2009) developed a Danger Assessment, which assesses lethality risk for intimate partner femicide.
Outcomes Identification	Supports use of clinical guidelines linked to positive patient outcomes	Retrospective audits of chart data, referrals to rape crisis centers, and adjudication of sexual assault cases can be used as objective measures for individual and program outcomes. Bechtel and colleagues (2008) found that when a SANE was present, more patients in a pediatric emergency setting received testing for sexually transmitted infections, rape crisis center referrals, pregnancy prophylaxis, and medical record documentation of a genitourinary examination. However, only 71% of patients with a SANE present had documentation of a genitourinary examination, indicating need for improvement.
Planning	Supports integration of clinical, human, medical-legal, social, and financial resources to enhance and complete decision making	There are over 500 SANE programs across the country. However, Patterson and colleagues (2006) demonstrated differences in program emphasis in three primary areas, with some programs focused more on prosecution; others attending to patients' needs, empowering patients, and changing community response to rape; and a third group with less focus on prosecution with average emphasis on other goals. Thus, forensic nurses have a role in identifying appropriate program goals for the delivery of comprehensive care to victims of sexual assault to ensure outcomes.

Element	Measurement Criterion Example	Practical Application From the Literature
Implementation	Fosters organizational systems that support implementation of the plan	Nurses can use safety net systems in order to ensure that vulnerable elders are discharged from hospitals into a safe home environment. Popejoy (2008) described the characteristics of health-care team members' use of adult protective services. The forensic nurse can be instrumental in identifying gaps in services that need to be incorporated into effective discharge planning to prevent elder abuse.
Evaluation	Includes patient and others involved in the care of situation in the evaluation process	The Domestic Violence Survivor (DVSA) is a tool developed with the input of survivors and practitioners, as well as a literature review, and is used to measure survivor movement toward a life free of violence (Dienemann, 2007). This instrument is being used by a county agency to evaluate program effectiveness. Forensic nurses can use scientifically sound measures to evaluate individual and program outcomes in the prevention and reduction of violence.

Adapted from American Nurses Association and the International Association of Forensic Nurses. (2009). *Forensic nursing: Scope and standards of practice.* Silver Spring, MD: American Nurses Association.

families, communities, and societies necessitate that the skilled and educated experts at the helm be aware and current in their knowledge base and clinical expertise. Specifically, the nature of forensic nursing and its intersection with other professional practices and potential impact on legal outcomes makes up-to-date knowledge related to forensic nursing practice mandatory.

Forensic nurses also have the responsibility to interact with nurses and members of other disciplines in a collegial, collaborative, and ethical manner to enhance patient care. Professional interaction with colleagues and mentorship of others require current knowledge, use of best practices, and dissemination of the science to promote improved patient outcomes.

For example, SANE programs in most communities are not teams practicing in isolation. They interact with other mental health and medical professionals, advocacy agencies, and law enforcement as part of a community sexual assault response team. They work in collaboration, which is essential to the provision of effective services. However, Cole and Logan (2008) found in a telephone survey of randomly selected SANE programs that the nurses at one-third of the programs ($N = 231$) had experienced conflicts with victim advocacy organizations related to professional autonomy, control, or "turf" issues. Addressing conflict to promote quality improvement of care is the professional responsibility of all health-care providers for effective care of all patients.

The professional performance standards also address forensic nurses' leadership roles. The evaluation of research and integration into practice are standard for the

nurse, whereas the advanced practice forensic nurse's responsibility is to conduct, synthesize, and disseminate research. Forensic nurses expect to take part in various leadership roles to advance the profession. The work of nursing, nursing education, professional organizational involvement, and advocacy are avenues for the forensic nurse to influence decision-making bodies and improve patient care through development of nursing standards. Nurses can take an active part in public policy and legislation related to health-care practices and delivery; prevention of trauma, violence, and abuse; victim rights; prisoner rights; Internet crime; bioterrorism; disaster-preparedness; and resources for forensic nurse education. Forensic nurses can become involved in addressing health care, health promotion, and forensic issues at the local, state, and national levels. Taking part in educational efforts to prevent violence is consistent with the forensic nursing practice standard related to the promotion of health and a safe environment. Membership in the ANA, IAFN, and the ANA constituent member associations, such as a state nurses associations, brings about an exchange of knowledge among practicing professional nurses. Being active in professional organizations gives nurses the opportunity to bring forensic issues to the attention of the larger group of nurses to solicit feedback and support when advocating for change. Conversely, awareness of current legislative and regulatory initiatives may be achieved by nurses while attending professional conference and political action meetings. Forensic nurses have made important contributions to the position statements of professional leadership and political action organizations, thus contributing to the strength of collective action of nurses improving health care.

Standards Supporting the Forensic Nursing Role

Additional standards specifically supporting the role of forensic nursing responsibilities in the institution include the Joint Commission accreditation criteria, which require that health-care organizations have written criteria in place for the assessment of forensic patients who might be victims of physical assault, sexual assault, sexual molestation, domestic abuse, or elder or child abuse or neglect. The Joint Commission delineates various forensic responsibilities for institutions regarding the care of forensic patients. Storage of evidence, staff education, internal reporting, and reporting suspected child abuse or elder abuse to external agencies are responsibilities that must be included in policies for nurses. In 1974, the Federal Child Abuse Prevention and Treatment Act required reporting of child abuse in all states. Furthermore, reporting elder mistreatment is mandated in most states. The Occupational Safety and Health Administration (OHSA) does not have regulations for violence prevention in the workplace, but it does have numerous documents that provide guidance on the implementation of strategies to prevent workplace violence.

Position statements and resolutions of the ANA and IAFN provide guidance for nursing action in specific situations. For example, the IAFN has a position statement on collaboration with victim advocates. The position indicates that each member of the team should have the opportunity to provide patients with information about their roles and that autonomy should be respected by affording patients the opportunity to choose which team members may provide services. The IAFN has also published standards for intimate partner violence nursing practice that provides guidance for nurses working with patients or clients who are the victims/survivors of intimate partner violence, including physical, sexual, psychological/emotional, and economic abuse. Similarly, the ANA has position statements on a wide variety of topics applicable across the broad spectrum of nursing practice. One such position statement of interest to forensic nurses is ANA's position statement, *Adapting Standards of Care under Extreme Conditions: Guidance for Professionals During Disasters, Pandemics and Other Extreme Emergencies*. This position statement is designed to provide guidance for nurses who are at the site of a disaster when it happens, who are working in settings that have been affected by disasters when typical resources for the provision of health care and nursing care are limited or absent, or who are at some other site because of relocation due to the disaster.

Well-designed forensic nursing research, once it has been published and disseminated, has the potential to become a practice standard. For example, McFarlane and colleagues (2006) were able to demonstrate that simple abuse assessment and the offer of referrals have the potential to interrupt and prevent recurrence of intimate partner violence and associated trauma. This research clearly illustrates the value of incorporating abuse assessment and referral into practice.

Standards guiding forensic nursing practice are derived from multiple sources. The forensic nurse needs to be aware of the standards and how to apply them to the individualized care of the patient in a sensitive, professional, and thorough manner. The case study, which describes a potential case of elder mistreatment, highlights some important considerations to be made in applying standards to forensic nursing practice.

Case Study

THE NURSE CARING FOR AN ELDERLY PATIENT AT RISK FOR MISTREATMENT

An 82-year-old woman is admitted to the emergency department for a possible myocardial infarction. She lives with her daughter and son-in-law. The mother had been complaining of feeling weak and too tired to even get out of bed upon awakening and did not get out of bed at all, which was in stark contrast to her usual routine. The daughter called 911 at 4 p.m., and the mother was transported to the ER via ambulance. Upon admission, an EKG was performed, and blood was drawn for troponin levels. The ER doctor made a preliminary diagnosis of inferior wall myocardial infarction. The patient was stabilized and transferred to the telemetry unit for further treatment. The patient met the criteria for a research study that involved examining patterns of treatment delay in myocardial infarction. The nurse researcher went into the patient's room to explain the

Case Study

THE NURSE CARING FOR AN ELDERLY PATIENT AT RISK FOR MISTREATMENT (continued)

study and request that the patient consider participation. When discussing why the patient was selected for possible inclusion in the study, the patient said that the daughter didn't want to call 911 for her because her husband was still home and that she had to wait until he went to work. Since she wasn't really sure what was going on and thought her fatigue might get better, she didn't say anything else. Subsequently, the patient declined to participate in the study stating that she herself would want to participate but that she had better not because her son-in-law would be upset with her and she didn't want to get her daughter in trouble. The nurse researcher asked the patient if there was anyone who was hurting her. The patient responded that she didn't want the nurse researcher to say anything to anyone else and wanted the nurse researcher to agree that she would not. Subsequently, the nurse researcher reported the patient's responses to the staff nurse.

Answer the following questions based upon the application of standards of practice relevant to forensic nursing:

1. What specifically about the dialogue between the patient and the nurse researcher might indicate a suspicion of abuse?
2. Should the nurse researcher have reported the patient's statements about her decision to take part in the study to the staff nurse? What information should be included and what should be excluded to protect the patient's confidentiality?
3. What tenets of the Code of Ethics for Nurses (ANA, 2001) provide guidance in addressing the issues raised in this case study?
4. What standards of the *Forensic Nursing: Scope and Standards of Practice* should be applied to this patient care situation?
5. What should be said to a patient who asks that confidentiality be preserved? What is the most appropriate action for health-care professionals who might not have the direct care responsibility for the patient in this regard?

6. What are the responsibilities of the staff nurse upon learning this information? The charge nurse? The nurse manager?
7. What should be communicated to the patient's health-care provider?
8. What strategies can be used in collaborating with members of different health-care disciplines?
9. What should the staff nurse say to the patient? What strategies can be used to elicit the appropriate information in a nonthreatening manner?
10. Should the nurse caring for the patient ask the daughter if anyone is hurting her or her mother?
11. What resources might be available within the institution to address the issues raised by the information obtained about the patient?
12. What are differences that might be observed when examining an elderly person who might be experiencing abuse in comparison to a younger person?
13. What are the laws or regulations in your state regarding elder mistreatment? Are nurses considered mandated reporters?

Resources

American Nurses Association and International Association of Forensic Nurses. (2009). *Forensic nursing: scope and standards of practice.* Silver Spring, MD: ANA.

Fulmer, T. (2008). Screening for mistreatment of older adults. *American Journal of Nursing, 108*(12), 52-59, quiz 59-60.

Wiglesworth, A., Austin, R., Corona, M., Schneider, D., Liao, S., Gibbs, L. et al. (2009). Bruising as a marker of physical elder abuse. *Journal of the American Geriatrics Society, 57*(7), 1191-1196.

Yaffe, M.J., Wolfson, C., & Lithwick, M. (2009). Professions show different enquiry strategies for elder abuse detection: Implications for training and interprofessional care. *Journal of Interprofessional Care, 2*:1-9.

Therapeutic Jurisprudence

A recent area of development that impacts forensic nursing practice is the application of therapeutic jurisprudence. **Therapeutic jurisprudence** is a legal reform theory, originally developed by Wexler and Winick in response to mental health laws, that considers how the well-being of those in the legal system is impacted by legal actors, legal rules, and legal procedures. Within this context, there are laws that are therapeutic and laws that are not therapeutic. Laws produce behavioral consequences. For example, the three strikes law implemented in many states has contributed to the tremendous growth of the prison population in the United States. Therapeutic jurisprudence focuses on the law's impact on emotional and psychological well-being, humanizing the law and the human, emotional, and psychological aspect of the law and legal processes. By understanding the impact of the law and the legal system, nurses can be more effective in using research to demonstrate the effects of health-care policies. The application of therapeutic jurisprudence is illustrated by Roberson and Kjervik's analysis of North Carolina laws related to the adolescents' competencies to provide consent for treatment.

ON BECOMING A FORENSIC NURSE

Forensic Nursing

Educational preparation for forensic nursing may be accomplished through a variety of means, depending on the role and specific specialization of the nurse. According to the ANA and IAFN, basic forensic nursing is a generalist practice, and the specifics of the practice are guided by protocols and standards for the care of specific forensic populations. Forensic nurses may become certified as SANE nurses, reflecting the nurses' specialized knowledge and competencies for the sexual assault nurse examiner's role and commitment to leadership in forensic nursing. According to the National Organization for Competency Assessment (n.d.) "certification represents a declaration of a particular individual's professional competence" and "certification of specialized skill-sets affirms a knowledge and experience base for practitioners in a particular field, their employers, and the public at large." Thus, SANE education guidelines help guide programs to ensure that what is taught is more standardized. A nurse must have 3 years of experience as a registered nurse and complete a SANE program, which includes supervised patient encounters, to qualify to take the IAFN-developed examination for SANE-A or SANE-P certification. The SANE certification can be renewed by documentation of related continuing education or by passing the examination every 3 years. There are SANE-A certification review courses conducted by sexual assault experts who teach participants what they need to know to pass the examination. The SANE certification examinations are administered by the Forensic Nursing Certification Board, an autonomous component of the IAFN.

Other subspecialty certifications, such as forensic nurse death investigator or forensic nurse generalist, may be developed in the future based on the competencies and standards. There are also examination-based certificates that have been developed by forensic nurses available through various forensic nurse organizations that attest to a nurse's knowledge and expertise in a particular area.

Advanced Practice in Forensic Nursing

Advanced practice forensic registered nurses are prepared at the graduate level in nursing as a nurse practitioner, certified nurse-midwife, or clinical nurse specialist.

Advanced practice forensic nurses may hold a master's or doctoral degree and have formal course work in forensic nursing and related courses. They are licensed, certified, and approved to practice in their advanced practice nursing role as a nurse practitioner, clinical nurse specialist, or certified nurse midwife. Often, whether their advanced practice education was specifically in forensic nursing or not, advanced practice forensic nurses hold a leadership role in their practice, institution, or community by way of their special education and role responsibilities.

In 2004, an international committee of IAFN advanced practice educators developed the advanced practice core curriculum based on forensic nursing competencies. However, this is a highly specialized area of practice. Therefore, experts in credentialing and forensic nursing have been exploring options for an advanced practice forensic nurse portfolio credential. The advanced practice forensic nurse portfolio would be a means of evaluating competencies for individuals who meet criteria detailed in the core curriculum. The forensic advanced practice registered nurse portfolio credential will evaluate transcripts of course work, continuing education, publications, research, and completed projects, which support the individual's attainment of the competencies for the practice specialization. A portfolio is used when the potential number of individuals taking the certifying examination is not sufficient to conduct appropriate analyses to ensure that the examination is valid and reliable. It is hoped that the forensic advanced practice registered nurse certification credential will be available in the future. As with other certifications, periodic renewal will be required to maintain the credential.

Advanced practice registered nurse (APRN) specialty education and practice build upon the education and practice focus of the APRN role and population focus. Generally, advanced practice nursing education programs grant a master's level certificate or post-master's certificate. Programs consist of from 12 to 18 graduate level credits and generally include at least one clinical practicum. Many programs are listed on the IAFN Web site (www.iafn.org). Programs prepare nurses to prevent violence, crime, and traumatic injuries as well as to provide crisis response. Nurses are also prepared to provide leadership in forensic nursing through the advancement of forensic science and evidence-based practice, influencing legislation and policy, as well as collaboration with health-care and related professionals, other social service agencies, and criminal justice systems to provide care for individuals, families, and communities who will benefit from forensic nursing services.

EVIDENCE-BASED FORENSIC NURSING PRACTICE

Forensic nurses are concerned with truth and accuracy and must consider the evidence, which tends to logically prove or disprove a fact at issue in a judicial case of controversy. Evidence is that which is used to determine the truth of a matter and may have the slightest bearing on the outcome of a case, provided there is a logical tendency to relate the evidence to the outcome of the case. Evidence serves to associate a suspect to a victim, a crime scene to a suspect, and a victim to a crime scene. Categories of evidence include information or testimonial evidence and physical or real evidence.

The Role of Evidence

Testimonial or oral evidence includes the statements of witnesses who observed an act or event that took place. The nurse does not know the facts. However, the routine conduct of nursing business, the nursing process, is initiated with the first-hand history obtained from the forensic patient/witness. Without a sufficient history of a chief complaint or event on which to base the nursing care, the forensic nurse cannot proceed with the performance of forensic nursing competencies: collection and preservation of real evidence that is biological or physical, that can be tested, and that is admissible in court to prove facts related in verbal information obtained from the patient.

Real evidence that is biological or physical may be transient or altered by drying or other natural conditions.

Therefore, real evidence requires a chain of custody to verify every person who has had the item in custody from its collection to the courtroom.

The standard for admissibility of evidence prior to 1993 was the *Frye* test and Federal Rules of Evidence Rule 702. However, the Frye test was considered to be inconsistent with the Federal Rules in 1993 in a case called *Daubert v. Merrell Dow Pharmaceuticals, Inc.* The Supreme Court delineated several criteria for determining admissibility of expert scientific evidence in court. Theories and techniques employed by scientists must have been tested and subjected to peer review and publication. There must be error rates associated with the techniques that indicate the theory or technique has been tested. From this information it is assumed that the trier of fact (finder of fact) could see the limitations. Standards and controls governing the application of the test are expected, along with others doing similar work. Theories and techniques must be presented and be relatively widespread and accepted in the field, even if results are not supported by all experts in the field. While all states do not have to adhere to the Federal Rules, many do use the higher standard of the *Daubert Rule* to admit scientific evidence in court. All of the considerations of the *Daubert Rule* do not need to be met, but the majority of them must meet the higher standard of admissibility of evidence. The ruling specifically addressed the value of science and evidence used for courtroom evidence, not just uninformed opinions and "junk science."

Research Evidence

The evidence of most importance for the nurse scientist is relevant, scientifically sound, and ethical research. The scientific evidence is the base on which experts develop an informed practice; these practices are based on the previously mentioned standards and competencies that support their expert opinion testimony for the courts.

The expert has no basis for forming, applying, and reaching an opinion without solid science behind his or her theories and actions. In forensic nursing practice, fact evidence is collected through careful observation, physical examination, documentation of all findings, and preservation of the physical evidence. Thus, the best evidence derived from research should be used to guide forensic nursing principles and practice of forensic nursing. Forensic nursing science and the expert opinions of the forensic nurse will then be admitted in court and evaluated according to *Daubert Rule* standards.

The mandate for the use of evidence is derived from the *Code of Ethics for Nurses* which indicates that nurses have an obligation to advance the profession through knowledge development, dissemination, and application to practice. Furthermore, the *Forensic Nursing Scope and Standards of Practice* indicates that the forensic nurse and advanced practice forensic nurse are obligated to use the best available scientific evidence to guide practice decisions and to inform their opinions. Evidence-based practice in forensic nursing is an important guide for nursing students, educators, researchers, and administrators. It provides a clear and succinct summary of current, relevant nursing and related multidisciplinary research.

Evidence-based nursing practice is derived from the work of Archie Cochrane, who emphasized the importance of using evidence from randomized controlled trials (RCTs) because they were more likely to provide more reliable information. Also, because resources for health care were limited, it was important to use them wisely. The term evidence-based medicine was coined by the work group of Gordon Guyatt at McMaster University. Since then, the emphasis on evidence-based practice for all health-care professionals and educators has expanded exponentially. The drive to use evidence for a more sound professional practice includes nurses in the development of various resources, work groups, and centers to examine the scientific foundation for various practices and provide recommendations for the best care in a given situation.

Evidence-based practice is the integration of the best research evidence with clinical expertise and the patient's unique values and circumstances (Strauss, et al., 2005). Fawcett and Garity (2009) integrate research as theory development, theory as evidence, and practice as research in their definition of evidence-based nursing practice: "the deliberate and critical use of theories about human beings' health-related experiences to guide actions associated with each step of the nursing process." In this definition, research provides the critical foundation for theory that guides practice.

Processes for Using Research Evidence

Determining an appropriate evidence-based practice for use in a particular clinical situation requires a systematic process. Quite often, there is no information on a best practice because there has been no research conducted on that particular area of practice. An example of this is research conducted by Sommers and her colleagues on anogenital injuries after consensual sex, as illustrated in the Research Exemplar (Box 1.2). Sometimes a standard that has been in place for many years is not an evidence-based standard. Nurses are encouraged not to perform nursing actions "because it was always done this way," but rather to take a leadership role, develop the clinical

---

Box 1.2 Research Exemplar

Sommers, M.S., Zink, T M., Fargo, J.D., Baker, R.B., Buschur, C., Shambley-Ebron, D.Z. et al. (2008). Forensic sexual assault examination and genital injury: is skin color a source of health disparity? *American Journal of Emergency Medicine, 26*(8), 857-866.

This study was designed to examine the types of anogenital injuries experienced by black and white women after consensual sex as well as to examine the relationships of skin color associated with the injury as observed during the sexual assault examination. The sample consisted of volunteers who had a forensic examination after consensual sexual intercourse. Of the white women, 68% had at least one anogenital injury, whereas 43% of the black women had at least one such injury. However, skin color confounded the relationship between race and ethnicity, and injury. A red and/or green appearance of the skin was associated with injury to the internal genitalia.

Implications: Health-care professionals completing forensic sexual assault examinations should be aware of the significance of skin color in relation to anogenital injuries. It is important that misconceptions about the relationship of injury to race and or ethnicity do not impede a thorough and comprehensive forensic sexual assault examination. Cultural competence is critical when completing a forensic sexual assault examination.

---

questions for inquiry, and assess the science for the best way to perform the nursing action. Forensic nurses have a critical role to play in asking the clinical questions about their practice. While not every forensic nurse will be directly involved in the conduct of research, forensic nurses have the responsibility and the clinical expertise to ask the right questions, search for the scientific truth to advance forensic nursing practice, and ultimately, enhance the forensic patient outcomes.

A number of guides and resources are available for identifying an evidence-based practice (EBP) solution to a clinical problem. The seven steps of evidence-based practice are described as follows: (1) cultivating a spirit of inquiry, (2) asking clinical questions in the PICOT format, (3) searching for the best evidence, (4) critically appraising evidence, (5) integrating the evidence with clinical expertise and patient preferences and values, (6) evaluating the outcomes of practice decisions or evidence-based changes, and (7) disseminating the EBP results (Melnyk, et al., 2010).

Melnyk and colleagues (2010) suggest using the widely used standard PICOT format—**P**opulation/**P**atient, **I**ntervention of Interest, **C**omparison intervention or group, **O**utcome and **T**ime—to formulate the answerable clinical question. It is important to define the question so that the search for evidence and the analysis of the results can be accomplished more effectively. Formulating the answerable clinical question serves as a guide for the subsequent activities in appraising the evidence and decision making as it is applied to patient care. An illustration of the PICOT question as applied to forensic nursing practice is illustrated in Table 1.4.

The clinical question may need to be refined and modified. Revisions to the outcome measure may be needed based on preliminary results of the search. For example, it might be discovered that criminal prosecutions are not consistently reported as outcome measures in studies evaluating the effectiveness of SANEs, since it is, in fact, a legal outcome and not a health-care outcome. However, there may be much research on nursing actions taken, such as psychosocial support, which is often and consistently reported for a variety of forensic patients and therefore might be a more appropriate outcome measure. The time frame may or may not be appropriate for the particular practice that is being evaluated. This is a matter of the forensic nurse's clinical judgment as well as evaluation of the information gathered from the research reviewed.

Searching for Evidence

It is often necessary to use multiple search strategies in multiple databases to locate suitable research studies. One of the first decisions will be to determine the appropriate search terms and the appropriate databases that will yield the relevant evidence to answer the clinical question. The clinical question provides direction for keywords and search terms. Commonly used databases are listed in Table 1.5.

These databases will provide abstracts of single research studies as well as selected synthesis of evidence. One may also need to look at the Medical Subject Headings (MeSH) headings in PubMed, the National Library of Medicine database. This will help identify standard terms. For example, sexual assault is not listed in the MeSH database, whereas sexual abuse is listed, with a number of related terms provided. However, it should be noted that searching with the term "sexual assault" will yield numerous publications. Thus, successful searching will usually consist of attempting a number of strategies to increase the yield of relevant studies. An example of a search is illustrated in the Evidence-Based Practice box for this chapter. The assistance of a librarian is valuable in identifying suitable search strategies and as well as navigating different databases.

Evaluating the Strength of Evidence

While a single well-designed study may be useful in providing direction for clinical practice, very often multiple studies and synthesized evidence provide stronger evidence. There are hierarchies for rating the strength of scientific evidence, type of studies, or reviews, as well as rating systems for individual studies. The 6S hierarchy as suggested by Straus and Haynes (2009) and illustrated in Figure 1.2 is useful as an approach for determining the strength of the evidence to address a clinical problem. In this particular system, the ideal would be clinical decision support systems embedded in an electronic health record system.

An example of such a system is illustrated in the incorporation of abuse screening tools into the electronic record and the subsequent transmission of the information to the appropriate social service agency by a visiting nurse association. However, the reality is that many organizations do not have an electronic health record, let alone a clinical decision support system, as a resource. However, a number of syntheses, synopses, and summaries are readily available on the Internet as well as in the databases that

---

TABLE 1.4   Case Example: The PICOT Question Applied to a Clinical Problem in Forensic Nursing Practice

Clinical Problem	Does evidence collection in rape examinations completed by SANEs improve prosecution of rape perpetrators compared to evidence collection completed by those who are not trained as SANEs?
Population/Patient	Patients who have had evidence collected with a sexual assault examination.
Intervention Evidence Collection	
Comparison	SANEs' collection of evidence in sexual assault examinations compared with non-SANEs collection of evidence in sexual assault examinations.
Outcome	Improved completeness of evidence collected; improved prosecution and conviction of perpetrators.
Time	When the expected change or increase is expected to be observed, in this instance, the time frame used by the prosecutor in filing the case in court, up to 6 months from the time of the examination.

TABLE 1.5 **Commonly Used Databases for Forensic Nursing Evidence-Based Practice Literature Searches**

Database	Description
Cumulative Index to Nursing and Allied Health Literature (CINAHL)	Indexes nearly 3000 journals in nursing and 17 allied health disciplines with records back to 1981. Includes ANA and National League for Nursing publications, educational software, audiovisuals and book chapters, research instruments, and legal cases.
EMBASE	Specialized abstract and indexing database that covers biomedical and pharmaceutical research, including drugs and toxicology, clinical medicine, biotechnology, health affairs, psychiatry, and forensic medicine in over 3500 journals.
Medline	The abstract database of the National Library of Medicine (NLM), with over 17 million references to articles in more than 5200 current biomedical journals from the United States and over 80 foreign countries. It can be accessed via PubMed or through commercial browsers such as OVID or First Search.
PsycINFO	An abstract database that covers the psychological literature from the 1800s to the present. Includes over 2400 journals, 99% of which are peer-reviewed, selected book chapters, and dissertations.
PubMed	The search engine maintained by the National Library of Medicine for accessing MEDLINE in addition to several other databases, in-process citations, and citations for articles that precede the date that a journal was included in Medline.
Virginia Henderson International Nursing Library	Registry of Nursing Research database of the Sigma Theta Tau International (STTI) Honor Society of Nursing. Includes research abstracts and conference abstracts as well as e-mail contacts for first authors.
SocINDEX	A sociology research database that includes criminology, criminal justice, marriage and family, sociology, social psychology, sociological research, substance abuse, addictions, violence, and others.

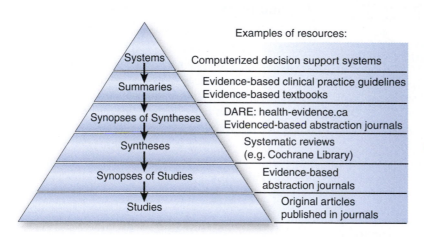

■ FIGURE 1.2 The 6S approach to finding useful evidence. (Reprinted with permission from Straus, S. & Haynes, R.B. (2009). Managing evidence-based knowledge: the need for reliable, relevant and readable resources. *Canadian Medical Association Journal.* 180(9), 942-945.)

are listed in Table 1.5. Examples of resources of synthesized evidence of interest to forensic nurses are illustrated in Table 1.6.

It is generally easier to use evidence that has been summarized, synthesized, or synopsized. However, regardless of the format, whether using a single research study, synopsis, synthesis, or summary, each still needs to be critically appraised. Generally, an RCT is usually considered the gold standard with regard to a single study. In an RCT, the recipients of the treatment are blinded, as are the individuals evaluating the outcome. However, an RCT cannot be used to answer all questions. Well-designed

TABLE 1.6   **Information Sources**

Evidence-Based Journals	▪ *Evidence-Based Nursing* ▪ *Worldviews on Evidence-Based Nursing* ▪ *Evidence-Based Medicine* ▪ *Evidence-Based Mental Health* ▪ *Evidence-Based Health Care Policy and Practice*
Evidence-Based Reviews	▪ Clinical Evidence (http://clinicalevidence.bmj.com) ▪ Physician's Information and Education Resource (http://pier.acponline.org) ▪ Evidence-Based Medicine Reviews (EBMR) (http://ovid.com) ▪ ACP Journal Club (http://acpjc.com)
Databases	▪ Database of Abstracts of Reviews of Evidence (DARE) ▪ Cochrane Database of Systematic Reviews (CDSR) ▪ Cochrane Database of Methodology Reviews (CDMR) ▪ Cochrane Register of Controlled Trials ▪ Health Technology Assessments (HTA) ▪ National Health Service (NHS) Economic Evaluation Database (NHSEED) ▪ National Clinical Guideline Clearinghouse (http://www.guideline.gov)
Evidence-Based Centers	▪ Cochrane Collaboration (http://cochrane.org) ▪ The Joanna Briggs Institute (http://joannabriggs.edu.au) ▪ Centre for Evidence-Based Medicine, Oxford (http://cebm.net) ▪ Center for Evidence-Based Corrections: University of California at Irvine (http://ucicorrections.seweb.uci.edu) ▪ University of Iowa College of Nursing Evidence-Based Practice Guidelines (http://nursing.uiowa.edu) ▪ Registered Nurses Association of Ontario (http://rnao.org) ▪ Center for Evidence-Based Crime Policy at George Mason University (http://gunston.gmu.edu/cebcp)
Governmental Agencies	▪ Agency for Healthcare Research and Quality (http://ahrq.gov) ▪ National Institute for Health and Clinical Excellence (NICE) (http://nice.org.uk) ▪ Scottish Intercollegiate Guidelines Network (http://sign.ac.uk)

descriptive, qualitative, or epidemiological studies (just to name a few) can provide important, accurate, and valuable information. For example, at the time this chapter was written, no RCT was located relative to the use of SANEs in emergency rooms. However, Bechtel, Ryan, and Gallagher (2008) examined outcomes related to the use of SANE nurses, and Campbell, Patterson, and Lichty (2005) reviewed the medical, legal, and community outcomes for SANE programs.

Critical appraisal of evidence requires determining whether the results are valid and whether the results can be applied to the patient population to improve outcomes. Evaluation of the strength of the design and the magnitude of the effect of the patient response is important. In reviewing the study, it is useful to have a guide that is specific to appraising the evidence derived from a particular study design, for example, a randomized clinical trial, a descriptive study, or a qualitative study. Guidelines are also available for appraising integrative reviews, summaries,

synopses, and clinical guidelines. For example, the *Appraisal of Guidelines for Research and Evaluation Instrument*, known as the Agree Collaboration (2001), provides a framework for the development, reporting, and assessment of clinical guidelines. This instrument is available from www.agreecollaboration.org.

Applying Evidence

Once it has been determined that the results of the study are valid and can be applied to a particular population, a practice decision can be made that integrates the evidence, the clinical population, and the values of the patient. Thus, the forensic nurse integrates scientific knowledge, clinical judgment, skills, and experience with the patient's preferences. For example, in providing evidence-based post–sexual assault counseling, it would be important to take the client's preferences into consideration in making a treatment recommendation. If a counseling program requires a woman to spend many hours on public transportation and to find child care, then some other option to obtain appropriate counseling should be considered.

Evaluating and Disseminating Outcomes

The last steps of the process are evaluating and disseminating the outcomes. An outcome measurement demonstrates the impact of the intervention upon the patient population, basically, the results of the care that was provided. These outcomes may have an impact upon the patient's health, use of health services, adherence to a treatment regimen, knowledge, psychosocial functioning, and quality of life. It is important to define the outcome in terms of how one will know whether the treatment or intervention was successful. Therefore, it is important to identify and choose the indicators to monitor so that an appropriate method is selected for the assessment of the outcome. And, the assessment of outcomes and disseminating information about them are important steps in advancing the recognition for the value of forensic nursing practice and advanced forensic nursing practice. For example, Bechtel and colleagues (2008) found that 98% of the pediatric patients admitted to an emergency room for sexual assault were referred to a rape crisis center when a SANE was involved in the care, compared to 30% of patients receiving such a referral when a SANE was not involved in the care. Another outcome measure for SANE nurses is completeness in evidence collection for sexual assault. Sievers and colleagues (2003) found that evidence collection by SANEs was more complete than evidence collection by non-SANEs.

The results of studies on the effectiveness of SANE programs provide strong evidence for establishing a SANE program within a hospital emergency department. However, once a program is adopted, for example, it is not sufficient to make the assumption that the forensic patient care outcomes have automatically improved. It is important to determine appropriate benchmarks or a standard by which the nursing actions or effectiveness of care is judged. One method of benchmarking is to submit data to a national database that then provides an analysis of comparative data to the organization. This is becoming increasingly important as the public demands data about health-care organizations and health-care providers. An example of such a database for forensic nurses is the National SANE-SART Database, which helps SANE programs to cooperate and share information. In addition, comparison of forensic program patient satisfaction, treatments, outcomes, referrals, and other nursing actions can be compared to existing national protocols and guidelines.

Translation Science

Identifying evidence-based practices to guide the care provided by forensic nurses is only one step in the process. More recently, emphasis has been placed on evidence-based practices to implement change and translate research into practice. Very often, there is a significant time lag between the publication of research results, the identification of its value for practitioners, and its ultimate use in practice. The entire process of implementing research into practice is referred to as **translation science.** The National Collaborating Centre for Methods and Tools provides a useful framework to guide the adoption of an evidence-based innovation. The Registered Nurses Association of Ontario (2002) has made a toolkit available for adoption on its Web site (http://rnao.org).

It takes a significant amount of time and effort to prepare for the implementation of an evidence-based practice using the latest findings of translation science. Implementation of an evidence-based practice requires the engagement of multiple stakeholders to achieve success in the process. Forensic nurses are in a unique position to provide leadership to facilitate the translation of research into practice because of their expertise in multidisciplinary collaboration.

CONCLUSIONS

In summary, as forensic medical issues have gained more public attention, clear evidence has emerged that the expertise of a forensic nurse is vital for optimal patient safety and care. With the implementation of forensic education programs that enhance the skills of nurses in all areas of practice, as well as establishment of standards of care in forensic cases, nurses will become part of the solution as patient advocates who are affected by the challenges we face in today's society. Finally, forensic nurses are uniquely positioned to advance the translation of research into practice to enhance the care of the populations they serve across the health-care continuum.

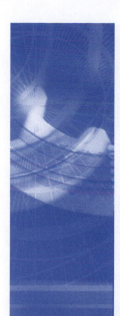

EVIDENCE-BASED PRACTICE

Reference Question: What are scope and standards of practice in forensic nursing?

Databases to Search: PubMed

Search Terms: When possible, it is best to use the standardized MeSH vocabulary. Searching for the appropriate search terms may be done in the MeSH database (http://www.ncbi.nlm.nih.gov/mesh). The search below demonstrates searching a topic broadly, "practice guidelines as topic" to more focused "practice guidelines as topic/*standards."

Selected References From Search:

1. Cashman, D.P. & Benak L.D. (2007). Preparing staff for testimony in sexual assault cases. *Journal of Forensic Nursing. 3*(1):47-49.
2. Ferguson, C.T. (2008). Caring sexual assault patients in the military: past, present, and future. *Journal of Forensic Nursing. 4*(4):190-198.
3. Pierce-Weeks, J. & Campbell, P. (2008). The challenges forensic nurses face when their patient is comatose: Addressing the needs of our most vulnerable patient population. *Journal of Forensic Nursing. 4*(3):104-110.
4. American Nurses Association and International Association for Forensic Nurses. (2009). *Forensic Nursing: Scope and Standards of Forensic Nursing Practice.* Silver Spring, MD: ANA. Available from: http://nursesbooks.org

Questions Used to Discern Evidence:

Choose two studies among the studies listed, read about them, and answer the following questions:

1. What are the differences between the two studies in the design, methods, and results?
2. What are the similarities between the two studies in the number of subjects, measures used, and interventions, if any?
3. What skills do you think you need to learn to practice forensic nursing?

REVIEW QUESTIONS

1. The mantra of forensic nursing is:
   A. Truth.
   B. Ethics.
   C. Trauma.
   D. Justice.

2. The International Association of Forensic Nurses adopted the definition of forensic nursing as a practice of nursing globally when:
   A. Health and illness intersect.
   B. Health and legal systems intersect.
   C. Disaster and health intersect.
   D. Violence and law intersect.

3. Nursing's *Social Policy Statement* defines nursing's obligations to society and includes six critical elements of nursing: provision of a caring relationship, attention to human experiences and responses to health and illness, integration of objective data with the patient's subjective experience, application of scientific knowledge, advancement of professional knowledge, and the promotion of:
   A. Health.
   B. Quality of life.
   C. Social justice.
   D. Well-being.

(review questions continued on page 24)

≡ R E V I E W   Q U E S T I O N S—cont'd ≡

4. The distinctive feature of forensic nursing practice is the nurses' knowledge and skill in navigating intersections of legal and social systems with:
A. Political systems.
B. Economic systems.
C. Ecological systems.
D. Health-care systems.

5. Well-designed forensic nursing research, once it has been published and disseminated, has the potential to become a practice standard as demonstrated in a randomized clinical trial by McFarlane and colleagues (2006) demonstrating that simple abuse assessment and the offer of referrals have the potential to:
A. Interrupt and prevent recurrence of intimate partner violence.
B. Escalate and magnify recurrence of intimate partner violence.
C. Protect and insulate the survivor of the intimate partner violence.
D. Reunite the abused and the abuser in a working relationship.

6. What is a legal reform theory that considers how the well-being of those in the legal system is impacted by legal actions, rules, and procedures?
A. General systems
B. Therapeutic intervention
C. Therapeutic jurisprudence
D. Complexity theory

7. According to the American Nurses Association and the International Association of Forensic Nurses, basic forensic nursing is a:
A. Generalist practice.
B. Specialist practice.
C. Mixed practice.
D. Legal practice.

8. Two general bodies of evidence are present in all potential litigation, fact evidence and:
A. Real evidence.
B. Tested evidence.
C. Expert opinion evidence.
D. Clear and convincing evidence.

9. To formulate an answerable clinical question, Melnyk and colleagues (2010) suggest the widely used standard PICOT format, **P**opulation/**P**atient, **I**ntervention of Interest, **C**omparison intervention or group, **O**utcome and:
A. **T**est.
B. **T**heory.
C. **T**herapy.
D. **T**ime.

10. The entire process of implementing research into practice is referred as:
A. Synergy science.
B. Complexity science.
C. Translation science.
D. Forensic science.

References

Advanced Practice Nursing Joint Dialogue Group. (2008). *Consensus model for APRN regulation: Licensure, accreditation, certification & education.* Retrieved August 18, 2009, from http://www.nursingworld.org

Agree Collaboration. (2001). *Appraisal of Guidelines for Research and Evaluation (AGREE) Instrument.* Retrieved August 15, 2009, from http://www.agreecollaboration.org

American Academy of Forensic Sciences. (n.d.). *Choosing a career.* Retrieved August 15, 2009, from http://www.aafs.org/

American Nurses Association (ANA). (2001). *Code of ethics for nurses with interpretive statements.* Washington, DC: ANA.

American Nurses Association (ANA). (2003). *Nursing's social policy statement* (2nd ed.). Washington, DC: ANA.

American Nurses Association (ANA). (2004). *Nursing: Scope and standards of practice.* Washington, DC: ANA.

American Nurses Association (ANA). (2006). *Legal nurse consulting; Scope and standards of practice.* Silver Spring, MD: ANA.

American Nurses Association (ANA). (2007). *Corrections nursing: Scope and standards of practice.* Silver Spring, MD: ANA.

American Nurses Association (ANA). (2008a). *Adapting standards of care under extreme conditions: Guidance for professionals during disasters, pandemics and other extreme emergencies.* Silver Spring, MD: ANA. Retrieved August 16, 2009, from http://www.nursingworld.org

American Nurses Association (ANA). (2008b). *Nurses voted the most trusted profession.* Silver Spring, MD: ANA. Retrieved August 29, 2009, from www.nursingworld.org

American Nurses Association (ANA) & International Association for Forensic Nurses (IAFN). (2009a). *Forensic nursing:
Scope and standards of practice*. Silver Spring, MD: ANA.

American Nurses Association (ANA) & International Transplant
Nurses Association. (2009b). *Transplant nursing: Scope
and standards of practice*. Silver Spring, MD: ANA.

Bechtel, K., Ryan, E., & Gallagher, D. (2008). Impact of sexual
assault nurse examiners on the evaluation of sexual assault
in a pediatric emergency department. *Pediatric Emergency
Care, 24*(7):442-447.

Bonnie, R.J., & Wallace, R.B. (Eds.). (2003). *Elder mistreatment,
abuse and neglect in an aging America*. Washington, DC:
National Academies Press, Committee on Law and Justice.

Bowring-Lossock, E. (2006). The forensic mental health nurse:
A literature review. *Journal of Psychiatric and Mental
Health Nursing, 13*(6):780-785.

Campbell, J.C., Webster, D., & Glass, N. (2009). The danger
assessment: Validation of a lethality risk assessment instrument for intimate partner femicide. *Journal of Interpersonal
Violence, 24*(4):653-674.

Campbell, R., Patterson, D., & Lichty, L.F. (2005). The effectiveness of sexual assault nurse examiner (SANE) programs: A review of psychological, medical, legal, and community outcomes. *Trauma Violence Abuse, 6*(4):313-329.

Canaff, R. (2009). Nobility in objectivity: A prosecutor's case
for neutrality in forensic nursing. *Journal of Forensic
Nursing, 5*(2):89-96.

Cochrane, A.L. (1972). *Effectiveness and efficiency: Random
reflections on health services*. London: Nuffield Provincial
Hospitals Trust.

Cole, J. & Logan, T. K. (2008). Negotiating the challenges of
multidisciplinary responses to sexual assault victims: Sexual
assault nurse examiner and victim advocacy programs.
Research in Nursing and Health, 31(1):76-85.

Coram, J.W. (2006). Psychiatric forensic nursing. In V.A.
Lynch (ed.), *Forensic nursing*. St. Louis: Elsevier Mosby,
pp. 505-520.

Daubert v. Merrell Dow Pharmaceuticals, Inc. (1993). 509
U.S. 579.

Dienemann, J., Neese, J., & Lowry, S. (2009). Psychometric
properties of the domestic practice in an organization. In
A. DiCenso, G. Guyatt, & D. Ciliska (Eds.), *Evidence-based
nursing: A guide to clinical practice*. St. Louis: Elsevier
Mosby, pp. 172–200.

Evidence-Based Medicine Working Group. Evidence-based
medicine. A new approach to teaching the practice of medicine. *Journal of the American Medical Association,
268*:2420-2425.

Fawcett, J., & Garity, J. (2009). *Evaluating research for
evidence-based nursing practice*. Philadelphia: F.A. Davis.

Fulmer, T. (2008). Screening for mistreatment of older adults.
American Journal of Nursing, 108(12):52-60.

Gilmore, J.H. & Pine, J.B. (2007). *Authenticity. What consumers
really want*. Boston: Harvard University Press.

Hawkins, J.W., Pearce, C.W., Skeith, J., Dimitruk, B., &
Roche, R. (2009). Using technology to expedite screening
and intervention for domestic abuse and neglect. *Public
Health Nursing, 26*(1):58-69.

International Association of Forensic Nurses (IAFN). (2002).
Standards of intimate partner violence nursing practice.
Arnold, MD: IAFN.

International Association of Forensic Nurses (IAFN). (2006).
What is forensic nursing? Retrieved August 17, 2009 from
http://www.iafn.org

International Association of Forensic Nurses (IAFN) &
American Nurses Association (ANA). (1997). *Scope and
standards of forensic nursing practice*. Washington, DC:
American Nurses Association.

International Council of Nurses (ICN). (2006). *The ICN code
of ethics for nurses*. Geneva: ICN. Retrieved August 18,
2009 from: www.icn.ch

Joint Commission. (2009). *Revised 2009 accreditation
requirements as of March 26, 2009. Hospital accreditation
program*. Retrieved August 18, 2009 from http://www.
jointcommission.org

Kent-Wilkinson, A. (2006). Forensic nursing education: Developments, theoretical conceptualizations, and practical
applications for curriculum. In R.M. Hammer, B. Moynihan,
& E.M. Pagliaro (Eds.), *Forensic nursing: A handbook for
practice*. Boston: Jones & Barlett, pp. 781-813.

Kerfoot, K. (2008). Patient satisfaction and high-reliability
organizations: What's the connection? *Medsurg Nursing,
17*(5):357-358.

Kettles, A.M., Byrt, R., & Woods, P. (2007). Forensic educational aspects of acute mental health care: Policy, characteristics, skills and knowledge. In National Forensic Nurses'
Research and Development Group, A. Kettles, P. Woods,
R., Byrt, M. Addo, M. Coffey, & M. Doyle. (Eds.), *Forensic
mental health nursing: Forensic aspects of acute care*.
London: Quay Books.

Kleinpell, R.M. (2009). Measuring outcomes in advanced practice nursing. In R.M. Kleinpell (Ed.). *Outcome assessment
in advanced practice nursing*. New York: Springer, pp.1-62.

Krug, E.G., Dahlberg, L.L., Mercy, J.A., Zwi, A.B., & Lozano, R.
(Eds.). (2002). World health report on violence and health.
Geneva: World Health Organization.

Ledray, L. (2005). The national sexual assault database: Can it
help you? *Journal of Forensic Nursing, 1*(1):36.

Ledray, L. (1999). *SANE: Development and operation guide*.
Office for Victims of Crime, Office of Justice Programs.
Washington, DC: U.S. Department of Justice. Retrieved
August 16, 2009, from http://www.ojp.usdoj.gov/ovc/
publications/infores/sane/saneguide.pdf

Lynch, V.A. (2013). Forensic nursing science. In: R.A.
Hammer, B. Moynihan, & E.M. Pagliaro (Eds.). *Forensic
nursing: A handbook for practice, 2nd ed.* Boston: Jones
& Bartlett, pp. 1-16.

Lynch, V.A. (2011). Evolution of forensic nursing science. In:
V.A. Lynch and J.B. Duvall (Eds.). *Forensic nursing science, 2nd ed.* St. Louis: Elsevier Mosby, pp. 1-9.

Lynch, V.A. (1993). Forensic aspects of health care: New roles,
new responsibilities. *Journal of Psychosocial Nursing,
31*(11):5-6.

Lyons, T. (2009). Role of the forensic psychiatric nurse. *International Journal of Forensic Nursing, 5*(1):53-57.

Mason, T., & Carton, G. (2002). Towards a "forensic lens"
model of multidisciplinary training. *Journal of Psychiatric
Mental Health Nursing, 9*(5):541-551.

McFarlane, J.M., Groff, J.Y., O'Brien, J.A., & Watson, K.
(2006). Secondary prevention of intimate partner violence:
A randomized controlled trial. *Nursing Research, 55*(1):
52-61.

McFarlane, J., Hughes, R.B., Nosek, M.A., Groff, Y., Swedlend, N., & Dolan Mullen, P. (2001). Abuse assessment screen-disability (AAS-D): Measuring frequency, type, and perpetrator of abuse toward women with physical disabilities. *Journal of Women's Health & Gender-Based Medicine, 10*(9):861-866.

McFarlane, J., Parker, B., Soeken, K., & Bullock, L. (1992). Assessing for abuse during pregnancy. Severity and frequency of injuries and associated entry into prenatal care. *Journal of the American Medical Association, 267*(23):3176-3178.

Melnyk, B.M., Fineout-Overholt, E., Stillwell, S.B., & Williamson, K.M. (2010). Evidence-based practice: Step by step: The seven steps of evidence-based practice. *American Journal of Nursing, 110*(1):51-53.

Merriam-Webster Online Dictionary. (2009). Forensic. Retrieved August 17, 2009, from http: //www.merriam-webster.com/dictionary/forensic

National Collaborating Centre for Methods and Tools. (2010). Framework for adopting an evidence-informed innovation in an organization. Hamilton, ON: McMaster University. Retrieved July 14, 2012 from http://www.nccmt.ca/registry/view/eng/47.html.

National Organization for Competency Assessment. (n.d.). *What is certification?* Retrieved August 18, 2009, from http://www.noca.org

Occupational Safety and Health Administration (OSHA). (2009). *Workplace violence.* Retrieved August 18, 2009, from http://www.osha.gov/SLTC/workplaceviolence/

Patterson, D., Campbell, R., & Townsend, S.M. (2006). Sexual Assault Nurse Examiner (SANE) program goals and patient care practices. *Journal of Nursing Scholarship, 38*(2): 180-186.

Peternelj-Taylor, C.A. (2005). Conceptualizing nursing research with offenders: Another look at vulnerability. *International Journal of Law and Psychiatry, 28*(4):348-359.

Pitts, R., Niska, R.W., Xu, J., & Burt, C. (2008). *National Hospital Ambulatory Medical Care Survey: 2006 Emergency Department Survey.* Washington, DC: U.S. Department of Health & Human Services, Centers for Disease Control & Prevention, National Center for Health Statistics, No. 7.

Plichta, S.B., Clements, P.T., & Houseman, C. (2007). Why SANEs matter: Models of care for sexual violence victims in the emergency department. *Journal of Forensic Nursing, 3*(1):15-23.

Popejoy, L.L. (2008). Adult protective services use for older adults at the time of hospital discharge. *Journal of Nursing Scholarship, 40*(4):326-332.

Rand, M.R. (2008). National Crime Victimization Survey, Criminal Victimization, 2007. *Bureau of Justice Statistics Bulletin, No. NCJ 224390.* U.S. Department of Justice, Office of Justice Programs. Retrieved August 15, 2009, from http://www.ojp.usdoj.gov/bjs/pub/pdf/cv07.pdf

Registered Nurses Association of Ontario. (2002). *Toolkit: Implementation of clinical practice guidelines.* Toronto, Canada: Author. Retrieved August 18, 2009, from http://www.rnao.org

Roberson, A.J., & Kjervik, D.K. (2007). Therapeutic jurisprudence: A theoretical model for research with adolescent psychiatric mental health populations. *Journal of Nursing Law, 12*(1):54-59.

Sabol, W.J., & Couture, H. (2008). Prison inmates at midyear 2007. *Bureau of Justice Statistics Bulletin, No. NCJ 221944.* U.S. Department of Justice, Office of Justice Programs. Retrieved August 15, 2009. from http://ojp.usdoj.gov/bjs/pub/pdf/pim07.pdf

Sampsel, K., Szobota, L., Joyce, D., Graham, K., & Pickett, W. (2009). The impact of a sexual assault/domestic violence program on ED care. *Journal of Emergency Nursing, 35*(4):282-289.

Schma, W., Kjervik, D., & Petrucci, D. (2005). Therapeutic jurisprudence: Using the law to improve the public's health. *Journal of Law, Medicine & Ethics, 33*(4):59-63.

Sievers, V., Murphy, S., & Miller, J.J. (2003). Sexual assault evidence collection more accurate when completed by sexual assault nurse examiners: Colorado's experience. *Journal of Emergency Nursing, 29*(6):511-514.

Smock, W.S. (2006). Genesis and development. In V.A. Lynch (Ed.). *Forensic nursing.* St. Louis: Elsevier Mosby, pp. 13-18.

Sommers, M.S. (2007). Defining patterns of genital injury from sexual assault: A review. *Trauma Violence Abuse, 8*(3):270-280.

Sommers, M.S., Zink, T.M., Fargo, J.D., Baker, R.B., Buschur, C., Shambley-Ebron, D.Z. et al. (2008). Forensic sexual assault examination and genital injury: Is skin color a source of health disparity? *American Journal of Emergency Medicine, 26*(8):857-866.

Straus, S. & Haynes, R.B. (2009). Managing evidence-based knowledge: The need for reliable, relevant and readable resources. *Canadian Medical Association Journal, 180*(9):942-945.

Straus, S., Richardson, W.S., Glasziou, P., & Holmes, R.B. (2005). *Evidence-based medicine: How to practice and teach EBM.* Edinburgh: Elsevier Churchill Livingstone.

Wexler, D.B. (1999). *Therapeutic jurisprudence: An overview.* International Network on Therapeutic Jurisprudence. Retrieved August 18, 2009, from http://www.law.arizona.edu/depts/upr-intj/

Wiglesworth, A., Austin, R., Corona, M., Schneider, D., Liao, S., Gibbs, L. et al. (2009). Bruising as a marker of physical elder abuse. *Journal of the American Geriatrics Society, 57*(7):1191-1196.

Williams, D. (2008). Forensic nursing and utilitarianism: The quest for being right. *Journal Forensic Nursing, 5*(1):49-50.

Yaffe, M.J., Wolfson, C., & Lithwick, M. (2009). Professions show different enquiry strategies for elder abuse detection: Implications for training and interprofessional care. *Journal of Interprofessional Care, 2*:1-9.

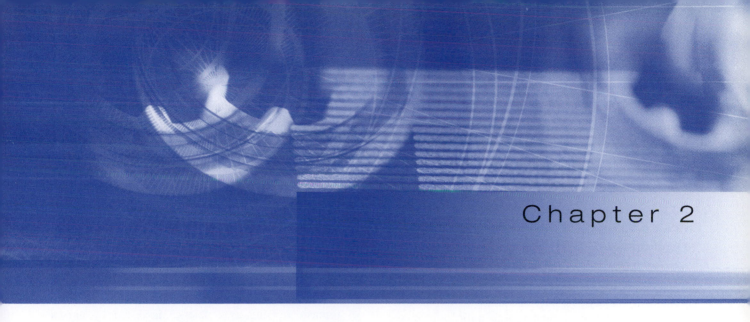

Chapter 2

THEORETICAL AND CONCEPTUAL FRAMEWORKS AND MODELS FOR UNDERSTANDING FORENSIC NURSING

Rose E. Constantino and Patricia A. Crane

"Science is organized knowledge. Wisdom is organized life."
Immanuel Kant

Competencies

1. Defining three theories: complexity, synergy, and systems.
2. Designing conceptual models for competent forensic nursing practice.
3. Discussing the importance of the theoretical framework in forensic nursing education, practice, research, and administration.
4. Differentiating between the three unifying theories of the complex synergistic system (CSS) theoretical framework and their applicability to evidence-based forensic nursing practice.
5. Synthesizing CSS theoretical framework in forensic nursing practice.

Key Terms

Complex adaptive systems
Complex synergistic systems
Complexity theory
Equifinality
Forensic nursing
General systems theory
Negentropy
Reverberation
Role behavior
Role clarification
Role expectation
Synergy theory

Introduction

As **forensic nursing practice** enters its third decade, a new integrated theoretical framework is needed. This chapter explains, defines, and synthesizes three transdisciplinary theories to form one such framework. There are three transdisciplinary theories:

- Complexity theory
- Synergy theory
- General systems theory

Integrating these theories to form the CSS helps you to understand the multifaceted nature of forensic nursing (complexity theory), its interrelatedness to various disciplines (synergy theory), and the permeability of its boundaries (systems theory).

Theoretical Framework Development

A forensic nurse (FN) is held to standards from a variety of sources, including the nursing practice act and the laws and regulations of the jurisdiction in which the nurse practices, the *Code of Ethics for Nurses*, the *Scope and Standards of Nursing Practice*, the *Scope and Standards of Forensic Nursing Practice*, accrediting organization standards, and institutional policies. It is expected that best-practice standards derived from research or evidence-based literature guide forensic nursing actions (see Chapter 1 for more information).

To begin developing a theory, it is important to review the origins of forensic nursing and to examine its background. The forensic nursing system has evolved substantially since its birth in 1991. In 1992, the International Association of Forensic Nurses (IAFN) was established in Minneapolis, Minnesota, by nurses who were caring for survivors of sexual assault. The nurses agreed that reducing human violence should be central to the mission and vision of the IAFN and a focus of the development of its members' competencies.

Competencies comprise the knowledge base with which all FNs need to be familiar so that they respond with accuracy and transparency. This includes when, why, and how the knowledge should be applied to improve health outcomes. When the American Nurses Association (ANA) approved forensic nursing as a specialty in 1995, there was an urgent need to develop a theoretical framework. Nursing is a very diverse profession: forensic nursing adds more layers of complexity. Lynch has described the theoretical foundation for forensic nursing as having connections with many mainstream nursing theories as well as with philosophy and sociology. Perhaps the most important aspect of forensic nursing is its connection with the law. This connection defines forensic nursing practice.

Theoretical development provides a way for FNs to express and test key ideas through rigorous scientific means, consisting of education, practice, research, and leadership. When forensic nursing is taught based on this theoretical framework, the ability of students to produce innovative leaps in knowledge is achieved. When knowledge is then transformed into evidence-based practices, stakeholders and communities of interest have a greater impact than do individuals alone. The global relevance of forensic nursing as a science is tested by nurses worldwide.

To explore the complexity, synergy, and systems aspects of forensic nursing, a qualitative method of data collection and analysis was used with a focus group of 10 graduate nursing students in advanced forensic nursing practice. Participants responded to the following discussion topics: the definition of forensic nursing, concepts that can be drawn from the sciences into forensic nursing, concepts and theories related to forensic nursing, and the definition of a "theoretical framework." Results showed that forensic nursing is a CSS of intersecting sciences including forensics, biology, psychology, sociology, law, medicine, and anthropology.

Unifying Theories for Forensic Nursing Practice

Complexity Theory

Complexity theory is a collection of scientific theories that attempt to explain complex behavior occurring in dynamic, nonlinear systems. Complexity theory is powerful and influences many areas of study and practice. It has great potential for use in forensic nursing. **Complex adaptive systems** (CAS) explore patterns of relationships, how they are sustained, how they are organized, and how outcomes emerge. It reinforces that, although interactions occur at a local level, they have an impact on the entire system, just by virtue of their influence on future interactions (Chafee, 2007).

Holden (2005) describes CAS as "the dynamic interactions of diverse agents who self-organize and produce adaptations that emerge in ways that can neither be predicted nor controlled." Paley (2009) characterizes CAS very pointedly: simple practitioners who follow simple rules could generate complex structures. Complexity theory is a collection of overlapping and complementary theories from various sciences, including chaos theory, organization theory, and general systems theory. The Plexus Institute considers complexity theory to be the intellectual successor of general systems theory; it combines the case study method and complexity science to create new ways for practitioners to understand **the complex synergistic systems** that are part of interpersonal relationships and interactions among practitioners.

Synergy Theory

Synergy theory is the study of organizations that form partnerships and that collaborate with other organizations to fulfill a unified mission and vision. Synergy theory may be applicable in unifying complex alliances, coalitions, and partnerships with forensic nursing.

The FN is suited to act as a leader in interdisciplinary relationships based on an understanding that today's practice environment requires partnership and collaboration between service providers and other professions to achieve desirable outcomes. In this environment, there is great potential for the FN to act as a catalyst to bring synergy to forensic practice. A synergistic system creates partnership capacity to address its mission, vision, roles, and goals. Synergy as a framework acts as a road map that lays out the pathways by which participatory collaborative processes create more effective community problem-solving and improvements in outcomes (Kerfoot et al., 2006).

Synergy specifies processes that are integral to collaboration that can be generalized across heterogeneous practice settings. Synergy is conducive to the cultivation of consequential leadership and management. It is a prerequisite in building a sense of empowerment among individual members and fostering stronger sociocultural ties among stakeholders and participants. Synergistic partnerships in forensic nursing are most likely to occur when leadership and management embody the following characteristics:

- Being inclusive by involving a broad array of people and organizations central to the cause
- Focusing on the processes of partnership engagement, such as who has influence and control
- Expanding to multiple issues as different areas begin to relate to each other

When leadership and management are based on a clear and transparent theoretical framework, they stimulate each other's ability to produce the creative leaps in thinking that Lasker and Weiss (2003) called synergy. Synergy is the creative blending of ideas; such ideas have a greater effect than do individual ideas that stand alone.

General Systems Theory

General systems theory considers interacting entities that form a unified functioning whole having permeable boundaries conducive to input, feedback, output, reverberation, equifinality, and negentropy. General systems theory was proposed in the 1940s by biologist Ludwig von Bertalanffy as a reaction to reductionism and as an attempt to revive the unity of science.

Input is information entering the system from the environment. Output is anything leaving the system, crossing the boundary, and entering the environment. Feedback occurs when output returns to the system (input), and it is used to regulate the system. Any change in the system or the environment can reverberate out from and into both the system and the environment. **Equifinality** is a principle that describes an open system as having the capacity to achieve outcomes through various mechanisms and processes. Similar results can be obtained by many different paths. **Negentropy** is the opposite of entropy. Entropy, in which a closed system falls apart and ceases to exist (death or entropy), is a measure of disorder, whereas negentropy, or negative entropy, maintains order and constant growth in open systems. Equifinality allows forensic nursing to achieve its goals through diverse and multidimensional activities and strategies. Forensic nursing lives, grows, adapts to challenges, and seizes opportunities to transform entropy into negative entropy. Negentropy sustains forensic nursing so that it survives and flourishes by transforming challenges into opportunities (Constantino, 1979 & 1984; Heylighen, 1992).

General systems theory is the transdisciplinary study of the abstract organization of phenomena, independent of their substance, type, and spatial or temporal existence. It explores the principles common to all complex entities and the models used to describe them. Systems theory is a theory of wholeness in which there is a general tendency toward integration and unification that can lead to transformation of scientific education and practice. Systems biology is an interdisciplinary science that studies complex systems using a holistic approach and that uses experimental and computational investigative methods. Systems biology can be integrated into forensic nursing because it can transcend how nursing affects and is affected by its own interventions (Founds, 2009).

Systems are either closed or open. Closed systems are considered detached and isolated from their environment, whereas open systems, which are connected and integrated with their environment, have permeable boundaries and maintain themselves by a continuous input and output of data and energy to and from their environment. *Feedback* is the constant give and take and breaking down and building up of data and energy. Feedback enhances systems' steady state or dynamic equilibrium (Constantino, 2007).

Complex synergistic systems, such as forensic nursing, are constantly buffeted by intentionally and unintentionally created challenges and opportunities that are created by intersections of theory and practice. Theoretical frameworks ground the professions so that they may withstand the challenge. A theoretical framework is a powerful tool that organizes, shapes, and guides thinking, feeling, and behavior in professional practice. It provides a lens through which ideas, vision, and mission come into focus.

FORENSIC NURSING AS A COMPLEX SYNERGISTIC SYSTEM

Forensic nursing is the application of the nursing process to public or legal proceedings. It is the application of health care in the scientific investigation of trauma or death related to abuse, violence, criminal activity, liability, and accidents. FNs work with other professional groups and systems (medicine, law, forensics, sociology, anthropology, behavioral science, and biology). It is the intersection with these professions and sciences that brings new depth to the practice of forensic nursing. All these fields form transdisciplinary theories that clarify the practice of forensic nursing as a specialty.

The scientific approach is by far the most advanced way to develop theoretical/conceptual frameworks. The scientific method is more reliable than tradition, authority, or experience. Scientists use this method to develop theories. The scientific method allows a more systematic explanation of how phenomena are related or interrelated. Concepts or conceptual models provide insight and understanding regarding relationships among phenomena. Frameworks are the skeleton upon which the theory or concept hangs. The frameworks are the foundation that explains how a phenomenon interacts and reacts within the environment. The importance of these frameworks to nursing in general and forensic nursing specifically is that they advance both the practice as a profession and the understanding of the practice and what it can be. The value of a framework is threefold:

1. It allows for the public debate of philosophical assumptions about the specialty, providing the opportunity for self-evaluation and accountability to the public and to the profession.
2. It provides a structure of theoretical statements and hypotheses that suggest appropriate and effective nursing interventions.

3. It allows hypotheses for systematic scrutiny and analysis of emerging care protocols.

Combining three theories—complexity, synergy, and (general) systems—to form one single theoretical framework for forensic nursing was not done lightly. Forensic nursing's framework was formed after a decade of discussion, thoughtful dialogue, deliberate questioning, and a search for answers to nagging questions that baffled students and educators alike.

The first concept that appeared was complexity. Forensic nursing is complex because it does not draw from one source of science but rather from several, including nursing, forensics, biology, psychology, sociology, law, medicine, and anthropology. Second, synergy, or collaboration, needs to occur to integrate these sciences. Third, this needs to be articulated and combined into one system or entity—forensic nursing. The IAFN promotes synergy among all complex intersecting domains and sciences related to forensic nursing by encouraging diverse theoretical frameworks. CSS is one newly suggested theoretical framework.

FACTORS INFLUENCING FORENSIC NURSING AS A COMPLEX SYNERGISTIC SYSTEM

There is no single encompassing theoretical or conceptual framework for forensic nursing. Kent-Wilkinson explored forensic nursing and factors influencing forensic nursing education. Through this research, she developed an important classification of common concepts as related and identified by the majority of FNs in her study. Findings identified social justice as a potential metatheory for forensic nursing.

Metatheory Development

Metatheory development focuses on questions that set forth a theory base. These questions concern the purpose, methods, and development of evaluation techniques of a theory. The metatheory is broadly focused and typically considers the meaning of nursing and how it relates as a profession and a science. Development of social justice as a metatheory is intriguing as it is in keeping with the central paradigm of forensic nursing, which is truth. Justice is served when truth is identified, verified, and magnified. The FN is the advocate of truth.

Population health (DeSouza et al., 2003) as another conceptual framework for forensic nursing education is discussed in the literature. Population health refers to the physical, social, cultural, and economic environment in which people work and live. Through population health, nurses obtain a greater understanding of macro-level trends in health status, such as lifestyle, attitudes, values, ethics, and behaviors; how social macro-systems (public policy, media, economy) and health are linked; and the performance of the health-care system in response to health-care needs. Population health (Radzyminski, 2007) incorporates health promotion, disease prevention, environmental influences, genetics, and culture for various groups of people. The goal of population health is to maximize the health of any given population. In doing so, it maximizes the development and evaluation of health-care policy, programs, and systems.

Tidal Model

The Tidal Model was developed in the 1990s and has been gaining support within psychiatric medicine, social work, and psychotherapy. The Tidal Model helps people recover from mental health distress. Its goal is to develop an alliance between the health-care provider and those needing support. In this way, an understanding of the problem is mutually achieved, personal meanings and relationships are defined, and the path to recovery from the mental distress event is illuminated. Published reports indicate that this model is used by forensic psychiatric nurses in Australia, Europe, and New Zealand. These reports are qualitative or descriptive in nature; they are not designed to evaluate the effectiveness of the technique, but rather to determine common themes. The Tidal Model focuses on the psychiatric component of forensic nursing, but it is useful in the other intersections and disciplines that FNs typically encounter.

Maternal Filicide

Maternal filicide is a theoretical framework developed to gain insight into how previous traumatic experiences may have affected a woman's relationship with her own children. The basis of this theory is the emphasis of childhood trauma on brain development, which may lead to effects on cognitive responses and on the individual's social and emotional development as she matures and eventually becomes a mother (Mugavin, 2008). This theory pulls from neurobiological development and Bowen's family system theory to help explain relationships and family dynamics. This theoretical framework assists in describing a particular type of individual quite specifically (the phenomenon of fatal and nonfatal abuse), especially in the areas of child abuse and neglect. Binder and others (2008) found that abuse and/or neglect in childhood combined with the *FKBP5* gene is a significant risk factor for the development of post-traumatic stress disorder in traumatized adults.

A CLOSER LOOK AT A COMPLEX SYNERGISTIC SYSTEM

Forensic nursing has added complexity and synergy to nursing theory and practice. As mentioned previously, forensic nursing intersects with many different disciplines and may adapt taxonomies and styles for its own use. Most important, characteristics of those disciplines are incorporated within the practice of forensic nursing itself. Integrating theories to form one theoretical framework will explain the complex nature of forensic nursing (complexity theory), its interrelatedness to various disciplines (synergy theory), and the permeability of its boundaries (systems theory). Forensic nursing is a CSS of intersecting sciences, including forensics, biology, psychology, sociology, law, medicine, and anthropology. The integration of complexity, synergy, and systems theories into one overarching theoretical framework for forensic nursing cultivates education, practice, research, and leadership in forensic nursing.

Forensic nursing as a CSS is an open system and maintains itself through continuous input and output of data and information to and from its environment. This constant give and take or breaking down and building up of data and energy is called "feedback." Feedback enhances systems' steady state or dynamic equilibrium (Fig. 2.1).

FORENSIC NURSING ROLES

Forensic nursing needs to set clear boundaries of the roles each area of concentration (education), practice (service), and research (scholarly work) plays because, as a system, it affects and is affected by its sheer complexity and synergy. As the community recognizes the Sexual Assault Nurse Examiner's (SANE's) knowledge and skills, FNs are rapidly branching out into new legal arenas, such as risk management, employee litigation, litigation in nursing education, and human rights violations.

Lynch and Duvall (2011) describe three components of roles: role clarification, role behavior, and role expectation. **Role clarification** is the shared and explicit knowledge, skills, boundaries, responsibilities, and accountability for each role player. **Role behavior** is the deliberate and careful performance and enactment of a differentiated or specific role. It includes accurate and evidence-based translation of knowledge, skills, rules, and procedures into practice. **Role expectation** is the acceptance of a contract (offer, acceptance, and performance) drawn between the professional and the professions, the community and society, and the role player. It is a promise for mutual respect, autonomy, and justice in the delivery of services.

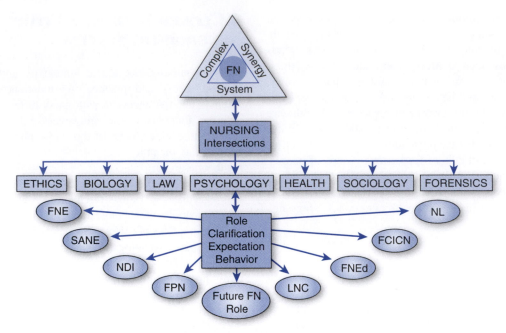

■ FIGURE 2.1 Forensic Nursing as a CSS: A Theoretical Framework.

The following roles are offered to illustrate the complexity and synergy that must be understood and applied by FNs in an array of settings and areas of concentration.

Forensic Nurse Examiner

Forensic nurse examiners (FNEs) are registered nurses who offer a combination of medical and legal care both to victims who have been physically or psychologically abused, neglected, traumatized, sexually assaulted, or injured as well as to the perpetrators of such crimes. FNEs conduct a comprehensive history and assessment and ensure that evidence is collected in a manner that ensures that the chain of custody is maintained. They also coordinate referrals for continuing care and work with crisis intervention teams. The FNE may also be asked to examine potential offenders and criminal suspects, provide a written or verbal report on the results of that examination, and testify as an expert witness in court. The special skills of the FNE include the ability to conduct and document a thorough, unbiased, and objective clinical forensic history and assessment (including digital imaging and laboratory specimens); collect and preserve evidence; and maintain the evidentiary chain of custody. Patients of the FNE also receive crisis intervention, medical treatment, education, and appropriate referrals for ongoing care.

Sexual Assault Nurse Examiner

A sexual assault nurse examiner (SANE) offers comprehensive care to survivors of sexual assault. Prior to the creation of this role, hospital emergency departments (EDs) were ill-equipped to handle such cases, and long waits, lack of privacy and sensitivity, as well as poor evidence gathering resulted in the continued victimization of survivors. SANEs provide prompt, caring, and culturally appropriate nursing care; they also collect evidence for use in legal proceedings.

The entrance to the health-care system for many survivors of sexual assault/rape/abuse (SARA) and their families remains the hospital ED. Whether in the ED or another setting, SANEs provide nursing care to survivors of SARA that is based on compassionate delivery of culturally and developmentally appropriate health care. SANEs are specially trained FNs who provide 24-hour first-response nursing care and crisis intervention, assessment of injuries, creation of a plan of care, and collection of evidence that will support future legal proceedings to survivors of SARA. The SANE attends to the survivor's related physical, emotional, and spiritual needs, including prevention and/or follow-up care for pregnancy and sexually transmitted diseases, evaluation and treatment of minor injuries, and referral to other providers.

The SANE's role has been validated through research. Research shows that SANEs collect forensic evidence more accurately than do non-SANE-trained nurses or physician colleagues. Better forensic evidence collection and documentation lead to more successful sexual assault prosecution. Additionally, more consistent follow-up care is provided by SANEs compared with the usual care providers.

Forensic Assessment and Consultation Team

The regional Forensic Assessment and Consultation Team (FACT) of Inova Fairfax Hospital in Falls Church, Virginia, is led by Suzanne Brown, MS, RN, SANE, CFN (certified FN). FACT comprises sexual assault and domestic violence team members who are available around the clock to provide sexual assault examinations and assessment of victims and/or suspects referred by law enforcement or child protective services. They use technology such as a binocular colposcope to document microscopic genital injuries, and they are able to conduct examinations in other hospitals or police departments if needed.

Nurse Death Investigator

Nurse death investigators (NDI) are also known as forensic nurse investigators, deputy coroners, or coroners in jurisdictions that do not require a physician to fill the role of coroner. NDIs assist the medical examiner in determining the cause and circumstances of death. NDIs work alongside law enforcement, social services, organ donor organizations, and other community service providers. They play an active role in ongoing communication with and education of the family. NDIs have the authority and responsibility to confirm or pronounce death, to establish decedent identification, and to notify next of kin. NDIs perform the critical components of death investigation, such as obtaining a thorough medical and social history of the decedent, examining the body, investigating the scene using evidence-based guidelines and procedures, and representing and reporting the decedent's right to justice. NDIs assist the medical examiner or coroner in determining the cause and manner of death. As a member of a response and investigative team, the NDI collaborates and consults with law enforcement, social services, organ and tissue procurement agencies, medical and legal advocates, the decedent's family, the media, and the community in all issues related to medical and legal aspects of a death.

Forensic Psychiatric Nurse

The role of the forensic psychiatric nurse (FPN) is defined not by where the patient is situated (psychiatric clinical setting) or the diagnosis but rather by the behavior or actions the FPN performs. The FPN interacts with those who have experienced emotional trauma, such as a child witnessing the murder of a parent or another family member, the aftermath of homicide or suicide, or a disaster or trauma survivor coping with post-traumatic stress disorder.

In trauma, the survivor is silenced. The survivor is robbed of the ability to communicate, whether orally or in writing. The role of the FPN is to aid survivors' sensory memory (what they saw, heard, and felt) and provide social support by listening to their stories and believing in them. An FPN may accept referrals from other nurses in nonpsychiatric settings, such as a patient referred from an ED or a parent grieving the death of a son or daughter in the military.

Forensic Nurse Educator

The forensic nurse educator (FNEd) sheds light on forensic nursing, dispels myths, and provides a foundation for incorporating principles and evidence into forensic nursing practice. FNEds often need to dispel myths about what forensic nursing entails (a result of television shows) by teaching students what the profession actually does through a variety of courses and training programs. Courses and programs include SANE training, education regarding domestic violence and elder and child abuse, and training in evidence collection. FNEds provide continuing education in forensics for nurses (both undergraduate and graduate), physicians, midlevel providers, teachers, lawyers, social workers, parents, and law enforcement personnel. National conferences on forensics also provide opportunities for learning about this field. FNEds emphasize the importance of protecting the health and welfare of underserved populations by networking with other forensic practitioners and selecting practicum experiences. Using case examples to highlight forensic principles is an important teaching strategy.

Legal Nurse Consultant

The legal nurse consultant (LNC), according to the American Association of LNC Consultants (AALNC), is a nursing specialty that uses an advocacy model. LNCs are included here because of the clear intersection and overlap between FN and LNC roles. The AALNC identifies two LNC domains: practice environment (PE) and practice area (PA). PE includes law firms, insurance companies, managed care organizations, risk management departments, state and governmental agencies, and independent legal nurse consulting practices. PA includes medical malpractice, personal injury, product liability, toxic tort, workers' compensation, and criminal, employment, administrative, educational, elder, health, and family law. These diverse practice environments also apply to FNs.

Forensic Correctional/Institutional/Custody Nurse

The forensic correctional/institutional/custody nurse (FCICN) is a registered nurse who specializes in the care, treatment, and rehabilitation of persons who have been sentenced to prisons, jails, or long-term care facilities for violation of criminal, civil, or constitutional laws and who require further assessment, treatment, and evaluation prior to adjudication. Functions for FCICNs vary from setting to setting.

Nurse Lawyer

A nurse lawyer (NL) is a registered nurse with a juris doctorate (JD) degree who practices as an attorney specializing in civil or criminal cases involving health-care law, policy development, and ethical/legal/sociocultural issues (ELSI) cases (Lynch & Duvall, 2011). The NL may hold and maintain both nursing and law licenses. In so doing, the NL enjoys the privileges of and accepts responsibilities required by both professions.

Future Forensic Nursing Role

In Figure 2.1, a space has been provided for a future FN role. Each FN today needs to embrace current challenges and transform them into opportunities. The FN's future is open to many more roles that will be discovered through education and research.

Capacity Elements of Forensic Nursing

Some of the capacity elements include the following:

- Acting as formal and informal leaders
- Interactive member participation
- Constructive engagement in group process, conflict resolution, collection and analysis of assessment data, problem solving and program planning, intervention design and implementation, evaluation, resource mobilization, policy, and media advocacy
- The ability to access, leverage, and share resources
- An understanding of the system's history as context for contemporary action
- The leveraging of power to create or resist change regarding community turf, interests, or experiences
- The expectation of desirable norms, standards, and attributes

The CSS as a theoretical framework for patient care in forensic nursing evolved from the following assumptions. Patients and the FN are:

- Biological, psychological, social, and spiritual beings who must be considered as a complex whole

- Members of a family, group, community, association, and society, and are multidimensional
- Synergistic with the context and ecology wherein each affects the other and is affected by the role and function of both
- Most productive when boundaries are permeable and conducive to input, feedback, output, reverberation, equifinality, and negentropy

Figure 2.2 shows the free flow of information in an open system through feedback and reverberation. Like systems theory, the CSS framework also shares characteristics of reverberation, permeable boundaries, equifinality, and negentropy.

Challenges and Opportunities Ahead

Although there are many more FNs than there were 10 or 20 years ago, forensic nursing is still addressing the challenges and opportunities of an evolving nursing specialty. One of these challenges is recognition of forensic nursing practice by the nursing profession itself. Although forensic nursing achieved official recognition by the American Nurses Association (ANA) in 1995, widespread understanding of the role of the FN has not yet been realized. Image building is all the more difficult because of the diversity of the roles and the patients found under the umbrella of forensic nursing.

Forensic nursing practice is a complex synergistic system. The purpose of the following case study is to discuss the FN as an expert witness for the defense in a case filed in court by a survivor of SARA. The FN in this case understands CSS and uses it as the theoretical framework of her practice.

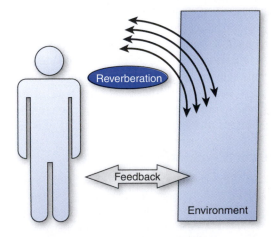

■ **Figure 2.2** Feedback and reverberation.

Case Study

WHOSE DNA CAME FIRST?

From: Constantino, R.E. (2007), Translation of ethical, sociocultural, and accountability issues in the nurse lawyer's practice. *Journal of Nursing Law*, 11(1): 27-33. The FN, who is also a SANE, agrees to testify in court as an expert witness for the prosecution of an alleged rapist. The FN was the SANE who examined the rape victim in the ED during the early morning hours of February 14. The accuser claims that she had consensual sex with her boyfriend at his apartment the night before the alleged rape by the accused.

After having consensual sex with her boyfriend, she returned to her apartment, where she showered and thoroughly washed her undergarments by hand using a liquid laundry detergent. She wore the same undergarments to work as a hotel receptionist the following morning. At work, she met a person who invited her to have dinner and movies in his suite. The person met her at the door and said, "Sorry, dinner and movies are the last things on my mind," proceeded to fondle her breasts, and slammed her to the bed. The accused chained her loosely to the bedpost as he raped and sodomized her repeatedly. She passed out. She woke up in the middle of the night while the perpetrator was sound asleep in another room. She escaped, returned home, and presented to the ED for care the following morning. In the process of the physical examination and collection of evidence in the ED by the FN, two sources of deoxyribonucleic acid (DNA) were found on the accuser's undergarments: one from the boyfriend and one from the accused.

The issue central to the case is whether DNA remains viable for collection and analysis (survives) after the garment has been washed by hand (as opposed to washed by machine) with soap and water. The accused claims he had consensual sex with the accuser. If the boyfriend's sample came first and survived after washing with soap and water, the accuser's story is believable. If the perpetrator's sample came first, questions of doubt can be raised about the accuser's story. Did she go home after the alleged SARA by the accused and have consensual sex with her boyfriend before coming to the ED for the examination? If the accused can tolerate two consensual sexual encounters with her boyfriend, once before and once after experiencing SARA, could the alleged SARA be consensual also?

The prosecution hires the SANE who examined the accuser in the ED as an expert witness to testify that washing undergarments (panties soiled with body fluids) by hand with soap and water would not completely remove DNA from the undergarments. The expert witness is to substantiate the accuser's account of the alleged SARA as true and accurate. SARA by the accused took place after she had consensual sex with her boyfriend the night before, after washing her undergarments by hand with soap and water, and after wearing them to work the following day.

The FN should understand that any expert testimony provided by the defense and the prosecution must meet the requirements of relevance and reliability. Relevance requires that the expert's testimony be based on science relevant to the case at hand and that the methodology or theory used to arrive at the opinion based on reliable science, as specifically enunciated in *Daubert v. Merrill Dow Pharmaceuticals, Inc.*, called the Daubert Rule. Other ways reliability can be established include presenting established professional opinion, peer-reviewed literature, known error rates, maintenance of standards and control, and acceptability in the scientific community. The FN's duty is to protect the client from further harm and to provide service for the good of the client, the accuser. According to the ethical principles of nonmalfeasance and beneficence, however, if the FN can do no "good" for the accused, then at least she should do no harm to the accused while maintaining her zeal in testifying for the accuser in finding the truth about whose DNA came first and whether both sexual encounters were consensual in the SARA incident.

Nurses are educated under a caring paradigm and are therefore taught to be caring to all patients, including those not assigned to them. CSS as a theoretical framework needs to be invoked by the SANE in her role as an expert witness. If a nurse identifies a patient needing immediate help on a unit, the nurse either gives the patient the necessary care or, if she is unable to give the care, calls for help to take care of the patient's immediate need. In FN practice, the FN is not obligated to help other parties, especially opposing parties. FNs are required only to be civil. Thus, the FN needs to balance her zeal to defend the accused through her testimony with empathy toward the accuser and all the other parties in the case.

Once the FN accepts the case, she needs to be thoughtful and proceed very carefully to respond to these searching questions: Is the ultimate issue of the case within the FN's specialty area, or should the attorney for the accused seek the services of another SANE? Is the FN prepared to assist the court in arriving

(case study continued on page 36)

Case Study

WHOSE DNA CAME FIRST? (continued)

at a fair, timely, and trustworthy outcome?

Upon responding to the questions truthfully, the FN proceeds to test the theory of the defense that washing undergarments with soap and water removes all traces of DNA. The FN performed a small randomized clinical trial to test whether or not washing undergarments with soap and water removes all traces of body fluids. Finding evidence of two different DNA donors (boyfriend and accused) on the accuser's undergarments supports the defense's argument for the accused that the accuser had consensual sex with her boyfriend after allegedly having experienced SARA by the accused.

The prosecution must demonstrate proof, by testimony of an expert witness, that washing a worn undergarment by hand with soap and water does not remove all traces of DNA, thus the presence of two sources of DNA. This argument supports the prosecution's theory that the accuser, after having been raped by the accused, went home in pain and great discomfort, rested, and waited until morning to report the crime without having consensual sex with her boyfriend.

Moreover, the prosecution would argue that finding two sources of DNA was due to the fact that the process of washing her undergarments by hand with soap and water did not remove all traces of the boyfriend's DNA and semen deposited before the alleged rape took place. The two sources of DNA were caused by the accuser's consensual intercourse with her boyfriend first, followed by the rape by the accused. On the other hand, the defense argues that the process of washing undergarments by hand with soap and water removes all traces of DNA

and that after her consensual sex with the accused, which she now claims as SARA, she went home and had consensual sex with her boyfriend. Thus, the two sources of DNA were products of two consensual sex acts.

The argument by the defense, when supported by facts and expert testimony, seems to be convincing to a reasonable person in that the accuser continued to fully comprehend her capacity and receptivity to consent to sexual intercourse with her boyfriend free of pain or other constraints after having sex with the accused earlier. Consenting to a sexual relationship with her boyfriend (just as she allegedly gave consent to have sexual intercourse with the accused earlier) is reasonable. This argument sounds favorable to the defense and meets the relevancy and reliability requirements; however, when sociocultural issues were explored, such as racial and ethnic background of the parties, mental capacity/disability of the parties, social standing of the parties in the community, and after the FN submitted her report to the prosecution, the case was settled out of court.

Discussion Questions

As illustrated in this case, any expert testimony provided by the defense and the prosecution must meet the requirements of relevance and reliability.

1. What does relevance require?
2. What does the Daubert Rule require?
3. How is reliability shown?
4. What are other ways that reliability can be established to meet the requirements of the Daubert Rule?

IMPLICATIONS IN FORENSIC NURSING PRACTICE

A theoretical framework provides organizations, health systems, and professional entities with a model to guide practice, inquiry, research, and evaluation. Theoretical frameworks provide an infrastructure that enhances efficiency and effectiveness of practice as well as reliability and validity of the research and evaluation process. Theoretical models that are simple and transparent serve as a powerful tool to separate professionals

from technicians. From a practice perspective, a theoretical framework serves as a guardrail, and from a research perspective, a conceptual framework serves as a frame that defines and demarcates the research aim and outcome.

The following case studies provide context for the forensic nurse so that she may put herself in the place of the patient Mary, observe for herself, and compare and contrast the treatment she received in the ED when staff did not use versus when staff did use CSS in their care of Mary. This is an account by the forensic nurse.

Case Study

MARY'S EXPERIENCE IN THE EMERGENCY ROOM WITHOUT USING CSS AS A CONCEPTUAL FRAMEWORK

Mary was sexually assaulted, raped, and abused by several individuals last weekend. The treatment she received after the assault is an example of what occurs outside the realm of forensic nursing and may make any reader of the report of the event feel sad and angry. The police phoned the hospital first to let them know Mary was coming. The nurses at the hospital were helpful to Mary, but they let too many things happen that were improper. She was left alone in the examination room by her nurse after being told the nurse would be "right back." The nurse never returned. The police detectives were very insensitive, asking her many questions making her feel it was her fault. They asked her why she did not push down on the gas (she was carjacked at a red light at gunpoint), why she did not try to run when the perpetrators took her out of the car to rape her (they dragged her out of the car by her hair), and why she did not scream for help (her mouth was duct-taped shut before she was dragged out of her car). They kept asking her questions, and at times it appeared that they did not listen to the answers. They saw her shake and rock in the chair, but these signs did not elicit any empathy from the interrogators.

Although the nurse put Mary in a private examination room right away, she was left alone for 30 minutes.

Mary was concerned that the physician who replaced the nurse didn't know what he was doing while collecting evidence with the rape kit. The physician kept asking the nurses in another room (on their break) what to do next. This made Mary question his competence to do the examination and whether or not evidence was being collected properly. Mary asked if pictures were taken, and they were not. Mary had many bruises and scratches from being held and pushed down. Lastly, no one called an advocate to be with Mary during this entire ordeal or even give her the option to have an advocate present during the examination: no counselor, no survivor's advocate, and no social worker was present.

Later, I heard that the nurse left Mary because she was called to a bigger emergency case in another room. What emergency could be bigger than Mary's situation? Mary was so traumatized she was unable to speak or show any emotion. She looked paralyzed. They discharged her from the ED with a phone number for counseling and that was it. They briefly did their duty to inform her of her need to be checked for sexually transmitted infections (STIs) and possible pregnancy, but it was merely a gloss over. They did not explain to her where she could get follow-up care and testing for sexually transmitted infections and pregnancy.

Case Study

MARY'S EXPERIENCE IN THE EMERGENCY ROOM USING CSS AS A CONCEPTUAL FRAMEWORK

In this case, the CSS framework is used to exemplify an entirely different experience for Mary. After Mary experienced SARA, she was sent to the ED for an examination. The police phoned the ED staff to provide them with an alert for Mary's arrival. Because the police had worked with the SANE nurses in the area, they also had contacted the nurse on call to let her know that Mary was on her way.

Once Mary arrived, the nursing staff performed their triage and assessments with care and efficiency. They had been educated in the past at a university SANE training center and understood Mary's needs and their

roles. Mary was taken to the examination room. The SANE nurse introduced herself and began to let Mary know about the process and procedures that were about to occur. Once the examination was completed, the SANE nurse conferred with the ED physician regarding wounds and injuries that were found. She also provided suggestions for STI prophylaxis. The police arrived to question Mary. The SANE nurse remained with Mary while they did so and also provided information to them regarding her findings.

Although their questions seemed to be cold and repetitive to Mary, the SANE nurse reinforced that it

(case study continued on page 38)

Case Study

was the police officer's job to be complete and clear about Mary's responses for Mary's benefit. The police officer may sound repetitive, but she needs to verify and confirm that Mary remembers clearly which side of her head hit the gravel road first and from which side of her car the perpetrators grabbed her. Before the police officer left, she reminded Mary she might be calling once the police find any leads and tips about the perpetrators. The SANE nurse contacted a local victim's advocate group and provided information, and they sent an advocate to be with Mary. She also provided Mary with an appointment at a local clinic, along with the clinic's phone number, where she can follow up for any issues related to STI transmission. As Mary already had a doctor, the SANE nurse offered to make follow-up arrangements for her with her physician. Once Mary was found to be physically stable and all injuries were addressed, Mary was discharged.

At Mary's request, the nurse notified a local counselor who worked with survivors of SARA and scheduled an appointment. The ED was a busy place that night, with a number of very critical patients. Because of the education SANE nurses provided to this ED,

Mary's care was not compromised because she was triaged at the same level of seriousness as those who were in car accidents or in an emergent physical condition. Synergy seems to reign over a complex system such as an ED.

In this instance, the CSS conceptual framework provides a roadmap for care for the random acts of violence that are not controlled nor can be explained away by the higher-level system. Mary survived a traumatic experience of violence and was totally dependent upon the health-care system to assist her. This theory shows the dynamics of individual interactions and their calming effects when it is in place and shows the dissatisfaction that ensues when it is misplaced.

It is the addition of the SANE who interacts with the ED staff—moving in and out of the environment, creating synergistic relationships with not only the ED staff, but also law enforcement and advocates—that is in the best interest of the patient. The SANE nurse transforms the situation seamlessly. Without the CSS framework, the situation was different, with each specialty remaining in its own silo, not truly helping the whole client or meeting all of her needs.

Forensic nursing is rooted in nursing science and, like other areas of concentration in nursing, must conduct the necessary research to support evidence-based practice. Research into the primary prevention of violence, the effects of violence, and the outcomes of forensic nursing practice is also needed, both in the United States and globally. A research exemplar of a study funded by the World Health Organization/Eastern Mediterranean Regional Office (WHO/EMRO) and conducted by Hamdan-Mansour and others (2011) evaluated the mental health consequences of intimate partner abuse (IPA) among Jordanian women using the "double open window" as a conceptual framework. They found Jordanian women experiencing IPA suffered anxiety, depression, suicide ideation, and substance use. Furthermore, the women indicated their need of social support from others (Safadi and others [2012]). This need could be met when another window is opened by health-care providers, hence the "double open window" concept in caring for IPA survivors.

The research exemplar for "Evaluating the Consequences of IPA Among Jordanian Women" is detailed in Box 2.1.

Elements of CSS

Defining the elements of a complex synergistic system is essential. The terms reverberation, permeable boundaries, feedback, equifinality, and negentropy, as they apply to forensic nursing, are important. **Reverberation** is a property of systems whereby a change in one part affects other parts of the system, like a ripple caused by a tiny pebble thrown into a pond. The ripple reverberates, expanding until it joins its boundaries. If its *boundaries* are *porous* or *permeable,* it mixes, blends, and transforms its properties into a complex synergy that continues to provide input and *feedback* to the pond, albeit in its transformed complex components.

Forensic nursing has *permeable boundaries* and is open to new ideas, theories, and principles. It accepts multiple intersections with and feedback from other disciplines and is transformed through the permeability of its

Box 2.1   Research Exemplar

Hamdan-Mansour, Constantino and others (2011) evaluated the mental health consequences of intimate partner abuse (IPA) among Jordanian women.

Background: IPA is a major contributor to illness of women worldwide. Most forms of IPA are not unique single incidents but rather are ongoing, continuing for years. IPA knows no borders. Globally, between 10% and 60% of women have at some time suffered abuse in their relationships, and about 5% have experienced or are experiencing some form of abuse currently. Women who experience IPA and do not seek or receive help suffer physical, psychosocial, and mental health problems. The aim of the authors was to explore the "double open window" as a conceptual framework in a research study with Jordanian women experiencing abuse. Walker describes three phases of IPA: tension building, assault, and honeymoon. Curnow suggests that between the assault and the honeymoon phases, a window of help-seeking and reality-testing behavior is opened in the IPA survivor. The authors conceptualized that a double open window synergy occurs when the survivor seeks help and the nurse provides it in a therapeutic relationship. Furthermore, IPA could escalate if the window from the health-care provider's side is not opened because the provider could further traumatize the abused by being judgmental or by giving inappropriate intervention. Evaluating participants' psychosocial, mental health, and coping skills needs to be followed with an intervention as planned by the authors of this study to test the feasibility of the double open window.

Literature on IPA in Jordan: In Arab countries, one third of the women experience IPA. As a result of IPA, women suffer significant physical, psychological, and mental health problems. IPA is a highly sensitive issue in Arab countries because of overlapping religious, legal, educational, and social structures. Previous studies showed that between 30% and 45% of the Jordanian women experienced at least one type of abuse, and physical abuse was the most reported type. In another study, the highest rate of abuse has been reported in women between 20 and 29 years of age, and batterers are mostly men between 30 and 39 years of age. IPA has been reported at a higher incidence rate in employed compared to unemployed Jordanian women.

Objectives: The purpose of this study was to evaluate the psychosocial and mental health consequences of abuse among Jordanian women seeking help from the Jordanian Women's Union (JWU). Research questions were as follows:

1. What is the level of mental health concepts, including depression, suicidal ideation, and substance use, and psychosocial concepts, including perceived social support from family and friends, self-efficacy, and coping strategies, among abused Jordanian women who seek help from JWU?
2. What is the relationship between the psychosocial and mental health variables of abused Jordanian women who seek help from JWU?
3. Is there any difference in the psychosocial and mental health variables in relation to selected demographic and personal characteristics?

Methods: A cross-sectional descriptive correlational design was used to collect data between November 2008 and February 2009 from 92 abused women who were seeking help from the JWU. Measures were taken after receiving informed consent from participants regarding form of abuse, depression, coping, suicidal ideation, substance use, social support, and self-efficacy.

Results: The most commonly reported form of abuse was psychological abuse. Analysis showed that a significant number of abused women had a moderate to severe level of depression, a low level of perceived social support, and a moderate to very high level of self-efficacy, and they used approach coping skills more frequently than avoidance coping. About 15% ($n = 14$) of them reported that the desire for death was stronger than the desire for life. Depression had a significant and negative correlation with self-efficacy ($r = -0.47$; $p > 0.001$). Perceived social support from family ($r = -0.27$; $p > 0.05$) and self-efficacy had a significant negative correlation with approach coping strategies ($r = -0.26$; $p > 0.05$).

Discussion: These findings indicate that the health of abused women in Jordan is compromised. Abused women in Jordan are in need of professional counseling and interventional programs. Larger studies need to be done to examine risk factors in Jordanian women who suffer physical, psychological, or sexual abuse and to explore through focus groups each participant's preference for intervention.

Discussion Questions

1. What is the purpose of this study?
2. Using Walker's three phases of IPA, when (between phases) did Curnow suggest that a window is opened by the IPA survivor?
3. Explain how the authors of this study further characterized the double open window as their conceptual framework from the three phases and the open window of IPA?
4. What are the implications of a theoretical framework in forensic nursing?

boundaries. Equifinality is another property of forensic nursing. Equifinality suggests that outcomes are achieved or reached using different paths. Equifinality allows forensic nursing to achieve its goal through diverse and multidimensional activities and strategies. Because of its equifinality, forensic nursing lives, grows, and adapts to challenges through negative entropy. Negative entropy, or negentropy, sustains forensic nursing so that it will thrive and flourish, not wither away.

As FNs function in a complex synergistic practice, they also provide care to a complex ecological domain represented by the client. The FN does not work with a patient alone because the patient belongs to a complex ecological system. Nursing interventions impact on the patient's entire ecological domain—individual, intrapersonal, interpersonal, family, and community—no matter the outcome (positive or negative) (Table 2.1). Therefore, it behooves every FN who comes in contact with a patient or client to consider the impact he or she will have on the patient's/client's complex ecological system.

CONCLUSIONS

Forensic nursing is a growing specialty, yet it struggles to define and clarify its role. Research on a national and global level is needed to support evidence-based practice and clarify the many facets of the profession. A theoretical framework upon which to base education, practice, and research will assist the profession to achieve its goals. The CSS framework serves as a useful foundation for beginning this process. No one knows what the future holds for forensic nursing, but this we know: as we enter the second decade of the 21st century, forensic nursing occupies the nursing stage front and center. It is up to current FNs to be visionaries and innovators.

TABLE 2.1 **An Example of Forensic Nursing Care Plan**

Problem: Difficulty in making decisions and the client's ecological system
Outcomes: Client will use the problem-solving process; client will make decisions appropriate to his or her own unique ecological system.

Intervention	Rationale	Goal
Individual Focus: Give limited choices when client is having difficulty making a decision (e.g., "Would you like to talk first or start the examination?")	Activity is directed while giving client limited control until decision-making ability is improved	Makes decision within limited context
Intrapersonal Focus: When client talks about being overwhelmed by all the decisions that have to be made, have him or her identify only one decision to work toward	Narrowing the focus to one decision at a time decreases feelings of helplessness	Focuses on one decision at a time
Interpersonal Focus: Teach and use the problem-solving process: explore previous problem-solving abilities; identify goals; choose and implement problem-solving strategy; evaluate on basis of goals	Rigid patterns of problem-solving decrease creativity in formulating alternatives	Uses new skills in problem-solving
Family Focus: Help client describe thoughts and feelings about family	Client may believe that all decision-making should be made by the family	Verbalizes feelings related to family values and expectations
Community Focus: Encourage client to consider how his or her experience can have an impact on the community	Major decisions require optimal functioning and social support	Delays major decisions until the entire ecological system domains are explored

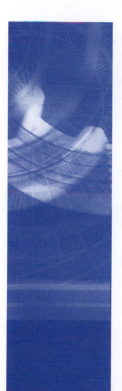

EVIDENCE-BASED PRACTICE

Reference Question: Examine other nursing specialties that use CSS as a conceptual/theoretical framework?

Database(s) to Search: PubMed, CINAHL

Search Strategy: Search each theory independently, then combine them with "AND" for an additional search. Search for the subject "Nurses" or "Nursing," depending on the database you are using, and combine the "nurse" term with the "AND" set. After searching both PubMed and CINAHL, the void in the literature for research combining all three theories is obvious.

Selected References From Search:

1. Chaffee, M.W., & McNeill, M.M. (2007). A model of nursing as a complex adaptive system. *Nursing Outlook, 55*(5):232-241.
2. Clancy, T.R. (2008). Control: What we can learn from complex systems science. *Journal of Nursing Administration, 38*(6):272-274.
3. Kaplow, R., & Reed, K.D. (2008). The AACN synergy model for patient care: A nursing model as a force of magnetism. *Nursing Economic$, 26*(1):17-25.

Questions Used to Discern Evidence:

Choose two studies among the studies listed, read about them, and answer the following:

1. What are the differences between the two studies regarding their design, methods, and results?
2. What are the similarities between the two studies regarding the number of subjects, measures used, and interventions, if any?
3. What skill do you think you need to acquire so that you may apply theory in your forensic nursing practice?

REVIEW QUESTIONS

1. The study of animate or inanimate entities' response to their surroundings, environment, or experiences is:
   A. Synergy theory
   B. Complexity theory
   C. General systems theory
   D. Developmental theory

2. The study of entities and organizations that form partnerships and collaborations to achieve a common goal is:
   A. Synergy theory
   B. Complexity theory
   C. General systems theory
   D. Developmental theory

3. The study of two or more intersecting animate or inanimate entities forming a unified functioning whole is:
   A. Complexity theory
   B. Synergy theory
   D. Developmental theory
   D. General systems theory

4. Lynch (2006) describes three components of roles. The role component that is described as a deliberate and careful performance and enactment of a differentiated or specific role is:
   A. Role clarification
   B. Role expectation
   C. Role behavior
   D. Role player

(review questions continued on page 42)

5. The offer and acceptance of a promise or contract between the professions, community, and society and the role player/professional is:
   A. Role expectation
   B. Role clarification
   C. Role behavior
   D. Role communication

6. The shared and explicit knowledge, skills, boundaries, responsibilities, and accountability placed on each role player is:
   A. Role clarification
   B. Role player
   C. Role behavior
   D. Role expectation

7. A property of general systems as translated into CSS whereby a change in one part affects other parts of the system like a ripple caused by a tiny pebble thrown into a pond is:
   A. Input
   B. Output
   C. Feedback
   D. Reverberation

8. According to Kerfoot (2006), from a practice perspective, a theoretical framework serves as a guardrail for the practitioner. and from a research perspective, a conceptual framework serves as a:
   A. Frame that defines and demarcates the research aim and outcome
   B. Signal that all is well
   C. Road map
   D. Consultant

9. A property of general systems theory as adapted in CSS that allows practitioners to achieve a common goal through diverse pathways and multidimensional activities and strategies is:
   A. Reverberation
   B. Negative entropy
   C. Equifinality
   D. Feedback

10. A property of general systems theory as adapted in CSS that allows the FN to grow and flourish while adapting to challenges and ceasing opportunities is called:
    A. Feedback
    B. Equifinality
    C. Reverberation
    D. Negentropy

References

Al-Hadidi, M., & Jahshan, H. (2001). Family violence. In *Handbook of family violence.* Amman, Jordan: Family Guidance and Education, the National Council for Family Affairs, pp. 31-48.

American Nurses Association (ANA). (2001). *Code of ethics for nurses with interpretive statements.* Washington, DC: ANA.

American Nurses Association (ANA). (2003). *Nursing's social policy statement* (2nd ed.). Washington, DC: ANA.

Anderson, R.A., Crabtree, B.F., Steele, D.J., & McDaniel, R.R. (2005). Case study research: The view from the complexity science. *Qualitative Health Research, 15*(5):669-685.

Barker, P. (2001). The tidal model: Developing an empowering, person-centered approach to recovery with psychiatric and mental health nursing. *Journal of Psychiatric and Mental Health Nursing, 8*:233-244.

Binder, E.B., Bradley, R.G., Liu, W.L., Epstein, M.P., et al. (2008). Association of FKBP5 polymorphisms and childhood abuse with risk of posttraumatic stress disorder symptoms in adults. *Journal of the American Medical Association, 299*(11):1291-1305.

Campbell, R., Patterson, D., & Lichty, L.F. (2005). The effectiveness of sexual assault nurse examiner (SANE) programs: A review of psychological, medical, legal, and community outcomes. *Trauma Violence Abuse, 6*:313-329.

Chafee, M.W., & McNeill, M.M. (2007). A model of nursing as a complex adaptive system. *Nursing Outlook, 55*:232-241.

Clements, P.T., & Sekula, L.K. (2005). Toward advancement and evolution of forensic nursing: The interplay of research, theory, and practice. *Journal of Forensic Nursing, 1*:35-38.

Constantino, R. (1979). Conceptualizing general systems theory for nursing students and clinicians. *Philippine Journal of Nursing, 49*(1):21-25.

Constantino, R.E. (1984). Beyond constitutional history. *Juris, 18*(3):19-21.

Constantino, R.E. (2007). Translation of ethical, sociocultural, and accountability issues in the nurse lawyer's practice. *Journal of Nursing Law, 11*(1):27-33.

Curnow, S.A. (1997). The open window phase: Helpseeking and reality behaviors by battered women. *Applied Nursing Research, 10*(3)128-135.

DeSouza, R.M., Williams, J., & Myerson, F. (2003). *Critical links: Population, health, and the environment*. Washington, DC: Population Health Bureau.

Family Guidance and Education Center. (2001). *Prevalence of family violence in Al- Zarqa City*. Zarqa, Jordan: Guidance and Education Center.

Founds, S. (2009). Introducing systems biology for nursing science. *Biological Research for Nursing, 10*(1):1-8.

Gharaibeh, M., & Al-Ma'aitah, R. (2002). The cultural meaning of violence against women: Jordanian women's perspective. *Guidance and Counseling, 18*:2-9.

Goodman, R.M., Speers, M.A., McLeroy, K., et al. (1998). Identifying and defining the dimensions of community capacity to provide a basis for measurement. *Health Education & Behavior, 25*(3):258-278.

Green, D.A. (2006). A synergy model of nursing education. *Journal for Nurses in Staff Development, 22*(6):277-283.

Haj-Yahia, M.M. (2000). Wife abuse and battering in the sociocultural context of Arab society. *Family Process, 39*:237–255.

Hamdan-Mansour, A.M., Constantino, R.E., Farrell, M., et al. (2011). Evaluating the mental health of Jordanian women in relationship with partner abuse. *Issues in Mental Health Nursing, 32*:614-623.

Hammer, R.M., Moynahan, B., & Pagliaro, E.M. (2005). *Forensic Nursing*. New York: Jones and Bartlett.

Holden, L.M. (2005). Complex adaptive systems: Concept analysis. *Journal of Advanced Nursing, 52*(6):651-657.

International Association of Forensic Nurses (IAFN). Retrieved June 10, 2009, from http://www. IAFN.org

International Association of Forensic Nurses and American Nurses Association. (2009). *Scope and standards of forensic nursing practice*. Washington, DC: ANA.

Iyer, P. (2003). *Legal nurse consulting principles and practice*. New York: CRC Press.

Kent-Wilkinson, A. (2009). Forensic nursing education in North America: An exploratory study. Dissertation, University of Saskatchewan.

Kerfoot, K.M., Lavandero, R., Cox, M., Triola, N., et al. (2006). Conceptual models and the nursing organization: Implementing the AACN synergy model for patient care. *Nurse Leader, 4*(4):20-26.

Lasker, R.D., & Weiss, E.S. (2003). Broadening participation in community problem solving: A multidisciplinary model to support collaborative practice and research. *Journal of Urban Health, 80*(1):14-47.

Lynch, V. (2007). Forensic nursing science and the global agenda. *Journal of Forensic Nursing, 3*(3 & 4):101-111.

Lynch, V.A., & Duvall, J.B. (2011). Forensic nursing science (2nd Ed.). St. Louis: Elsevier Mosby.

Mugavin, M. (2008). Maternal filicide theoretical framework. *Journal of Forensic Nursing, 4*:68-79.

Paley, J. (2009). Complex adaptive systems and nursing. *Nursing Inquiry, 14*(3):233-242.

Plexus Institute. (2009). Complexity science. Retrieved March 3, 2010, from http://www.plexusinstitute.com

Plsek, P.E., Zimmerman, B., & Lindberg, C. (2007). Nine emerging and connected organizational and leadership principles.

Polit, D.F., & Beck, C.T. (2008). *Nursing research: Generating and assessing evidence for nursing practice*. Philadelphia: Lippincott.

Radzyminski, S. (2007). The concept of population health within the nursing profession. *Journal of Professional Nursing, 23*(1):37-46.

Rask, M., & Brunt, D. (2007). Verbal and social interactions in the nurse patient relationship in forensic psychiatric nursing: A model and its philosophical and theoretical foundations. *Nursing Inquiry, 14*(2):169-176.

Safadi, R., Swigart, V., Hamdan-Mansour, A.M., et al. (2012). An ethnographic-feminist study of Jordanian women's experiences of domestic violence and process of resolution. *Health Care for Women International 10*:3-14.

Simon, R.I., & Gold, L.H. (2004). *Textbook of forensic psychiatry*. Washington, DC: American Psychiatric Publishing.

Stokowski, L.A. (2008). Forensic nursing. Part 2. Inside forensic nursing. *Medscape Medical News*.

Walker, L.O., & Avant, K.C. (2005). *Strategies for theory construction in nursing*. New York: Pearson/Prentice Hall.

Walker, L.E. (2000). The battered woman (2nd ed). New York: Springer.

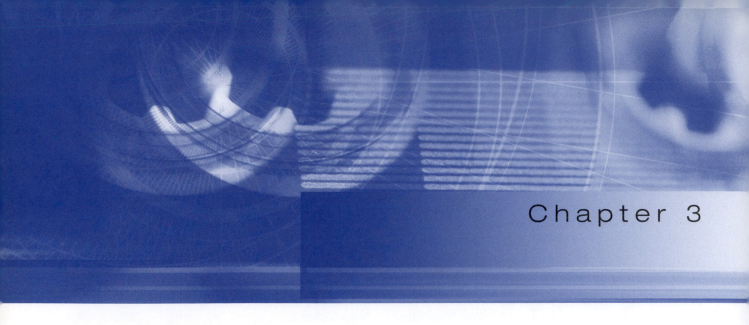

Chapter 3

THE ETHICAL, LEGAL, AND SOCIOCULTURAL ISSUES IN FORENSIC NURSING

Rose E. Constantino, Margarete L. Zalon, and Susan E. Young

"All the great things are simple and many can be expressed in a single word: freedom, justice, honor, duty, mercy, hope."

Winston Churchill

Competencies

1. Explaining the ethical and legal dilemmas encountered by nurses in diverse practice settings.
2. Defining the sociocultural issues encountered by nurses in diverse practice settings.
3. Analyzing the differences and similarities among ethical, legal, and sociocultural issues (ELSI) as they apply to diverse aspects of clinical nursing.
4. Discussing the basic premise of various ethical, legal, and sociocultural principles.
5. Synthesizing the principles for establishing practices in a socioculturally diverse health-care system.

Key Terms

Assault
Autonomy
Battery
Beneficence
Breach of duty
Community level
Consequentialism Damages
Defense of others
Deontologism
Deterrence
Duress
Duty
Entrapment
Fidelity
Incapacitation
Informed consent
Insanity
Intentional torts

Key Terms (continued)

Involuntary intoxication
Justice
Mistake
Necessity
Negligence
Nonconsequentialism
Nonmalfeasance
Patient-level
Proximate cause
Quasi-intentional torts
Rehabilitation

Respondeat superior
Restitution
Retribution
Self-defense
Sociocultural
Tort
Unintentional torts
Utilitarianism
Veracity
Voluntary intoxication
Whistle-blowing

INTRODUCTION

This chapter examines the roots of forensic nursing by using an ethical, legal, and sociocultural issues (ELSI) approach.

The past decade has witnessed an explosion of horrific incidents and disasters: the attacks of September 11, 2001; Hurricane Katrina, and unending wars. Adding to these calamities is the ongoing global economic and financial instability.

Whether an event is natural or by human design, the resulting loss of life, health, wealth, and property carries with it an obligation to fully and properly investigate. The collection, examination, and analysis of all physical evidence are paramount when assisting survivors of traumatic events to become as close as possible to being whole again. The critical work of saving lives, healing wounds, and restoring physical, mental, spiritual, and financial health is heightened by the intersecting demands of ethical, legal, and sociocultural responsibilities. The forensic nurse (FN) in an emergent environment is frequently in the best position to observe and gather significant data. Forensic nursing practice comprises many opportunities and challenges that require thoughtful, deliberate application of ethical, legal, and sociocultural principles.

ETHICS IN ELSI

Ethical Theories of Consequentialism and Nonconsequentialism

Two ethical theories from which ethical principles flow are **consequentialism** and **nonconsequentialism.** In the first, acts are right to the extent that they produce good results and wrong to the extent that they produce bad results. Acts are right by weighing the net of good consequences minus bad consequences for each person affected and adding them up to arrive at the total net good. This theory is also called **utilitarianism.** Utilitarianism encourages the FN to base decisions on what provides the greatest good for the greatest number of people.

Ethical principles are also derived from the opposing ethical theory of nonconsequentialism, also known as **deontologism,** or duty-based ethical theory. Deontologism is the idea that rightness and wrongness are inherent in an act or duty, independent of the consequences. Immanuel Kant described deontologism as the rightness or wrongness of one's actions based on the codified duty of care. An example of nonconsequentialism in forensic nursing is performing all rape case examinations on a pro bono basis.

Ethical Principles

Ethical theories provide a framework for ethical decision making but do not provide specific direction for translation into practice. However, ethical principles do provide direction for translation into practice. Among these principles are nonmalfeasance and beneficence (derived from the theory of consequentialism) and autonomy, justice, and veracity (derived from the theory of nonconsequentialism). Understanding these principles is crucial to the translation of ethical theories into actual forensic nursing practice.

Ethical Principles of Nonmalfeasance and Beneficence

Nonmalfeasance is illustrated by the saying *primum non nocere* (first, do no harm). Beneficence is captured in the Golden Rule: "Do unto others as you would have others do unto you." The ethical duty of FNs is protecting others (staff, clients, and patients) from harm (nonmalfeasance) and providing service for the good of the patients (**beneficence**). These two ethical principles operate together, one in a passive or inactive way (nonmalfeasance), the other in an active or assertive way (beneficence). Nonmalfeasance denotes a negative obligation requiring the FN to not engage in actions that injure or harm others, and beneficence requires the FN to act as to prevent or remove existing or potential harm (Matt, 2012). Forensic nursing practice, therefore, is not just another business and that good outcomes are driven by more than technological or procedural proficiency. To provide for nonmalfeasance and beneficence, the FN must value the physical, emotional, and spiritual needs of colleagues and patients, respect individuality, and focus on the multidisciplinary approach to advocacy (Constantino & Privitera, 2011).

Ethical Principles of Autonomy, Justice, Veracity, and Fidelity

These four principles guide the mission and vision of the FN. **Autonomy** is respect for the right of all persons to self-determination, independence, and goal setting. Autonomy requires all professionals to respect, protect, and keep in confidence important relationships and communications of all people in the community of interest to preserve the uniqueness of each person. Self-determination includes self-governance and the opportunity to live one's life freely without interference from others (Grace & Willis, 2012). Autonomy confers self-determination on all human beings, including individuals with diminished capacity by reason of age (children and frail elders) or illness (mental, psychological, or physical disorder; unconscious or semiconscious state; or under the influence of a mind-altering substance). It also includes those who are imprisoned. For those with little or no capacity for self-determination, a parent, guardian, or adult who holds only the best interest of the dependent should be vested with the dependent's right to self-determination. In such cases, autonomy or respect for the accused needs to be balanced with respect for all (Constantino & Privitera).

Violation of the ethical principle of autonomy is a violation of the right to be human. Only with a sincere and genuine respect for persons will the FN fulfill the requirements of the ethical principle of autonomy. When the FN applies the principle of autonomy, the principles of justice, veracity, and fidelity naturally follow.

Justice is an ethical principle and a moral concept (Grace and Willis). It demands that the FN be fair in all interactions and communications. Justice means making certain that policies and procedures in the forensic nursing practice are consistently and equitably applied without selective dispensation. Selective dispensation would occur, for example, if an alleged sex offender is not

prosecuted because the forensic examiner (physician, nurse, psychologist, social worker, or first responder) failed to collect important evidence or perform a thorough physical or psychological examination of the victim or the offender is not prosecuted in deference to a very influential defense team. Injustice is the outcome of failed justice.

Veracity includes truthfulness, trustworthiness, and transparency. To apply the ethical principle of veracity, or truth-telling, an environment of openness, honesty, and transparency must consistently be shown. In veracity, the FN makes certain that those involved in consultation and collaboration at all levels have all the information they need to make an informed decision about the case and to participate actively in an efficient and effective outcome. **Fidelity** means loyalty and faithfulness to persons or entities who place their trust in the FN. Trust serves as a foundation for the FN role. It is this trust that allows others to defer to the FN for guidance in decision making, safety, and well-being. Maintaining fidelity also implies that the FN will uphold commitments to all parties involved, including colleagues, patients, family members, health-care organizations, insurance providers, and the government. Affected by issues of fidelity and trust is the FN's degree of support to others. A lack of loyalty to another or an entity corrupts previous relationships, commitment, and loyalty.

CODE OF ETHICS FOR NURSES

The American Nurses Association *Code of Ethics for Nurses* (2001) serves as a guide for nurses in carrying out their professional responsibilities. The Code incorporates ethical principles as a standard for actions and addresses nurses in their responsibilities to individual patients and as members of the health-care team, the community, and the medical profession. The provisions of the Code as they can be applied to forensic nursing practice are illustrated in Table 3.1.

ETHICAL REASONING

Forensic nursing is complex because it takes place in the context of a health-care system as it intersects with the criminal justice system. Given this complexity, nurses need a model of ethical reasoning in order to provide care sensitive to needs of patients and in keeping with the *Code of Ethics for Nurses* and nursing practice standards. Fairchild's (2010) *Nursing Ethical Reasoning Skills*

TABLE 3.1   The ANA Code of Ethics for Nurses as Applied to Forensic Nursing

Focus of Code Provision	Forensic Nursing Application
Respect for human dignity	When caring for a patient who is a prisoner accused of murdering his wife who was a nurse at a local hospital, the nurse is obligated to provide care regardless of the patient's circumstances.
Commitment to patients	Advocating for a teenager who does not want his parents to know that he was in a minor accident, but who was driving under the influence of alcohol.
Protecting patient rights	Advocating for the respectful treatment of a pregnant prisoner who needs in-patient obstetrical services.
Accountability	When caring for an elderly patient who does not speak English and who may have been abused, the forensic nurse obtains the appropriate translation services, although the family indicates a translator is not necessary.
Professional growth	Improving knowledge, through continuing education and other means, of cultural factors influencing care for immigrant groups whose population has experienced recent growth in the community.
Improving health-care environments	Identifying best practices for providing services to victims of sexual assault and advocating for a revised model of care designed to provide quality services to patients who have experienced sexual assault.
Advancing the profession	Participating in a research study designed to improve documentation of care for patients who may have experienced abuse.
Promoting efforts to meet health needs	Advocating for making Sexual Assault Nurse Examiner training available to emergency department nurses in the community.
Participating in the profession's goals	Actively participating in the American Nurses Association, a state/constituent nurses association, and the International Association of Forensic Nursing.

(NERS) Model can be used as a framework for addressing forensic nursing ethical dilemmas. This model, which is based on a review of ethical reasoning skills and metacognition literature and how nurses think through ethical dilemmas, includes the metacognition skills of reflections, reasoning, and review of competing values (see Table 3.2). The NERS model is designed to assist nurses in engaging in systems thinking in order to reflect on and manage the competing values in complex patient care situations while being mindful of nurses' individual or collective actions in the context of professional practice. Use the NERS Model of ethical reasoning in the two case studies that follow to address an ethical issue in the context of a complex forensic nursing practice dilemma.

WHISTLE-BLOWING

Whistle-blowing is a situation in which the ethical or legal conflicts that arise in a particular situation are so egregious, that is, harmful or illegal, that the individual who knows about the situation is forced to take action in order to prevent harm. Generally, whistle-blowing refers to measures taken outside the established authority of an organization and making the situation public because of a failure of those in leadership positions to take action. The *Code of Ethics for Nurses* (ANA, 2001) requires that the nurse "promotes, advocates for and strives to protect the health, safety and rights of the patient." Additionally, nurses are to take action in the case of incompetent, unethical, illegal, or impaired practice by a health-care team member. The responsibilities of the nurse in relation to whistle-blowing are grounded in beneficence, doing good for others, and the fact that health care should result in a good outcome for patients.

FNs may face enormous challenges in speaking up about and reporting such behaviors. Numerous situations in health care could lead to whistle-blowing. These include concerns about patient care quality, incompetence, impaired practice, and health-care fraud, such as provider billing practices. Whistle-blowing is not without its risks. Nurses who are whistle-blowers may risk loss

TABLE 3.2   **Nurses Ethical Reasoning Skills (NERS) Model**

Metacognitive Skill	Description	Forensic Nursing Example
Reflection	Critical reflective consciousness. Awareness of how one's own values might influence care.	Providing nursing care to undocumented immigrants who were injured in a street fight regardless of their individual circumstances and what may or may not be known about them.
Reasoning	Dialectical reasoning. Examination of opposing forces within the health-care system.	Needing to respect the autonomy of a teenager who has been raped and does not want treatment, and the need for parents to know what happened to their child.
Review of competing values	Examination of competing values of patient, family, health-care providers, health-care organization, and the criminal justice system.	Providing care for a dangerous prisoner in an emergency department setting in a humane manner while providing for the safety of self and others.

Adapted from Fairchild, R. M. (2010). Practical ethical theory for nurses responding to complexity in care. *Nursing Ethics, 17*:353-362.

of employment, ostracism, or other forms of informal or formal sanction. They need to weigh the benefits of speaking out against the very real consequences of those actions. Whistle-blower protections vary by state and according to the whistle-blowing subject matter. A number of states have passed whistle-blower legislation designed to protect individuals who speak out against unsafe, unethical, or illegal practices. This legislation is designed to prevent employers from taking reprisals against individuals who report poor quality of care or questionable business practices. Such reprisals might include suspension, harassment, demotion, or termination of employment. At least 20 states have whistle-blower protections in place for nurses.

The federal Whistleblower Protection Act of 1989 applies to federal employees. In 1994, it was expanded to include certain Veterans Administration and government contractor employees. However, military nurses are prohibited from taking legal action against the federal government for harms caused by persons working for the Defense Department. The Supreme Court decided these protections do not apply to someone speaking out in their official capacity (*Garzetti v. Ceballos*, 547 U. S. 410, 2006). Thus, the patchwork of state and restricted federal legislation provides limited protection for whistleblowers. The FN must carefully weigh the alternatives, the potential consequences of whistle-blowing, and the patient's best interests.

Whistle-blowing in nursing is reflective of larger issues in nursing related to the power and voice of nurses in advocating for their patients. In 1994, a group of Canadian nurses made sustained efforts to report the incompetence of a pediatric cardiac surgeon that went unheeded. It was not until an inquiry into the death of 12 children that the lack of attention given to the nurses' concerns was recognized as an important problem (Ceci, 2004). The consequences of whistle-blowing is illustrated by the case of two nurses in Winkler County, Texas, who reported their

Case Study

A TEMPTING OFFER

Ms. Jones, an FN, has been hired by both the defense and prosecution in the past. In this high visibility rape case, the prosecution asked her, for a fee, to review medical records and verify the lack of evidence collection. The prosecution wanted to know whether the lack of evidence collection was due to the patient's refusal to give informed consent (as charted) or if it was due to the premature departure of the sexual assault nurse examiner (SANE) from the patient's room. The patient overheard the SANE say to another nurse that the SANE was "done with her" while the SANE was waiting for the patient to give her consent to a pelvic exam and collection of evidence. The SANE left the room abruptly to see another patient (her husband's boss) in the intensive care unit. The next day (before the SANE could respond to the prosecution's request), the defense in the same high visibility case called the SANE to ask her to do exactly the same task for triple the prosecution's fee.

Case Study

concerns about a physician's medical care, which included examples such as suturing a rubber cap to a patient's finger, to the Texas Medical Board using patient record numbers in their complaint. The county sheriff, a friend of the physician, learned that the complaint was filed by the two nurses. The nurses were arrested, charged, and indicted for failure to properly execute a public servant role (Yoder-Wise, 2010). They were also fired from their jobs at the county's 15-bed critical access hospital. The charges against one nurse were dismissed. The second nurse stood trial and was acquitted. The Texas Nurses Association and the American Nurses Association provided strong support to the nurses during this process.

Despite the outcome of the Winkler county legal proceedings, the case has forever changed the lives of these nurses and has cast a chilling pall over the ability of nurses to advocate for their patients. Fortunately, the jury in this instance understood the importance of the advocacy role of the nurses. The nurse's important patient safety role was in the national spotlight.

Nurses, by virtue of their 24-hour accountability for patient care, are in the position to observe actions that are hazardous and may place patients at risk for harm. It is incumbent upon the FN to explore all the appropriate options and resources in making decisions about the necessary actions. The *Code of Ethics for Nurses* provides guidance for actions. The professional associations at the state level, the ANA, and the International Association of Forensic Nurses (IAFN) are important resources for the nurse confronted with these dilemmas.

THE LAW IN ELSI

Laws govern contractual relations, ownership, and transfer of real and personal property; they establish definitions of crimes against society, protect individual citizens from harm created by others, guard the safety of workers, allow for the provision of health care, and influence most aspects of human existence (Constantino & Privitera, 2011). This section discusses criminal and tort laws as applied to forensic nursing. A "tort" is a crooked or wrongful act, not involving a breach of contract, for which civil action can be brought (*Black's Law Dictionary,* 2004).

The Theory of Law

The law is a social contract among members of a group that creates a binding rule of conduct or a system of rules established and enforced by an authority to bring order to society as well as to safeguard it. The creation of a system of laws naturally places limits upon the rights of citizens and creates obligations for them. As society has grown and become more complicated, the body of law, which sustains civilization, has also grown.

Sources of the Law

There are four major sources of the law:

1. Common law, or judicially created law, derived from the English system and developed by the U.S. judicial system
2. The Constitution of the United States
3. Statutes passed by Congress
4. Regulations promulgated by executive branch agencies through the authority granted them by the legislative branch

Areas of Law

There are three general areas of law: (1) criminal law includes federal and state laws that relate to society as a whole and deals with felonies and misdemeanors; (2) tort law, also known as civil law, deals with individuals and their relationships with each other; and (3) public law is associated with direct government involvement.

Criminal Law

Criminal laws protect society as a whole, are adopted by a legislative body, and prescribe specific punishment upon violation. Crimes are prosecuted by states' attorneys general or by the office of the U.S. attorney, if the crime is a violation of a federal law. Forensic nurses in emergency departments or other acute clinical services are most likely to be the first health-care professionals to attend to victims who have suffered bodily harm, the alleged perpetrator if also injured, or both. The U.S. population has become the most litigious in the world, and health-care systems are considered by plaintiffs' lawyers to be "deep pockets" ready for suing.

Crime has always been present in civilized society. Motives to commit crimes, such as greed, jealousy, political zeal, and lust, have generally remained constant. However, the means to commit crimes have changed drastically. According to Constantino and Privitera (2011), in the 21st century unparalleled, sophisticated Internet applications have altered the criminal playing field. Criminals no longer need face-to-face interaction when planning or conspiring to commit a crime, nor do they need physical access to their victim(s) to commit the crime.

Criminal prosecutions are different from civil prosecutions because a crime is an offense against people of the state, jurisdiction, or federal government. The attorney general and/or district attorney's office prosecutes the crime. The accused or alleged perpetrator of the crime is called the "defendant," and the victim of the crime, "a witness."

In criminal litigation, the standard of proof is beyond a reasonable doubt, whereas in civil litigation, proof of guilt is by a preponderance of the evidence. For cases related to the violation of administrative laws, the standard of proof is clear and convincing. "Reasonable doubt" means an honest and reasonable uncertainty about the guilt of the defendant. Another difference between civil and criminal prosecution is that penalties for civil wrongs include fines, damages, and legal admonishments to refrain from certain acts, whereas penalties for criminal violations can include incarceration and, in some jurisdictions, the death penalty.

Nurses, including FNs, occupy a special position of trust because they provide complete and seamless care to patients and their families. Despite this special position of trust, some nurses, including FNs, commit crimes or are accused of committing crimes. Below is a brief presentation of the elements, classification, and defenses of selected crimes in which FNs might be involved and the objectives of punishment.

The elements of a crime. The elements of a crime are as follows (Ormerod, 2010):

1. *Actus reus,* which is Latin for "guilty act," also referred to as the physical element of committing prohibited conduct, may be accomplished by an action, by threat of action, or by omission of an act or failure to act.
2. *Mens rea,* which is Latin for "guilty mind," is the intent to commit a crime, as seen in the mental state of the accused at the time the crime was committed.
3. *Causation* is when criminal conduct produces a criminal result, as in murder, which produces death, or in theft, which results in a loss of property by the owner.
4. *Strict liability crimes* are created by statute and impose liability in the absence of intent or mens rea.

Types of crimes. *Crimes against persons* are fatal offenses and personal offenses. Fatal offenses include murder or felony murder (a killing that occurs while in the process of committing a felony, as in an HIV-positive nurse injecting herself with a patient's pain medication, then using the same needle to draw up a saline solution and injecting it into the patient, thereby exposing the patient to the virus). Murder or felony murder in the first degree requires intent with malice aforethought. Manslaughter is a lesser charge because it is committed in the absence of malice. Involuntary manslaughter or negligent homicide is a killing that lacks guilty intent but involves gross and wanton neglect and extreme recklessness. Personal offenses include **assault** (creating a fear of imminent battery), **battery** (unlawful touching), false imprisonment, kidnapping, and sexual assault, rape, or abuse (SARA).

Crimes against property include trespass, conversion, embezzlement, theft, robbery, fraud, extortion, false pretenses, and larceny. The FN could commit or be accused of committing crimes against property if the FN possesses the mens rea and actus reus. *Participatory crimes* include aiding, abetting, and conspiracy.

Crimes against justice comprise compounding (receipt of some consideration in return for a promise not to prosecute the crime), misprision (failure of a duty to prevent the commission of a crime as to conceal a crime), obstruction (preventing, hindering, or delaying the progress of the prosecution of a crime), perverting the course of justice, and perjury. Perjury is swearing willfully, absolutely, and falsely in a judicial proceeding. Perjury is the most common among crimes against justice. In addition, Northrop and Kelly (1987) describe in detail, with case examples, other offenses an FN may commit or be accused of committing, such as *reporting statutes* and *willful failure to provide emergency services.* Misdemeanor charges are often provided by statute for failure to report certain injuries and willful failure to provide emergency services.

Five purposes of crime punishment. Criminal law stands alone in its distinctively serious potential consequences for or punishment of the accused when found guilty of the crime. Punishment ranges from incarceration for a day to life in prison (federal or state) or jail (county or local) to death by various methods, depending upon the death penalty jurisdiction. There are five purposes for punishment: (1) deterrence, (2) retribution, (3) incapacitation, (4) restitution, and (5) rehabilitation (DRIRR). **Deterrence** is meant to prevent the criminal from reoffending or to prevent others from committing a crime. **Retribution,** as one of the purposes of punishment, is traced to the Latin word *retribo*, which means "I pay back," in that the individual causing the harm deserves to, and in fact must, be harmed. This approach is referred to as *lex talonis*, the law of retaliation that is exacted in the words "an eye for an eye, a tooth for a tooth, an arm for an arm, a life for a life." **Incapacitation** is placing the criminal away from society through confinement in a secure environment to prevent future criminal acts against those who remain free. The ultimate form of incapacitation is death. **Restitution** means to repair the injustice that was done to the victim, such as an embezzler being required to pay back the amount taken. **Rehabilitation** aims at transforming a criminal into a valuable member of society through education, training, and counseling programs. Some people believe the only true punishment for all serious crimes is removing offenders from society through incapacitation, specifically death.

Selected defenses. Because of the gravity of punishment, several types of defenses are made available to the accused. However, several of these defenses depend on the defendant's intent or beliefs at the time of the alleged crime (such as self-defense or defense of others) and do not apply to strict liability crimes. Northrop and Kelly provide a list of defenses that might be applicable to the accused. **Insanity** is a defense unlike any other; if successful, the defendant is not acquitted of the crime, but rather a special finding is made of "not guilty by reason of insanity" or "guilty but insane." The defendant is sent to a mental health facility for treatment until recovered from the mental illness. **Voluntary** or **involuntary intoxication** with alcohol or drugs is a defense to a crime when it negates an element of the crime such as intent or knowledge.

Mistake is another defense whereby an honest mistake of fact negates intent as an element of the crime. For example, an FN fails to check a patient's identification band and administers an antibiotic that was not ordered to an elderly patient with renal insufficiency who has the same last name as another patient. The patient then develops nephrotoxicity requiring dialysis. The standard of care is to use two means of identification. The FN in this case did not verify the patient's identity. The patient suffered a serious complication. This is a case of an honest mistake of fact, in that the patient was not identified properly. This mistake of fact may negate intent or result in consideration of the FN's mental state because the FN did not intend to harm the patient.

Entrapment is a defense to a crime in which a government or private citizen acting as a government agent or a private citizen acting as a government agent forced the accused to perform an illegal act or when an informer provides an idea for the crime, inducing another to commit the crime. For example, an FN in a large clinic is induced by the clinic manager to falsify billing records. For the entrapment defense to be successful, the accused must not be predisposed to commit the crime. The defense of **duress** requires that an unlawful threat be made to the defendant so that the only way to avoid death or serious bodily injury to self and/or another is to commit the crime. **Necessity** is a defense that requires an emergency that induces the defendant to choose between the lesser of two wrongdoings. Northrop and Kelly provide an example of the usefulness of the defense of necessity in a nurse speeding to an emergency in the early hours of the morning, in violation of the law. The nurse's act is justified by the necessity to drive over the speed limit so that he or she may provide the necessary emergency care.

Self-defense applies when the defendant uses a reasonable amount of force against the aggressor, believing that (1) he or she is in an immediate danger of bodily harm and (2) use of such force is necessary to avoid bodily harm. **Defense of others** may be justified if reasonable force is necessary to defend a third person who is not the aggressor (or may even be a stranger) from suffering bodily harm at the hands of the aggressor. Deadly force is reasonable when the attack of the aggressor upon the other reasonably appears to be a deadly attack (Northrop & Kelly; Constantino & Privitera).

Tort Law

A **tort** is a wrongful act that harms and is classified as an (1) intentional tort, (2) a quasi-intentional tort, or (3) an unintentional tort—professional negligence. In tort law, the common principle is that injuries are to be compensated, and antisocial behavior is to be discouraged. The torts concept evolved from the principle that an individual should not injure a person or a person's property or infringe on a person's rights. The same act may constitute both a tort and a crime; however, a crime is an offense against the public that is prosecuted by the state or federal government, whereas a tort is a private injury that may be pursued in civil court by the injured party. The focus of tort law is to compensate individuals for injuries sustained due to the conduct of another (Constantino & Privitera).

Intentional torts are intentional or willful acts that violate another person's property rights. The distinction between an intentional tort and a negligent tort is the intent of the person committing the act. An intentional tort requires that the person committing the act has the requisite knowledge and will to commit the wrong.

The basis of an intentional tort focuses on intent and consent. Intentional torts include assault, battery, false imprisonment, intentional infliction of emotional distress, and trespass to land. Types of intentional torts are as follows:

(1) *assault,* intentionally placing someone who is conscious in immediate fear or apprehension of an immediate bodily harm or a noxious event without that person's consent; (2) *battery,* a harmful or offensive touching of another (who may be conscious or unconscious) without his or her consent or without a legally justifiable reason; (3) *false imprisonment,* the unlawful detention of a person through chemical, physical, or emotional means without consent; (4) *intentional infliction of emotional distress,* conduct toward a third party plaintiff (a spouse of an elderly patient with Alzheimer's disease watched his wife being raped by a staff member who fainted and fell hitting and breaking his head) that is outrageous and beyond the bounds of common decency (actions must be egregious); and (5) *trespass to land,* the entrance, without the consent of the landowner, onto another's land or that causes anyone or anything to enter the land or premises (Northorp & Kelly; Constantino & Privitera).

Quasi-intentional torts include defamation (libel and slander), invasion of privacy, and breach of confidentiality. Defamation is an oral or written communication to a third party about the plaintiff that is false and that tends to injure the plaintiff's reputation. Two kinds of defamation are (1) libel, which is a written defamatory statement, and (2) slander, which is a spoken defamatory statement. Other quasi-intentional torts include (1) breach of confidentiality, which occurs when someone who has legitimate access to a patient's health information shares it (without the patient's consent) with others who have no legitimate reason to know or discusses a patient's specific medical information and diagnosis in an elevator within the hearing of others, and (2) invasion of privacy, which

involves unjustifiably intruding on another's right of privacy by appropriating his or her name or likeness, unreasonably interfering with his or her seclusion, publishing private facts, or publicly placing a person in a false light (Constantino & Privitera).

Unintentional torts include personal injuries suffered as a result of the commission of an act without permission or the omission of an act. Unlike crimes and intentional or quasi-intentional torts (which generally require the alleged perpetrator to have the specific intention to cause injury), unintentional torts do not require intent to harm. An unintentional tort requires that an individual "tortfeasor" act in a manner in which a reasonable person would not act under similar circumstances and that the commission of the act result in injury to another person. Under limited circumstances, a person may be personally liable for *not acting* under circumstances that require action to prevent harm to another person. The law does not require a person generally to act or intervene in a dangerous situation to prevent the injury of another unless there is a "special relationship" between the parties. The parent-child relationship and health-care provider–patient relationship are among those recognized by the law as a "special relationship" imposing a duty to act. Therefore, forensic nurses have a duty to act to prevent any harm to their patients and may be held liable if they fail to do so (Northrop & Kelly; Constantino & Privitera).

The duty to act or the duty to refrain from acting is an example of a legal principle or a basic rule, law, or doctrine. Legal principles are applied to the facts of a case, and the principles determine the legal standard by which the acts or the omission of an act of an individual or legal entity is governed. The principles of malpractice law enable forensic nurses to assess current practices and take action or respond to issues and questions to provide quality care and achieve optimal patient outcomes.

Professional **malpractice** or **negligence** is the act or the omission of an action by a professional individual or legal entity that constitutes failure to exercise care in the performance of professional duties. The underlying legal theory is that since the practice of a learned profession requires specific education, learning, and/or experience beyond that of the average person, and the profession is required to set its own standards, the law holds professionals (including nurses) to the minimum standard of care that would be required of a competent professional in the same field under similar circumstances. Proof of professional malpractice or negligence requires that a patient (or personal representative, if deceased) prove (1) that the defendant had the *duty* to provide care based on the applicable standard of care; (2) that there was a *breach of duty* or the standard of care by the defendant; (3) that the breach was the *proximate, direct, or legal cause* of the injury to the patient; and (4) that compensable *damages* for loss exist (Northorp & Kelly; Constantino & Privitera).

The standard of care in all health-care fields, and its breach, can generally be proved only through the testimony of another individual in the same profession, known as an "expert witness," who is familiar with the alleged facts of the case. In most courts, physicians may be allowed to testify to the standard of care and breach by a defendant nurse. This is gradually changing; for example, in *Edwards v. Sullivan Hospital* the Illinois Supreme Court held that a physician was not competent to testify to the standard of care required by a nurse or to its breach. A physician, however, is required to testify to the cause of injuries in most cases because determining the cause of an illness or injury requires a diagnosis, which nurses are not licensed to perform.

Other legal principles or doctrines frequently seen in malpractice cases include informed consent and respondeat superior. **Informed consent** is often raised in malpractice cases involving an error in a procedure requiring patient consent, such as surgery or other invasive procedures. The consent requirement arises from the laws recognizing the sanctity of one's physical body, which another person may not touch without permission. The informed consent doctrine arose late in the development of malpractice law as the "physician knows best" attitude fell by the wayside. The first two cases to which an informed consent doctrine was applied were *Canterbury v. Spence* (464 F.2d 772 C.A.D.C., 1972) and *Karp v. Cooley* (93 F.2d 408 5th. Cir., 1974). These decisions were "judge-made" law based on the rights of an individual to control what happens to his or her body and the principle that an individual cannot validly consent to a procedure without being advised of the options and the material risks. Informed consent is now generally governed by laws passed by state legislatures and differ from state to state (Northrop & Kelly; Constantino & Privitera).

Respondeat superior is a well-established legal principle that varies little from state to state. It is a Latin term meaning "let the master answer." It is a legal doctrine that makes an employer indirectly liable for the consequences of his or her employee's wrongful conduct while the employee is acting within the scope of the employment or agency. Respondeat superior is also known as the "master-servant rule." In malpractice cases, a jury is allowed to hold the employer liable for the negligence of its employees but only if the act was "within the scope of employment." The scope of employment legal issue is frequently litigated as the plaintiff attempts to hold a hospital or other employer with a greater ability to pay a judgment and the defendant's employer tries to prove that its employee's act was not within the employee's job description. A "legal issue" is an unsettled question of law or law needing examination to achieve a resolution or conclusion in the case.

Professional standards in corrections nursing. The standards of practice in corrections nursing (ANA, 2007) and forensic nursing standards (ANA & IAFN, 2009) provide guidance for the FN's action as seen in the case study specifically when the patient is in the prison system and when a prisoner is transported and receives care in a health-care facility. In the pregnant prisoner case study, the corrections nurse who began her shift made the necessary

Case Study

A PREGNANT PRISONER

A 22-year-old Hispanic female has been incarcerated in a state prison since the fifth month of her first pregnancy, and she is now at 37 weeks gestation. Two weeks ago, she was complaining of severe abdominal pain and was taken to the emergency room of a local community hospital where she was examined by an obstetrician. There was no evidence of abnormality or complication, and the pain subsided.

This evening, she calls out to the guard to indicate that she is having a severe headache. The guard reports the situation to the nurse, who examines the woman and decides that the prisoner is faking it since the last time she had a trip out of the prison nothing was wrong. Therefore, the woman is taken back to her cell and a security camera is directed toward her cell. For the next several hours, the woman cries out that she has a severe headache, but the nurse did not return to the cell. The shift changes, and the nurse on the next shift checks on the patient and notes the prisoner's vital signs are BP 180/90, HR = 110, R = 24, 4+ pitting edema. It is apparent that she has had spontaneous rupture of membranes. The prisoner is now experiencing contractions every 4 minutes for approximately 30 seconds in duration.

(case study continued on page 54)

Case Study

The nurse has a guard call 911. When the paramedics arrive, the guards place the woman in shackles and transport her to the local hospital maternity unit. Upon arrival at the labor and delivery suite, the guard insists on keeping the shackles around the woman's waist. The woman was convicted of second-degree theft and therefore was a medium security prisoner who was not considered a threat.

The labor and delivery nurses admitted the woman to the unit and instituted fetal monitoring. In the interim, the guard left the unit, presumably for the restroom. The fetal monitor reading was interpreted to indicate late decelerations, a sign of fetal distress. The obstetrician was called and it was decided that an emergency cesarean section was needed. The nurses were unable to immediately locate the guard to remove the shackles from the woman's waist and legs so that preparations for the cesarean section could be made in a timely manner.

Subsequently, the woman had the caesarean section. When the baby was born, the Apgar score was a 5. The baby was whisked away to a neonatal intensive care unit. The mother was taken back to the prison 2 days later. It was then determined that the baby had severe developmental delays, most likely due to hypoxia at birth.

assessments resulting in the transfer of the patient who was in labor and at risk for developing toxemia demonstrated commitment to the patient. The ethical principle of justice is applied in that the nurse must treat the patient with fairness and ensure that the patient has access to the appropriate care. Ensuring access to care is a critical responsibility of the corrections nurse.

Additional questions are raised about reporting the lack of care received by the prisoner when the headache was reported. In this instance, the first nurse may not have realized that the prisoner, late in her pregnancy, was exhibiting symptoms that might be related to toxemia. Regardless of the cause of the symptoms, the patient, in this instance the pregnant prisoner, has the right to treatment for pain. Also at issue may be the first nurse's competency to care for a prisoner who is pregnant. However, with the growth of the prison population, particularly with the increase of young women in prison, the numbers of women who are pregnant and then deliver while serving a prison sentence have increased.

Pregnant women in prisons are at greater risk for adverse outcomes. According to Knight and Plugge (2005), they are more likely to be single, an ethnic minority, less likely to have completed high school, less likely to receive antenatal care, more likely to have a medical condition affecting the pregnancy outcome, and more likely to smoke, drink excessively, or use illegal drugs.

Standards of practice require that the nurse obtains and maintains current knowledge and competency in nursing practice. Therefore, nurses working with women in correctional facilities need to be prepared not only to address sociocultural issues in this population but also to provide care that is compassionate, respectful, and adheres to professional practice standards.

Shackling women in labor and delivery is not only inhumane but can also interfere with the safe delivery of the baby. The U.S. Federal Bureau of Prisons ended its policy of shackling pregnant women. Some states have legislated bans on shackling pregnant women. However, there is variation in the time period when shackling is prohibited.

This case study illustrates the conflicts that may occur when the criminal justice system intersects with the health-care system. The health-care professional in the hospital did not override the guard's action and did not insist that the shackles be removed, resulting in a delay in the baby's delivery.

Health-care facilities need to be prepared to take care of patients who are prisoners. Clear policies need to be in place to ensure access to care. The FN can advocate for the adoption of a facility policy prohibiting the use of shackles for pregnant women. Having such a policy in place would be an important first step in providing support for the staff. The FN can be instrumental in setting the tone for staff's responses to actions that may place patients at risk. In addition, the FN can advocate for change in legislation and policy in his or her jurisdiction. The Rebecca Project for Human Rights is a national legal and policy organization focused on training mothers recovering from violence, trauma, and addiction to be leaders and policy advocates within their communities.

Understanding legal requirements of negligence. Was the nurse providing care to the patient in the case study negligent? The law does not expect that nurses who come to court as defendants be perfect. The law requires only that they be *reasonably:* as reasonably trained professionals they follow the standards of care enunciated by the profession for which they have been educated. Negligence is an unintentional wrongdoing in the form of failure to meet a standard of care that any *reasonably* prudent health-care provider would meet, possessing similar knowledge and skills under comparable circumstances. As discussed above, negligence is present if the case includes the following elements: the nurse's *duty* is established, there was a *breach of duty*, the breach was *proximate*, and *damages* for the loss exist.

1. *Duty.* The element of **duty** is established when the nurse accepts direct care and treatment of an individual. In accepting an assignment, the nurses in the case study had the responsibility to care for the patient. Duty was established when the nurses accepted the responsibility to provide care and treatment for the patient.

2. *Breach of duty.* The element of **breach of duty** occurs when the nurse fails to provide an expected standard. The prison nurse may have been negligent because of her failure to recognize that a severe headache might be a symptom of preeclampsia. The nurses at the hospital failed to take appropriate action to provide the patient with timely intervention to mitigate the effects of toxemia and provide for the safe delivery of her baby. In this instance, standards of care as established by the ANA, IAFN, and others would guide such a determination. The weight given by the courts to clinical standards, guidelines, and other such documents depends on the (1) degree of acceptance and authority of the practice parameter, (2) the fit between the clinical situation and the practice parameter, and (3) the validity of the research and evidence for the practice parameter.

3. *Proximate Cause.* The element of **proximate cause** requires that the act of negligence be identified as the proximate (legal) and direct cause of the patient's injury or loss. Although this is by far the most difficult element to prove, it appears that inaction by the nurse (doing nothing when the prisoner had potential symptoms of toxemia and failure to insist upon the removal of shackles) can be considered the proximate cause.

4. *Damages.* There are three types of **damages:** special, general, and punitive. Special damages provide monetary compensation for expenses incurred by the plaintiff as a consequence of the negligence. General damages recompense for damages on which a monetary value cannot be placed, such as pain and suffering. Punitive damages are imposed to punish the defendant, set a representative example, and act as a

deterrent for future negligent behavior. In this case, the damages do exist and fall under the type of special punitive damages specifically compounding the developmental delays suffered by the baby.

The actions of the nurses in this case study meet the legal requirements of negligence. The nurses had a duty to provide effective care for the pregnant patient and when the patient was in active labor. The first nurse breached that duty by failing to act on a common symptom of toxemia of pregnancy. The nurse who did not insist on removing the shackles breached that duty by not advocating for the patient so that care could be delivered in a safe and effective manner. Proximate cause is proved by the baby, who is developmentally delayed. Proof of damages, special, general, and punitive, can be shown through current and future care needs of the baby.

In this case study, the FN and the agencies involved face a complex legal dilemma regarding failure to provide the appropriate standard of care. Furthermore, the nurses may have violated the ANA *Code of Ethics for Nurses* and accepted practice standards. The case study illustrates the complexity of the application of standards of care to a specific situation and the challenges of dealing with a complex situation. To prevent a situation such as that described in this case, health-care institutions can adopt policies for the appropriate treatment of prisoners, provide opportunities for training FNs, and provide administrative support for the implementation of evidence-based policies.

Criminal negligence. Criminal negligence occurs when a licensed professional, for example a forensic nurse, is not only negligent but has also committed a crime. The key feature of criminal negligence is intentionality. Criminal charges have been brought against nurses in the United States and abroad for their actions (Cady, 2009; Lin & Wang, 2008). Criminal negligence is defined by a jurisdiction's statutes. Generally, charges can be filed against a health-care professional when the person's actions were such that the result was serious harm or death and the actions could have been foreseen and therefore are considered to be reckless and a wanton disregard for safety. Increased public awareness of the consequences of errors may contribute to the willingness of prosecutors to press criminal charges against health-care professionals. In 2006, a 16-year-old patient in labor was given, via a peripheral intravenous line, a fentanyl and bupivacaine infusion intended for the epidural route instead of the ordered antibiotic. Within 5 minutes, the patient began having a seizure and ultimately died, although the infant survived (Smetzer et al., 2010). Criminal charges were filed against the nurse and subsequently dropped. In 1996, a newborn died after receiving a 10-fold intravenous dose of penicillin G benzathine that was to have been administered via the intramuscular route (Smetzer, 1998). Two registered nurses and one nurse practitioner had criminal charges filed against them. Two pled to a lesser charge, and the third was acquitted after a trial.

Criminal charges were filed against 10 Filipino nurses who resigned from a nursing home because of poor working conditions. Even though their shifts were covered, the nurses were charged with endangering the welfare of a child and the welfare of a physically disabled person. The nurses, along with their attorney, were charged with conspiring to commit the offenses (Keepnews, 2009). Ultimately, the charges were dismissed by the state's appellate court (*Matter of Vinluan v. Doyle*, 2009).

The aforementioned criminal cases received a great deal of publicity. The nurses garnered support from the professional community, and ultimately, the nurses did not receive criminal sentences. However, nurses are at risk for criminal charges being filed against them not only if they have seriously breached a standard of practice or are believed to have breached a standard but also if they destroy evidence or deliberately deceive a patient. Failure to report child or elder abuse, assault and battery, and physical abuse of patients may also result in criminal charges. Malpractice insurance generally does not cover the costs of a defense of criminal charges. In addition, a health-care professional may be subject to sanctions from the licensing board up to and including revocation of one's license to practice stemming from the incident and/or conviction of the crime (Cady, 2009).

The FN may have a number of roles in a criminal negligence case. These may include conducting an investigation, conducting a root-cause analysis to identify factors contributing to the situation, providing counseling to family members, providing counseling to nurses who are involved in such incidents, and instituting corrective measures depending on the circumstances.

Public Law

Public law refers to the laws and ordinances promulgated by states and other jurisdictions to protect the public and keep its citizens safe. They vary from one jurisdiction to another. An example of public law is the Nurse Practice Act of each state, which generally includes a definition of nursing and certain requirements for individuals who are allowed to take the licensure examination and the composition and qualifications of individuals serving on nursing boards. In addition, regulations, which contain more detail, are promulgated to implement the law. Regulations

carry the force of law because each jurisdiction has a well-defined process that includes public comment and oversight before implementation.

The patchwork of laws and regulations in different jurisdictions results in a lack of common definitions for advanced practice registered nurses (APRNs), creating confusion and limitations for APRNs in their ability to practice within the full scope of their abilities. The *Consensus Model for APRN Regulation: Licensure, Accreditation, Certification and Education* (2008) is a consensus document for the four recognized advanced practice roles: nurse practitioners, nurse midwives, nurse anesthetists, and clinical nurse specialists. It provides consistency and clarity of licensure, accreditation, credentialing and education (LACE) for APRNs. States or jurisdictions will introduce legislation and regulations to implement the model. The Center to Champion Nursing in America (2011) tracks the progress on consumer access and barriers to primary care as evidenced by physician–nurse practitioner restrictive collaboration requirements by state. This resource can inform forensic nurses about the challenges and opportunities in advanced practice roles. The implication for advanced practice in specialties such as forensic nursing is that competence will not be assessed by licensing boards, but rather by professional organizations and/or certifying bodies.

Public law is very broad in scope at the state and federal level and includes laws on a wide range of topics relevant to the health of the public, including protections for patient privacy such as the Health Insurance Portability and Accountability Act (HIPAA), reimbursement for advanced practice, helmet legislation, regulations related to water pollution, and whether nurses may pronounce death.

SOCIOCULTURAL ISSUES IN ELSI

According to the **sociocultural** perspective, a social practice, such as forensic nursing, develops as a result of the linguistic and physical tools of the practice that are available for its members to interact with and use for their work. These tools both make possible and limit what can be done, and they also help FNs to formulate viewpoints and define reality. Sociocultural factors such as nationality, race, ethnic background, religious beliefs, beliefs about health and illness, sexuality, mental and physical disability status, and traditions also impact the thoughts, affect, and behavior of the FN as well as his or her clients. The obligation of the FN is to sort out which behaviors or thought processes stem from these factors rather than from objectivity.

Sociocultural theory states that human cognition and learning are social and cultural phenomena. They are applicable to forensic nursing because language and cultural issues with clients/patients can present barriers to receiving health care and can lead to disparities and inequities in health outcomes and quality of care. This theory provides a concise and systematic framework for providing care based on four principles in sociocultural competence known as A-B-C-D: *A* is for accommodating specific population needs, *B* for building a foundation, *C* for collaborating with internal and external resources, and *D* for diversifying resources, data collection, and data analysis (Constantino & Privitera, 2011).

A is for accommodating specific population needs. To deliver safe quality care and reduce health disparities, services and activities should be designed to meet the needs of diverse populations. FNs should work to accomplish this goal by increasing their own awareness of cultural issues and incorporating culturally competent care into training and educational programs that they deliver. Additionally, they can take training courses in cultural competence or use self-study materials and seek out additional opportunities to increase their knowledge about commonly encountered cultures. FNs could also enhance their communication skills by learning how to work with an interpreter and by learning a second language. This may involve designing the waiting room to ensure accessibility, using bilingual signage, and having neutral decor. Patients need help navigating the health-care system and should be provided with educational and training materials that are appropriate to their language, culture, and literacy competencies. The spiritual and religious needs of patients should also be considered. FNs can use these guidelines to help ensure that the needs of specific patient populations are met. Accommodation is the basic internal and personal precept to follow if FNs desire true and lasting sociocultural competence (Constantino & Privitera).

B is for building a foundation. Developing mission and vision statements and creating policies and procedures that make meeting the needs of diverse patient populations a priority are integral components of a socioculturally competent health-care system. Organizations should also become familiar with community demographics to determine appropriate service provision as well as areas for improvement or growth. Wilson-Stronks (2008) and others strongly suggest that the role of leadership is central to building a foundation. Strong leadership that guides the development of a supportive infrastructure for sociocultural competence is the cornerstone of the foundation, and it starts with the health system's mission, vision, and values. Every health system policy, procedure, and regulation must be mission-, vision-, and values-driven. The Joint Commission has specifically proposed requirements to advance effective sociocultural competence for the hospital accreditation program. Under these proposed requirements are elements of performance specifying that health-care systems provide patient education and training based on each patient's needs and abilities. Furthermore, the health-care system staff should assess each patient's understanding of the education and training provided. The Joint Commission suggests that understanding and other outcomes may be assessed and evaluated using mixed methods of assessment: quantitative (question and answer) or qualitative (teach back or return demonstration) methods. Building a foundation may sound like a tall order for FNs to follow; however, by collaborating with a multidisciplinary group, synergy is accomplished (Constantino & Privitera).

C is for collaborating with internal and external resources. Partnerships within and across health-care organizations provide an opportunity for FNs to share information and pool resources. Constantino and others believe that the outcome of collaboration is synergy, and synergy begets diversity. Community leaders can also be enlisted to assist in recruiting a diverse workforce, act as cultural brokers, and bridge cultural and/or religious barriers to accessing care. FNs can form or sit on cultural diversity committees within their organizations and become actively involved in their communities. Leadership is instrumental to the success of such collaborations, and FNs can play an important role in ensuring that productive internal and external partnerships are initiated and maintained (Constantino & Privitera).

D is for diversification of resources, data collection, and data analysis. Diverse human and technological resources are crucial in diversification. To monitor and evaluate the quality and effectiveness of linguistically and culturally appropriate services, data must be collected and analyzed at various levels. Such data may include **community-level** standard demographic information such as age, race, and gender, as well as more specific information on cultural and dietary needs, health literacy, sexual orientation, disability, and religious practices. Various populations that compose the service community can thereby be identified, and the health-care facility can respond to their specific health-care issues and needs. **Patient-level** data such as demographics and family membership can also help. FNs identify the frequency with which certain populations use specific services and tailor care accordingly. For example, data on how often Spanish language interpreters are used can provide a basis for assessing effectiveness, allocating resources, evaluating patient satisfaction and determining clinical outcomes for the population that uses the service. FNs can play an instrumental role in the collection of data and ensure that they are used to guide culturally appropriate services for diverse populations (Constantino & Privitera).

THE SOCIOCULTURAL NATURE OF MENTAL ILLNESS

Imagine a case study in which Mary is brought to the ED in a dazed and confused state and diagnosed as mentally incompetent because she "hears voices." At a preliminary hearing, the court orders that she be admitted to a psychiatric hospital for treatment and remain there until further evaluation of her mental health. Ironically, the FN/expert witness/nurse practitioner treated the patient for schizophrenia with symptoms of hearing voices 5 years ago and was aware of her long history of schizophrenia. Upon realizing their past nurse-patient therapeutic relationship, the expert witness immediately informed the defense attorney. The sociocultural factor that must be explored is the accused's mental illness and whether or not her mental illness interferes with her capacity to assist in her defense, make informed decisions and consent for a treatment plan.

Bias and discrimination based on sociocultural factors is an uncomfortable subject for many because the topic gives rise to difficult conversations and different responses. The subject matter challenges personal assumptions and conjures up the concepts of powerlessness, weakness, disparity, and lack of control. Sometimes a FN is tempted to be indifferent to his or her own biases or fails to acknowledge personal stereotypes (e.g., regarding mental illness or HIV/AIDS status). Consequently, such biases and stereotypes remain dormant, unexamined, and unresolved. They sometimes become manifested in the FN's nonverbal interactions and interfere with the ability to maximize his or her own growth, development, and capacity to lead.

The FN needs to keep a vision of fairness and equality and to eliminate disparities in the provision of legal and/or nursing services. This can be achieved by (1) collecting data to assess and improve service delivery to under-represented and diverse clients; (2) enhancing personal and staff knowledge, skills, and competence in understanding mental health and mental illness; (3) developing policies and standards of practice from which all groups can benefit equitably; and (4) performing qualitative and quantitative studies that support the analysis and integration of sociocultural equity and diversity.

Sociocultural equity is evident in forensic nursing practice when staff members and clients of diverse ethnicity, race, gender, sexual orientation, religious beliefs, age, and physical or mental disability status are integral members of the organization led by the FN. When principles of fairness, equality, and elimination of disparities are discussed and become a part of the mission, vision, and worldview, sociocultural competence is evident. The FN should replace outdated care plans with evidence-based strategies, identify areas in which disparities occur, and assist others' efforts in monitoring compliance with human rights laws and regulations.

Accountability and ELSI

Accountability is internalized responsibility. To be accountable, each FN agrees to be morally responsible for the consequences of his or her own actions. No one can claim accountability for another. Society holds each person accountable for his or her actions and the execution of assigned tasks and duties. Integrating sociocultural competence and personal, professional, and organizational accountability into ELSI should be an ongoing goal for all practitioners.

To achieve personal accountability and cultural competence, the FN must be consciously aware of the impact of his or her actions, words, and decisions. The FN needs to be equipped with the tools and skills of cultural competence that are gained by training and education. Furthermore, FNs must empower clients to be active partners in legal or health encounters and dialogue. These goals can be accomplished by participating in cross-cultural and quality improvement training. Such training should include programs that focus on developing process and outcome measures that reflect the needs of multicultural and diverse clients as well as "train the trainer" programs for educating clients on navigating the legal system effectively and efficiently.

To achieve professional accountability and cultural competence, it is essential for the FN to conduct community/client assessments, develop client input and feedback mechanisms, implement quality measures for diverse populations, and ensure the availability of culturally and linguistically appropriate legal materials and brochures. Developing legal information for clients that is written at an appropriate literacy level and that is targeted to the language and cultural norms of specific client populations facilitates professional accountability and cultural competence. Furthermore, the FN needs to maximize diversity in his or her own organization. This can be accomplished by establishing programs for leadership development and strengthening existing programs, hiring and promoting diverse employees, and involving community representatives in practice planning and quality improvement meetings.

Accountability is crucial to the growth and progress of individuals, professions, and organizations. The FN has fiduciary responsibility for the resources of the practice. Stakeholders, clients, and the government all hold the right to an accurate and transparent accounting and review of the practice assets. Accountability means recognizing one's own limitations and resources and promoting policies that ensure continued availability and equitable distribution of resources. Accountability related to the forensic nursing role can be categorized as personal, professional, and organizational.

As seen in Table 3.3, each form of accountability has six realms of responsibility. Each realm has its own source, and problems can arise when the FN confuses the source of each responsibility. For example, a conflict may arise when FNs in an organization act as if their position and power base come from family or their position in the community and not from a legitimate position of authority.

Some of the most difficult tasks of FNs are envisioning goals, affirming values, and motivating self and others. In envisioning goals, the FN needs to point others to the mission of the practice and resolve tension between long-term and short-term goals among self and staff. Affirming

values means regenerating and revitalizing the beliefs, values, purposes, and wishes shared by staff. In this process, conflicting values held by some who may have digressed from the vision of the practice must be identified and discussed, without being judgmental. Motivating includes unlocking or challenging existing motives, having and promoting positive attitudes, being creative and innovative, and encouraging others to become passionate about the future and to be stakeholders in that future.

CONCLUSIONS

Forensic nursing practice is not a team sport; rather, it resembles cross-country running. FNs can glide along with the pack and blend with either the nursing or the paralegal group as they pursue ELSI and strive for excellence in their work. FNs are in an excellent position to translate principles of nonmalfeasance, beneficence, autonomy, justice, veracity, diversity, and accountability into practice to expand their worldviews.

Forensic professionals must be cognizant of the cultural beliefs that influence individuals affected by sex crimes and their families. Definitions of sexual violence may be equivocal in various countries. The importance of multiple intersecting factors impact the management of sex crimes in different cultural groups. Within one's own culture and country of origin, vast variations, attitudes, and opinions

TABLE 3.3   Realm of Responsibility Related to Issues of Personal, Professional, and Organizational Accountability

Realm of Responsibility	Personal Accountability	Professional Accountability	Organizational Accountability
Position	Allowed by family/community	Appointed by someone in the organization hierarchy	Selected by members of the same profession
Power base	Comes from age or consensus	Comes from knowledge, skills, credibility, and ability	Comes from legitimate position of authority
Goals/vision	Arise from personal interest and wishes of family and community	Arise from the mission/vision of the profession and may not be synonymous with that of the individual	Arise from mission/vision prescribed by the organization
Innovation	Taught, learned, discussed, suggested	Encouraged among all members	Allowed and tested
Focus	Family members, especially the elder, youth, infirm	Autonomy and competence of members	Systems, structure, and human resources
Action	Does things well	Does things right	Does the right thing

Adapted with data from Grossman, S. C. & Valiga, T. M. (2005). *The new leadership challenge*. Philadelphia: F.A Davis.

evolve. Differences exist within and among culturally defined populations as well. Among cultures, factors that may vary extremely include attitudes toward the human body, sex and gender, level of understanding and acceptance of the sexual activities and practices of other cultures, individual survival, and victims of crime as well as criminals.

FNs should convey respect for the values, beliefs, and customs of a culturally diverse people. It is necessary to recognize cultural distinctions of the diverse groups and at the same time focus on similarities to reduce stereotyping.

Every individual and each distinct culture is enriched by features and practices that are unique and valued positively. Cultural awareness, along with incorporation of the A-B-C-D of sociocultural issues into research and development, leadership and management, results in cultural competence. Expanded awareness for professionals in practice may offer ample opportunity to institute individual and organizational change. An increase in cultural competence can promote more effective management of ELSI in forensic nursing practice.

Some of the most difficult tasks of the FN include envisioning goals, affirming values, and motivating self and others. In envisioning goals, the FN should uphold and direct others to support the mission of the practice. Affirming values means regenerating and revitalizing the beliefs, values, purposes, and wishes shared by staff. Motivating includes unlocking or challenging existing motives, having and promoting positive attitudes, being creative and innovative, and encouraging others to become passionate about the future and to be stakeholders in that future.

Suzanne Gordon was asked what nurses really do. Part of her answer reflects our belief about the role of the FN as well: "What they do is a form of rescue," she said. When FNs develop a relationship with clients or their families, they are rescuing them from social isolation, terror, or stigma. Translating ethical, sociocultural, and accountability issues and the principles derived from these issues into forensic nursing practice does not add to the workload but rather lightens it. They are not time-consuming; instead, they are time-savers because they enable the FN to make optimal use of available time and resources. By viewing these principles as a bundle of privileges, the FN is free to reach into the bundle and pick one or several principles at a time to rekindle his or her vision and passion for the work at hand.

FNs are faced with an array of possible "futures." FNs are shapers of futures and occupy a special place in society as the first responders to health as well as ethical, legal, and sociocultural events that baffle communities, law enforcement, and the judiciary. Shaping more hopeful futures requires FNs to go beyond translating ethical, legal, and sociocultural issues into practice. It requires tough choices and the energy to play an active role in hedging against the inevitable technological, legal, and social changes that may undermine opportunities for progress. FNs are among the first providers of services to the lost, abused, accused, terrorized, and, often, the underserved. They must become champions of ethical, legal, sociocultural, and accountability issues as a means to enhance personal, organizational, and professional growth and development.

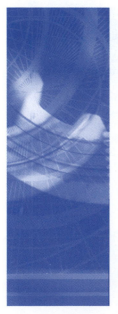

EVIDENCE-BASED PRACTICE

Reference Question: Does an awareness of culture and ethics help the FN provide high-quality care?

Database(s) to Search: CINAHL, PubMed

Search Strategy: "Forensic nursing" is both a MeSH term and CINAHL term. Because this question asks if FNs make a difference in quality of care, the type of research used to discover the answer is the comparative study research method. Thus, using "comparative study" as a MeSH and CINAHL term helps find the appropriate articles.

Selected References From Search:

1. Jacob, J.D., Holmes, D., & Buus, N. (2008). Humanism in forensic psychiatry: The use of the tidal nursing model. *Nursing Inquiry, 15* (3):224-230.
2. Lech, R. (2008). Getting inside their skin—Improving SANE's cultural competence. *On the Edge, 14* (3):6.
3. Williams, D. (2009). Forensic nursing and utilitarianism: The quest for being right. *Journal of Forensic Nursing, 5* (1):49-50.

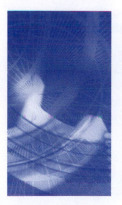

EVIDENCE-BASED PRACTICE (continued)

Questions Used to Discern Evidence:

Choose two studies among the studies listed, read about them, and answer the following questions:

1. What are the differences between the two studies in the design, methods, and results?
2. What are the similarities between the two studies in the number of subjects, measures used, and interventions, if any?
3. What skill do you think you need to learn to create a culturally competent practice environment?

REVIEW QUESTIONS

1. The duty of the FN is to protect the client from harm, which is enunciated by the ethical principle of non-malfeasance. The duty to provide service for the good of the client is enunciated in the ethical principle of:
   A. Beneficence
   B. Malfeasance
   C. Consequentialism
   D. Nonconsequentialism

2. The ethical principle that confers respect and self-determination on all human beings, including individuals with diminished capacity by reason of age or illness due to mental, psychological, or physical disorder; unconscious or semiconscious state; or under the influence of a mind-altering substance is:
   A. Veracity
   B. Justice
   C. Autonomy
   D. Fidelity

3. The ethical principle that demands that the FN is fair in all of his or her interactions and communications, making certain that policies and procedures are consistently and equitably applied without selective dispensation, is:
   A. Fidelity
   B. Justice
   C. Veracity
   D. Autonomy

4. Laws are derived from four major sources on the national level in the United States and in several states and territories: common law, administrative law, legislative law, and:
   A. Treaties
   B. Policies
   C. Regulations
   D. Constitutional law

5. For the accused to be found guilty in criminal litigation, the prosecution must prove:
   A. Guilt beyond a reasonable doubt
   B. Guilt beyond all doubts
   C. Clear and convincing guilt
   D. Guilt based on preponderance of the evidence

6. An unintentional wrongdoing such as the failure to meet a standard of care, as performed by any *reasonably* prudent health-care provider possessing similar knowledge and skills under comparable circumstances, is:
   A. Battery
   B. Assault
   C. Negligence
   D. Kidnapping

(review questions continued on page 62)

REVIEW QUESTIONS—cont'd

7. In this chapter, crimes are classified in several ways. The crime that comprises uncommon terms such as compounding, misprision, obstruction, perverting the course of adjudication, and perjury is:
   A. Crimes against persons
   B. Crimes against property
   C. Crimes against justice
   D. Participatory crimes

8. There are several purposes or objectives for punishing crime. The purpose that exacts equal payback, as in the words "an eye for an eye, a tooth for a tooth, an arm for an arm, a life for a life," is:
   A. Incapacitation
   B. Retribution
   C. Restitution
   D. Deterrence

9. The sociocultural theory presented in this chapter provides a concise and systematic framework for providing care based on four principles known as A-B-C-D. *A* is for accommodating specific population needs, *B* for building a foundation, *C* for collaborating with internal and external resources, and *D* for:
   A. Duty to others
   B. Dedication to moral values
   C. Diversifying data collection and analysis
   D. Due diligence

10. Internalized responsibility is:
   A. Diversity
   B. Compatibility
   C. Diligence
   D. Accountability

References

Aiken, T.D. (2004). *Legal, ethical, and political issues in nursing* (2nd ed.). Philadelphia: F.A. Davis.

American Nurses Association (ANA). (2001). *Code of ethics for nurses with interpretive statements*. Washington, DC: ANA.

American Nurses Association (ANA). (2007). *Corrections nursing: Scope and standards of practice*. Silver Spring, MD: Nursesbooks.org

American Nurses Association (ANA). (2003). *Nursing's social policy statement*. Washington, DC: ANA.

American Nurses Association & International Association for Forensic Nurses. (2009). *Scope and standards for forensic nursing practice*. Silver Spring, MD: Nursesbook.org.

Amnesty International Inc. (n.d.). *Excessive use of restraints on women in US prisons: Shackling of pregnant prisoners*. Retrieved May 15, 2010 from http://www.amnestyusa.or/violence against women.

APRN Consensus Workgroup & the National Council of State Boards of Nursing National Advisory Committee. (2008). *Consensus model for APRN regulation: Licensure, accreditation, credentialing and education*. Retrieved May 1, 2010, from http://www.nursingworld.org/consensusmodeltoolkit

Baldwin, D. (2003). Disparities in health and healthcare: Focusing efforts to eliminate unequal burdens. Washington, DC: ANA.

Betancourt, J.R., Green, A.R., & Carillo, J.E. (2002). *Cultural competence in healthcare: Emerging frameworks and practical approaches*. Washington, DC: The Commonwealth Fund.

Black's Law Dictionary (8th ed.). (2004). St. Paul: West Publishing.

Cady, R.F. (2009). Criminal prosecution for nursing errors. *JONA's Healthcare Law, Ethics, and Regulation, 11*(1): 10-6; quiz 17-8.

Ceci, C. (2004). Nursing, knowledge and power: A case analysis. *Social Science & Medicine, 59*(9):1879-1889.

Center to Champion Nursing in America. (2011). *Consumer access and barriers to primary care physician-nurse practitioner restrictive collaboration requirements by state*. Retrieved November 21, 2011, from http://championnursing.org/aprnmap

Constantino, R.E. (1996). *Legal issues in psychiatric mental health nursing* (2nd ed.). New York: Lippincott-Raven.

Constantino, R.E. (2007). Translation of ethical, sociocultural, and accountability issues in the nurse lawyer's practice. *Journal of Nursing Law, 11*(1):27-33.

Constantino, R.E., Boneysteele, G., Gesmond, S., et al. (1997). Restraining an aggressive suicidal paraplegic patient: A look at ethical and legal issues. *Dimensions of Critical Care Nursing, 16*(3):144-151.

Constantino, R.E., & Jackson, N.S. (2005). Psychiatric nursing: The crossroads of ELSI. *LNC Resource, 2*(2):21-2.

Constantino, R.E., & Privitera, M.R. (2011). Understanding the ethical, legal, and sociocultural issues in workplace violence. In M. R. Privitera (Ed.), *Workplace violence in mental and general health care settings*. Boston: Jones and Bartlett.

Daubert v. Merrill Dow Pharmaceuticals, Inc. 509 US 579, 113 S. Ct. 2786, 125 L. Ed. 2d 469.

Doyle, R. (2009). *Evidence-based nursing guide to legal and professional issues*. Philadelphia: Wolters Kluwer/Lippincott Williams & Wilkins.

Diamond, J.C., & Jacobs, E.A. (2010). Let's not contribute to disparities: The best methods for teaching clinicians how to overcome language barriers to health care. *Journal of General Internal Medicine, 25*(Suppl 2):S189-193.

Fairchild, R.M. (2010). Practical ethical theory for nurses responding to complexity in care. *Nursing Ethics, 17*(3): 353-362.

Farmer, L. (2000). Reconstructing the English codification debate: The criminal law commissioners, 1833-45. *Law and History Review, 18*(2).

Gabriele, E. (2005). Shifting the emphasis. In Protecting human subjects. Washington, DC: Office of Biological and Environmental Research.

*Garzetti v. Ceballo*s, 547 U. S. 410 (2006). Retrieved May 15, 2010, from http://www.supremecourt.gov/opinions/05pdf/04-473.pdf

Gordon, S. (2006). What do nurses really do? *Topics in Advanced Practice Nursing* eJournal, *6*(1).

Grace, P.G. & Willis, D.G. (2012). Nursing responsibilities and social justice: An analysis in support of disciplinary goals. *Nursing Outlook,* 60:198-207.

Greiner, A.C., & Knebel, E. (2003). *Health professions education: A bridge to quality*. Washington, DC: National Academies Press.

Grossman, S.C., & Valiga, T.M. (2005). *The new leadership challenge*. Philadelphia: F.A. Davis.

Keepnews, D.M. (2009). Welcome news in the Sentosa nurses case. *Policy, Politics & Nursing Practice, 10*(1):4-5.

Knight, M., & Plugge, E. (2005). Risk factors for adverse perinatal outcomes in imprisoned pregnant women: A systematic review. *BMC Public Health, 112*(11):1467-1474.

Lewin, S., Munabi-Babigumira, S., Glenton, C., Daniels, K., et al. (2010). Lay health workers in primary and community health care for maternal and child health and the management of infectious diseases. *Cochrane Database of Systematic Reviews* (Online), 3, CD004015. doi:10.1002/14651858.CD004015.pub3

Light, P.C. (2005). *Facing the futures: Building robust nonprofits in the Pittsburgh region*. Pittsburgh: Forbes Fund.

Lin, J.C., & Wang, T. (2008). Criminal liability research in vaccine administration by public health nurse: A case study of the Nantou vaccine administration case. *The Journal of Nursing Research: JNR, 16*(1):1-7.

Matt, S.B. (2012). Ethical and legal issues associated with bullying in the nursing profession. *Journal of Nursing Law, 15*(1): 9-13.

Marquis, B.H., & Hudson, C.J. (2009). *Leadership roles and management functions in nursing* (6th ed.). Philadelphia: Lippincott Williams & Wilkins.

Matter of Vinluan v. Doyle. 2009 NY Slip OP 219. [60 AD3d 237] New York State Supreme Court Appellate Division. (2nd Dept. Jan. 13, 2009).

Murray, J.S. (2010). There is no evidence that military nurses participated in torture and abuse of detainees. *Nursing Outlook, 58*(1):6-7.

Northrop, C.E., & Kelly, M.E. (1987) *Legal issues in nursing*. Washington, DC: Mosby.

Ormerod, D. (2005). *Smith Hogan: Criminal law*. London: Oxford University Press.

Pennington, K. (1993). The prince and the law, 1200-1600: Sovereignty and rights in the Western tradition. Los Angeles: University of California Press.

Privitera, M.R. (Ed.). (2011). *Workplace violence in mental and general healthcare settings,* Sadbury, MA: Jones and Bartlett Learning. www.iblearning.com

The Rebecca Project for Human Rights. (n.d). *Who we are*. Retrieved June 28, 2010, from http://www.rebeccaproject.org.

Saljo, R. (2000). Learning and practice: A sociocultural perspective. Stockholm: Prisma.

Scott, C.L., & Gerbasi, J.B. (2005). *Handbook of correctional mental health* (1st ed.). Washington, DC: American Psychiatric Publishing.

Shin, H.B., & Bruno, R. (October 2003). *Language use and English speaking ability: 2000* (Census 2000 brief). U.S. Census Bureau, U.S. Department of Commerce, Economics and Statistics Administration. Retrieved April 11, 2010, from www.census.gov.

Simon, R.I., & Gold, L.H. (2004). *Textbook of forensic psychiatry*. Washington, DC: American Psychiatric Publishing.

Smetzer, J., Baker, C., Byrne, F.D., & Cohen, M.R. (2010). Shaping systems for better behavioral choices: Lessons learned from a fatal medication error. *Joint Commission Journal on Quality and Patient Safety/Joint Commission Resources, 36*(4):152-163.

Smetzer, J.L. (1998). Lesson from Colorado. Beyond blaming individuals. *Nursing Management, 29*(6):49-51.

Veatch, R.M., & Fry, S.T. (2000). *Case studies in nursing ethics* (2nd ed.). Boston: Jones & Bartlett.

Wilson-Stronks, A., Lee, K.K., Cordero, C.L., et al. (2008) *One size does not fit all: Meeting the health care needs of diverse populations*. Oak Brook Terrace: The Joint Commission.

Yoder-Wise, P.S. (2010). More serendipity: The Winkler county trial. *Journal of Continuing Education in Nursing, 41*(4):147-148.

Zalon, M., Constantino, R., & Andrews, K.L. (2008). The right to pain treatment. *Dimensions in Critical Care Nursing, 27*(3):93-103.

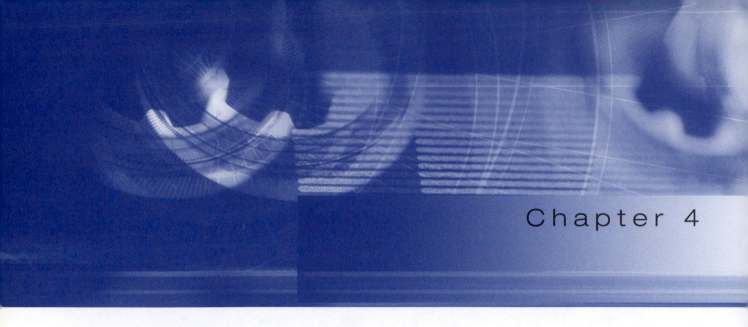

Chapter 4

The Anatomy and Physiology of a Lawsuit for the Forensic Nurse

Rose E. Constantino

"If I asked people what they wanted, they would have said faster horses."
Henry Ford

Competencies

1. Naming accurately the parties in a lawsuit.
2. Understanding the anatomy (structure) and physiology (function) of a lawsuit.
3. Identifying the purpose of pleadings and motions.
4. Comparing various forms of discoveries and disclosures.
5. Contrasting a fact witness from an expert witness.
6. Analyzing the four requirements of negligence.
7. Synthesizing the structure and function of a lawsuit.

Key Terms

Adverse witness
Complaint
Cross-examination
Defendant
Deposition
Discovery
Expert witness
Fact witness
Hearing
Hostile witness
Impeach
Interrogatories
Leading questions
Moral turpitude
Plaintiff
Trial
Trial by jury

INTRODUCTION

On the author's first day of law school, she was assigned to read *Anatomy of a Lawsuit*. She read all 152 pages that evening. The book was interesting but incomplete because the author did not compare and designate which body parts (anatomy) corresponded to the parts of the lawsuit. The book related a lawsuit between two women who had been in an auto accident, one of them the driver and the other the passenger. The author described the lawsuit as it moved from the pretrial procedures to the trial and through the appellate courts. The book left readers no choice but to relate human body parts to each aspect of the lawsuit and to compare the function of the body part with each step of the legal process.

The purpose of this chapter is to provide a simple anatomy of a lawsuit to serve as a guide for understanding the complex role forensic nurses (FNs) play in the legal arena.

Case Study

A QUESTION OF PROXIMATE CAUSE

This case illustrates the anatomy of a lawsuit between a plaintiff (Ann Roe), who brings a complaint against a defendant (Nurse Web), a Sexual Assault Nurse Examiner (SANE). The lawsuit is filed by Attorney Joseph Jones on behalf of Ann Roe against Nurse Web and the University General Hospital in a state court in Certain County/Parish in Any State. Nurse Web and the hospital are represented by Attorney Oliver Ott.

Ann Roe presents in the emergency room (ER) disheveled, crying, and complaining of unbearable pain while a man supports her as she clutches her abdomen. Ann introduces the man to the security guard and the triage nurse as her brother. Although hunched over, her pace is urgent, and within moments she reaches for the arm of the triage nurse. The triage nurse is taken by surprise and immediately notices blood on Ann's pants. When the triage nurse questions Ann, she becomes hysterical, causing disruption in the ER. The triage nurse immediately takes Ann away as her brother goes to the waiting area. Nurse Web leads Ann to a curtained bay and assists Ann to a treatment table. Ann confides to Nurse Web that she was raped by the man who brought her in, that the man in the waiting room is not her brother.

Nurse Web immediately moves Ann to a secure private room and quiet environment. Once Ann became calm, Nurse Web asked her if she was having any active bleeding. When Ann responds she is not bleeding, Nurse Web asks if Ann will consent to a physical examination, with the intent of collecting evidence. Ann hesitates momentarily and then verbally consents to the exam. Nurse Web again asks if there are any injuries she needs to know about immediately, and once again Ann denies any urgent physical injuries. Nurse Web, a SANE, explains the procedure for the physical examination and evidence collection. Nurse Web then explains that, as part of the procedure, she must call both the county police for an investigator to interview Ann and the rape center for an advocate for Ann's emotional support. Although upset and crying, once again Ann agrees.

Nurse Web, realizing she has to retrieve a camera from another department, tells Ann not to move from the table, go to the bathroom, wash herself, or rinse her mouth, as this will degrade or destroy any evidence Nurse Web will have to collect. Ann nods that she understands. Nurse Web leaves the room to get the camera and to get the assistance of another nurse to contact the police department and rape center for an advocate.

Nurse Web returns to Ann's room in 15 minutes. She notices the door to Ann's room is ajar, and Ann, still on the table, is splinting the left side of her abdomen and bleeding profusely. As Nurse Web approaches, Ann screams, "He just stabbed me!" The security guard, hearing the screams, enters the doorway to Ann's room while Nurse Web pushes the page for the physician STAT. The security guard asks Ann who stabbed her, and Ann replies, "That man with me is not my brother. He was the one who raped me in my apartment, and now he stabbed me." Nurse Web forgot that Ann confided in her earlier that the man in the waiting room was not Ann's brother because she was intent on proceeding with the collection of evidence.

The alleged perpetrator is noted to have left the ER moments after the triage nurse gave him access to the back of the ER to "check on his sister." Ann is taken to the operating room for emergency surgery as the knife pierced her spleen and caused massive hemorrhaging.

Discussion Questions

1. Is the hospital responsible for providing a safe environment?
2. Did Nurse Web breach a standard of care in any way?
3. Who is responsible for notifying or knowing who accompanied the patient?
4. Is the hospital still liable if the patient lied about the "brother"?
5. What should be documented by Nurse Web?
6. Should Nurse Web have left the patient unattended? What are the policies, procedures, or protocols?

The following discussion concerns only the issue of professional negligence.

The threshold question in this professional negligence lawsuit is whether Nurse Web breached the standard of care. Although the nurse did not know that the assailant, posing as her brother, came to the ER with the patient, Ann confided in her once they were in the examination room that the man in the waiting room was not her brother. The nurse forgot because she did not see the alleged rapist. The nurse was thinking only of the patient's best interest as she gathered the necessary supplies and equipment to conduct an examination and collect evidence. Although the nurse was informed, somehow she forgot to inform Security or another nurse about the presence of the man who raped Ann.

PROFESSIONAL NEGLIGENCE

Professional negligence as an unintentional tort occurs when the health-care professional fails to meet the standard of care. The professional fails to perform the duties as would another nurse with the same knowledge or experience under similar circumstances.

CIVIL LIABILITY AND THE FN

Civil liability in forensic nursing practice mainly falls in the area of tort law. Torts are classified as (1) intentional torts: assault, battery, false imprisonment, and intentional infliction of emotional distress; (2) quasi-intentional torts: defamation (slander is defamation by oral communication; libel is defamation by written communication), malicious prosecution, breach of confidentiality, and invasion of the right to privacy; and (3) unintentional torts, including professional negligence and special negligence doctrine: respondeat superior, independent contractor, captain of the ship and borrowed servant, and ostensible agency (Doyle, 2009; Northrop & Kelly, 1987).

Although the FN may be involved in intentional and/or quasi-intentional torts as a consultant, employer, employee, or independent contractor, the focus of this case is on unintentional tort in professional negligence. The FN may be found negligent if a standard of care is breached by omitting a procedure or committing error in computation, recording, charting, timing, counting, observing, providing care, assessing, reporting, testifying, and behaving unreasonably. For example, failing to provide a safe environment for a patient in the ER may be held by a judge or jury to be a negligent act.

PRELITIGATION PROCESSES/ PANELS

Ann, with the support of her family and through her attorney, Mr. Jones, files a lawsuit against Nurse Web and the University General Hospital 22 months after her discharge from a month-long hospital stay and only after fully recovering from her injuries. Before filing a complaint against Nurse Web on behalf of Ann, the attorney consults Nurse Smith to determine if Ann's case has merit. Nurse Smith determines whether Nurse Web's action (leaving patient Ann Roe unattended in the examination room and on the examination table) meets the four legal elements/requirements of negligence: duty, breach of duty, proximate cause, and damages.

Nurse Smith is qualified to review Ann's case because of her knowledge, skills, and practice as an emergency department (ED) nurse, as a certified SANE, and as a legal nurse consultant (LNC). She has practiced for 15 years and has cared for thousands of patients. She is also a legal nurse consultant specializing in professional negligence cases.

Most malpractice cases are tried in state courts, not federal courts. Prior to litigation of a case, in many states the plaintiff has to present the case to a prelitigation panel, medical tribunal, medical review panel, or arbitration panel to determine if the case has merits.

If a prelitigation panel is required, the plaintiff typically submits the evidence to a group of health-care providers, attorneys, and/or judges (depending on the state law) who prove how the injury was caused by the defendant and the extent of the injury and damages. Evidence can include medical records, affidavits, expert reports, treatises, authoritative texts, journal articles, photographs, medical illustrations, depositions, medical or legal memoranda, and position papers. A preliminary opinion is rendered whether the defendant is negligent and has breached a standard of care or questions of fact that must be decided by the jury at trial.

Filing a complaint is a serious undertaking. Lawsuits have multidirectional effects, are stressful, and may consume much time, effort, and financial resources from the attorneys, the individual parties, and the organizations and health-care systems named in the lawsuit. Therefore, some jurisdictions safeguard the rights of the parties with the certificate of merit rule.

To comply with this rule, Mr. Jones consulted Nurse Smith for the specific purpose of writing a report in support of the certification. Mr. Jones received a letter from Nurse Smith stating that the complaint has merits, and she attached a 50-page report of her findings. Nurse Smith used a chronological system that outlined the incident to support a complaint of negligence.

Nurse Smith reviewed Ann's medical and forensic records provided to Mr. Jones by the University General Hospital. Nurse Smith reviewed the records to be certain that the four requirements of negligence were met: duty, breach of duty, proximate cause, and damages. Nurse Smith wrote, "I have completed my review of the *Roe v Web* case and found the following breaches of the standard of care. It is my opinion that such breaches have caused and/or contributed to the plaintiff's injuries/damages. Attached is my complete and detailed report."

The report pages are numbered accurately, the records are clearly reviewed and placed in an appendix, and no additional records are requested. States and the Federal Tort Claims Act have specific statutes for filing medical malpractice claims. Timing is crucial. A delay in filing the complaint could cause the time limit defined by the statute of limitations to run out, depending on when the statute of limitations started to toll. In Pennsylvania, for example, the statute of limitations for negligence cases is 2 years. The statute of limitations starts to toll when the plaintiff knows or has reason to know that the injury is the direct cause of action was serious.

Mr. Jones and Nurse Smith agreed on an hourly rate of pay for the review and report and a slightly higher fee for time spent testifying at depositions and trial. The statute of limitations is not an issue in this case. The complaint was filed on the 23rd month after the injury occurred, when Ann realized that the injury she suffered was directly caused by Nurse Web's action of leaving her unattended in the examining room.

The Lawsuit

The central goal of civil lawsuits is the resolution of disputes. Lawsuits have complex procedures; thus, only a professional who is educated and skilled in the law can represent a person in a civil lawsuit; sometimes, however, people attempt to act as their own attorney (pro se). Also, an attorney may volunteer pro bono services for those who cannot pay hourly fees. Because of the contingency fee structure allowed in civil cases, in which an attorney receives a percentage of the amount awarded to the plaintiff, pro se is uncommon.

The Issue

The issue is whether Nurse Web was negligent in failing to provide safe nursing care and a safe environment when she left Ann unattended in the examination room, at which time the alleged perpetrator stabbed Ann with a knife. Did Nurse Web's actions satisfy all four elements of negligence: duty, breach of duty, proximate cause, and damages?

Understanding Negligence

The law does not expect nurses to be perfect; it only requires that they act reasonably under the circumstances and not deviate from the acceptable professional standard so as to injure a patient under their care. This means that, as an FN, Nurse Web is expected to follow the standards of care upheld by the nursing profession and the forensic nursing specialty.

Negligence is an unintentional wrongdoing caused by the failure to meet a standard of care that any reasonably prudent health-care provider who possesses similar knowledge and skills would provide under similar circumstances. Negligent behavior is an act that falls below a professional standard for protecting others from unreasonable risks of harm.

Duty was established when Nurse Web accepted the responsibility to provide nursing care and treatment of Ann. Even though Nurse Web did not choose Ann as a patient, duty was established when she accepted the assignment.

Breach of duty occurred with the act of omission or commission. Nurse Web breached her duty by failing to take appropriate action to provide Ann with safe nursing care once she was informed that the rapist may have been in the waiting room. The hospital may be held liable for failing to provide a safe environment under the theory of *respondeat superior,* which is to let the employer answer for the negligent acts of its employees.

In this instance, standards of care established by the American Nurses Association (ANA) and the Emergency Nurses Association (ENA) indicate that nurses must provide patients with competent nursing care, including safety and appropriate freedom from pain and harm. Furthermore, ENA indicates that patient safety, confidentiality, and privacy are priorities in the assessment and treatment of patients and families who present to the health-care setting with a history of interpersonal violence, as Ann Roe did in this case.

Proximate cause requires that Nurse Web's act (leaving Ann alone) was the legal and direct cause of Ann's injury or loss. Proximate cause is by far the most difficult element to prove in a lawsuit. In this case, however, Nurse Web failed to provide a safe environment for her patient by leaving Ann Roe alone and unattended in an examination room, even though Nurse Web had a suspicion that the "brother" might be involved as the proximate, legal, and direct cause of Ann's injuries. Nurse Web neglected Ann's need for a safe environment by leaving Ann alone for an unreasonably long time (15 minutes) when she left to retrieve the camera for the collection of evidence. The length of time Ann was alone allowed time for the person posing as her brother to stab her.

The prudent and reasonable action for Nurse Web would have been to ask another person to retrieve the camera for her. The law does not assume that the assailant waited for Nurse Web to leave Ann alone in the room; however, in this case the timing was, by coincidence, perfect.

Damages can be compensatory, special, or punitive. Compensatory damages can be addressed by awarding money for expenses incurred by the plaintiff as a consequence of the negligent act of the defendant. Special damages compensate when exact monetary value cannot be placed, such as for pain and suffering. Punitive damages are imposed to punish the wrongdoer, set a representative example, and act as a deterrent for future wrongdoers. In this case, the plaintiff sought all three types of damages. In some states a plaintiff cannot receive punitive damages for medical malpractice claims. The plaintiff argued that all of Ann Roe's injuries, pain, and suffering were caused by Nurse Web's action (leaving Ann unattended). Table 4.1 presents the elements of liability, explanation, and example of professional negligence.

Pleadings

The first phase in proceeding with a lawsuit is to file a **complaint**. A lawsuit is also known as a civil action. A civil action in professional negligence begins with the plaintiff filing a complaint or petition for damages. Ann Roe filed a complaint with the state court of Certain County/Parish in the United States. The complaint states the plaintiff's version of the facts, the legal theory under which the case is brought (in this case, professional negligence), describes the allegations of the breaches of the standard of care against Nurse Web and the University General Hospital, and describes what Ann plans to seek to recover in the lawsuit in the form of damages. Along with the complaint, the plaintiff also files a notice with the court clerk that a lawsuit has been filed against the defendant.

The Parties

Most lawsuits involve a plaintiff and a defendant. The **plaintiff** is the party filing the lawsuit, the injured person. The **defendant** is the person or entity who is alleged to have directly caused the injury and is the party against whom the case is filed. The parties in a lawsuit (plaintiff and defendant) are the most important individuals because, as "reasonable persons," they bring their irreconcilable perceptions or their own version of

TABLE 4.1 Elements of Professional Negligence

Elements of Liability	Explanation	Example: Leaving the Patient Unattended
1. Duty	To provide a safe environment and prevent additional harm.	Nurse Web breached her duty by leaving the patient unattended even though she suspected that Ann might have been in danger.
2. Breach of Duty	Failure to meet the standard of care as a reasonable prudent nurse would have done under similar circumstances or because of an act of omission.	Nurse Web and the hospital failed to provide a safe environment.
3. Proximate Cause	The direct and legal connection between a professional person's action or inaction (breach of care) to the patient's injuries.	Leaving Ann Roe unattended for 15 minutes provided ample time for the assailant to enter the examination room and stab Ann with a knife.
4. Damages	Actual injury including pain and suffering to the patient resulting from the professional's action or inaction (other types of damages can include loss of love and affection; emotional distress; mental anguish; loss of consortium; loss of nurturance; decreased life expectancy; loss of a chance of survival; decreased enjoyment in life; past, present, and future medical expenses; and lost wages).	Ann Roe suffered a stab wound that punctured vital organs and necessitated surgery, medications, and rehabilitation; long-lasting pain and suffering; emotional distress; mental anguish; past, present, and future medical expenses; and lost wages.

Data adapted from: Marquis, B. L. & Huston, C.J. (2012). Leadership and management tools for the new nurse, p. 75. Philadelphia: Lippincott, Williams, and Wilkins.

a set of facts of the dispute to court, a public forum. In short, they are going to tell their own version of the story. They bring others to add facts and experts as witnesses to bolster their story as the version the jury or the judge should hold as true. Whether there was a duty and that duty was breached, the proximate cause of the injury and the amount of damages of the injury will be argued.

The function of a civil lawsuit is to resolve disputes, stabilize the relationship of the parties, place the injured party back at the position where she or he was before the incident, and teach the defendant and other health-care providers a lesson: to be careful and vigilant in following the scope and standard of practice set by the nursing profession. Plaintiffs must always be aware of the heavy burden they bear by initiating a lawsuit. The four requirements of negligence must be met; meeting only one, two, or three of the four requirements will cause the lawsuit to fail. Also, the plaintiff needs to overcome being viewed as an opportunist marked by greed. Furthermore, the community and the media may have notions of the plaintiff as persona non grata or may overreact with negative reports of the case, bringing unwelcome notoriety that is beyond anyone's control. Recalling the metaphor of anatomy, the plaintiff is the lower right extremity.

The defendant, likewise, can be viewed as the left lower extremity and must respond to the complaint filed by the plaintiff. If the defendant does not answer the complaint, serious consequences will follow in a form of a sanction, fine, or loss of the lawsuit by default. Furthermore, throughout the duration of the lawsuit, the plaintiff's and the defendant's families are involved as well. The families bear the burden and stress of supporting their loved one who is involved in the complaint, sustaining the belief that he or she will prevail in the end. They may harbor lingering doubts and fears regarding the competence of the attorney who represents the family member. They may not have confidence in a fact or expert witness who was recruited to clarify and amplify the case for the judge and jury. Witnesses are required to tell the story of the party they represent, tell the truth, and balance their enthusiasm with accuracy. After the complaint is filed and the defendant is served, the defendant must respond to the allegations. The plaintiff then files a reply to the defendant's answer. This completes the pleadings phase of a lawsuit.

Hearing Motions

At the completion of the pleadings phase, if the defendant is convinced there are no disputed facts and that the plaintiff failed to state a claim that entitles plaintiff to recovery in damages, the defendant in a **hearing** could file a motion to dismiss for failure to state a claim. A hearing is held in court in front of a judge, with only the attorneys and respective parties of the lawsuit. The judge may deny or grant the defendant's motion to *dismiss*. If the defendant's motion to dismiss is denied, the next step is to proceed with discovery. The motion to dismiss can be granted by the judge in two ways: *dismiss with prejudice* or *dismiss without prejudice*. In the former, the case has ended, and the only process left for the plaintiff is to appeal the case to a higher court. In the latter, the plaintiff may amend or restate the claim in the complaint, and the parties start all over again with the pretrial phase of the complaint, answer, and reply.

In *Roe v Web,* there is a central fact that cannot be denied. That central fact is that the plaintiff's physical injury was not inflicted by Nurse Web. Nurse Web was not present when someone entered the room and stabbed Ann Roe. Nurse Web's action or absence was not the direct cause of Ann's injury. Ann claims to be stabbed by someone who accompanied her to the ER, misrepresenting himself and claiming to be her brother. The truth of that claim and the guilt of the assailant will be determined in a criminal trial at another time. The focus of this argument is the action of Nurse Web, who is being sued by Ann Roe for professional negligence.

Discovery

The discovery phase was handled by the attorneys Jones and Ott. In the anatomy metaphor, they are the upper extremities. The attorneys manage the discovery phase with precision, professionalism, and transparency. Their duty is to produce all available witnesses and to extract all testimony or evidence to support their argument and to discredit or even destroy that of their opponent. Litigants pursue discovery in three ways: deposition, interrogatories, and request for production of documents.

The function of **discovery** is to allow the parties to prepare for trial. Discovery offers the parties the opportunity to learn more about the other's case. This discovery period includes learning about the witnesses called to testify: witnesses' personal and professional background; fact and expert witnesses called by each party; and what documents, testimony, and evidence each witness will bring, or disclose. Most important, the parties will be searching for an opportunity to discredit the opposing witnesses or bolster their own witnesses by using fact or expert witnesses.

A **fact witness** is one who testifies about his or her individual knowledge regarding the case. The fact or lay witness must testify as to first-hand observations or knowledge about the case. For example, in this case, the ED staff who allowed the "brother" access to the area of the ER to "check on his sister" may testify as fact witnesses as to what was heard and seen during the encounters with Ann Roe and her visitor. An **expert witness** is one who, by reason of education or specialized training or experience, possesses a particular knowledge of the subject in question and forms an opinion to assist the jury in understanding the subject in dispute. For example, Nurse Smith could testify as an expert witness for the plaintiff.

Fact or expert witnesses and all the evidence they bring, oral or written, are the vital organs in the abdominal cavity. They are the vital parts and function of a lawsuit. In this case, a three-pronged discovery (deposition, interrogatories, and production of documents) was used as a tool by Mr. Jones (for the plaintiff) and Mr. Ott (for the defendant). Without the vital parts in discovery, the attorneys would be left without bases and evidence to support their arguments. Without the vital organs, there is no lawsuit.

There are several ways discovery is accomplished. For this scenario, the focus is on interrogatories, depositions, and production of documents. Each party may start the discovery phase with interrogatories. Either the defendant's or the plaintiff's attorney may start the discovery phase by serving written interrogatories, notice of the time and place where the deposition will take place, and request the production of documents.

Interrogatories are written statements or questions served by one party upon any other party during a discovery. Interrogatories should not exceed 25 statements or questions, including all discrete subparts to be answered by the party being served. Attorneys may at times get carried away and neglect to keep an accurate count of the discrete subparts in their interrogatories. The use of countless interrogatories may be due to a party's lack of understanding and organization of the process or as retaliation against the party who first served a longer set of interrogatories. Each item on the interrogatory must be accepted or denied by the party being served. Every denial is explained and the rationale for the denial provided as the volley of interrogatory items goes back and forth.

A **deposition** is an oral testimony taken from any person who is a party to a lawsuit, and it is conducted before a court officer or the attorney for the party designated to take the deposition. The party seeking to take the deposition should give notice in writing to every other party to the lawsuit, including the name, address, and telephone number of all individuals to be deposed and the time, place, and the method by which the testimony will be recorded. The witnesses present their talent and skills for screening by the attorneys. Attorneys take meticulous notes during the deposition regarding whether a deponent's participation will strengthen or weaken the case. Another more important function of depositions is to preserve and memorialize the fresh memory and recollection of witnesses of the events for presentation at trial when memories may be more clouded by the passage of time and occurrence of subsequent events.

Request for **production of documents** may be served upon any party. The request for production is to permit the party making the request to inspect and copy documents, including writings, drawings, graphs, charts, photographs, phone records, and other recordings from which information can be obtained. Items may be inspected and copied. Items that may be tested or sampled include any tangible thing that relates to the possession, custody, or control of the party upon whom the request is served. Many items included in a patient's records, such as special laboratory results, radiography films, MRI discs, and other imaging results, generally may not be produced without being specifically requested or if not provided by request, with a subpoena.

Once the discovery phase is complete, the trial follows. After the discovery phase, the plaintiff, Ann Roe, and her attorney, Mr. Jones, felt confident regarding the strength of their case. They felt that the testimony of the defendant's fact witnesses was weak, and the expert witnesses were equivocal in their responses to the questions posed to them by Mr. Jones. Ms. Roe was convinced that she would prevail at trial. To this effect, Mr. Jones asked the judge to decide in her favor even before and without a trial by jury. Ms. Roe through Mr. Jones filed a motion for summary judgment. If the judge were to grant the motion, judgment would be entered, and the case would be ended. However, the plaintiff's motion for summary judgment was denied, and the case proceeded to trial. In some jurisdictions, when the plaintiff seeks money damages less than $50,000, the case will by law proceed to mandatory arbitration. Ann Roe sought more than $100,000 in damages; therefore, the case proceeded to a trial by jury.

Analysis of the Anatomy and Physiology of a Lawsuit

The elements of a lawsuit may be easily understood by matching them to parts of the human body (Fig. 4.1). The plaintiff and the defendant of the lawsuit are the lower extremities because they take the first steps to commence the lawsuit. The plaintiff starts the lawsuit by walking into a lawyers' office and accepting the lawyer's promise or explanation of the contingency fee arrangement.

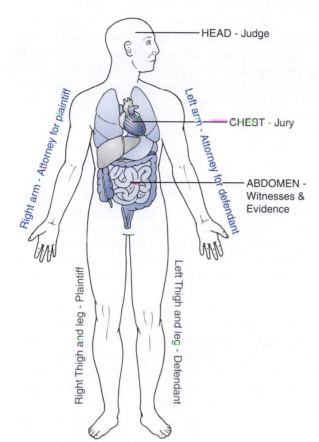

HEAD - Judge

Right arm - Attorney for plaintiff

Left arm - Attorney for defendant

CHEST - Jury

ABDOMEN -
Witnesses &
Evidence

Right Thigh and leg - Plaintiff

Left Thigh and leg - Defendant

■ **FIGURE 4.1** Schematic representing the anatomy and physiology of a lawsuit.

THE TRIAL

A **trial** is the examination of evidence, presentation of arguments and applicable law, and their synthesis into a coherent whole by a competent advocate in front of a competent court to determine the issue of specified claims. Trials are expensive. They wear down witnesses and juries physically and emotionally. Witnesses may die or relocate to faraway places; worse, they may forget the facts or recant their knowledge of the case. The discovery phase allows depositions and witnesses' testimony to be preserved and the fresh memory and recollection of the events to be recorded. Therefore, during the trial phase, it behooves witnesses to refresh their memory by reviewing their deposition statements so that the opposing attorney will not find any discrepancy and thus not have the opportunity during cross-examination to ask such questions as "When were you telling the truth Nurse Web, at your deposition or at trial?"

A **trial by jury** is a right preserved to the parties as declared by the Seventh Amendment of the Constitution.

Any party may demand a trial by jury in writing and by serving the demand on the other parties. The failure to demand a trial by jury constitutes a waiver by the party. In *Roe v Web*, the demand for a trial by jury was made in writing by plaintiff Ann Roe in her complaint through her attorney Mr. Jones.

The Jury

In the anatomy analogy, the members of the jury are the vital organs of the chest. The jury is the "heart" of the trial. The jury is the trier of fact. The jury absorbs all information presented in court. Jury members must balance all they have learned on an individual subjective scale and determine which side has the preponderance of evidence. In criminal trials there is a burden of proof that requires that the jury be convinced beyond a reasonable doubt. In administrative cases, clear and convincing evidence must be presented. In negligence cases, such as the Ann Roe case, the jury must be persuaded that a preponderance of the evidence is in favor of the party who bears the burden of proof, Ann Roe. Despite a belligerent fact witness, disorganized attorney, or elaborate exaggerations by an expert witness, the jurors must make a decision. Jurors may be persuaded by skillful questioning or cross-examination by an attorney who acts with calm precision and clarity. Jurors may appear passive, bored, or disinterested, but an onlooker would be warned not to misinterpret their appearance. The jurors' feelings, trust, and understanding of court presentations are all being sifted together to help form their opinions. FNs and other experts specialize as jury consultants to observe, take notes, describe, and report to their employer information gained from observation, the nonverbal communication of jurors at trial, and the impact of potential relationships, behaviors, and attitudes toward the verdict.

Jury Selection

A trial by jury begins with jury selection. A pool of jurors (45 to 50) is summoned into a courtroom, each with a number. In a process known as *voir dire*, each attorney asks the potential jurors questions to determine if they have relationships with any of the parties, attorneys, and witnesses involved in the case. The attorneys need to elicit all potential jurors' feelings about a similar situation or discover if they have experienced a similar situation that would preclude their being chosen for this trial. Questions put forth by the attorneys are called "peremptory challenges." Once the questioning is complete, each attorney may request that specific jurors be stricken from the jury pool if they appear to disclose bias or prejudice.

Each attorney may then eliminate other potential jurors if it appears they would favor one side or the other. Once peremptory challenges are complete, the first 12 remaining jurors comprise the jury panel for the trial.

Opening Statements

Opening statements are presented to the jury by the attorneys for each party. In terms of anatomy, the attorneys are the upper extremities: the plaintiff's attorney is the right upper extremity, and the defendant's attorney is the left upper extremity. They are the lifters of the heavy load a lawsuit generates. The expectation of winning placed upon them by the respective parties is heavy.

Cases may be won or lost with an opening statement, which is often referred to as the crux of a case. Through the opening statement, each attorney gives the jury a map or a framework of the trial. They describe how the facts align with the testimony and evidence that they will present through fact or expert witnesses and documents.

After Mr. Jones completes his opening statements, the defense attorney, Mr. Ott, commences his opening statements. Mr. Ott could have chosen to defer his opening statements until the end of the plaintiff's case, but he chose to follow Mr. Jones' opening statements.

The first part of the opening statement by Mr. Jones may be as follows: "Ladies and gentlemen of the jury, we are gathered here today to right the wrong done by Nurse Web and the hospital to Ms. Ann Roe. Nurse Web was employed by the University General Hospital and assigned to take care of Ms. Roe, who was a patient in the hospital. Instead of receiving emergency care at the hospital, Ann was left alone unattended in an examination room of the UGH Emergency Department, where she was stabbed by her assailant who had also raped her earlier that morning."

Mr. Jones names Nurse Smith as one of the expert witnesses he will bring to support his theory that Nurse Web was negligent in leaving Ann Roe unattended. Nurse Smith has provided expert testimony regarding forensic nursing practice and emergency nursing practice in other trials. She has been qualified by judges in past trials because she meets the conditions of giving expert testimony. She has completed a post-master's certificate program in forensic nursing and legal nurse consulting in addition to her training and certification as a Sexual Assault Nurse Examiner and emergency room nurse. She is well prepared to testify regarding the scope and standards of emergency nursing practice and the policies and procedures for the ED.

Mr. Ott, in turn, provides his opening statement, which is short and precise: "The person who injured Ann Roe in the UGH ED was not Nurse Web. Ms. Roe was injured by an assailant who had previously hurt her, whom she introduced as her brother, and who accompanied her to the hospital. Ms. Roe did not inform Ms. Web that the person who raped her accompanied her to the hospital and was, in fact, in the waiting room posing as her brother. When Ms. Roe and Nurse Web were alone in the examining room, Ms. Roe revealed to Nurse Web that the person who accompanied her and waited for her in the emergency waiting room was her assailant. Witnesses who were on duty when Ann Roe was admitted to the ED, Mr. Burns, the ED security guard, and Nurse Dunn, who was the ED triage nurse, will testify as to hospital procedures and privacy and safety regulations that protect patients in the ED. They will inform us and show records and procedure manuals that attest to their actions being in accordance with the hospital policy." Mr. Ott briefly described the elements of negligence, and he implants into the judge and jury's minds the fact that the single, most-important element of negligence was not present in this case, which is proximate, legal, or direct cause.

As soon as the opening statements are completed, Mr. Jones presents his testimony and evidence for the plaintiff. By rule, the attorney representing the plaintiff presents the case first. Mr. Jones presents the plaintiff's case by calling his witnesses and offering exhibits to make sure that every witness, piece of evidence, and exhibit build to the weight of the preponderance of the evidence being in the plaintiff's favor. During the plaintiff's case, Mr. Ott has the opportunity to cross-examine every witness after they were questioned by Mr. Jones. Mr. Jones presents all of his witnesses, including expert witness Nurse Smith. The examination and cross-examination proceed until Mr. Jones rests his case.

Mr. Ott presents the case for the defendant Nurse Web and UGH by questioning his witnesses, who may then be cross-examined by Mr. Jones. His goal is also to instill in the jurors that he has presented the preponderance of the evidence. His witnesses are well prepared. Each of them testify as though the event happened recently and was fresh in his or her memory. Their testimony is reflected in the documentation of events from the medical and security guard notes from that day. The jury heard that Nurse Dunn and Mr. Burns offered refreshments to the man who posed as Ms. Roe's brother because he said he was a family member of Ann Roe. Ms. Roe was the only person who knew that he was her assailant. Ms. Roe exposed the emergency department staff, patients, and innocent visitors to a dangerous and violent person who roamed freely among them. This is the central theme of the defendant's argument: Nurse Web's action was not the *proximate cause* of Ms. Roe's injury. Proximate cause was the single element of negligence in this case that no reasonable person could say is met by the evidence presented on behalf of the plaintiff because Nurse Web did not injure Ms. Roe. This is a critical point that has to be impressed upon each juror.

The Examination and Cross-Examination

The drama begins as the witnesses are sworn one by one to "tell the truth and nothing but the whole truth. . . ." Direct examination is done by the lawyer for the plaintiff or the lawyer who called the witness first. Witnesses are asked questions to elicit both direct and circumstantial evidence. Witnesses may testify to matters of fact (fact witnesses) and, in most professional negligence cases, provide opinions (expert witnesses). They also may be called to identify documents, pictures, or other items introduced into evidence. Only expert witnesses state opinions or give conclusions. Witnesses qualified in a particular field as **expert witnesses** may give their opinion based on the facts in evidence and may give the reason for that opinion. Lawyers may not ask leading questions of their own witnesses. **Leading questions** are those that are framed in such a way as to suggest the answers desired, in effect prompting the witness. An example is "Isn't it true that you saw Ann Roe doing the belly dance at a party?" Objections may be made by the opposing counsel for many reasons under the rules of evidence, such as objecting to leading questions, questions that call for an opinion or conclusion by a witness, or questions that require an answer based on hearsay.

Cross-Examination

When the lawyer for the plaintiff has finished questioning a witness, the lawyer for the defendant may then cross-examine that witness. **Cross-examination** is generally limited to questioning only on matters that were raised during direct examination. Leading questions are allowed to be asked during cross-examination because the purpose of cross-examination is to test the credibility of statements made during direct examination. Another reason for allowing leading questions on cross-examination is that the witness is usually being questioned by the lawyer who did not originally call him or her, so it is likely that the witness will resist any suggestion that is not true. When a lawyer calls an **adverse** or **hostile witness** (a witness whose relationship to the lawyer's client is such that his or her testimony is likely to be prejudicial) on direct examination, the lawyer can ask leading questions as on cross-examination.

On cross-examination, the attorney might try to question the witness's ability to identify or recollect information or try to impeach the witness or the evidence. To **impeach** the witness means to question or reduce the credibility of the witness or evidence. This is done by trying to show prejudice or bias in the witness, such as his or her relationship or friendship with one of the parties or his or her interest in the outcome of the case. Witnesses may be asked if they have been convicted of a felony or a crime involving **moral turpitude** (dishonesty), since this is relevant to their credibility.

Opposing counsel may object to certain questions asked on cross-examination if the questions violate the state's laws on evidence or if they relate to matters not discussed during direct examination.

Impeached Expert Witness

The witnesses (fact or expert) play very important roles in a lawsuit. Mr. Jones presents Nurse Smith as his expert witness. Most of the work with an expert actually takes place prior to the trial. Nurse Smith is sworn in as a witness and promises to "tell the truth and nothing but the whole truth, so help me God." The first stage of Mr. Jones' questioning of Nurse Smith is to review her knowledge, skill, and training for the court to qualify her as an expert witness.

Nurse Smith provides insight into the standards of practice for Nurse Web in her role in the ED and how adherence to the standards of nursing practice and hospital policies and procedures in the ED were related to Ann Roe's injury. The expert must be aware of the theoretical and clinical explanations as well as alternative explanations for the injury and how events took place. The expert must be without bias and emotion in his or her presentation, letting the truth of the testimony speak for itself, and answer without defensive and argumentative statements.

Sometimes, when attorneys least expect it, expert witnesses commit errors. An expert witness may make a mistake before and during the trial. Nurse Smith as expert witness did not take the responsibility lightly. She realized the significance of her role as an expert witness and the implications for affecting the jurors' decisions. Her role was to make the trial come alive and transport the jury into the time and place of the event when human emotions and actions related to Ann Roe occurred. Witnesses can evoke emotions and awe from jurors. However, witnesses also make mistakes or commit an error in carrying out their duties. Reflect on the questions in Box 4.1 related to Nurse Smith's role.

After Nurse Smith is qualified as an expert by the judge, Mr. Jones starts the direct questioning of Nurse Smith. She is well prepared. Nurse Smith has testified as an expert witness in sexual assault and negligence cases many times and has a routine list of questions and practiced

Box 4.1 Discussion Questions

1. What courses or clinical experiences are relevant to the case?
2. What documents should she review to prepare for trial?
3. How should she respond to the allegations of perjury?
4. How should she respond to the question "Were you paid to testify on behalf of the plaintiff?"

answers that she prepared for attorneys with whom she worked. When Mr. Ott's cross-examination begins to review her precise certifications, he discovers that Nurse Smith has lied under oath. She claimed that she was certified by the state forensic nursing certification board as a sexual assault nurse and worked as a FN examiner at a hospital. Upon review of the records presented at cross-examination by Mr. Ott, it is noted that Nurse Smith's certification expired 4 years ago. Furthermore, Nurse Smith did not mention when asked by Mr. Ott upon cross-examination that she had testified 2 weeks ago in the same court in another case for the prosecution regarding child abuse injuries. The revelation in court under oath of Ms. Smith's expired certification is surprising information that had been overlooked by the plaintiff's attorney. The outcome of such a revelation during the trial is shocking to all present, including the judge who had qualified Ms. Smith as an expert. The effect of her failure to renew her certification and update her list of qualifications may have negative effects at multiple levels of the trial. (See Box 4.2.)

Nursing Error

Mr. Ott also found administrative records from another hospital regarding the fact that Nurse Smith had been dismissed 5 years ago from a University Health System's facility based on her refusal to follow a doctor's order. The cause for the termination was gross negligence by failure to follow

direction from a treating physician. The discharge memorandum that supported the termination stated that Nurse Smith interfered with the physician's ability to perform an intubation by refusing to obey the physician's order.

Nurse Smith had refused to carry out a physician's order, and according to the Code of Ethics for Nurses and general standards of competent nursing practice, a professional nurse serves as a vigilant advocate for the health, safety, and rights of a patient. Public policy addresses the disciplinary measures to be taken against a nurse who acts in accordance with the guidelines that are believed to be in good faith but may endanger a patient.

Nurse Smith countermanded the doctor's order to intubate a patient in the patient's room. Nurse Smith's rationale was that the staff and equipment on the floor were not adequate for intubation. She documented that the patient was awake but lethargic, breathing spontaneously, and had palpable pulses. There was no cardiac monitor on the floor, and if intubation were attempted in the patient's room, there was further risk of complications due to the patient's condition. Calling a code would compromise all patients in the unit during a shift change.

The doctor wanted to carry out the intubation in the patient's room immediately. Nurse Smith unplugged the electric bed and maneuvered it out of the room to the cardiac care unit (CCU). The patient was transported without any device for monitoring cardiac status or vital signs but was receiving oxygen from a portable tank. The patient was stable with a normal sinus cardiac rhythm and blood pressure of 128/86 upon arrival at the CCU. The doctor successfully secured the patient's airway with an endotracheal tube that was attached to a ventilator. (See Box 4.3.)

Box 4.2 Discussion Questions for Perjured Testimony

1. What is perjury?
2. Is forgetting the expiration date of certification perjury?
3. What is negligence?
4. What are the elements of negligence?
5. Was the issue an error?
6. What could several effects of the error be on the trial?
7. Should Nurse Smith have told Mr. Jones (plaintiff's lawyer) that 2 weeks earlier in the same court and in another case she testified for the prosecution?

Box 4.3 Discussion Questions Related to Nurse Smith's Qualification to Act as an Expert Witness in the *Roe v. Web* Case

1. How should it be determined if Nurse Smith lied in her presentation of herself and the certification? Does it matter? How might the case for the plaintiff be affected?
2. Would it be ethical for Ms. Smith to give the attorney the name of another expert witness equally qualified to take her place upon giving this new expert all her work product on the case?
3. Is it permissible for a registered nurse to disobey an order that is inaccurate or unsafe?
4. What standard of nursing practice, if any, did Nurse Smith violate in refusing to follow doctor's order?

Consider the arguments that could be made regarding this nurse's errors and the negative impact on her career. The nurse's expertise and her past actions that caused her to lose her previous job take up much time in court and detract from the defense of Nurse Web. The real issue before the court relates only to outcomes related to negligence and the damages to Ann Roe and the separate, but perhaps more important issue of the trial of the assailant accused of crimes against her. It may be unlikely that a jury will respect the opinions of Nurse Smith and view her testimony as trustworthy and believable.

The Judge

The judge is the head in the anatomy of a lawsuit. In trials by jury, the judge is the trier of the law. In trials without a jury, the judge is the trier of fact and of the law. The function of the judge is to rule on matters of fact (without the jury) and of law, including subject matter jurisdiction, personal jurisdiction, venue, statutes of limitation, motions, hearings, jury instructions, qualifying expert witnesses, and testimonies. There are three initial aspects of the court's decision to accept a lawsuit: subject matter jurisdiction, personal jurisdiction, and venue. In most jurisdictions, a case in negligence can be brought to the courts only in the county of the state. County courts in any state are the only courts with subject matter jurisdiction and personal jurisdiction competent to try a case in professional negligence.

The specific county court has personal jurisdiction over the parties in *Roe v Web* because the plaintiff and the defendant are residents of the county in which the court is located. Even if the plaintiff and/or the defendant reside in another county, the county court will still have subject matter jurisdiction of the parties because the hospital in which the events occurred is located in the same county in which the court is located. The venue is proper in the county court because both parties are residents and accept the venue as being proper. A defendant may file a motion for a change of venue if the present venue is deemed improper and incapable of conducting a fair trial. Change of venue seldom happens in negligence cases. Even if the plaintiff and/or defendant reside in another county, the venue would still be proper because the defendant hospital is located and is doing business where the court is located.

The judge as the head includes the skull, which protects the brain and all its complex and synergistic facets and functions. The brain is the origin of all cognitive, affective, and executive functions that come into play in the time frame leading up to the judge's ruling in a trial. The judge exemplifies the balance between the two parties and the jury's vision of fairness, decency, and respect for persons. The life of a lawsuit comes to an abrupt end without a judge, just as decapitation of a human body results in its demise.

CONCLUSIONS

The anatomy and physiology of a lawsuit through the case example of *Roe v. Web* provides a simple but comprehensive way of introducing the complex interactions of a lawsuit and the synergistic functions of the anatomical parts.

With their closing statements, each of the attorneys has an opportunity to summarize the evidence presented by their witnesses during the trial, to assert the value or implications of the tangible, trace, and transient evidence presented, and to restate key points made by the witnesses. The closing statements of the attorneys are the final attempt to clarify, shape, and influence the thinking of the jury.

In essence, the points made in the opening statements are maintained, and the attorney reviews key evidence used to support the opening statements. Attorneys also take this opportunity to pointedly note what their opposition did not do.

The nurse as an expert witness has an opportunity as a respected leader in health care to fill a critical need in a lawsuit. As the most highly respected professionals in national public polls, nurses are held to a high standard of ethics and honesty as caretakers of the ill and infirm. Plaintiffs and defendants involved in lawsuits, juries of their peers, and other persons involved in trials hold nursing professionals in high regard and assume that they will conduct themselves in a worthy manner, providing dependable and honest testimony.

When one part of the anatomy (here a witness, or a vital organ such as the liver) fails to function as expected (perjured testimony), other organs are markedly impacted. The ineffectiveness of a witness has an impact on the perceptions of the judge and jury related to the events in question. The outcome of a case depends on the evidence presented. Evidence that is trustworthy, relevant, and complete influences judges and juries and could factor heavily into their deliberations in weighing the preponderance of the evidence. The efficiency of a lawsuit is threatened or reduced by the errors made by the nurse. Diminished effectiveness of evidence or a witness may have a significant impact on outcomes. Therefore, it is incumbent upon each party and all players in a lawsuit to perform according to expectations and at maximum ability to support the entire (anatomy and physiology) lawsuit.

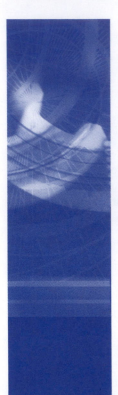

EVIDENCE-BASED PRACTICE

Reference Question: What are the best practices in reducing medication errors in hospital settings to reduce malpractice lawsuits?

Database(s) to Search: Cochrane Database, PubMed

Search Strategy: Any number of terms can be used for this search. Use, in the order of your choice, terms such as the following: hospitals, medication errors, guideline adherence, patient safety, lawsuits, reduce*(use appropriate wildcard for selected database), prevent*, and best practice.

Selected References From Search:

1. Cusano, F.L., Chambers, C.R., & Summach, D.L. (2009). A medication error prevention survey: Five years of results. *Journal of Oncology Pharmacy Practice,* *15*(2):87-93.
2. Momtahan, K., Burns, C.M, Jeon, J., Hyland, S., & Gabriele, S. (2008). Using human factors methods to evaluate the labelling of injectable drugs. *Healthcare Quarterly, 11*(3 Spec No.):122-128.
3. Reid-Searl, K., Moxham, L., Walker, S., & Happell, B. (2008). Shifting supervision: Implications for safe administration of medication by nursing students. *Journal of Clinical Nursing, 17*(20):2750-2757.

Questions Used to Discern Evidence:

Choose two studies among the studies listed, read about them, and answer the following questions:

1. What are the differences between the two studies in the design, methods, and results?
2. What are the similarities between the two studies in the number of subjects, measures used, and interventions, if any?

REVIEW QUESTIONS

1. In a civil case, the litigant who files the complaint to commence a lawsuit is the:
   A. Plaintiff
   B. Defendant
   C. Witness
   D. Consultant

2. In certain jurisdictions, the statute of limitations in a professional negligence case is:
   A. 5 years
   B. 4 years
   C. 2 years
   D. 6 months

3. In a professional negligence case, the burden of proof is:
   A. Clear and convincing
   B. Preponderance of the evidence
   C. Beyond all reasonable doubts
   D. Beyond a reasonable doubt

4. In a jury trial, the judge is the trier of the law and the jury is the trier of:
   A. Proof
   A. Fact
   B. Truth
   C. Evidence

REVIEW QUESTIONS—cont'd

5. To prevail as a plaintiff in a lawsuit under the theory of professional negligence, the plaintiff must meet four requirements or elements. Which requirement calls for the plaintiff to show evidence that the defendant's action did not meet the standard of care established by the profession?
   A. Duty
   B. Breach of duty
   C. Proximate cause
   D. Damages

6. When a lawsuit is "dismissed with prejudice," the case has ended and the only step the opponent of the motion must take is to:
   A. Appeal
   B. Move for a change of venue
   C. Move for jury deliberation
   D. Revise the complaint

7. When a lawsuit is "dismissed without prejudice," the case has ended and the next step the opponent of the motion must take is to:
   A. Appeal
   B. Move for a change of venue
   C. Move for jury deliberation
   D. Revise the complaint

8. In a jury trial, who declares or qualifies an expert witness to testify based on his/her expertise?
   A. Attorney for the plaintiff
   B. Judge
   C. Jury
   D. Attorney for the defendant

9. Bias is a common human characteristic and sometimes colors jury verdicts. In jury selection, this human characteristic is tempered by:
   A. Jury nullification
   B. Peremptory challenge
   C. Jury randomization
   D. Jury dismissal

10. The goal of all lawsuits is to:
    A. Resolve disputes
    B. Punish the wrongdoer
    C. Unite families
    D. Provide work for attorneys

References

Ackley, B., Swan, B.A., Ladwig, G.B., & Tucker, S.J. (2008). *Evidence-based nursing care guidelines* (1st ed.). New York: Mosby Elsevier.

Aiken, T. (2004). *Legal, ethical, and political issues in nursing.* Philadelphia: F.A. Davis.

American Bar Association (ABA). (2010). *How courts work.* Retrieved March 8, 2010, from www.abanet.org

American Nurses Association (ANA). (2001). *Code of ethics for nurses with interpretive statements.* Washington, DC: ANA.

American Nurses Association (ANA). (2003). *Nursing social policy statement.* Washington, DC: ANA.

Constantino, R.E. (1996). *Legal issues in psychiatric mental health nursing* (2nd ed.). Suzann Lego (Ed.). New York: Lippincott-Raven.

Constantino, R.E., & Zalon, M. (2008). Legal issues in emergency pain management. *Nursing Management.*

Doyle, R. (2009). *Evidence-based nursing guide to legal and professional issues.* Philadelphia: Lippincott Williams & Wilkins.

Emergency Nurses Association (ENA). (2008). *Code of ethics.* Washington, DC: ENA.

Emergency Nurses Association (ENA). (2008). *Position Statement: Intimate partner and family violence, maltreatment, and neglect.* Washington, DC: ENA.

George Mason American Inn of Court. (2000). Examination of expert witness. Retrieved March 11, 2010 from http://www.law.gmu.edu/org/assets/site/innofcourt/files/pubs/expert.pdf

Greene, E., Heilbrun, K., Fortune, W.H., & Nietzel, M. (2007). *Wrightsman's psychology and the legal system* (6th ed.). Belmont: Thomson Wadsworth.

International Association of Forensic Nurses (IAFN). (2009). http://iafn.org/displaycommon.cfm?an=1&subarticlenbr=137

Iyer, P. (2003). *Legal nurse consulting principles and practice.* New York: CRC Press.

Joel, L. (2001). Education for entry into nursing practice: Revisited for the 21st century. *Online Journal of Issues in Nursing Practice, 7*(2).

Marquis, M.L. & Huston, C. J. (2012). Leadership and management tools for the new nurse. Philadelphia: LWW.

Melnyk, B. & Fineout-Overholt, E. (2005). *Evidence-based practice in nursing and healthcare*. Philadelphia: Lippincott Williams & Wilkins.

Prosser, W. (1988). *Prosser and Keaton on torts* (5th ed.). St. Paul.

Rayne, T. (2008). Anatomy of a lawsuit-Part 2. Retrieved September 12, 2009 from http://EzineArticles.com/? Anatomy-of-a-Lawsuit—-Part-Two&id=1308083

Rowe, T.D., Sherry, S., & Tidmarsh, J.H. (2008). *Civil Procedure* (2nd ed.). New York: Thomson West.

Services HaH. 2008. 45 CFR 46.102. Retrieved July 6, 2008, from http://www.hhs.gov/ohrp/humansubjects/guidance/ 45cfr46.htm

Simon, P.N. (1984). *The anatomy of a lawsuit*. Charlottesville, VA: The Mitchie Company.

Stark, E., & Pagliaro, E.M. (2006). Expert witness testimony and a domestic violence paradigm. In R.M. Hammer, B. Moynihan, & E.M. Pagliaro (Eds.), *Forensic nursing: A Handbook for practice*. Sudburry, MA: Jones and Bartlett, pp. 667-688.

Taylor, R. (2006). *Civil procedure: Continuing legal education*. Pittsburgh: Duquesne University School of Law.

Waltz, J.R., & Park, R.C. (1999). *Evidence: Cases and materials*. New York: Foundation Press.

Warlick, D. (2008). Amicus curiae for The American Association of Nurse Attorneys. *TAANA Newsletter, 1*.

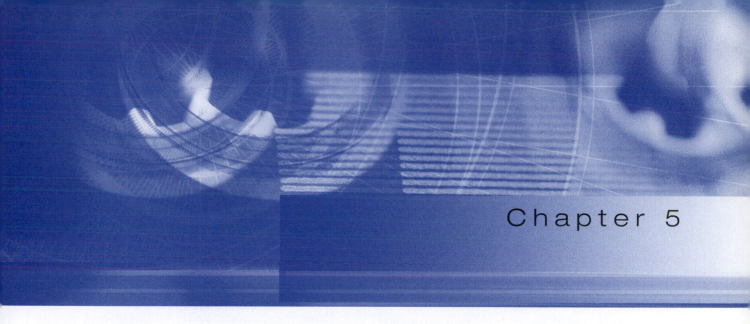

Chapter 5

INFORMATICS AND SIMULATIONS IN FORENSIC NURSING

Karen A. Monsen and Patricia R. Messmer

"Any sufficiently advanced technology is indistinguishable from magic."
Arthur C. Clarke

Competencies

1. Defining health information literacy and skills.
2. Assessing health informatics skills related to forensic nursing and the electronic health record.
3. Analyzing privacy and confidentiality of health information.
4. Synthesizing health information and data technical security.
5. Evaluating basic computer literacy skills in collaboration with others.

Key Terms

Electronic health record
Health-care quality
High-fidelity simulation
Interdisciplinary collaboration
Low-fidelity simulation
Nursing informatics

Introduction

There have been significant advances in forensic nursing science in the last few years, yet not enough of this knowledge has been put to work in daily clinical practice. There is a gap between what is known and what is done. One consequence of this gap is the wide variation in the quality of care from one clinician to another and from one area of the country to another. It is imperative that forensic nurse clinicians provide the best patient care and address legal and medical needs of victims while promoting a safety-first environment.

This chapter provides an overview of informatics and simulations in forensic nursing. To illustrate the major concepts, several examples from advanced women's health nursing practice are presented, with particular examples from Sexual Assault Nurse Examiner (SANE) practice.

Health information management and informatics core competencies have been developed by a joint task force of the American Medical Informatics Society and the American Health Information Management Association for individuals working with electronic health records. The core competencies are available online in the *EHR Core Competencies Matrix Tool* at www.amia.org, in five domains, or categories: (I) health information literacy and skills, (II) health informatics skills using the EHR, (III) privacy and confidentiality of health information, (IV) health information/data technical security, and (V) basic computer literacy skills.

There are no core competencies for simulation, but simulation competencies for specialties include oncology nursing, end of life care, emergency nursing, neonatal nursing, operating room nursing, and other disciplines such as respiratory care.

Informatics and Simulations in Nursing

Nursing Informatics

Nursing informatics is a specialty that integrates nursing science, computer science, and information science to manage and communicate data, information, and knowledge in nursing practice and outcomes. Outcomes are the end results of particular health-care practices and interventions.

An assumption underlying nursing informatics is that nurses working in collaboration with information resources can provide better care and make fewer mistakes than nurses who do not have access to such resources. Based on this premise, information technology has been widely adopted in a broad range of clinical practice settings. Computerized clinical information systems are now being employed to guide practice by providing timely decision support and by translating standards of care and best practices. When used for clinical documentation, these information systems gather, store, aggregate, and disseminate clinical data. Efforts are under way in forensic nursing to create usable information systems to enhance forensic nursing practice and improve outcomes of care. Informatics applications in forensic nursing provide new avenues for interdisciplinary collaboration across health care and the judicial system. The coordination of evidence in an electronic format is a best practice that improves services and outcomes for patients, advocates, health-care providers, and law enforcement.

Simulations in Nursing

Simulations have been noted to improve learning, retention, overall performance, and communication skills and to foster the development of consistently competent new graduates and experienced nurses. Participants who use simulations rather than reading a book feel they are better able to learn how to handle a live patient.

High-fidelity and **low-fidelity simulation** have their own feasibility and usability in clinical settings. High-fidelity simulators change and respond to the users and are:

- Immersive (provides realistic system-like training environment with visuals)
- Connected (able to conduct long-term training)
- Integrated (able to conduct debriefings among all participants).

Low-fidelity simulation is characterized by a simulator that remains static, such as a CPR task trainer or a pelvic model.

High-fidelity simulation has been found to be an effective teaching, learning, and evaluation tool in healthcare for nurses and for interdisciplinary health-care teams. Hoadley (2009) reported that health-care providers, including physicians, nurses, respiratory therapists, and advanced practice nurses, adamantly recommended using human patient simulation to complete the advanced cardiac life support (ACLS) course. LeFlore and Anderson (2008) demonstrated that expert-model learning using high-fidelity simulation for neonatal transport team members was as effective as self-paced modular learning. Messmer (2008) found that nurses and pediatric residents using human patient pediatric simulation could learn cohesiveness and collaboration while decreasing medical errors and improving patient outcomes. Participants in simulation consistently indicate they value the opportunity to make mistakes and learn from them in a safe educational environment. Overall, simulation enhances professional education while reducing safety risks for patients.

Electronic Health Records and Standards

The **electronic health record (EHR)** is a longitudinal electronic record of patient health information generated by one or more encounters in any care delivery setting. Included in this information are patient demographics, progress notes, problems, medications, vital signs, past medical history, immunizations, laboratory data, and radiology reports. The EHR automates and streamlines the clinician's work flow. The EHR has the capacity to generate a complete record of a clinical patient encounter as well as to support other care-related activities directly or indirectly via interface, including evidence-based decision support, quality management, and outcomes reporting.

Nursing's work within an electronic health record requires the use of standards to support data entry and data retrieval. Several standardized terminologies representing nursing practice have been developed, starting in the 1970s with the North American Nursing Diagnosis Association (NANDA) and the Omaha System. Currently, 12 terminologies are recognized by the American Nurses Association (ANA). Data generated through standardized nursing documentation are beginning to be used in program evaluation and research to demonstrate the effectiveness of nursing care.

Informatics and Simulations Tools for Forensic Nursing

Health-care quality is the extent to which health services increase the likelihood of desired health outcomes and that are consistent with current professional knowledge.

Health-care quality is achieved through **interdisciplinary collaboration.** Effective collaboration is exemplified by the ability of those in different disciplines, including nurses, physicians, respiratory therapists, pharmacists, and computer scientists, to work together to improve patient safety, reduce medical errors, and ensure provider competency.

Standards for simulation competencies are established along with consensus among several organizations to record and exchange data within and across information systems. The organizations with the most influence include the Society of Academic Emergency Medicine (SAEM), Society for Simulation in Healthcare, Advanced

Initiatives in Medical Simulation, Society in Europe for Simulation Applied to Medicine, and the National League for Nursing.

Nursing education and continuing education is changing at a phenomenal pace. Cannon-Deihel stresses that the state of the science of simulation in nursing and health care is influenced by driving forces, including consumers of education having higher expectations for curricula at the same time that health care is evolving with fewer resources and more complex roles. Advancing technology is creating a dependence on simulation as a teaching and learning strategy. Current, present, and future research will determine if simulation becomes assimilated into nursing and health-care education.

Informatics solutions specifically for forensic nursing are rapidly being developed and adopted. For example, a nonproprietary computer-based system for documenting sexual assault reports has been developed with direct input from forensic nursing experts. Use of the form generates data on forensic patients of all types and enables practitioners to securely house and send data from the bedside to the researcher, attorney, or law enforcement. These rich assessment data offer unparalleled opportunities to conduct research on evidence from forensic patients. Researchers using the system can access hundreds of independent multipage electronic forms and extract up to 1000 separate data fields and columns into an open-format comma-separated value (CSV) text file. Case-related de-identified high-quality digitized images are also secured and transmitted with the collected data through a secure file portal. The electronic forms are available for use by forensic nurses across diverse facilities and locations throughout the United States.

Standardized nursing terminologies are the interface between nursing's work and the electronic health record. As such, they are an essential informatics tool. One standardized terminology, the Omaha System, has been recognized by the ANA since 1992. It exists in the public domain, has passed the Healthcare Information Technology Standards Panel (HITSP) selection criteria in 2007, and is registered (recognized) by Health Level Seven (HL7). It is integrated into the National Library of Medicine's Metathesaurus; Logical Observation Identifiers, Names, and Codes (LOINC); and SNOMED CT. The Omaha System was originally adopted in community practice settings, and has been used more recently by case managers in hospital-based managed care, acute care, and long-term care.

The Omaha System provides standardized terms for client problems, practitioner interventions, and problem-specific client outcomes (Martin, 2005). Some Omaha

System problems that are particularly applicable in forensic nursing are Abuse, Pregnancy, Sexuality, Family planning, Interpersonal relationship, Mental health, and Communicable/infectious conditions. Nursing interventions consist of four actions (called "Categories") that address these problems:

- Teaching, guidance, and counseling
- Treatments and procedures
- Case management
- Surveillance

Additional standardized terms (called "Targets") are combined with the "Problem" and "Category" terms to add specificity to the intervention. Client outcomes consist of problem-specific five-point Likert-type ordinal scales for three concepts: Knowledge, Behavior, and Status (KBS).

Data regarding nursing interventions and client outcomes are an essential component of health-care quality research. In conjunction with forensic assessment data described above, standardized nursing terminologies are integral components of comparative effectiveness research and program evaluation studies.

Standardized Care Plans

The role of standardized care plans in support of evidence-based practice cannot be overestimated. Electronic health records deliver information in the form of data entry requirements to nurses as they document client assessments and nursing interventions. These data entry requirements implicitly communicate standards of care from the administration and management to the nurse. Such standards ensure that patients receive evidence-based care, and nursing documentation generates appropriate data to meet regulatory requirements and evaluate programs. Thus it is essential that standardized care plans are thoughtfully and purposefully incorporated into electronic health records and reviewed regularly to ensure that they remain current.

Data regarding nursing interventions and client outcomes are an essential component of health-care quality research. In conjunction with the forensic assessment data described above, standardized nursing terminologies are integral components of comparative effectiveness research and program evaluation studies. An example of using simulation would be to demonstrate the prone knee-chest position used by the patient during a sexual assault examination, as discussed by Kellogg (2010). This position is useful to confirm clefts. Small, obscure submucosal hemorrhages often are better found when the patient is in this position, as well. The SANE nurse can also examine the vaginal vault for foreign bodies (see Fig. 5.1). The finding of a foreign object (condom)

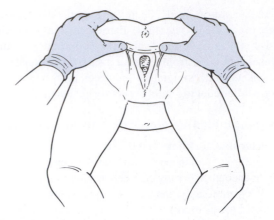

■ **Figure 5.1** The prone knee-chest position. (Reprinted with permission from the Christus Santa Rosa Children's Hospital Forensic Nurse Examiner Program and Nancy Kellogg, MD, Professor, Division Chief of Child Abuse, University of Texas Health Science Center, San Antonio, Texas.)

using the prone knee-chest position is illustrated in Figure 5.2.

Four standardized care plans developed for SANE practice are presented in Tables 5.1 through 5.4. Each care plan addresses a single Omaha System problem (Martin, 2005), as given at the top of the table. Columns in the table detail the intervention category, target, and additional care descriptions to guide practice. Physical assessment and evidence documentation are critical components of SANE practice; however, the forensic nurse must also provide

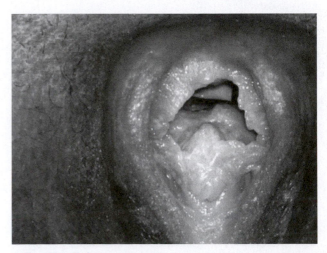

■ **Figure 5.2** A foreign body (condom) found by examining the patient who is in the prone knee-chest position. (Reprinted with permission from the Christus Santa Rose Children's Hospital Forensic Nurse Examiner program and Nancy Kellogg, MD, Professor, Division Chief of Child Abuse, University of Texas Health Science Center, San Antonio, Texas.)

TABLE 5.1   **Sexual Assault Nurse Examiner Care Plan for Abuse**

Category	Target	Care Description
Teaching, guidance, counseling	Legal system	Options (would include options around consent for examination and reporting)
Teaching, guidance, counseling	Legal system	Procedures to obtain services
Teaching, guidance, counseling	Legal system	Benefits (would include benefits of reporting vs. not reporting)
Teaching, guidance, counseling	Safety	Safety plan (such as safe place to go to or known abuser)
Teaching, guidance, counseling	Sickness/injury care	Routine/emergency care plans (explanation of what sexual assault examination consists of and what to expect)
Teaching, guidance, counseling	Support system	Active listening (encouraging client to share details of assault and empathetic listening)
Teaching, guidance, counseling	Support system	Emotional support (safe, nonjudgmental environment, reassurance)
Teaching, guidance, counseling	Support system	Realistic expectations (related to healing and legal process)
Treatments and procedures	Other	Physical exam (see attached examination report)
Case management	Home	Options (if client is unable to return home or homeless)
Case management	Legal system	Legal assistance (legal advocate groups)
Case management	Nursing care	Coordination among providers (r/t follow-up appointment with general practitioner)
Case management	Other community services	Resource options (support groups)
Case management	Other community services	Referral process (referral to specific group)
Case management	Sickness/injury care	Recognize need for care and follow-up (r/t a specific injury or condition)
Case management	Social work/counseling	Coordination among providers (r/t counseling services)
Case management	Support group	Age/cultural/condition-specific group for those who were abused, have special needs, etc.
Case management	Support group	Community- or facility-based services
Case management	Support group	Telephone information/reassurance
Surveillance	Continuity of care	Coordination among providers (ensuring follow-up appointment is set up)
Surveillance	Safety	Monitor safety plan
Surveillance	Signs/symptoms–mental/emotional	Behavioral extremes
Surveillance	Signs/symptoms–mental/emotional	Other (consent issues, intoxication)

Data from Omaha System care plans developed by Anne C. Tatro, MS, PHN, SANE, and Emily A. Robb, RN, PHN, SANE.

TABLE 5.2   **Sexual Assault Nurse Examiner Care Plan for Family Planning**

Category	Target	Care Description
Teaching, guidance, counseling	Anatomy/physiology	Reproductive system
Teaching, guidance, counseling	Family-planning care	Methods (plan B contraception)
Teaching, guidance, counseling	Medication action/side effects	Important to take as prescribed (r/t Plan B)
Teaching, guidance, counseling	Medication action/side effects	Purpose/benefits (r/t Plan B)
Teaching, guidance, counseling	Screening procedures	Pregnancy testing
Surveillance	Medication action/side effects	Takes as prescribed (r/t Plan B)

TABLE 5.3 Sexual Assault Nurse Examiner Care Plan for Mental Health

Category	Target	Care Description
Teaching, guidance, counseling	Coping skill	Crisis intervention (emotional responses, healing)
Teaching, guidance, counseling	Signs/symptoms–mental/emotional	Affect
Teaching, guidance, counseling	Signs/symptoms–mental/emotional	Suicidal tendencies
Teaching, guidance, counseling	Support group	Emotional support (importance of)
Teaching, guidance, counseling	Support group	Others' experiences (normalizing feelings and responses)
Case management	Other community resources	Mental health services

TABLE 5.4 Sexual Assault Nurse Examiner Care Plan for Communicable/Infectious Condition

Category	Target	Care Description
Teaching, guidance, counseling	Anatomy/physiology	Disease process
Teaching, guidance, counseling	Anatomy/physiology	Transmission
Teaching, guidance, counseling	Medication action/side effects	Important to take as prescribed (r/t antibiotics)
Teaching, guidance, counseling	Medication action/side effects	Purpose/benefits
Teaching, guidance, counseling	Screening procedures	Other: Follow-up care and screening for sexually transmitted infection
Teaching, guidance, Counseling	Signs/symptoms physical	Evidence of disease/infection (r/t what to watch for in future)
Case management	Medication coordination	Multiple medications (ordering from pharmacy or elsewhere)
Surveillance	Medication action/side effects	Take as prescribed

highly sensitive, culturally competent, comprehensive care. These care plans reveal the complex, holistic nature of forensic nursing practice.

New techniques and new technology can be disseminated into practice by incorporating them into academic and continuing education simulations. For example, there is new evidence that an alternative light source (ALS) should be used in a sexual assault examination to detect semen instead of using the Wood's lamp.

High-fidelity human patient simulation can be incorporated into competency testing so that forensic nurses can experience the same scenario and have their competencies validated. The METI Pelvic Exam SIM is invaluable for testing the forensic nurses' competencies. The forensic nurses can receive a printout of their examination and receive feedback on their technique. By videotaping the forensic nurse interacting with the human patient simulator, the nurse can learn what steps are correct and which steps can be improved. Moulage should be incorporated, such as makeup for bruising and avocado juice for semen, to enhance the reality of the simulated experience.

It is important to have a culturally diverse group of simulators, including one with a disability, since Newton and Vandeven (2009) report that children with disabilities are at higher risk for abuse. In addition, Fredland and colleagues reported that youth are exposed to many forms of violence, so one could use a young adult simulation such as METIman or SimMan 3G.

Campbell and colleagues (2009) and Mayer and Coulter (2002a; 2002b) remind forensic nurses that the most vulnerable period in the cycle of violence is when the abused prepares to leave the abuser/partner. The potential loss and legal consequences to be faced by the abuser may lead or escalate to murder. Patient interviewing therefore needs to be conducted in a controlled environment. Simulation training could prepare the novice forensic nurse to safely conduct effective interviews.

Ferguson and Faugno indicate that a common problem for many forensic nurses who perform sexual assault examinations is that sexual assault cases may be infrequent; thus, simulation may be the answer to maintaining these unique and special competencies. In addition, since there may be several forensic nurses using the human patient simulator during a session, nurses can be benchmarked against each other for peer review. See Table 5.5 for case scenario applications relevant to SANE nursing. In addition, the Society for Academic Emergency Medicine (SAEM) Simulation Case Library provides complete case studies and scenarios for child abuse, with learning objectives and competencies

TABLE 5.5   Examples of Case Scenarios, Simulators, and Competencies

Situation	Simulator	Competency
A pregnant woman presents in the emergency room with signs of domestic abuse.	The Noelle Maternal and Neonatal Simulator, Susie, made by Gaumard.	Using a colposcope and taking swabs in all involved areas, including the mouth, genital, and anal areas, along with fingernail clippings and pubic hair. Every move is recorded via twin cameras located inside NOELLE; movements and an overhead camera capture actions of the forensic nurse.
A 14-year-old presents in the emergency room with signs of sexual abuse.	Safe Care models, such as Resusci-Anne mannequins or pelvic models or human patient simulators made by Gaumard, Laerdal, and METI. The simulators can be programmed so clinicians have to recall the steps involved in the interviewing process.	Adams (2008) advises a protocol wherein children with acute presentations are seen urgently if they are within 24 hours of the assault for forensic evidence collection; if it is past that time they should be scheduled to be seen promptly by an expert clinician.
An infant presents in the emergency room with signs of shaken baby syndrome.	Pediatric and newborn simulators made by Gaumard, Laerdal, and METI, removing the outer skins and replacing them with skins showing subtle signs of abuse or by using moulage to achieve the effect.	Assessment of the child to be followed by x-rays.

The authors acknowledge Ms. Tammie Wingert, RN, BSN, CPST, SANE-A, CARE Clinic, Children's Mercy Hospitals and Clinics, Kansas City, Missouri, for her review of the case studies.

As in any human patient simulation center, it is important to schedule time for debriefing and showing the videotape of the forensic nurses completing the scenarios. Debriefing is an essential element and should include:

- Critique
- Correction
- Evaluation of performance
- Discussion of the experience
- An environment that provides a safe space for discussion

Examples of Data Analysis and Reporting

Statistics regarding sexual assault, rape, and abuse (SARA) are sobering. These health statistics and research findings describe the prevalence and implications of SARA for various populations. It has been estimated that one out of every six American women has been the victim of attempted or completed rape in her lifetime (14.8% completed rape, 2.8% attempted rape). The rate of SARA for all women is 17.6%; for White women, 17.7%; African American women, 18.8%; Asian or Pacific Islander women, 6.8%; American Indian or native American Alaskan, or Inuit, women, 34.1%; and mixed racial or ethnic women, 24.4%. About 3% of American men, or 1 in 33, have experienced an attempted or completed rape in their lifetime. As for children, 15% of

sexual assault and rape victims are under the age of 12, and 44% are under 18, with girls 16 to 19 years old four times more likely than the general population to be victims of rape, attempted rape, or sexual assault.

Despite the high occurrence of SARA, it remains one of the most underreported crimes, with 60% of SARA crimes in the general population left unreported; fewer than 5% of college women report SARA to police. However, approximately two-thirds of the survivors of SARA eventually will tell someone, a trusted friend or confidant, immediately after the event or several years after the event. Fisher and others (2008) found over 40% of survivors of SARA who did not report the incident said they did not do so because they feared reprisal by the assailant or others. In addition, some survivors of SARA may fear the emotional trauma of the legal process itself. Other reasons for low reporting of SARA events by survivors are (1) embarrassment and shame, (2) fear of publicity, (3) fear of being retraumatized, (4) fear of social isolation from the assailant's friends, (5) fear that the police will not believe them, (6) fear that the prosecutor will not believe them or will not bring charges, (7) self-blame due to drinking or using drugs before the rape, (8) self-blame for being alone with the assailant, perhaps in their own or the assailant's residence, (9) mistrust of the campus judicial system, and (10) fear that their family will find out. Past studies found the importance of testing new and efficient use of technology and evidence-based practices prior to its dissemination for use by the target population.

Surviving SARA is a health-shifting event. Survivors of SARA are:

- Three times more likely to suffer from depression
- Six times more likely to suffer from PTSD
- Thirteen times more likely to abuse alcohol
- Twenty-six times more likely to abuse drugs
- Four times more likely to contemplate suicide

Most of them will experience multiple, co-occurring symptoms, related to SARA, mental health and physical symptoms, or both. Past research has clearly linked occurrence and severity of multiple symptoms with impairments in functioning and quality of life in survivors of SARA. More than 50% of survivors will suffer multiple physical and mental sequelae: shock, humiliation, anxiety, sadness, substance abuse, suicidal thoughts, loss of self-esteem, social isolation, anger, distrust, and failure in school, work, or social roles.

Clinical informatics data provide another avenue for investigating the SARA problem and SARA-related services. Electronic health records or evidentiary electronic forensic medical records are the primary sources of detailed data about forensic patients. These data are necessary to understand masses of forensic patients with similar intentional injuries or pathology, presentation, and descriptions of assaults. The goal of such research is the improvement and development of evidence-based diagnostic, assessment, and management interventions.

Using Informatics and Simulations to Guide Practice and Policy

Injury resulting from violence is one of the nation's top health concerns. The economic cost of SARA is estimated to be $159 million in the United States annually, with 79% of this cost due to quality-of-life factors, lost earnings and productivity, and legal and medical costs. Although treatment-related cost as a single factor is seldom studied, one study estimated the cost per survivor to be $85,000 per SARA incident, including physical injuries and psychological harm. In addition, violence against women in developing countries has emerged as a growing concern among researchers and policy makers. Clearly, these statistics argue on behalf of governmental agencies and payer policies to reduce SARA through law enforcement and crime prevention efforts and improving services for SARA victims through research and expanding access to care.

The health informatics agenda is advancing rapidly due to governmental mandates and incentives, and electronic health records have been adopted in many forensic

Case Study

FORENSIC MEDICAL RECORD DATA ANALYSIS

One sample of cases ($n = 85$) that were entered into an online forensic medical form by Jill Crum, RN, SANE, was used to demonstrate the successful use of data from an electronic forensic medical records database. Data entry into forensic medical records was performed at the time of the patient encounter at the bedside by forensic nurses in a California clinic that provides services to patients reporting sexual assault or abuse. Digital images for identification of the patient and images associated with the forensic case are stored on a secure server.

The database was accessed via a secure server and downloaded into an Excel file that was transferred into SPSS 14.0. Specific variables were chosen for descriptive purposes only in an initial trial of the process. The sample ($n = 85$) included only two males, and the rest were females. Almost 16% were under 18 years of age, and 56.6% were 18 to 24 years of age. Only five women

45 years and older were in the sample. Age groups of patients in the sample were consistent with other research on large databases of patients reporting sexual assault and abuse. Almost half of the sample were Caucasian, and 41% reported being Hispanic, which is typical for many southern California communities. However, the percentage is double the number of Hispanics (21%) reported in a sample from another California city.

Use of weapons and abundant intentional injury is often considered to be commonplace with crimes of violence. However, the use of weapons was reported in only 10 cases. No injuries intentionally caused by the weapons were reported, although about 10% of the patients reported other bodily injuries. Specific genital injuries were reported by 14 patients (16%). The subjective data percentages on injury reports are consistent with what the forensic nurses documented from objective assessment.

Research Exemplar

Bakken, S., Currie, L.M., Lee, N-J., Roberts, W.D., et al. (2008). Integrating evidence into clinical information systems for nursing decision support. *International Journal of Medical Informatics, 77*:413-420.

Randell, R., & Dowding, D. (2010). Organizational influences on nurses of clinical decision support systems. *International Journal of Medical Informatics,* epub15 March 2010.

Randell and Dowding (2010) state that nurses are increasingly using computerized decision support systems (CDSSs) to support their practice. Bakken et al (2002) integrated three types of clinical information systems for decision support function (information management and patient-specific attention) focusing attention on screening and guideline-based management of depression, obesity, or smoking cessation. The unit of analysis was clinical encounters by nurses in an advanced practice nurse program with the subjects. PDAs and cellular phones were used, and the hypothesis was that decision support compared to no decision support resulted in greater adherence to guidelines implementing informatics when caring for a sample of predominately Hispanic or African American patients. Of the 30,845 encounters for obesity (experimental group = 10,938; control group = 19,907), the screening rate was 43.7% (>age 2), with missed diagnosis at 4.5% for the experimental group versus 66.5% for the control group; the number of diagnoses and number of interventions was significantly greater for the experimental group than for the control group. Of 23,625 encounters for smoking cessation (E = 7874; C = 15,751), screening rate was 75.6% for ages greater than 8, and the number of diagnoses was significantly greater for the experimental group than for the control group. Of 10,779 encounters for adult depression (E = 4343; C = 6436), screening rate was 51.5% for ages greater than 17, and the number of diagnoses for the experimental group was significantly greater than for the control group. Of 7085 encounters of pediatric depression (E = 2832; C = 4253), screening rate was 22.5% for ages 8 to 17, and the number of diagnoses was significantly greater for the experimental group than for the control group.

nursing settings. As nursing documentation systems are incorporated into electronic health records, forensic nursing data are becoming available. Research employing forensic nursing documentation data will enable the description and analysis of forensic nursing services for the purposes of improving forensic nursing care and patient outcomes. See the following diagram.

CONCLUSIONS

This chapter illustrates:

- How technologies in nursing informatics and human patient simulations are emerging as powerful new approaches to enhance forensic nursing care quality.

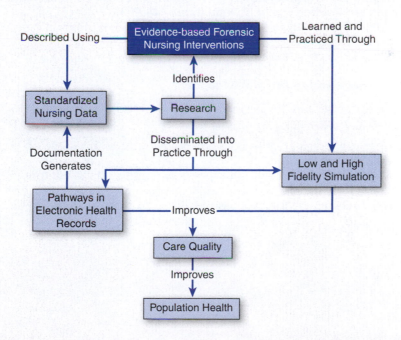

- How information is becoming available to support and improve practice, enhance the legal process, and guide policy.
- Why education no longer depends on the type of patient available because simulation provides access to many rare or emergent conditions.

As forensic nurses adopt these technology solutions, forensic nursing practice will continue to advance and will benefit vulnerable patients, systems of care, and the health of the public.

EVIDENCE-BASED PRACTICE

Reference Question: In forensic health-care training, does the use of high-fidelity simulation as compared to low-fidelity simulation improve interdisciplinary collaboration immediately after simulation training?

Population: Interdisciplinary collaborators

Intervention: High-fidelity simulation

Comparison Group: Low-fidelity simulation

Outcome: Improved collaboration

Time: Immediately after simulation training

Databases to Search: ERIC, InSpec, PubMed

Selected References From Search:

1. Freeth, D., Ayida, G., Berridge, E.J., et al. (2009). Multidisciplinary obstetric simulated emergency scenarios (MOSES): Promoting patient safety in obstetrics with teamwork-focused interprofessional simulations. *Journal of Continuing Education in the Health Professions, 29*(2):98-104.
2. Mili, F., Barr, J., Harris, M., & Pittiglio, L. (2008). Nursing training: 3D game with learning objectives. Advances in Computer-Human Interaction, Piscataway, NJ. http://ieeexplore. ieee.org/xpl/freeabs_all.jsp?arnumber=4455988.
3. Osmani, V., Balasubramaniam, S., & Botvich, D. (2008). Human activity recognition in pervasive health-care: Supporting efficient remote collaboration. *Journal of Network and Computer Applications, 31*(4):628-655.

Questions Used to Discern Evidence:

Choose two studies among the studies listed, read about them, and answer the following questions:

1. What are the differences between the two studies in the design, methods, and results?
2. What are the similarities between the two studies in the number of subjects, measurements used, and interventions, if any?
3. What skills do you think you need to learn to practice forensic nursing?

REVIEW QUESTIONS

1. Advanced technology is creating a dependence on simulation as a/an:
   A. Enculturation into nursing and health-care education
   B. Replacement for clinical experience
   C. Self-paced learning module
   D. Teaching and learning strategy

2. Low-fidelity simulation is:
   A. Connected
   B. Immersive
   C. Integrated
   D. Static

3. Alternative light source (ALS) should be used to detect:
   A. Gonorrhea
   B. Human papilloma virus
   C. Pelvic inflammatory disease
   D. Semen

4. Simulation for the forensic nurse should not be conducted:
   A. In a team
   B. Alone or with a partner
   C. In a classroom
   D. Without videotaping

5. Debriefing as a component of simulation should be conducted:
   A. Prior to the scenario
   B. During the scenario
   C. After the scenario is completed
   D. One week after the simulation has been completed

6. Forensic nursing data from the electronic health record should not be used as:
   A. A source of evidence for prosecution
   B. Press release material
   C. Quality improvement evaluation information
   D. Formal research datasets

7. The Omaha System provides standardized terms for client problems, practitioner interventions, and problem-specific client outcomes. Some Omaha System problems that are particularly applicable in forensic nursing are:
   A. Abuse, Skin, Communicable/infectious condition
   B. Speech and language, Vision, Hearing
   C. Respiration and Circulation
   D. Personal care, Medication regimen

8. Electronic forensic medical record data do not provide information on the:
   A. Type and location of provider
   B. Race/ethnicity of victims
   C. Type of assault
   D. Narrative notes of the encounter

9. Informatics solutions specifically for forensic nursing do not include:
   A. Generating data
   B. Warehousing data
   C. Data to attorneys and law enforcement
   D. Vital statistics data

10. Forensic nurses cannot use data to:
    A. Reduce assault through law enforcement and crime prevention efforts
    B. Improve services for assault victims through research
    C. Identify perpetrators
    D. Expand access to care for assault victims through health systems policy

References

Adams, J.A. (2008). Guidelines for medical care of children evaluated for suspected sexual abuse: An update for 2008. *Current Opinion Obstetrics Gynecology, 20*:435-441.

Advanced Initiatives in Medical Simulation (AIMS). Retrieved August 1, 2009, from http://www.medsim.org

Agency for Health Care Research and Quality (AHRQ). (2009). *Outcomes research fact sheet.* Retrieved August 1, 2009, from http://www.ahrq.gov/clinic/outfact.htm

American Medical Informatics Association (AMIA). (2008). *Health information management and informatics core competencies for individuals working with electronic health records.* Report of Joint AHIMA and AMIA Work Force

Task Force. Retrieved August 1, 2009, from http://www.amia.org/files/shared/Workforce_2008.pdf

American Nurses Association (ANA). (2006). *ANA recognized terminologies and data element sets.* Retrieved August 1, 2009, from http://nursingworld.org/npii/terminologies.htm

American Nurses Association (ANA). (2008). *Nursing informatics: Scope and standards of practice.* Silver Spring, MD: ANA.

American Nurses Association/International Association of Forensic Nurses. (2009). *Forensic nursing: scope and standards of practice.* Silver Spring, MD: ANA.

Anderson, M., & Leflore, J. (2008). Playing it safe: Simulated training in the OR. *Association of periOperative Registered Nurses Journal, 87*(4):772,774-776, 778-779.

Bakken, S., Currie, L.M., Lee, N-J., et al. (2008). Integrating evidence into clinical information systems for nursing decision support. *International Journal of Medical Informatics, 77*:413-420.

Beyea, S.C., & Kobokovich, L.J. (2004). Human patient simulation: A teaching tool. *Association of periOperative Registered Nurses Journal, 90*(4):738-742.

Beyea, S.C., von Reyn L.K., & Slattery, M.J. (2007). A nurse residency program for competency development using human patient simulation. *Journal for Nurses in Staff Development, 23*(2):77-82.

Bracken, M.I., Messing, J.T., Campbell, J.C., et al. (2010). Intimate partner violence and abuse among female nurses and nursing personnel: Prevalence and risk factors. *Issues in Mental Health Nursing, 31*(2):137-148.

Brett-Fleegler, M.B., Vinci, R.J., Weiner, D.L., et al. (2009). A simulation-based tool that assesses pediatric resident resuscitation competency. *Pediatrics, 12*(3):e597-e603.

Bruce, S.A., Scherer, Y.K., Curran, C.C., et al. (2009). A collaborative exercise between graduate and undergraduate nursing students using a computer-assisted simulator in a mock cardiac arrest. *Nursing Education Perspectives, 30*(1):22-27.

Btoush, R., Campbell, J.C., & Gebbie, K.M. (2009). Care provided in visits coded for intimate partner violence in a national survey of emergency departments. *Women's Health Issues, 19*(4):253-262.

Btoush, R., Campbell, J.C., & Gebbie, K.M. (2008). Visits coded as intimate partner violence in emergency departments: Characteristics of the individuals and the system as reported in a national survey of emergency departments. *Journal of Emergency Nursing, 34*(5):419-427.

Campbell, J.C., Webster, D.W., & Glass, N. (2009). The danger assessment: Validation of a lethality risk assessment instrument for intimate partner femicide. *Journal Interpersonal Violence, 24*(4):653-274.

Campbell, R. (2005). What really happened? A validation study of rape survivor's help-seeking experiences with the legal and medical systems. *Violence and Victims, 20*(1):34-40.

Cannon-Deihel, M.R. (2009). Simulation in healthcare and nursing: State of the science. *Critical Care Nursing Quarterly, 32*(2):128-136.

Crane P.A. (2006). Predictors of injury associated with rape. Doctoral dissertation. Pittsburgh, PA: University of Pittsburgh.

Dongilli, T., DeVita, M., Schaefer, J.J., et al. (2005). The use of simulation training in a large multi-hospital health system to increase patient safety. *Anesthesia and Analgesia, 98*(Suppl.):S22.

Dreifuerst, K.T. (2009). The essentials of debriefing in simulation learning: A concept analysis. *Nursing Education Perspectives, 30*(2):109-114.

Ferguson, C., & Faugno, D. (2009). The SAFE CARE model: Maintaining competency in sexual assault examinations utilizing patient simulation methods. *Journal of Forensic Nursing, 5*:109-114.

Fisher, B.F., & Turner, M. (2008). *The sexual victimization of college women.* US Department of Justice, National Institute of Justice and Bureau of Justice Statistics. Retrieved September 11, 2008 from Fisher, B.S., Daigle, L.E., Cullen, L.E., et al. (2003). Reporting sexual victimization to the police and others: Results from a national-level study of college women. *Criminal Justice and Behavior, 30*(1):6-38.

Fredland, N.M., Campbell, J., & Han, H. (2008). Effect of violence exposure on health outcomes among young urban adolescents. *Nursing Research, 57*(3):157-165.

Friedman, C.P. (2009). A "fundamental theorem" of biomedical informatics. *Journal of the American Medical Informatics Association, 16*(2):169-170.

Glass, N., Perrin, N., Hanson, G., et al. (2008). Risk for reassault in abusive female same-sex relationships. *American Journal of Public Health, 98*(6):1021-1027.

Healthcare Information and Management Systems Society (HIMSS). (1999). *Electronic health record.* Retrieved August 1, 2009, from http://www.himss.org/ASP/topics_ehr.asp

Healthy People. (2010). Retrieved August 3, 2009, from http://www.healthypeople.gov/LHI/ihiwhat.htm

Hoadley, T. (2009). Learning advanced cardiac life support: A comparison study of the effects of low and high fidelity simulation. *Nursing Education Perspectives, 30*(2):91-95.

Institute of Medicine (IOM). (1998). *IOM definition of quality.* Retrieved August 1, 2009 from http://www.iom.edu/CMS/8089.aspx

Issenberg, B.S., McGaghie, W.C., Petrusa, E.R., et al. Features and uses of high-fidelity medical simulations that lead to effective learning: A BEME systematic review. Retrieved August 6, 2009, from www.bemecollection.org/. . ./beme%20guide%204%journal%text.pdf

Jeffries, P.R. (Ed.). (2007). *Simulation in nursing education: From conceptualization to evaluation.* New York: National League for Nursing.

Koenig, M.A., Stephenson, R., Ahmed, A., et al. (2006). Individual and contextual determinants of domestic violence in North India. *American Journal of Public Health, 96*(1): 132-138.

Kuhrik, N.S., Kuhrik, M., Rimkus, C.F., et al. (2008). Using human patient simulation in the oncology clinical practice setting. *The Journal of Continuing Education in Nursing, 39*(8):345-355.

LeFlore, J.L., & Anderson, M. (2008). Effectiveness of 2 methods to teach and evaluate new content to neonatal transport personnel using high fidelity simulation. *The Journal of Perinatal & Neonatal Nursing, 22*(4):319-328.

Lincoln, C., McBride, P., Turbett, G., et al. (2006). The use of an alternative light source to detect semen in clinical forensic medical practice. *Journal of Clinical Forensic Practice, 13*:215-218.

Martin, K.S. (2005). *The Omaha System: A key to practice, documentation, and information management* (2nd ed.). St. Louis: Elsevier.

Mayer, B.W., & Coulter, M. (2002a). Part one: Psychological aspects of partner abuse. *American Journal of Nursing, 102*(5):24MM-24WW.

Mayer, B.W., & Coulter, M. (2002b). Part two: Psychological aspects of partner abuse. *American Journal of Nursing, 102*(6):24AA-24GG.

Messmer, P.R. (2008). Enhancing nurse-physician collaboration using pediatric simulation. *The Journal of Continuing Education in Nursing, 39*(7):319-327.

Monsen, K.A., Fulkerson, J.A., Lytton, A.B., et al. (2009). Comparing maternal child health problems and outcomes across public health nursing agencies. *Maternal Child Health Journal* Epub.

Monsen, K.A., Neely, C., Oftedahl, G., et al. (2012). Feasibility of encoding the Institute for Clinical Systems Improvement Depression Guideline using the Omaha System. Journal of Biomedical Informatics. www.ncbi.nlm.nih.gov/pubmed/22742937

Nelson, D.G., & Santucci, K.A. (2002). An alternate light sources to detect semen. *Academy of Emergency Medicine, 9*(10):1045-1048.

Newton, A.W., & Vandeven, A.M. (2009). Update in child maltreatment. *Current Opinion in Pediatrics, 21*:252-261.

National League for Nursing Simulation. Articles highlighted in *Nursing Education Perspectives Journal.* Retrieved August 1, 2009, from http://www.nln.org

O'Donnell, J.M., Rodgers, D.L., Lee, W.W., Edelson, D.P., et al. (2009). Structured and Supported Debriefing (Computer Software). Dallas, TX: American Heart Association.

Omaha System. (2009). *The Omaha System: Solving the clinical data-information puzzle.* Retrieved August 1, 2009, from http://omahasystem.org

Patow, C.A. (2005). Medical simulation makes medical education better and safer. *Health Management Technology, 26*(12):39-40.

Pugh, L.C., Eldredge, K., & Huggins, E. (2009). *Evidence-based practice in forensic nursing: A collaborative effort.* Poster presentation at STTI Nursing Research Congress. Book of Proceedings, Vancouver, Canada, July 13-15, 2009.

Simulation Interest Group (SAEM). Retrieved August 1, 2009, from http://www.saem.org

Randell, R., & Dowding, D. (2010). Organizational influences on nurses of clinical decision support systems. *International Journal of Medical Informatics,* epub15 March 2010.

Rape Abuse Incest National Network (RAINN). (2010). *Rape, abuse and incest: Who are the victims?* Retrieved February 2, 2011, from www.rainn.org

Saied, N. (2005). Virtual reality and medicine—From the cockpit to the operating room: Are we there yet? *Missouri Medicine, 102*(5):450-455.

Sampson, R. (2002). Acquaintance rape of college students. *Problem-oriented guide for police series.* Volume 17.

Schmid-Mazzooccoli, A., Hoffman, L.A., Wolf, G.A., et al. (2008). The use of medical emergency teams in medical and surgical patients: Impact of patient, nurse, and organizational characteristics. *Quality Safe Health Care, 17*(5):377-381.

Secure Digital Forensic Imaging (SDFI). (2009). SDFI®-TeleMedicine: A complete colposcope replacement. Retrieved XXX from http://www.sdfi.com

Smith-Stoner, M. (2009). Using high-fidelity simulation to educate students about end-of-life care. *Nursing Education Perspectives, 30*(2):115-125.

Society of Academic Emergency Medicine (SAEM). Retrieved August 3, 2009, from http://www.saem.org/saemdnn

Society for Academic Emergency Medicine (SAEM). *Take care of my kids.* Simulation Case Library. Retrieved August 1, 2009, from http://www.emedu.org/simlibrary/

Society for Simulation in Healthcare. Retrieved August 1, 2009 from http://www.ssih.org

Society in Europe for Simulation Applied to Medicine. Retrieved August 1, 2009, from http://www.sesam-eb.org

Sportsman, S., Bolton, C., Bradshaw, P., et al. (2009). A regional simulation center partnership: Collaboration to improve staff and student competency. *The Journal of Continuing Education in Nursing, 49*(20):67-73.

Steadman, R.H., Coates, W.C., Huang, Y.M., et al. (2006). Simulation-based training is superior to problem-based learning for the acquisition of critical assessment and management skills. *Critical Care Medicine, 34*(1):252-253.

Tuttle, R.P., Cohen, M.H., Augustine, A.J., et al. (2007). Utilizing simulation technology for competency skills assessment and a comparison of traditional methods of training to simulation-based training. *Respiratory Care 52*(3):263-270.

U.S .Department of Justice (USDJ). (2005). *National crime statistics.* Washington, DC: USDJ.

Wasco, S.M. (2004). Conceptualizing the harm done by rape. *Trauma, Violence & Abuse 4*(4):309-322.

Westra, B.L., Delaney, C.W., Konicek, D., et al. (2008). Nursing standards to support the electronic health record. *Nursing Outlook, 56*(5):258-266.

Xu, X., Zhu, F., O'Campo, P., et al. (2005). Prevalence of and risk factors for intimate partner violence in China. *American Journal of Public Health 95*(1):78-138.

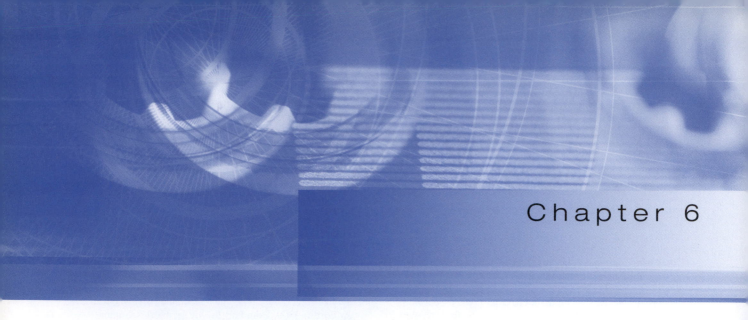

Chapter 6

FORENSIC NURSING EDUCATION

Nancy Martin

"Knowing is not enough; we must apply. Willing is not enough; we must do."
Johann Wolfgang von Goethe

Competencies

1. Discussing forensic nursing education at the undergraduate and graduate level.
2. Describing a forensic nursing conceptual framework.
3. Identifying core competencies for forensic nursing education.
4. Describing the components of competency-based forensic nursing education.

Key Terms

Competency-based education
Evidence-based education
Forensics
Forensic aspects of nursing care
Forensic environment
Forensic populations
Forensic nursing
Nurse generalist

INTRODUCTION

As a consequence of domestic and social violence, societal changes, and increased emphasis on forensic issues in the media, forensic nursing has become a specialty at the forefront of education and practice. Higher education in nursing has begun to incorporate forensic nursing into curricula, most commonly in advanced practice. However, there has been a need for core competencies for undergraduate forensic nursing education, which can help guide the development of instructional programs and enhance student competencies in assessing and responding to violence.

ISSUES AND CHALLENGES FOR FORENSIC NURSING UNDERGRADUATE EDUCATION

Violence and its associated trauma are now regarded as a major public health problem and a threat to the health and well-being of persons of all ages. Screening for violence is a minimum standard of health care, and it is expected that health-care providers be prepared to recognize and treat victims of violence. In 1992, the Joint Commission Accreditation of Healthcare Organizations required every emergency department to have staff skilled in the identification of crime victims and the collection and preservation of evidence.

Nurses interact with victims of violence in all practice settings and witness the effects of violence on patients and their families. Forensic cases often go undiscovered due to lack of knowledge and skills required to identify and manage clients with forensic needs. A nurse can be a patient's first line of defense and can affect the outcome of violence. A patient's injuries can become the basis for criminal action, and documentation can be used as evidence in a court of law. Thus, nurses need basic forensic knowledge and skills that can enhance their practice.

Domestic violence has been increasingly recognized as a major concern by criminal justice, health, and professional organizations. Growing pressure to include domestic and other violence content in nursing curricula initially resulted in a fragmented approach in attempts to provide students with the knowledge and skills for patient care. Woodtli and Breslin published findings that examined changes in violence-related content in bachelor of science in nursing (BSN) curricula. Those findings indicated little change in nursing curricula over 4 years.

Need for Basic Forensic Nursing Knowledge and Skills

The term "forensic" means "pertaining to the law," and **forensics** is the application of science in the resolution of legal issues. The American Nurses Association (ANA) and the International Association of Forensic Nurses (IAFN) describe **forensic nursing** as the application of nursing practice to public and legal proceedings. It is part of the scientific investigation and treatment of victims (and perpetrators) of violence, criminal activity, and accidents. Forensic nursing addresses health-care issues that also have a medicolegal component. The role incorporates a new identity, language, terms, and definitions.

There is a need for forensic nursing education. The establishment of formal education programs is recognized as an important component of antiviolence strategies. However, despite this need, forensic nursing education is not widely available. Only recently have colleges and universities begun to embrace forensic education and to offer courses ranging from elective and credit courses to certificate and specialty programs. Forensic content means going beyond the behavioral and physical indicators of abuse and adding family dynamics, assessment, and intervention strategies. New graduates in nursing are prepared as generalists, but the reality is that as new graduates they are increasingly required to function in a more complex health-care environment with an increasingly broad continuum of care and responsibilities.

COMPETENCY AND COMPETENCY-BASED EDUCATION

Competency Components for Nursing Practice

The definition of competency is varied and depends on many factors, including context and setting. The literature regarding competency in nursing is controversial and confusing, with little agreement on its definition. Many definitions of competency consist of knowledge, performance skills, and values and attitudes. There is agreement that complex nursing practice requires these three competencies.

In nursing, core competencies mean an integration of knowledge, skills, and attitudes to meet established standards of performance. The ANA and the IAFN have provided a standard of education in which the registered nurse (RN) and forensic nurse attain competency in the knowledge and skills that reflect current nursing practice. Competence in nursing is ensured by licensing examinations for practice entry, state licensing laws, the National Council of State Boards of Nursing (NCSBN), and professional standards such as those developed by the ANA.

Competency-Based Education in Nursing

Educational competencies provide the foundation that enables graduates to meet workplace competencies. **Competency-based education** is also directed at defining, teaching, and assessing competencies. Many accreditation organizations in nursing and nursing education, including the Commission on Collegiate Nursing Education, an accrediting arm of the American Colleges of Nursing (AACN), identify core competencies or standards for education and practice. Competency-based learning can be incorporated directly into nursing fundamentals instruction and the initial health assessment courses. It fosters critical thinking and self-direction that allows a learner to build on previous knowledge.

Core competencies and standards for education have also been the focus of national reports and national nursing organizations, including those of the Institute of Medicine (IOM) and the ANA. The IOM reports identify core competencies for health-care education. Nurse educators are finding the IOM reports relevant for guiding decisions involving curriculum and clinical learning experiences. The ANA has developed standards of nursing practice that are considered standards of basic competency that apply to all nurses.

At the senior level of education, forensic content can be added into the curriculum. Forensic projects and the use of case studies are excellent ways to incorporate forensic critical decision making.

Determining the level of nursing competence in transition from the educational setting to the practice setting is difficult and often discussed concurrently with competencies. Senior nursing students are still considered novices, with knowledge, performance skills, individual differences, and practice at the novice level until they have additional experience. But competence at the novice level is a prerequisite for performing in the real practice setting.

Evidence-Based Education in Nursing

Evidence-based education is "the integration of professional wisdom with the best available empirical evidence in making decisions about how to deliver instruction." This definition describes a process that values both research and professional educational experiences.

Evidence-based practice is new to nursing; it is primarily focused on clinical nursing practice. The NCSBN identified evidence-based elements of nursing education that are characteristic of curricula, faculty, and teaching methods associated with better learning outcomes and safe entry-level practice. The NCSBN characterized the elements as adjunctive teaching methods, assimilation to the role of nursing, deliberate practice with actual patients, and faculty-student relationships. Identification of evidence-based elements of nursing education can guide decisions to improve educational programs in the preparation of nurses for practice.

CONCEPTUAL FRAMEWORK FOR UNDERGRADUATE FORENSIC NURSING EDUCATION

The definition of undergraduate competency-based nursing education was the foundation for developing a conceptual framework for undergraduate forensic nursing education. The definition contained the three components of knowledge, performance skills, and values and attitudes.

A conceptual framework groups related ideas in order to organize knowledge. Models and theories in nursing science usually contain four concepts that are considered central to nursing: (1) person, (2) health, (3) nursing, and (4) environment. These concepts were also identified and described for a forensic nursing framework by Lynch and Hufft. The concepts were further modified for an undergraduate level of forensic nursing education by Martin (Box 6.1).

Box 6.1 Conceptual Framework for Undergraduate Forensic Nursing

- **Forensic populations** include patient, victim, suspect, and perpetrator, as well as groups, families, and communities.
- Health involves persons in relation to the environment or potential environment or context in which violence or abuse occurs.
- Nursing includes nursing science, forensic nursing science, and nursing practice using the nursing process and essential skills for forensic nursing.
- A **forensic environment** is an event or location in which violence or potential for violence occurs or where forensic populations receive health care or are involved in medicolegal issues.

Case Study

DISCUSSION QUESTIONS FOR A CURRICULUM COMMITTEE

A faculty member is part of a curriculum committee of an undergraduate nursing program that is charged with ensuring that key concepts and principles of competency-based undergraduate forensic nursing instruction are incorporated throughout nursing courses. The curriculum committee is responsible for evaluating courses to ensure that students will have essential knowledge and skills for best practice of aspects of forensic nursing upon graduation.

Discussion Questions

1. What decisions must be made before implementing competency-based undergraduate forensic nursing instruction?

2. What are the central problems that may be identified?
3. What courses in the curriculum would be appropriate for integration of undergraduate forensic nursing core competencies, instructional objectives, and content outline?
4. What resources might be used to help integrate aspects of forensic nursing instruction into courses?
5. What are the resources for faculty who may not be qualified to teach aspects of forensic nursing?
6. How will core competencies for undergraduate forensic nursing be evaluated?

CORE COMPETENCIES FOR UNDERGRADUATE FORENSIC NURSING EDUCATION

Criteria for Core Competencies

These criteria are provided by professional nursing education and accreditation organizations, scope and standards of professional nursing practice, and an undergraduate forensic nursing conceptual framework. The criteria incorporate the definition of competency-based nursing education and a description of the conceptual framework for undergraduate forensic nursing. Other defined terms are **nurse generalist** and **forensic aspects of nursing care** (Box 6.2).

Box 6.2   Definitions

- Competency-based nursing education includes the three components of knowledge, performance skills, and values and attitudes for undergraduate education and practice.
- Forensic aspects of nursing care are forensic nursing concepts of knowledge, performance skills, and values and attitudes appropriate for the undergraduate nurse generalist.
- A nurse generalist is an undergraduate senior nursing student who is at the novice level of competency regarding knowledge, performance skills, and individual differences.

Core competencies include the knowledge, performance skills, and values and attitudes appropriate for the nurse generalist. Specialty competencies usually represent knowledge and skills required to provide appropriate nursing care to a specific population. A core competency consists of a competency statement and performance criteria. The statement describes a general level of performance. Performance criteria are the essential aspects of skill needed to be demonstrated. Criteria are statements that identify the variables that need to be examined when evaluating a standard.

Core Competencies for Undergraduate Forensic Nursing

These are the knowledge, performance skills, and values and attitudes required for undergraduate forensic nursing education and practice (Box 6.3).

COMPETENCY-BASED UNDERGRADUATE FORENSIC NURSING INSTRUCTION

Elements of the Undergraduate Forensic Nursing Instructional Program

The competency-based undergraduate instructional program for forensic nursing is based on the development of a conceptual framework and core competencies. The undergraduate forensic nursing instructional program design

Box 6.3 Core Competencies for Undergraduate Forensic Nursing

1. Core Competency 1 is knowledge. The nurse generalist will demonstrate understanding of essential knowledge about forensic aspects of nursing that affect violence, interpersonal violence, trauma, and injury in a forensic environment.
2. Core Competency 2 is performance skills. The nurse generalist will demonstrate mastery of essential forensic aspects of nursing skills delivered to forensic populations in a forensic environment.
3. Core Competency 3 is values and attitudes. The nurse generalist will influence and model professional behavior essential to the forensic aspects of nursing care for forensic populations in a forensic environment.

was guided by a model that consists of instructional objectives, content outline, and delivery strategies.

Instructional objectives are guided by core competencies. They are broad and outline the program content for future courses or integration into an existing curriculum. Instructional objectives guide appropriate instruction, evaluation of outcomes, and the learner. The instructional objectives and content outline are based on recurrent topics and concepts in forensic nursing education and are organized and presented in sequence for mastering the body of knowledge.

The need to consider learners for whom the program is being developed is a key element of instructional design. Nursing students are adult learners, and practice settings include patients and families across the life span who have varying cultural, ethnic, and socioeconomic status.

Delivery strategies are general and include a variety of approaches. Using several approaches is more effective than using a single one.

The core competencies and elements of the instructional design developed by Martin are presented in Boxes 6.4 to 6.6. Box 6.4 incorporates core competency 1 (knowledge); Box 6.5 incorporates core competency 2 (performance skills); and Box 6.6 incorporates core competency 3 (attitudes and values).

The following terms are defined by Martin to enhance clarification and understanding: competency-based nursing education, forensic aspects of nursing, forensic environment, forensic populations, and nurse generalist.

Concepts of multiculturalism and ethnicity are usually found in the mission, philosophy, and statements of beliefs and values of individual nursing education programs. The mission and goals should address the healthcare needs of patient populations and the learning needs of students. The undergraduate competency-based forensic nursing instructional program incorporates ethical and cultural considerations into its objectives. For instance, the mission of one Texas university "is to provide scholarly teaching, innovative scientific investigations, and . . .

Box 6.4 Core Competency 1: Knowledge

The nurse generalist will demonstrate understanding of essential knowledge about forensic aspects of nursing affecting violence, interpersonal violence, trauma, and injury in a forensic environment.

Instructional Objectives	Content Outline	Delivery Strategies
1. Describe the history and development of forensic nursing.	1. Introduction and overview of forensic nursing	Lecture
2. Examine the problem of violence and the impact on society.	2. Violence and victimology	Written assignments
3. Identify roles and responsibilities of the generalist in the forensic aspects of nursing.	3. Forensic aspects of the nursing process and forensic populations	Group discussion
4. Describe the legal and ethical issues for the forensic aspects of nursing.	4. Injury identification, interpretation, and documentation	Case review
5. Discuss current forensic nursing research and forensic issues.	5. Evidence recognition, collection, preservation, and documentation instruction	Multimedia
	6. Multidisciplinary collaboration and care of forensic populations	Guest speakers
	7. Legal and ethical issues in the forensic aspects of nursing	Virtual reality
	8. Research and evidence-based nursing practice related to forensic issues	Computer-assisted instruction

Box 6.5   Core Competency 2: Performance Skills

The nurse generalist will demonstrate mastery of essential forensic aspects of nursing skills to forensic populations in a forensic environment.

Instructional Objectives	Content Outline	Delivery Strategies
1. Practice the forensic aspects of communication skills, including interviewing, listening, and documenting, in interacting with persons experiencing violence or trauma. 2. Demonstrate forensic aspects of nursing using the nursing process. 3. Recognize various types of injury and documentation using body diagrams. 4. Describe methods of evidence collection and preservation. 5. Demonstrate the forensic aspects of nursing using teaching methods, including prevention strategies, safety measures, referrals, and resources. 6. Investigate learning experiences that operationalize the forensic aspects of nursing in a variety of settings. 7. Complete predetermined guided clinical care directed to undergraduate forensic core competencies.	1. Communication skills in the forensic aspects of nursing 2. Forensic aspects of nursing and the nursing process 3. Health promotion and prevention 4. Environmental settings for forensic learning experiences	Case review Multimedia Simulation Field trips Demonstration Laboratory practice Clinical observation

Box 6.6   Core Competency 3: Values and Attitudes

The nurse generalist will influence and model professional behavior essential to the forensic aspects of nursing care for forensic populations in a forensic environment.

Instructional Objectives	Content Outline	Delivery Strategies
1. Examine personal values and beliefs about interpersonal violence and trauma. 2. Analyze the effects of values and beliefs on the forensic aspects of nursing care for forensic populations. 3. Recognize the implications of professional nursing practice regarding human rights. 4. Demonstrate professional nursing behavior and responsibilities appropriate to the forensic aspects of nursing care occurring in forensic populations. 5. Identify resources that further educational needs of forensic aspects of nursing. 6. Recognize the evolving competence of the generalist in the forensic aspects of nursing.	1. Violence issues that affect nurses and the provision of nursing care 2. Concepts involving professional nursing behavior 3. Forensic resources for education and research	Lecture Written assignments Group discussion Case review Multimedia Guest speakers Computer-assisted instruction Laboratory experience Clinical observation

state-of-the-art culturally relevant patient care and [to] contribute to the health of the community. . . ."

National and international surveys indicate that the characteristics of ethnicity, race, and age in patient profiles are related to differences in prevalence of health conditions, health outcomes, responses to treatments, and so on. The findings are used to develop new treatments and programs that focus on the individual differences in response to illness and health-care problems specific to the needs of a population. Individual differences in a community's dynamic population can also be fitted to the recruitment, outreach, and retention strategies for students in order to develop and educate a nursing body that mirrors the population.

Components of the Competency-Based Undergraduate Instructional Program

The components of competency-based undergraduate instructional education consist of instructional objectives, content outline, and delivery strategies that lend themselves to course development or integration in an undergraduate nursing curriculum, and they are based on core competencies of knowledge, performance skills, and values and attitudes. (Table 6.1. and Box 6.7.) Integration paths could include physical and psychosocial assessment classes and labs, mental health courses, communication skills, and community courses.

Finkelman and Kenner identified a framework, with safeguards for building patient safety, that could be used for undergraduate forensic nursing education. The appropriate safeguards for the competency-based undergraduate forensic nursing educational components include those that will ensure high-quality content with measurable outcomes that can advance evidence-based forensic nursing education.

Nurse educators should be cognizant of the safeguards and guided by them as forensic nursing curricula are developed and the education programs flourish. Box 6.8 is an example of an introductory undergraduate course in which the course description and objectives address Martin's competencies.

Practice Applications

The competency-based undergraduate educational program in forensic nursing should be applied as evidence-based nursing education. Although such a program could be used to develop an individual course or several courses, or be integrated throughout a curriculum, it would need to be congruent with the individual nursing education program philosophy, mission, and goals. In addition, each nursing program varies with faculty turnover and transitions and

Box 6.7 Components Useful for Evidence-Based Forensic Nursing Education

- Core competencies for student evaluation
- Quality faculty teaching and clinical expertise
- Faculty collaboration and clear communication between faculty and students
- Consistent and current content
- Current curriculum based on evidence-based practice
- Competency evaluation that includes aspects of forensic nursing
- Knowledge of available clinical resources

the faculty's ability to teach forensic nursing; the student populations, their interest, and their need for forensic nursing within the curriculum; and local community agencies and resources.

GRADUATE EDUCATION IN FORENSIC NURSING

Forensic nursing has been a specialty recognized by the ANA since 1994. For years, nurses and other health-care providers depended on continuing education course offerings in various formats. By 2000 several universities had formalized programs of study for nurses that included forensic science. Most programs included four didactic courses and varying hours of clinical practice. A nurse could have a specialty focus in forensic nursing at the graduate level. Content varied from university to university. Content was built on the core advanced practice nursing content at the individual institutions.

The numbers of nurses with varying educational levels, forensic course work, and professional responsibilities

TABLE 6.1 **Forensic Aspects of Nursing: Basic Forensic Nursing Competency Using the Nursing Process**

Competency: Knowledge	Competency: Skill	Competency: Values and Attitude	Evaluation
Objective 1: Identify roles and responsibilities of the generalist in the forensic aspects of nursing.	Injury identification, interpretation, and documentation.	Aware of vulnerable population groups and their risk factors.	Collects pertinent data in the health assessment regarding physical findings on the skin. Documentation reflects differentiation in blunt and sharp injuries, patterned injury and pattern of injury; acute and old injury in a forensic case review. Accurate documentation using nonbiased language.

Box 6.8   School of Nursing Forensic Nursing Syllabus Example

Course Number: Nursing XXXX
Course Title: Introduction to Forensic Nursing
Placement in the Curriculum: Variable
Credits: 3 credits
Faculty:
Prerequisites:
Course Description: The purpose of this course is to build on nursing knowledge, skill, and experience and advance the students' competencies of knowledge, performance skills, and values related to aspects of forensic nursing. Students will explore the history of forensic nursing and a variety of forensic nursing specialty roles. Skills needed for competent and holistic forensic nursing practice will be presented. The application of patient teaching, prevention, and intervention, long-term health effects, and referral resources will be defined for multiprofessional practice. Risks and vulnerabilities will be explored related to forensic populations throughout the life span, their families, and communities. Participation in case study analysis will promote examination of personal views, open discussion on ethical and legal dilemmas, human rights, and application of critical thinking. A group project with a population will incorporate knowledge, skills, and values for basic forensic nursing practice.

Course Objectives: Upon completion of the course, the student will be able to:

1. Define forensic nursing practice and various specialty roles.
2. Define forensic concepts, principles, and terminology.
3. Examine risks and vulnerabilities for victim and criminal populations across the life span.
4. Demonstrate forensic skills of collection, documentation, and preservation of physical and psychological evidence.
5. Analyze prevention and intervention strategies.
6. Discuss the role of the forensic nurse as a courtroom witness.

7. Synthesize ethical, legal, social, and cultural issues that guide forensic nursing practice.

Teaching/Learning Strategies: This course will use a variety of teaching and learning methods, including online seminar and lectures, small group discussions, and independent readings related to forensic nursing roles and responsibilities. Group discussions will address ethical issues and population-specific prevention and intervention strategies and will guide community project development and application.

Evaluation: Quizzes, professional interviews, group community project, discussion group/seminar participation, brief research-based paper, demonstration of forensic skills.

Topical Outline:

I. **Knowledge**
  A. Introduction and overview of forensic nursing
  B. Victimology and criminology
  C. Forensic aspects of the nursing process and forensic populations
  D. Injury identification, interpretation, and documentation
  E. Evidence recognition, collection, preservation, and documentation
  F. Multiprofessional collaboration
  G. Ethical, legal, cultural, and social issues
  H. Research and evidence-based nursing practice

II. **Skill Performance**
  A. Communication skills
  B. The nursing process with forensic populations
  C. Health promotion and prevention
  D. Environmental settings for forensic learning experiences

III. **Values and Attitudes**
  A. Personal issues that impact nurses and provision of care
  B. Professional nursing behavior
  C. Forensic resources for referral, education, and research

---

continued to expand globally. Undergraduate forensic nursing education was not the priority of educators because the undergraduate degree is considered to be a generalist degree. Specialty courses of study are more appropriate for the graduate level of education. Competency development for the forensic advanced practice nurse (APN) originated when a group of forensic nurse educators convened in 2003 at the International Association of Forensic Nursing (IAFN). The committee operated through 2007 as the IAFN Core Curriculum Committee (CCC). The assumptions of the CCC for framing forensic nursing competencies were as follows:

1. Core curriculum and competencies to be identified in the *Scope and Standards of Advanced Practice*

Registered Nursing and *The Essentials for Master's Education for Advanced Practice Nursing* were the foundation of the forensic APN; translation of competencies needed to be developed only in relation to forensic aspects of nursing care.

2. Competencies would apply to all subspecialties in which the forensic APN works.
3. Competencies and core curriculum must be able to be subsumed into existing curricula at different types of institutions.

The CCC used the draft revision of the *Scope and Standards of Forensic Nursing Practice*, currently under review by ANA, and compiled the *Core Competencies for*

Advanced Practice Forensic Nursing, which is currently under review as well.

In line with all APN education, it builds on the competencies that are expected for the undergraduate curriculum. Additional measurement criteria for the forensic APN follow measurement criteria for the forensic nurse under each of the standards of practice. Furthermore, the provided supporting curriculum content and exemplars are consistent with the new ANA template.

Graduate Forensic Nursing Competencies

The forensic APN is expected to develop, implement, and promote knowledge and theory related to nursing care of forensic patients and their families. The forensic APN should be able to develop and oversee care for complex forensic health-care issues from a systems perspective. This represents a leadership role within the health-care structure. Education on forensic nursing concepts, skills, and health care is an expectation of the APN; however, graduate students are expected to learn and apply knowledge and skill beyond the basic nursing competencies. The APN is expected to be involved in research and policy related to forensic patient outcomes. Evidence-based practice patient-outcomes approaches are expected at the undergraduate and graduate levels. The APN, however, is responsible for evaluating the level of evidence related to practice issues and interventions. The APN with leadership responsibilities would be expected to synthesize the comparative scientific research evidence and articulate protocol or institutional policy changes that reflect contemporary best practices. Translation of current research into practice assures that the patients will not only benefit from the health-care perspective, but also from health-care and legal policy issues that may influence funding and care.

While there are few manuscripts in publication regarding the incorporation of research into forensic nursing practice, the forensic APN is ideally positioned to develop an evidence-based practice for patient care. Translation of complex research findings into nursing practice requires evaluating methods and results for application to a particular patient population and setting. The APN uses a transformational theoretical perspective to relate science to patient preferences and to choices for the unique culture and vulnerabilities of special population groups. The most common practices, "what has always been done," may not be the best practice. A practice may not be appropriate or applicable to all population groups, sex groups, or age, racial, or cultural groups. Evidence-based practice may not give a clear answer for every clinical question the forensic nurse is confronted with daily. However, the

framework of evidence-based practice will be a guide toward making the most informed clinical decisions. In the leadership role, the forensic APN has the authority and the ability to transform the thinking of others and to transform the care provided for the patient populations, which should lead to the final responsibility—to maximize the improvement of health outcomes.

In the educational milieu, an example of a forensic APN competency builds on other nursing skills, such as reading and evaluating evidence-based literature. Knowledge can be used to address real issues and improvement of care. Workers can be transformed and clinical care and health of forensic patients improved.

The forensic APN faculty can address the competency of the promotion and implementation of knowledge and theory related to forensic health care. A forensic nursing course can have as a priority goal the application of research into practice. APN students can write clinical questions of interest for their practice area. A variety of tools and Web sites with instructions that explain clinical levels of evidence, the types of clinical questions, study methods, and how to search for evidence-based articles are available for students. Students can compare a number of research studies, rate the levels of evidence, and report on the article with the highest level of evidence. Research findings regarding the similar and related questions, situations, and solutions can be used by the students to generate a change in their practice setting. An evidence-based research critique can be useful to answer the clinical question of interest and to create best practice guidelines in the work setting.

CONCLUSIONS

Educators at all levels of nursing education will be better able to incorporate forensic concepts into basic and advanced knowledge acquisition when guidelines for education are clearly delineated, documented, published, and accessible. The proliferation of forensic nurses globally and the impact of media that influences the public to demand forensic evidence or proof, often called the "CSI effect," have resulted in a demand for forensic nursing knowledge and education at all levels. For the past 20 years, the supply of qualified forensic nursing educators has not met the demands of the learners, partly because the specialty is still in its infancy. Course development and programs of study in nursing are based on specific content designed to maintain a safe and legal practice by developing the consistent ethical thinking of nurses. The state of forensic nursing education is related primarily to the novelty of the practice area; few forensic nursing experts are experienced educational development experts, and fewer still are leaders in education who are qualified as experts in forensic nursing. Therefore, the forensic nursing standards, competencies, and programs are in developmental transition. However, many educational professionals are now setting the stage for evidence-based education and scholarly educational endeavors. All should emphasize the use of the highest levels of evidence into clinical decision making and best practices.

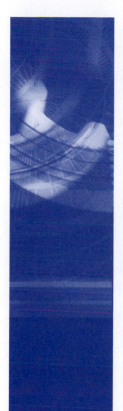

EVIDENCE-BASED PRACTICE

Reference Question: What are the master competencies in forensic nursing education?

Databases to Search: ERIC

Search Strategy: There are a few databases that can be used for this question, but because it is primarily about education, ERIC is one of the better sources. Since ERIC is a database of education materials, only the primary subject needs to be entered for the search. By entering "forensic nursing," the materials searched will all be education based.

Direct Resources: The American Association of Critical-Care Nurses: http://www.aacn.org; The International Association of Forensic Nurses: http://www.iafn.org

Selected References From Search:

1. Campbell, R., Adams, A.E., & Patterson, D. (2008). Methodological challenges of collecting evaluation data from traumatized clients/consumers: A comparison of three methods. *American Journal of Evaluation, 29*(3):369-381.
2. Mannynsalo, L., Putkonen, H., Lindberg, N., & Kotilainen I. (2009). Forensic psychiatric perspective on criminality associated with intellectual disability: A nationwide register-based study. *Journal of Intellectual Disability Research, 53*(3):279-288.

Questions Used to Discern Evidence:

Choose two studies among the studies listed, read about them, and answer the following questions:

1. What are the differences between the two studies in the design, methods, and results?
2. What are the similarities between the two studies in the number of subjects, measures used, and interventions, if any?
3. What competencies do you need to acquire to practice forensic nursing?

REVIEW QUESTIONS

1. A minimum standard of care in forensic nursing would be:
   A. Forensic nursing expertise
   B. Violence-screening intervention
   C. Referral for forensic cases
   D. Basic emergency room skills

2. A concept of the undergraduate forensic aspects of nursing care for new graduates is:
   A. Nursing diagnosis
   B. Forensic pathology
   C. Performance skills
   D. Legal issues

REVIEW QUESTIONS—cont'd

3. Which of the following is the best description of evidence-based nursing education?
   A. Use of research results approved by the AACN
   B. Application of research-based nursing practice
   C. Integration of professional wisdom and empirical evidence in instructional decisions
   D. Publication of nursing research

4. Which of the following is considered to be a component of core competencies for undergraduate forensic nursing education?
   A. Safety
   B. Values and attitudes
   C. Nursing diagnosis
   D. Care plans

5. The practice of forensic nursing requires:
   A. Essential skills that compare to those of law enforcement
   B. Elimination of the nursing process
   C. Occasional breach of confidential information
   D. Working with families

6. Forensic nursing addresses health-care issues that have a:
   A. Medicolegal component
   B. Research component
   C. CSI component
   D. DNA component

7. What factor is a barrier to undergraduate forensic nursing education?
   A. Major health-care problems are the only subjects that should be taught
   B. The market is saturated with proclaimed experts
   C. Students have enhanced competency
   D. Nurse educators possess insufficient forensic knowledge

8. Competency-based undergraduate forensic nursing education includes:
   A. All basic nursing competencies
   B. Nursing diagnoses
   C. Research components
   D. Forensic practice experience

9. Forensic APNs should possess leadership skills that prepare them to:
   A. Prosecute the guilty
   B. Collaborate with police to investigate crimes
   C. Refer all forensic health care issues
   D. Evaluate relevant clinical forensic questions

10. Ethical and social issues in forensic nursing:
    A. Play a minor part in the investigative role
    B. Are overshadowed by evidence collection
    C. Are the base of forensic nursing practice
    D. Rarely impact nursing care in general

References

American Association of Colleges of Nursing (AACN). (2007). Draft revision of: *The essentials of baccalaureate education for professional nursing practice.* Washington, DC: AACN.

American Association of Colleges of Nursing (AACN). (1996). *Essentials of master's education for advanced practice nursing.* Washington, DC: AACN.

American Nurses Association & International Association of Forensic Nurses (ANA & IAFN). (1997). *Scope and standards of forensic nursing practice.* Washington, DC: ANA.

Barber, J.M. (2002). Raising the forensic antenna. *Forensic Nurse, 1:*38.

Bastable, S.B. (2003). *Nurse as educator: Principles of teaching and learning for nursing practice* (2nd ed.). Sudbury, MA: Jones & Barlett.

Beecroft, P.C., Kunzman, L.A., Taylor, S., et al. (2004). Bridging the gap between school and workplace: Developing a new graduate nurse curriculum. *Journal of Nursing Administration, 34:*338-345.

Blair, M. (2002). Violence in society: Nursing faculty respond to a health care epidemic. *Journal of Nursing Education, 41:*360-361.

Burgess, A.W., Berger, A.D., & Boersma, R.R. (2004). Forensic nursing. *American Journal of Nursing, 104*(3):58-64.

Burns, H.K., & Foley, S.M. (2005). Building a foundation for an evidence-based approach to practice: Teaching basic concepts to undergraduate freshman students. *Journal of Professional Nursing, 21:*351-357.

Commission on Collegiate Nursing Education. (2003). *Standards for accreditation of baccalaureate and graduate nursing programs.* Retrieved November 4, 2004, from http://www.aacn.nche/Accreditation.com

Cowan, D.T., Norman, I., & Coopamah, V.P. (2005). Competence in nursing practice: A controversial concept. A focused review of literature. *Nurse Education Today, 25:*355-362.

Dalley, K., Candela, L., & Benzel-Lindley, J. (2008). Learning to let go: The challenge of de-crowding the curriculum. *Nurse Education Today, 28*(1):62-69.

Davies, B., & Hughes, A.M. (2002). Clarification of advanced nursing practice: Characteristics and competencies. *Clinical Nurse Specialist, 16*:147-152.

Evans, A.M., & Wells, D. (2001). Scope of practice in forensic nursing. *Journal of Psychosocial Nursing, 39*(1):38-54.

Fawcett, J., Newman, D.M., & McAllister, M. (2004). Advanced practice nursing and conceptual models of nursing. *Nursing Science Quarterly, 17*:135-138.

Fey, M.K., & Miltner, R.S. (2000). A competency-based orientation program for new graduate nurses. *Journal of Nursing Administration, 30*:126-132.

Field, D.E. (2004). Moving from novice to expert—The value of learning in clinical practice: A literature review. *Nurse Education Today, 24*:560-565.

Finkelman, A., & Kenner, C. (2007). *Teaching IOM: Implications of the IOM reports for nursing education.* Silver Spring, MD: American Nurses Association.

Foss, G.G., Janken, J.K., Langford, D.R., et al. (2004). Using professional specialty competencies to guide course development. *Journal of Nursing Education, 43*:368-388.

Freedberg, P. (2005). Domestic violence in same-sex relationships. *On the Edge, 11*:1, 4-10.

Freedberg, P. (2008). Integrating forensic nursing into the undergraduate nursing curriculum: A solution for a disconnect. *Journal of Nursing Education, 47*(5):201-207.

Fulton, J.S. (2003). It's about practice competencies. *Clinical Nurse Specialist, 17*:176-177.

Fulton, J.S. (2006). In search of advanced clinical nurse specialist education. *Journal for Advanced Nursing Practice, 20*:114-115.

Henry, T. (2004). Forensic nursing. *Alaska Nurse, 54:*6.

Hood, L.J., & Leddy, S.K. (2003). *Conceptual bases of professional nursing* (5th ed.). Philadelphia: Lippincott Williams & Wilkins.

Hoyt, K.S., & Warner, C.G. (2005). Introduction. *Topics in Emergency Medicine, 27*:1-2.

Hufft, A.G. (2006). Theoretical foundations for advanced practice forensic nursing. In R.M. Hammer, B. Moynihan, & E.M. Pagliaro (Eds.), *Forensic nursing.* Sudbury, MA: Jones & Barlett, pp. 41-58.

International Association of Forensic Nurses (IAFN). (2004). *Core competencies for advanced practice forensic nursing.* Retrieved May 31, 2008, from http://www.iafn.org

International Association of Forensic Nurses (IAFN). (2004). *International Association of Forensic Nurses 12th annual scientific assembly.* Program book. Chicago: IAFN.

International Association of Forensic Nurses (IAFN). (2005). *Scope and standards for forensic nursing practice.* Manuscript in preparation.

Iwasiw, C.L., Goldenberg, D., & Andrusyszyn, M. (2005). *Curriculum development in nursing education.* Sudbury, MA: Jones & Barlett.

Janssen, P.A., Keen, L., Soolsma, J., et al. (2005). Perinatal nursing education for single-room maternity care: An evaluation of a competency-based model. *Journal of Clinical Nursing, 14*:95-101.

Keating, S.B. (2006). *Curriculum development and evaluation in nursing.* Philadelphia: Lippincott Williams & Wilkins.

Keating, S.B., Rutledge, D.N., Sargent, A., et al. (2003). A test of the California competency-based differentiated role model. *Managed Care Quarterly, 11*(1):40-46.

Lynch, V. (1993). Forensic nursing: Diversity in education and practice. *Journal of Psychosocial Nursing, 31*(11): 7-14.

Lynch, V. (1995). Clinical forensic nursing: A new perspective in the management of crime victims from trauma to trail. *Critical Care Nursing Clinics of North America, 7*:489-507.

Lynch, V. (1997). *Clinical forensic nursing: A new perspective in trauma and medicolegal investigation of death.* Ft. Collins, CO: Bearhawk Consulting Group.

Lynch, V. (Ed.). (2006a). *Forensic nursing.* St. Louis, MO: Elsevier Mosby.

Lynch, V. (2006b). Forensic nursing science. In R.M. Hammer, B. Moynihan, & E.M. Pagliaro (Eds.), *Forensic nursing.* Sudbury, MA: Jones & Barlett, pp. 1-40.

Lynch, V., Roach, C.W., & Sadler, D.W. (2006). Education and credentialing for forensic nurses. In V. Lynch (Ed.), *Forensic nursing.* Sudbury, MA: Jones & Barlett, pp. 593-604.

Markenson, D., DiMaggio, C., & Redlener, I. (2005). Preparing health professional students for terrorism, disaster, and public health emergencies: Core competencies. *Academic Medicine, 80*:517-526.

Martin, N. (2007). *Development of a competency-based, undergraduate instructional program for forensic nursing with plans for implementation and evaluation.* Unpublished doctoral dissertation. Nova Southeastern University, Ft. Lauderdale, FL.

McKay, Y.D. (2002). Forensic nursing: A challenge for nursing education. *Forensic Nurse, 1*:34-35.

McLean, C., Monger, E., & Lally, I. (2005). Assessment of practice using the National Health Service knowledge and skills framework. *Nursing in Critical Care, 10:*136-142.

Meretoja, R., Isoaho, H., & Leino-Kilpi, H. (2004). Nurse competence scale: Development and psychometric testing. *Journal of Advanced Nursing, 47*:124-133.

Morrison, G.R., Ross, S.M., & Kemp, J.E. (2004). *Designing effective instruction* (4th ed.). Hoboken, NJ: John Wiley & Sons.

National Council of State Boards of Nursing. (2005). *Clinical instruction in prelicensure nursing programs.* Retrieved November 1, 2006, from http://www.ncsbn.org

National Council of State Boards of Nursing. (2006). *Evidence-based nursing education for regulation (EBNER).* Retrieved November 1, 2006, from http://www.ncsbn.org

Pyrek, K.M. (2003). Forensic nursing pioneers ponder the future (Electronic version). *Forensic Nurse.* Retrieved March 5, 2003, from http://www.forensicnursingmag.com/articles/3blcover.html

Ramritu, P.L., & Barnard, A. (2001). New nurse graduates' understanding of competence. *International Nursing Review, 48*:47-57.

Sekula, K.L. (2005). The advance practice forensic nurse in the emergency department. *Topics in Emergency Medicine, 27*:5-14.

Stevens, S. (2004). Cracking the case: Your role in forensic nursing. *Nursing, 34:*54-56.

Suling, L., & Kenward, K. (2006). *A national survey on elements of nursing education.* Retrieved March 28, 2008, from http://ncsbn.org

Tanner, C.A. (2001). Competency-based education: The new panacea? *Journal of Nursing Education, 40*:387-388.

U.S. Department of Health and Human Services. (2000). Injury and violence prevention. In *Healthy people 2010: Understanding and improving health* (2nd ed.), pp. 5-61. Retrieved December 28, 2005, from http://www.healthypeople.gov/Document/html/uih/uih_4.htm#injviol

Utley-Smith, Q. (2004). Five competencies needed by new baccalaureate graduates. *Nursing Education Perspectives, 25*:166-170.

Whitehurst, J. (2006). *Evidence-based education.* Retrieved March 24, 2008, from http://www.ed.gov/offices/OERI/presentations/evidencebase.html

Woodtli, M.A. (2000). Domestic violence and the nursing curriculum: Tuning in and tuning up. *Journal of Nursing Education, 39*:173-182.

Woodtli, M.A., & Breslin, E.T. (2002). Violence-related content in the nursing curriculum: A follow-up national survey. *Journal of Nursing Education, 41*:340-348.

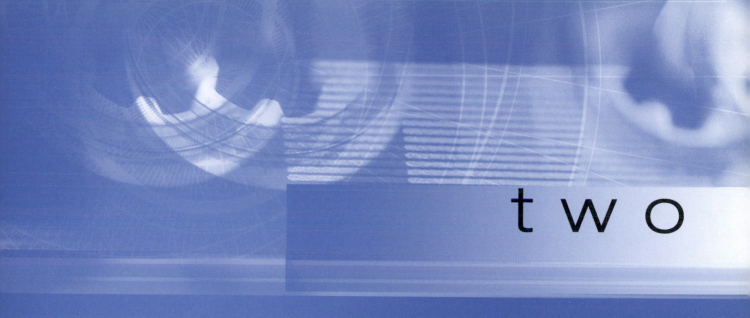

two

FORENSIC NURSING IN INTERPERSONAL VIOLENCE

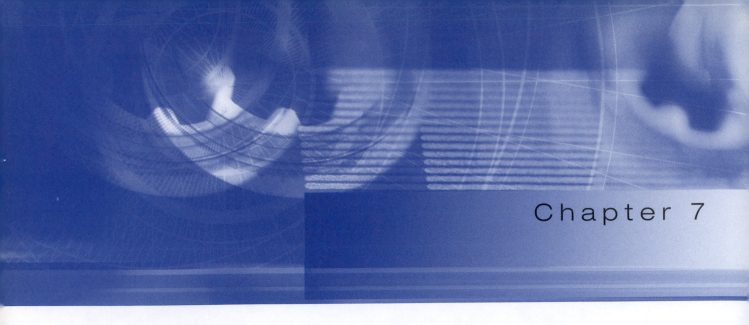

Chapter 7

Typology of Violence: A Global Challenge

Louanne Lawson and Sara Rowe

"For knowledge too is itself a power."
Bacon

Competencies

1. Articulating the need for clear definition of the concept of violence.
2. Discussing the theories of violence.
3. Delineating the critical attributes and characteristics of violence.
4. Discussing the role of context in relation to violence.
5. Exploring the fluid dynamics of violence over time.
6. Defining consequences of violence.

Key Terms

Aggression
Context
Control
Destruction
Domestic violence
Prevention
Violence

INTRODUCTION

Violence is a violation of the fundamental human need for safety. All people, whatever their age, gender, sexual orientation, or place of residence, are at risk, and the consequences are dire. Females' lifetime exposure to partner violence, for example, is estimated to be 20% to 50% worldwide. Violence in the workplace is both physical and psychological, and males are only slightly less exposed to violence than females. Health-care providers, in particular, are subjected to verbal abuse, threats, and physical assault, making violence a serious personal as well as professional issue. The high cost of violence is drained from multiple system resources, including criminal justice, health care, and mental health. Violence also affects child services, housing, and employment, making it a social and economic problem as well.

Efforts to prevent violence include attempts to reduce or control access to weapons, attempts to increase public awareness of the nature and impact of violence, and officially sanctioned intervention guidelines. **Prevention** efforts are widespread and passionate, but few have evaluated outcomes. Thus, which attempts have value will remain unclear until concerted efforts address audience, impact, cost, and accountability; coordinate systematic efforts; and examine the predictive factors.

UNDERSTANDING THE CONCEPT: DEFINING VIOLENCE

A clear understanding of violence is crucial. The purpose of this chapter is to define the concept of violence; clarify the related antecedents, consequences, and critical attributes; and discuss the role of the forensic nurse.

The antecedents, consequences, and critical attributes of violence change over time. In 1990, for example, war was ranked 16 in a list of the 19 leading causes of death. However, it is projected that by 2020 it will be ranked as 8 in the leading causes of death. Interpersonal violence and self-inflicted injuries are also going up in ranking, from 19 to 12 for interpersonal violence and from 17 to 14 for suicide. Furthermore, new forms of violence are being identified. For example, the National Center on Health Statistics developed the classification of "terrorism death" after the September 11, 2001, terrorist attacks.

As the phenomenon of violence changes, so must the nursing response. Without a clearly articulated definition, it is virtually impossible to measure violence, identify and test interventions, or develop guidelines for clinical practice.

Violence is an observable phenomenon as well as a private experience. The evolutionary method of concept analysis is particularly useful for developing nursing knowledge because it helps nurses identify the characteristics of the problems that violence causes. Furthermore, the need for clinically relevant background questions lays the foundation for evidence-based research to support timely prevention efforts, clinical interventions, and promotion of clear communication among disciplines, as well as contribute to theory development and facilitate categorizations of the fluid phenomenon of violence.

Myriad societal issues make it necessary to identify how the concept of violence has changed over time. Some issues that contribute to the shifting definition of violence include current events; war; abuse of elders, persons with disabilities, and vulnerable populations; and the rise of forensic nursing care of victims and others exposed to violence. The shifting definition results in challenges for professionals working on the development of clinical guidelines, research programs, administrative frameworks, and educational curricula that guide professional practice.

Without a clearly articulated definition, it is virtually impossible to measure violence, generate potential interventions, or develop evidence-based guidelines for clinical practice. Violence is a violation of fundamental human need for safety. All people, whatever their age, gender, sexual orientation, or place of residence, are at risk, and there are far-reaching after-effects of violence in all groups.

Violence is characterized by behavior intended to cause harm. Context is a key feature of violence. Two major changes took place related to the concept from 1990 to 2006: (1) criteria used to classify the circumstances leading to injury were expanded to include legal intervention, unintentional firearm death, terrorism death, and events of undetermined intent, and (2) nursing interventions were refined to include cultural considerations, the relationships between intimate partner violence and child maltreatment, and the mental health–care needs of victims and aggressors.

METHODOLOGY

The identification of aspects of violence that are particularly relevant to nursing is critical. Health-care literature was examined during two periods, 1990 to 1995 and 2000 to 2005. For the years 1990 to 1995, a convenient sample of articles and book chapters on the Cumulative

Nursing and Allied Health Literature (CINAHL) selected. For 2000 to 2005, articles that were indexed on Medline, the Cochrane Databases, CINAHL, PsycInfo, and Psychology and Behavioral Sciences Collection were identified. All were English-language articles published in peer-reviewed journals. Dissertations were excluded.

Search results included 55 articles and book chapters, of which 27 were published between 1990 and 1995, and 28 were published from 2000 to 2005. All included "violence" and "definition" as subject terms. References to definitions of violence were included in the abstracts of 22 of the articles.

CONTEXT AS AN ATTRIBUTE OF VIOLENCE

Context includes aggressor characteristics, culture, the setting in which the violence occurs, and systems designed to identify or prevent violence. Violent aggressors were identified as bullies or persons operating under the influence of illicit drugs. They were responding to some level of perceived provocation or intrusion.

Culture determines what constitutes violence, and cultural influences can be paradoxical. In China, for example, "aggression is disapproved in general because the Chinese culture emphasizes harmony, discipline, and self-restraints [sic] in interpersonal relationship. On the other hand, traditional Chinese culture also embraces rigid gender norms and patriarchal values conducive to the exploitation of women and even VAW (Violence Against Women)." In the United States, in some states women are prosecuted for allowing their children to remain in violent households, but adequate protection and support for extricating these women from abusive situations are often unavailable. A culture that holds an abused woman responsible for the safety of her children while ignoring the aggressor's actions or the victim's needs is operating paradoxically, leaving victim with limited options. This cultural paradox makes women particularly vulnerable to violence because it offers no way to find a solution.

Violence occurs in multiple settings, including the victim's or aggressor's home or other residence; fast-food restaurants; bars, taverns, or other commercial locations; the workplace; outdoors; in a variety of institutional settings for children, the elderly, and the mentally ill; and in correctional facilities. Violence also occurs in the context of relationships. There are instances of violence between strangers; however, it is far more common that the victim and aggressor are at least acquainted with one another.

The systems designed to identify and track violence include the Uniform Crime Reporting Program, managed by the Federal Bureau of Investigation (FBI); the ICD-10, managed by the International Classification of Diseases; and the National Vital Statistics System (NVSS), a mortality reporting system used throughout the United States. Prevention systems include those in the public health system, the individual workplace, and schools. Such systems recognize that violence is not an individual, episodic issue but rather is a global problem rooted in social, economic, and organizational contexts. Social systems organize efforts to prevent violence associated with urbanization, housing problems, stigmatization, educational disparities, employment, family life, women's equity, alcohol and drug abuse, firearms, prejudice, and poverty. For example, one school-based violence prevention system "attempts to alter the climate of a school by teaching students and staff simple rules and activities aimed at improving child social competence and reducing aggressive behavior."

CRITICAL ATTRIBUTES

The critical attributes of violence are behavior, intention, and harm. Violent behavior includes hitting, intimidation, strong-arming, and the use of a weapon, including threats made with a weapon in hand. Other behaviors are biting, kicking, mobbing, punching, scratching, squeezing, attacks by animals that are instigated by humans, sabotage of machinery with the intent of causing injury, stabbing and shooting, rape, and pushing, shoving, grabbing, or throwing something (Table 7.1).

Harm may take the form of physical, psychological, or emotional injury. For instance, persons who experience intimate partner violence often claim that the multiple episodes of demeaning, insulting, and trivializing statements made by their partners over the years are much more painful than being physically injured with a fist or an object. Other forms of harm include educational difficulties, deteriorating health status, and rage, guilt, and hatred. One family member, in discussing the family's responses to the murder of a loved one, said, "I want him dead, but I want him never to stop suffering." The harm may be experienced by a third person, as is the case when a child witnesses the beating or murder of a parent.

Intent is defined as "the plan and will to act in a particular way." The aggressor's intent may be to harm a person directly through targeted individual action; indirectly, by exposure to a violent act intended for another; or by proxy, as is the case when victims of violence engage in

TABLE 7.1 **Critical Attributes and Examples**

Critical Attribute	Example	
Behavior	Attacks by animals that are instigated by humans	Sabotage of machinery
	Biting	Scratching
	Grabbing	Shooting
	Hitting	Shoving
	Intimidation	Squeezing
	Kicking	Stabbing
	Mobbing	Strong-arming
	Punching	Threats made with a weapon in hand
	Pushing	Throwing something
	Rape	Use of a weapon
Intention	Direct, indirect, or by proxy	
	Rationalized	
Harm	Physical, psychological, or emotional injury	
	Educational difficulties	
	Deteriorating health status	
	Rage, guilt, and hatred	
	May be experienced by a third person or entity	

assaultive behavior themselves. The nature of the intent may be rationalized. A parent may injure a child and say that the intent was to discipline, rather than harm, the child. In some contexts it is possible to understand violence as a type of action that "fulfils a particular psychological function, namely the ridding of unwanted mental contents" or that serves the purpose of achieving something desirable, such as fighting a war for freedom.

Behavior and harm are objective and therefore observable. Intent, however, is a subjective phenomenon and can only be inferred. For instance, the intent of a parent may not be to cause harm but to stop a child's dangerous behavior. The child runs toward the street and so the parent spanks the child, thereby preventing the greater harm. Therefore, the action cannot be called violent. Conflict emerges when an interested party not directly involved in the behavior, such as a victim rights advocate, considers an act violent but the aggressor does not. Before interventions can be successful, an agreement must be reached in regard to whose perception is to be considered definitive: that of the aggressor, the victim or victims, or the third-party observer. It is tempting to modify the definition, as Rippon has done, to read, "Violence is an act carried out with the intention or perceived as having intention of physically hurting another person." Even though Rippon's definition is useful from a theoretical perspective, it is less

useful from a practical point of view. Where there is conflict regarding the nature of the intention, it must be resolved among the parties directly involved before progress can be made toward resolution of the problem.

The global society also allows for a variety of cultural practices and valued norms to be called into question. When there are actions taken with no intention to harm, but there is a perception of harm by the dominant society, the actions may be actually against the law. When cultural practices and behaviors that are illegal are carried out, there may be significant repercussions on all persons involved: the actor, the recipient of the harmful act, the family, and community. One example is the tradition of female genital cutting (circumcision or mutilation). Some cultural groups will not allow a woman to return home after childbirth unless the vagina has been "closed," or sutured, afterward. She may be harmed by the procedure or harmed by being an outcast from her family.

ANTECEDENTS

The antecedents of violence include aggression and power imbalance. **Aggression** may be directed toward self, others, or objects. Other forms of aggression, particularly in the workplace, include aggressive posturing; deliberate silence; denigration/harassment based on age, class, disability, ethnicity, gender, race, religion, or sexual orientation; exclusion from the social community; hostile behavior; innuendo; interference with work; irrational and/or unreasonable demands; name calling; offensive messages by telephone, e-mail, fax, or text message; ostracism; rude gestures; shouting; swearing; and threats.

Antecedents of violence also include hopelessness and fearlessness, especially in instances of youth violence. Hopelessness comes from the sense that there is no place for many young people in the community. Fearlessness comes from the sense that there is nothing to lose by being violent. The result is that those young people perceive that a certain amount of recognition and material goods stand to be gained and little of value is to be lost when they act violently.

The most common power imbalance identified in the review of literature from 1990 to 1995 was economic. Youth violence flourished in conditions of high unemployment, depressed economic conditions, and high population density. Nelson compared the social response to economic conditions in the 19th century with that of modern times. The economic power imbalance was said to arise in the 1800s, when the benefits of mechanization went to the owners of factories rather than to the workers.

There was an influx of cheap immigrant labor that enabled employers to hire adult male workers rather than less reliable younger ones.

In contemporary times, a large proportion of teenage males find no place for themselves in the workplace. **Control** is the primary emphasis, in the form of intermediate youth detention facilities, also known as "boot camps," which were popular in the 1980s. Welfare benefit cuts and emphasis on mandatory employment are other forms of control with no resolution of problems or imminent meaningful work.

CONSEQUENCES

The consequences of violence are injury, continuation of the cycle of violence, and prevention efforts. Direct or more immediate effects of violence include intentional injury, death, and fear of future violence. Also, war, captivity, personal attack, abduction, and torture result in fear, helplessness, and horror. Further consequences of violence include long-term effects such as the potential or actual continuation of the cycle of violence and post-traumatic stress disorder (PTSD).

The *International Classification of Diseases*, Ninth Edition (ICD-9), which was the system used in hospitals to delineate medical disorders in the early 1990s, included a section for injuries called external cause of injury (E-code). E-codes for injuries caused by violence were divided into two main categories: homicide and suicide. Homicide was defined as "injuries inflicted by another person with intent to injure or kill by any means"; suicide was defined as "self-inflicted injuries specified as intentional." Injuries categorized with homicide included assault, rape, and child abuse. The ICD-10 expanded the E-code to include legal intervention, unintentional firearm death, terrorism death, events of undetermined intent as well as the extended repercussions of violent injury.

Repercussions include disruption of the work environment and interpersonal relationships, costs associated with lost work time, and the inability to function in a role, including work-related and intimate relationship roles. Violence experienced in childhood may result in isolation, alcoholism, criminality, low self-esteem, self-destructive behavior, and difficulty asking to have needs met and meeting the personal needs of others. Children exposed to war and other forms of political violence demonstrate behavioral disorders; impaired social, educational, and emotional development and disordered development of speech accompanied by a longing for a safe place. Adverse childhood experiences such as abuse, neglect, and household dysfunction place the child at higher risk for co-occurring health problems.

A second consequence of violence is the potential for the continuation of the cycle of violence. The tension-violence-contrition cycle has been reported as characteristic in the context of intimate partner violence. Less familiar but equally important is the problem of children carrying weapons to school in an effort to protect themselves from violent age-mates. Youths who have been assaulted or have adverse experiences are at greater risk for toxic stress that leads to higher rates of self-directed violence and to developing assaultive behavior within a year of their initial injury.

Violence-prevention efforts are a direct consequence of violence, especially youth violence. Violence-prevention efforts include health education, home visits, and mentoring programs set in primary care clinics, school-based health centers, full-service schools, and visiting nurse associations. Some prevention programs focus on the skills and attitudes needed for growth-enhancing social interactions.

The Centers for Disease Control and Prevention consider violence to be a preventable public health problem. Their Violence Prevention page features a variety of funded projects, resources, and lists of evidence-based prevention programs for various populations and types of violence. Social structures considered to be less vulnerable to the threat of violence are those that consider health as a collective responsibility as well as a personal good; that use democratic-style decision making within an egalitarian atmosphere; and that take the future into account in decision making. Reactive interventions, including on-site security, metal detectors, and surveillance cameras in the emergency department (ED), have been instituted to protect ED staff from patients' violent responses to power imbalance. More proactive interventions have included skill building, mentoring programs, decision control, professional competence, risk assessment, and community-based decision making.

AN EXEMPLAR

The familiar story of Cain and Abel illustrates the context within which violence takes place and the aggression, hopelessness, fearlessness, and power imbalance that precede a violent act. It shows the behavior intended to cause harm that must be present and the injury, potential for continuation of the cycle of violence, and efforts at preventing further violence that follow.

Case Study

Adam lay with his wife Eve, and she became pregnant and gave birth to Cain. She said, "With the help of the Lord I have brought forth a man." Later she gave birth to his brother Abel.	Antecedents, consequences, and critical attributes
Now Abel kept flocks, and Cain worked the soil. In the course of time Cain brought some of the fruits of the soil as an offering to the Lord. But Abel brought fat portions from some of the firstborn of his flock.	Context
The Lord looked with favor on Abel and his offering, but on Cain and his offering he did not look with favor.	Power imbalance
So Cain was very angry, and his face was downcast.	Aggression
Then the Lord said to Cain, "Why are you angry? Why is your face downcast? If you do what is right, will you not be accepted? But if you do not do what is right, sin is crouching at your door; it desires to have you, but you must master it."	Hopelessness Fearlessness
Now Cain said to his brother Abel, "Let's go out to the field." And while they were in the field, Cain attacked his brother Abel . . .	Intention to cause harm
. . . and killed him.	Injury
Then the Lord said to Cain, "Where is your brother Abel?"	Continuation of the cycle of violence
"I don't know," he replied. "Am I my brother's keeper?"	
The Lord said, "What have you done? Listen! Your brother's blood cries out to me from the ground. Now you are under a curse and driven from the ground, which opened its mouth to receive your brother's blood from your hand. When you work the ground, it will no longer yield its crops for you. You will be a restless wanderer on the earth." Cain said to the Lord, "My punishment is more than I can bear. Today you are driving me from the land, and I will be hidden from your presence; I will be a restless wanderer on the earth, and whoever finds me will kill me."	
But the Lord said to him, "Not so; if anyone kills Cain, he will suffer vengeance seven times over." Then the Lord put a mark on Cain so that no one who found him would kill him.	Prevention efforts

NURSING RESPONSE TO VIOLENCE

Nurses play a significant role in violence remediation and prevention because they provide health care in every social context. The nursing response to violence takes the form of interventions that target both the victim and the aggressor in every age group. Interventions can also include nursing action in every environmental context at all levels of society and in all systems. Nurses should help promote community-based decision making and all members of the family.

The nursing response to violence includes the context within which the victim and aggressor interact. Clinicians, educators, administrators, and researchers should address the factors that influence violence, including the type of violence, the populations involved, and its etiology, so that they may identify violent situations, plan appropriate activities, and carefully evaluate the results of their efforts. Violence prevention is preferable to violence remediation. It costs less in terms of human suffering, lost wages and productivity, health-care costs, and costs to the criminal justice system.

Clinicians who intervene to alter individual aggressor characteristics, such as cognitive appraisal, affective response, and intrinsic motivation, are addressing a critical issue, but it is not sufficient. Nurses must create a context that supports the development of autonomy, self-efficacy, and self-control to effectively prevent violence and its repercussions. Nurses may be involved in therapeutic interactions with the aggressors, with the staff in correctional communities or schools, or with families of the aggressor.

Recognizing that aggressive behavior does not generally follow a simple, linear trajectory is crucial. It is a mistake to focus exclusively on individual factors. Clinicians must come to terms with this unfamiliar responsibility. They may feel unprepared, both personally and professionally, to address a problem for which they have ed training and administrative support. Nurses should develop an understanding of the sociocultural context.

Nurses in the school system are an integral part of activities designed to prevent violence, especially when the activities are contextualized rather than situation-specific. In one school-based program, for example, children and staff all learn the same pro-social rules and use the same terminology, thus incorporating praise for other people, avoiding put-downs, having wise people as advisers and friends, taking notice and correcting hurtful behavior, and making right the wrongs done.

School violence, and, by extension, school violence prevention, takes place in the context of the larger community. Nurses can help promote community-based decision making, strength-focused interventions, carefully crafted goals, and involvement of all members of the school community. Prevention programs should indicate zero tolerance for violence, along with clear guidelines for intervening in aggression and other precursors to violence, carefully delineated lines of authority and responsibility, and procedures for balancing communication with confidentiality. Nurses who develop after-school programs for potentially violent youth should provide information designed to promote hope by enhancing nonviolent problem-solving skills. Also included must be emotional support that recognizes the personal characteristics and capacity for decision making by the students.

At another system level, such as the workplace, nurses are in key positions to create health promotion and violence prevention. Nurses recognize that it takes everyone involved to support pro-social behaviors. Workplace health promotion can go beyond responding to violent incidents and toward empowering both employers and employees to focus their efforts on taking responsibility for all facets of violence prevention.

Prevention efforts are maximally effective when a multiprofessional effort is the focus. Nurses in the school and work settings need to know about the types of weapons being brought onto the campus or workplace to prepare for emergency management of injuries in case a violent incident occurs.

Victims of political violence may be seen in a variety of contextual settings: school, work, health care, legal, correctional, and others. Skilled nursing interventions may be needed. Victims should be supported as they express their sense of loss, identify the meaning of strength and weakness, adjust to being in a safe place, and reexperience negative past events. They should be encouraged to tell their stories within a safe and supportive environment. They should have the opportunity to examine, and perhaps redefine, the nature of their own strength. Those who feel paralyzed by the threat or memory of their experiences may benefit from sharing how they have learned to cope with uncertainty. A place that symbolizes safety because it cannot be destroyed can be created within their memory or situation.

Nurses in educational settings should teach nursing students to be conversant in the laws and regulations that guide identification of violent behavior, reporting, and testimony. Educators must carefully evaluate frameworks for providing postgraduate education about violence, such as that developed by the International Society for Education and Research in Psychiatric and Mental Health Nursing (SERPN) and that being developed by Martin and others. Integration into nursing education of concepts that can help screen, evaluate, and prevent violence and its negative impact will empower educators and advance knowledge in future generations of nurses.

Nursing administrators recognize the importance of context in everyday nursing activities and are familiar with involving patients in the care-planning process. They are responsible for providing structural support and adequate resources. In long-term care settings, recognition of the residents' need for autonomy in decision making opens the door to innovative approaches to violence prevention. Work groups with the representation, resources, and authority to address violence in the workplace can be formed. In the workplace, a policy group including representatives from management and the workforce, along with violence prevention experts, can be created. The policy group should identify the factors within the workplace that can lead to violence, including attitudes toward violence, likely sources of violence, and the current response when violence occurs. The worker-on-worker violence, worker-patient violence, and worker-visitor violence should be considered. A policy group can anticipate situations antecedent to violence, develop prevention policies, provide support when violence occurs, develop reporting mechanisms, and identify ways to prevent future events.

The work group should develop policies to guide clinicians, educators, students, families, and patients when a violent event occurs. Work groups should comprise credible and nonbiased workers who represent all potentially involved groups and who are not personally or professionally invested in a situation. Ethical, legal, social, cultural, and health-care issues should be considered for all stages of anticipation, policy development, prevention, assessment, and reporting to ensure a comprehensive approach. If appropriate, methods of maintaining patient, student, visitor, and other confidentiality, as well as reporting to the appropriate authorities inside and outside the institution, should be considered and should also address conflicts of interest.

Those developing programs of research in violence may struggle with the need for explicit definitions of terms, sound theoretical frameworks that are appropriate for the phenomenon of interest, the area of nursing practice, and reliable measurement instruments. Clinical judgment enhances predictive theoretical model design. Sound, sensible, and well-grounded protocols with valid instruments for individual and contextual factors, their relationships, and evaluation outcomes will lead to reproducible research studies that expand knowledge. Nursing research in violence and prevention must take into account both individual and universal factors because effective prevention efforts will depend on incorporation of both.

DISCUSSION

The major elements of violence are (1) an aggressor, (2) aggressor behavior that is intended to cause harm, (3) intent, (4) harm from physical, psychological, or emotional injury, and (5) a recipient of the aggression. The aggressor forms intent to behave in a specific way to cause interpersonal, systemic, or global harm to the subject of the aggression. The intent may be direct, indirect, or enacted by proxy to cause physical or psychological injury. Injury that results from violence alerts the social structure to respond with attempts to ameliorate the injury and prevent the behavior, intention, and harm in the future.

If the elements are not met, then the phenomenon is not violence, although it may be a phenomenon related to violence. Aggression is necessary for violence to occur, but it is not sufficient in and of itself to meet all the critical attributes of violence. Other phenomena that are commonly, but mistakenly, considered synonymous with violence or aggression are intimidation, **destruction,** and hostility. However, destruction may occur due to violence or aggression, but if intent is missing, then prevention efforts may not be adequate. Nursing interventions must be examined for appropriateness, and the focus may need to be directed toward prevention of physical or mental illness of individuals, or its exacerbation, as in the role of a forensic mental health nurse.

Macro forces such as social and cultural background, socioeconomic conditions, urbanization, and political and legal circumstances affect local settings. Local settings, including the home, the school, neighborhood, and workplace, influence individual behavior. Individuals who lack characteristics such as resilience and social skills are more likely to engage in violent behaviors, including self-directed, interpersonal, and group violence. Violent acts have an impact on social morbidity, mortality, and general individual well-being. The high cost of violence can only be estimated and is absorbed by legal, health-care, social, and political systems.

All systems must participate in anticipating, preventing, and intervening with all types of violence. Prevention efforts depend on health-care, community, school, and government systems, and a multiprofessional approach must be used to continue to improve the quality of life and strive for life without violence. Violence is always influenced by the context in which the aggressor and victim interact. Violence is not only an individual, episodic issue, but also is a global problem rooted in social, economic, and organizational contexts. The nature and characteristics of the context must be made explicit so that nurses and nursing systems will recognize that patient-specific interventions, while necessary, are insufficient to solve the problem.

EVIDENCE-BASED PRACTICE

Nursing interventions for violence currently focus on identification and treatment of injuries caused by violence. Between 1995 and 2005, nursing interventions were refined to incorporate cultural considerations, address the complex relationships between **domestic violence** and child maltreatment, and identify the mental health-care needs of victims and aggressors. Administrators are beginning to recognize and address safety considerations that arise when screening policies are implemented. Nursing research is being conducted to find ways to intervene with women who are living in abusive situations and to support women who have removed themselves and their children. Nurse educators are beginning to develop continuing education opportunities and evaluate the results. Evidence-based education and evidence-based forensic nursing research courses are being developed to help students access literature and evaluate the current state of knowledge so that they may answer clinical questions in forensic nursing subspecialties.

Multiple disciplines, especially education and business professionals, published position papers, studies, and program outlines that identified prevention strategies. Violence research is more well-developed in fields other than nursing, and the contribution of nursing to research on violence and injury is appropriate and inevitable and will be valuable to the future of forensic nursing.

Violence occurs universally, but the literature reviewed for this analysis was limited to English-language publications. Because of the subtle relationships between language and the experience of people exposed to violence in different cultures, the application of violence research globally is limited, which reduces its applicability globally as well. Furthermore, it can be argued that using the term "violence" to "cover such an array of experience is confusing, ultimately self-defeating, and may create more problems than it resolves." There is such a wide range of behaviors, intentions, and harmful results that investigators and others often stipulate a definition to be used in the particular instance rather than try to use a universal definition. While it may be expedient, this practice makes it difficult to build a program of violence-focused research. The definition, antecedents, critical attributes, and consequences of violence are relatively arbitrary. While they are grounded in published material, other equally grounded and rigorously conducted analysis might result in a different set of characteristics.

CONCLUSIONS

The findings of this evolutionary concept analysis of violence are consistent with the definition of violence published by the World Health Organization in 2002: "The intentional use of physical force or power, threatened or actual, against oneself, another person, or against a group or community, that either results in or has high likelihood of resulting in injury, death, psychological harm, mal-development or deprivation." (Krug et al, 2002, p. 5)

By designating violence a public health issue, the World Health Organization implies, but does not state explicitly, that violence is always influenced by the context within which the aggressor and victim interact. The nature and characteristics of the context must be made explicit so that nurses and nursing systems will recognize that patient-specific interventions, while necessary, are insufficient for addressing the problem. Possessing a firm knowledge of the concept through its antecedents, attributes, and consequences allows for directed studies, research and prevention, and intervention efforts that will improve the health outcomes of persons exposed to violence.

EVIDENCE-BASED PRACTICE BOX

Reference Question: What are the current (within the last year) tested interventions for pedophilia?

Database(s) to Search: PubMed

Search Strategy: Using the MeSH term "pedophilia" works best when limiting the search to the last year. "Treatment" or "therapy" could be used with "AND" to get more specific results.

Selected References From Search:

1. Cohen, L.J., Grebchenko, Y.F., Steinfeld, M., Frenda S.J., et al. (2008). Comparison of personality traits in pedophiles, abstinent opiate addicts, and healthy controls: Considering pedophilia as an addictive behavior. *Journal Nervous & Mental Dieases, 196*(11):829-837.
2. Guay, D.R. (2009). Drug treatment of paraphilic and nonparaphilic sexual disorders. *Clinical Therapeutics, 31*(1):1-31.
3. Seto, M.C. (2009). Pedophilia. *Annual Review of Clinical Psychology, 5*:391-407.

Questions Used to Discern Evidence:

Choose two studies among the studies listed, read about them, and answer the following questions:

1. What are the differences between the two studies in the design, methods, and results?
2. What are the similarities between the two studies in the number of subjects, measures used, and interventions, if any?
3. What skills do you need to learn to practice forensic nursing with this specific population?

REVIEW QUESTIONS

1. Attributes of violence include which one of the following groups?
   A. Aggression, harm, prevention
   B. Violence, harm, intent
   C. Behavior, direct or indirect intent, harm
   D. Aggression, behavior, injury

2. Violence takes place in a:
   A. Societal context
   B. Macro-level deficit
   C. Cultural system
   D. Vacuum

3. Defining the concept of violence is necessary because:
   A. There is no universally accepted definition.
   B. Violence is equivalent to aggression and harm.
   C. The public understanding of a concept is critical.
   D. The current definition is not consistent with that of the World Health Organization.

4. Antecedents of violence include:
   A. Behavior, intent, harm
   B. Aggressor, victim, cost
   C. Aggression, lack of hope, fearlessness
   D. Hopelessness, fearlessness, imbalance of power

5. Which of the following include consequences of violence?
   A. Intentional injury, unintentional injury
   B. Unintentional injury, cycle of violence
   C. Perpetuation of the cycle of violence, prevention efforts
   D. Unintentional injury, accidental death

6. One description of the context in which violence occurs is defined as:
   A. Aggression
   B. Behavior
   C. Culture
   D. Prevention efforts

7. Consequences of violence include which one of the following?
   A. Prevention efforts
   B. Culture
   C. Relationships
   D. Will to act

8. Intent to cause harm is:
   A. A focus of prevention efforts
   B. A target for intervention
   C. The will to act
   D. Aggressive behavior

9. Conceptual ambiguity:
   A. Enhances global acceptance of a concept
   B. Is necessary for an enduring definition
   C. Confuses the focus research and intervention efforts
   D. Creates a clear pathway for evidence-based practice

10. Harmful injury related to violence may be:
    A. Intentional or unintentional
    B. Direct or indirect
    C. Psychological or emotional
    D. Culturally acceptable

References

Heuermann, W.K., & Melzer-Lange, M.D. (2002). Developing community coalitions in youth violence prevention. *Wisconsin Medical Journal, 101*(6):30-33.

Hickey, G. (1996). A multi-stage approach to the coding of data from open-ended questions. *Nurse Researcher, 4*(1):81-91.

Hootman, J., Houck, G., & King, M. (2002). A program to educate school nurses about mental health interventions. *Journal of School Nursing, 18*(4):191-195.

Howells-Johnson, J. (2000). Verbal abuse. *British Journal of Perioperative Nursing, 10*(10):508-511.

Huskinson, L. (2002). The Self as violent Other: The problem of defining the self. *Journal of Analytic Psychology, 47*(3):437-458.

Johnson, R., & Larkin, G. (2001). Emergency department screening for domestic violence: Effect of an administrative intervention on rates of screening for domestic violence in an urban emergency department. *American Journal of Public Health, 91*(4):651-652.

Kane, M., & DiBartolo, M. (2002). Complex physical and mental health needs of rural incarcerated women. *Issues in Mental Health Nursing, 23*(3):209-229.

Karaffa, M.C. (1992). *International classification of diseases* (9th ed.). Los Angeles: Public Management Information Corporation.

Krug, E.G., Dahlberg, L.L., Mercy, J.A., et al. (2002). *World Report on Violence and Health*. Geneva: World Health Organization.

Laaser, U., Donev, D., Bjegovic, V., et al. (2002). Public health and peace. *Croatian Medical Journal, 43*(2):107-113.

Lawson, L., & Rowe, S. (2009). Violence. *Journal of Forensic Nursing, 5*(3):119-123.

Little, L., & Kantor, G.K. (2002) Using ecological theory to understand intimate partner violence and child maltreatment. *Journal of Community Health Nursing, 19*(3): 133-145.

MacArthur Research Network (MRN) on Mental Health and the Law. (2005). *MacArthur Risk Assessment Study.* Retrieved November 11, 2006, from http://www.macarthur.virginia. edu/risk.html

Martinez-Schallmoser, L., MacMullen, N., & Telleen, S. (2005). Social support in Mexican-American child-bearing women. *Journal of Obstetric, Gynecologic, & Neonatal Nursing, 34*(6):755-760.

McFarlane, J., Groff, J., O'Brien, J., et al. (2005). Behaviors of children exposed to intimate partner violence before and 1 year after a treatment program for their mother. *Applied Nursing Research, 13*(1):7-12.

McKay, I., Paterson, B., & Cassells, C. (2005). Constant or special observations of inpatients presenting a risk of aggression or violence: Nurses' perceptions of the rules of engagement. *Journal of Psychiatric and Mental Health Nursing, 12*(4):464-471.

Mizen, R. (2003). A contribution towards an analytic theory of violence. *Journal of Analytic Psychology, 48*(3):285-305.

Monahan, J., Steadman, H.G., Robbins, P.C., et al. (2005). An actuarial model of violence risk assessment for persons with mental disorders. *Psychiatric Services, 56*(7):810-815.

Nelms, T. (1999). An educational program to examine emergency nurses' attitudes and enhance caring intervention with battered women. *Journal of Emergency Nursing, 22*(1):59-66.

Nelson, K. (1995). The child welfare response to youth violence and homelessness in the nineteenth century. *Child Welfare, 74*(1):56-70.

Nugent, K.S. (n.d.) *Library and Legal Glossary.* Retrieved January 15, 2007, from http://www.attorneykennugent.com/ library/i.html

Paley, J. (1996). How not to clarify concepts in nursing. *Journal of Advanced Nursing, 24*(3):572-578.

Perry, C., Shams, M., & DeLeon, C. (1998). Voices from an Afghan community. *Journal of Cultural Diversity, 5*(4): 127-131.

Prevention Institute (PI). (n.d.). *Violence Prevention.* Retrieved October 27, 2007, from http://www.preventioninstitute.org/ violenceprev.html

Rivara, F.P., Shepherd, J.P., Farrington, D.P., et al. (1995). Victim as offender in youth violence. *Annals of Emergency Medicine, 26*:609-614.

Rodgers, B.L. (1989). Concepts, analysis and the development of nursing knowledge: The evolutionary cycle. *Journal of Advanced Nursing, 14*(4):330-335.

Rodgers, B.L. (1993). Concept analysis: An evolutionary view. In B.L. Rodgers & K.A. Knafl (Eds.), *Concept development in nursing: Foundations, techniques, and applications.* Philadelphia: W.B. Sanders, pp. 73-92.

Rodgers, B.L., & Knafl, K.A. (Eds.). (2000). *Concept development in nursing: Foundations, techniques, and applications.* Philadelphia: W.B. Saunders.

Rollins, J.A. (1993). Nurses as gangbusters: A response to gang violence in America. *Pediatric Nursing, 19*:559-569.

Sanko, D.J., & Vellman, W.P. (1994). Security measures: What can be done? *Topics in Emergency Medicine, (3)*:61-69.

Schnitzer, P.G., & Runyan, C.W. (1995). Injuries to women in the United States: An overview. *Women & Health, (1)*:9-27.

Sells, C.W., & Blum, R.W. (1996). Morbidity and mortality among U.S. adolescents: An overview of data and trends. *American Journal of Public Health, 86*:513-519.

Serra, P. (1993). Physical violence in the couple relationship: A contribution toward the analysis of the context. *Family Process, 32*(1):21-33.

Shamai, M. (2003). Using social constructionist thinking in training social workers living and working under threat of political violence. *Social Work, 48*(4):545-555.

Sheehan, K., Kim, L.E., & Galvin, J.P. (2004). Urban children's perceptions of violence. *Archives of Pediatrics and Adolescent Medicine, 158*(1):74-77.

Srnec, P. (1991). Children, violence, and intentional injuries. *Critical Care Nursing Clinics of North America, 3*:471-478.

Stern, P.N. (1991). Are counting and coding a cappella appropriate in qualitative research? In J.M. Morse (Ed.), *Qualitative nursing research: A contemporary dialogue.* Newbury Park, CA: Sage Publications, pp. 147-162.

Strauss, A., & Corbin, J. (1990). *Basics of qualitative research: Grounded theory procedures and techniques.* Newbury Park CA: Sage Publications.

Stuart, G.W., & Sundeen, S.J. (1995). *Principles and practice of psychiatric nursing.* St. Louis: Mosby.

Tang, C.S., Tang, F.M., Chen, R., et al. (2002). Definition of violence against women: A comparative study of Chinese societies of Hong Kong, Taiwan, and the People's Republic of China. *Journal of Interpersonal Violence, 17*(6):671-688.

Townsend, M.C. (1997). *Nursing diagnoses in psychiatric nursing: A pocket guide for care plan construction.* Philadelphia: F.A. Davis.

Trickett, P.K., Duran, L., & Horn, J.L. (2003). Community violence as it affects child development: Issues of definition. *Clinical Child and Family Psychology Review, 6*(4):223-236.

Varcarolis, E.M. (1994). *Foundations of psychiatric-mental health nursing.* Philadelphia: W.B. Saunders.

Varvaro, F.F., & Lasko, D.L. (1993). Physical abuse as cause of injury in women: Information for orthopaedic nurses. *Orthopaedic Nursing, 12*(1):37-41.

Waddington, P.A.J., Badger, D., & Bull, R. (2005). Appraising the inclusive definition of workplace violence. *British Journal of Criminology, 25*(2):141-164.

Walby, S. (2004). *The cost of domestic violence.* Leeds, England: University of Leeds.

Walker, L.O., & Avant, K.C. (2005). *Strategies for theory construction in nursing* (4th ed.). East Norwalk, CN: Appleton & Lange.

Weil, J., & Lee, H. (2004). Cultural considerations in understanding family violence among Asian American Pacific Islander families. *Journal of Community Health Nursing, 21*(4):217-227.

Weiner, M.D., Sussman, S., Sun, P., et al. (2005). Explaining the link between violence perpetration, victimization and drug use. *Addictive Behaviors, 30*(6):1261-1266.

Yegidis, B.L. (1992). Family violence: Contemporary research findings and practice issues. C*ommunity Mental Health Journal, (6)*:519-530.

Zink, T., Kamine, D., Musk, L., et al. (2004). What are providers' reporting requirements for children who witness domestic violence? *Clinical Pediatrics, 43*(5):449-460.

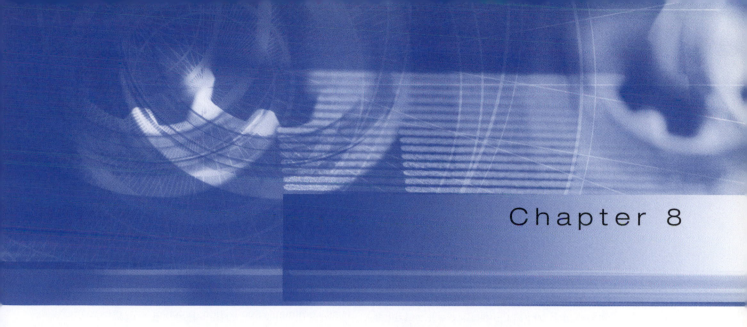

Chapter 8

Intimate Partner, Child, and Elder Violence and the Three Levels of Prevention

Patricia M. Speck and Diana K. Faugno

"When we long for life without . . . difficulties, remind us that oaks grow strong in contrary winds and diamonds are made under pressure."

Peter Marshall

Competencies

1. Recognizing the effects of violence across the life span.
2. Delineating the dynamics of intimate partner violence, child, and elder abuse.
3. Explaining the three levels of prevention.
4. Describing the role of the health-care provider (HCP) in the recognition and response to violence in three levels of prevention.
5. Reducing HCP fatigue through self-awareness and care for those affected by violence.

Key Terms

Acquaintance violence
Abandonment
Child maltreatment
Collective violence
Community violence
Elder maltreatment
Emotional abuse
Exploitation
Family violence
Financial abuse
Interpersonal violence
Intimate partner violence
Neglect
Physical abuse
Property crimes

(key terms continued on page 118)

Key Terms (continued)

Psychological abuse
Self-directed violence
Sexual abuse

Stranger violence
Workplace violence
Youth violence

INTRODUCTION

Violence occurs across the life span everywhere in the world. Adverse childhood events are associated with violence and are correlated with high-risk behaviors, poor health, and early death. Violence is not related to socioeconomic status, but it is consistently associated with illicit drug use, addictions, and conflict, including war and other types of violence. Categories of violence fall into age- and target-specific groups. Health-care providers have a critically significant role to play in prevention and early intervention in the effects of violence. Early intervention reduces the negative long-term negative health consequences of violence and is cost-effective.

Nursing Competencies

Health-care providers must have competencies that include extensive knowledge about biological, psychological, social, and spiritual aspects of health and evidence-based interventions for improvement of health. Competencies are demonstrated by performance measures that include use of critical-thinking skills, development of a plan for the identified health threat; implementation of an evidenced-based intervention; and evaluation of the process throughout the patient encounter. This is called the nursing process: it is a basic and ever-recurring tenet of nursing education at all levels and is applied through the use of ADPIE—assessment, diagnosis, plan, intervention, and evaluation. Each step of the nursing process reflects other steps as the assessment is continuous and requires maximum critical thinking skills from the registered nurse.

For the forensic nurse, the domains of practice and core competencies are contained in *The Forensic Nursing Scope and Standards of Practice.* Specialty activities borrow from forensic science and public health core competencies as well as require knowledge about intentional and unintentional wounds and the healing process; ethical dilemmas of forensic nurses, their patients, and the interface with the legal community; collection, procurement, preserving, and handling of evidence important to the legal community, including records, photographs, and other items generated in the process of a patient's medical evaluation; and legal systems processes and outcomes. This knowledge base is commonly referred to as WHEEL (wounds and healing, ethical dilemmas, evidence, and legal systems).

Overview of the Problem

Violence occurs on a continuum beginning with emotional distancing and verbal abuse and ending with murder (Fig. 8.1). Violence in all forms affects the health of an individual and shortens the life span. Violence is "the intentional use of physical force or power, threatened or actual, against oneself, another person, or against a group or community, that either results in or has a high likelihood of resulting in injury, death, psychological harm, mal-development, or deprivation."

VIOLENCE AND CHILDREN

Child maltreatment is any act or series of acts of commission or omission by a parent or other caregiver that results

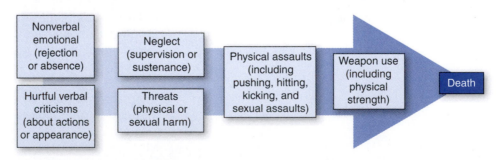

■ **FIGURE 8.1** Continuum of Violence. ("Continuum of family violence," n.d.)

in harm, potential for harm, or threats of harm to a child. Acts of commission include physical maltreatment or abuse, sexual abuse, and psychological or emotional abuse. Acts of omission include a failure to provide or supervise, resulting in neglect that can be physical, emotional, medical/dental, educational; inadequate supervision; or exposure to violent environments.

Physical abuse is the intentional use of force against a child that results in or has the potential to result in physical injury. Sexual abuse is any completed or attempted sexual act, sexual contact with, or exploitation of a child by a caregiver. Psychological abuse is the continual or episodic intentional caregiver behavior that conveys that the child is worthless, flawed, unloved, unwanted, endangered, or valued only in meeting another's needs. Child trafficking is movement of a child within a country or across borders, whether by force or not, with the purpose of rendering the child vulnerable to exploitation.

Children experience victimization throughout their childhoods. The number of children exposed to at least one type of violence and the percentage of children exposed to four or more types of violence increase annually and more frequently as children age. In early childhood, the experiences include neglect and physical and sexual abuse, as well as witnessing violence against their siblings, mothers, fathers, and extended family members. As children enter school, rejection and emotional abuse, bullying, and physical assaults are witnessed and experienced. Boys and girls are exposed to sexual violence in school, with girls experiencing increasing victimization in the adolescent years. Boys experience increased bullying and physical assaults. Both boys and girls are vulnerable to cyber-bullying in addition to sibling, parental, and extended family abuse. Poly-victimizations during the early and critical developmental stages result in diverse patterns of adaptation that are just beginning to be understood.

Children are exposed to violence internationally through global conflict and learn conflict resolution through witnessing violent acts against the women and men in their lives. They also watch television laced with violence. Violent or antisocial music can increase aggressive thinking, whereas the violence on television results in more aggressive behaviors in children and teens (as opposed to their peers who do not watch violence on television). Video games have not yet been studied, but 17% of the games have been designed with violence as the focus and only 48% of parents supervise video games. In all media, depictions of violent acts are attractive, humorous at times, and do not associate punishment

with the violent or aggressive behaviors. This can result in disbelief when violent children are eventually held accountable by systems outside their families; for example, law enforcement and criminal justice.

Children witnessing violence in families or at school are considered victims of child maltreatment. Children exposed to maternal intimate partner violence (IPV) are at risk of behavior problems as well as poor performance. These victimized children often have higher levels of anxiety, which can be traced to elevated cortisol levels.

ECOLOGICAL FRAMEWORK

The ecological framework states that no one factor can explain why one person is at risk and others are protected from becoming victims of or offenders who perpetrate violent acts. Research has identified some factors that influence a person becoming a victim or a perpetrator. They include a person's relationships, his or her community, and the sociocultural factors noted in Figure 8.2. Others have created models to help the community understand that there are many factors that explain one's vulnerability to violence, noted in Figure 8.3.

The ecological factors operate with equal importance, the model can only explain the result after careful consideration of all the experiences, influences, vulnerabilities, and choices made by the victim or offender. It is still not understood why some persons experience multiple victimizations throughout childhood and never become a victim or perpetrator as an adult.

The types of violence vary according to age, gender, relationships, community standards, and societal beliefs. **Interpersonal violence** refers to violence between individuals and is subdivided into family and IPV and community violence. The category of **family violence** includes child maltreatment and elder maltreatment or abuse, and **community**

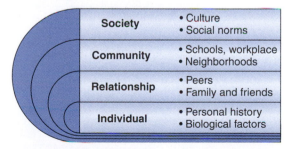

■ **FIGURE 8.2** Ecological framework for understanding why a person is at risk of interpersonal violence or becoming a perpetrator of violent acts.

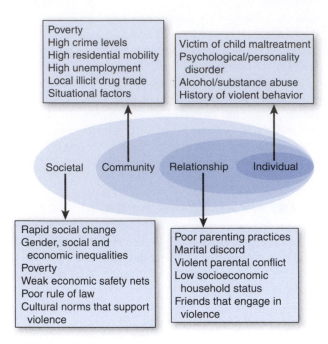

Poverty
High crime levels
High residential mobility
High unemployment
Local illicit drug trade
Situational factors

Victim of child maltreatment
Psychological/personality
  disorder
Alcohol/substance abuse
History of violent behavior

Societal   Community   Relationship   Individual

Rapid social change
Gender, social and
  economic inequalities
Poverty
Weak economic safety nets
Poor rule of law
Cultural norms that support
  violence

Poor parenting practices
Marital discord
Violent parental conflict
Low socioeconomic
  household status
Friends that engage in
  violence

■ **Figure 8.3** Ecological approach to violence.

violence is broken down into acquaintance and stranger violence, including youth violence, assault by strangers, violence related to property crimes, and violence in workplace and other institutions.

Community Violence

Community violence can be defined as exposure to acts of interpersonal violence committed by individuals who are not intimately related to the victim. Such acts include sexual assault, burglary, use of weapons, muggings, and such

social disorder issues as teen gangs, drugs, and racial divisions. Community violence includes the following.

- **Stranger violence** is assault by strangers or someone you have seen but do not know.
- **Acquaintance violence** is assault by someone known to the victim.
- **Youth violence** is interpersonal violence of children between the ages of 10 and 24, although patterns of youth violence can begin in early childhood.
- **Collective violence** refers to violence committed by larger groups of individuals and can be subdivided into social, political, and economic violence.
- **Property crimes** are the offenses of burglary, larceny-theft, motor vehicle theft, and arson. The object of the theft-type offense is the taking of money or property, but there is no force or threat of force against the victims. Property crime includes arson because it involves the destruction of property.
- **Workplace violence** and violence in other institutions is both community and interpersonal violence. Workplace violence includes stranger, acquaintance, and youth violence, collective violence, and property crime, as well as rape and sexual assault, robbery, and homicide.

The World Health Organization's typology of violence demonstrates the interpersonal nature of violence, how it occurs in communities, and the relationships between members of the family and community (Fig. 8.4).

International Scope of the Violence Against Women

Violence against women perpetrated by intimate partners occurs internationally but varies country to country

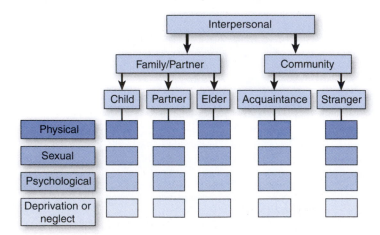

■ **Figure 8.4** Typology of interpersonal violence.

(Box 8.1 and 8.2). Worldwide, 52% of women report physical abuse, and up to 30% report sexual violence by their intimate partner. Overall, 27% report sexual abuse in their childhood. When sexual initiation was before age 15, 30% report it was forced. In some countries, the forced initiation was likely related to marriage at an early age. The physical violence against women varied among countries such as Bangladesh, Ethiopia, Samoa, and provincial Peru, where significant numbers of women report loss of consciousness as a result of IPV. Although the WHO study asked about general health, it was noted that women who had *ever* experienced violence reported poor or very poor health. The prevalence of research documenting the association between violence in women's lives and poor health outcomes is increasing.

In the United States, 1.3 million women and 835,000 men report physical assault annually. At some time in their lives, 25% women and 7.6% men report having been raped by an intimate partner. In 2001, 20% of nonfatal crime was IPV, and 33% of all murdered females are killed by their intimate partners.

INTIMATE PARTNER VIOLENCE

Intimate partner violence (IPV) is abuse that occurs between two people in a close relationship. The term "intimate partner" includes current and former spouses and dating partners. IPV includes four types of behavior that may co-occur, including physical abuse, sexual abuse, threats, and emotional abuse.

IPV physical abuse occurs when a person hurts or tries to hurt a partner by hitting, kicking, burning, or other physical act. IPV sexual abuse occurs when a partner is forced (does not consent) to take part in a sex act. IPV threats of physical or sexual abuse include the use of words, gestures, weapons, or other means to communicate the intent to cause harm. IPV emotional abuse is threatening a partner or his or her possessions or loved ones or harming a partner's sense of self-worth. Examples include stalking, name-calling, intimidation, or not letting a partner see friends or family.

Durose reports that the U.S. Department of Justice found:

- 3.5 million violent crimes were committed against family members.
- 49% of these were crimes against spouses.
- 84% of spouse abuse victims were females.
- 86% of victims of dating partner abuse were female.
- 83% of spouse murderers were male.
- 75% of partner murders were committed by the dating partner.
- 50% of offenders in state prison for spousal abuse had killed their victims.
- Wives were more likely than husbands to be killed by their spouses.
- Wives are half of all spouses in the population in 2002, but 81% of all persons killed by their spouse.

When women are able to leave the abusive relationship, the male may choose to stalk the female. Stalking is a method used to harass a person, and in the case of domestic violence, it is initiated to force the partner back into a relationship. It is a crime in over 30 states, but legislation varies. The crime occurs with a credible threat to another person. Credible threat is determined when a "reasonable person" would be in fear that the threat would cause harm, either to self or others, including family members and pets. Harassment can include language (e.g., obscene comments); gestures (e.g., signs, hand gestures); or technology

---

Box 8.1   Difficult Choices

"So I take a blanket and I spend the night with my children out in the cold because he is hitting me too much and I have to take the kids to stop him hitting them, too. I would go up the mountain, and sleep there all night. I've done that more than 10 times."
Woman interviewed in Peru.

(Taken from Garcia-Moreno, C., Jansen, H., Ellsberg, Heis, L., & World Health Organization. (2005). WHO multi-country study on women's health and domestic violence against women. Retrieved November 7, 2009, from http://www.who.int/gender/violence/who_multicountry_study/en/)

Box 8.2   Leaving or Staying?

"A woman I know was recently killed by her live-in partner. Now I am very fearful and hardly sleep at night. I keep watch because when my partner is drunk or has smoked marijuana, he sharpens his knife before going to bed. He regularly warns me that he will kill me if I leave him, or do not please him in any way."
Woman interviewed in Namibia.

(Taken from Garcia-Moreno, C., Jansen, H., Ellsberg, Heis, L., & World Health Organization. (2005). WHO multi-country study on women's health and domestic violence against women. Retrieved November 7, 2009, from http://www.who.int/gender/violence/who_multicountry_study/en/)

(e.g., texting, telephone, e-mails). A single threat is not harassing; however, repeated threats and activities associated with furthering the threat are considered stalking. The following statistics reflect the incidence and prevalence of the problem:

- 1,006,970 women and 370,990 men are stalked annually in the United States.
- 1 in 12 women and 1 in 45 men will be stalked in their lifetime.
- 77% of female and 64% of male victims know their stalker.
- 87% of stalkers are men.
- 59% of female victims and 30% of male victims are stalked by an intimate partner.
- 81% of women stalked by a current or former intimate partner are also physically assaulted by that partner.
- 31% of women stalked by a current or former intimate partner are also sexually assaulted by that partner.
- The average duration of stalking is 1.8 years, increasing to 2.2 years when the stalking involves intimate partners.
- 61% of stalkers made unwanted phone calls; 33% sent or left unwanted letters or items; 29% vandalized property; and 9% killed or threatened to kill a family pet.
- 28% of female victims and 10% of male victims obtained a protective order against their stalker.
- For 69% of female victims and 81% of male victims, the protection order was violated.

Lethality increases for the woman entangled in domestic violence when she tries to leave. Nurses should be aware and anticipate that voluntary separation could place the woman's life at risk. Counseling the patient about the potential lethal outcome could save her life. In the event of separation, the partner's beliefs of entitlement and ownership expressed through power and control can result in stalking by the intimate partner. The stalking literature reveals the potential outcomes:

- 76% of femicide victims had been stalked by the person who killed them.
- 67% had been physically abused by their intimate partner.
- 89% of femicide victims who had been physically abused had also been stalked in the 12 months before the murder.
- 79% of abused femicide victims reported stalking during the same period that they reported abuse.
- 85% of attempted femicide cases involved at least one episode of stalking within 12 months prior to the attempted femicide.

- 54% of femicide victims reported stalking to police before they were killed by their stalkers.

Understanding the intersection of the neurobiology of trauma and the roots of health disparity during childhood is emerging. In response to trauma, the hormonal chemical levels change and disrupt the architecture of the brain. Once the architecture of the brain is repatterned, the developing brain is changed in the child. Exposure to violence has lasting physical, mental, and emotional effects. This is particularly concerning for the developing brain of infants and toddlers who are sensitive to the stresses in the family. If the parents have also been victimized as children, they are ill-equipped to address the needs of their own children. Many adult diseases can be traced to experiences in childhood, and children exposed to adverse events in childhood experience health risk for increased morbidity and early mortality.

Recognition of the impact of violence on adult health began with a simple analysis of a cohort enrolled in Kaiser Permanente Health Center in California. Two physicians from the Centers for Disease Control and Prevention (CDC), Robert Anda and Vincent Feletti, developed a tool that asked about adverse childhood events (ACE), in order to provide a score. They found that the higher the ACE score, the more likely it is that the adult will have major health complications.

ELDER MALTREATMENT

At the other end of the age continuum is **elder maltreatment,** which is any abuse, neglect, and/or exploitation of persons 60 years and older by a caregiver or another person in a relationship involving an expectation of trust. Forms of elder maltreatment include physical abuse, sexual abuse or abusive sexual contact, psychological or emotional abuse, neglect, abandonment, financial abuse, or exploitation.

Physical abuse occurs when an elder is injured (e.g., scratched, bitten, slapped, pushed, hit, burned, and so on), assaulted or threatened with a weapon (e.g., knife, gun, or other object), or inappropriately restrained.

Sexual abuse or abusive sexual contact is any sexual contact against an elder's will. This includes acts in which the elder is unable to understand the act or is unable to communicate. Abusive sexual contact is defined as intentional touching (either directly or through the clothing) of genitalia, anus, groin, breast, mouth, inner thigh, or buttocks.

Psychological or **emotional abuse** occurs when an elder experiences trauma after exposure to threatening acts or coercive tactics. Examples include humiliation or embarrassment; controlling behavior (e.g., prohibiting or limiting access to transportation, telephone, money, or other resources); social isolation; disregard for or trivialization of needs; or damage or destruction of property.

Neglect is the failure or refusal of a caregiver or other responsible person to provide for an elder's basic physical, emotional, or social needs, or failure to protect him or her from harm. Examples include not providing adequate nutrition, hygiene, clothing, shelter, or access to necessary health care or failure to prevent exposure to unsafe activities and environments.

Abandonment is the willful desertion of an elderly person by a caregiver or other responsible person.

Financial abuse or **exploitation** is the unauthorized or improper use of the resources of an elder for monetary or personal benefit, profit, or gain. Examples include forgery, misuse or theft of money or possessions, use of coercion or deception to force surrender of finances or property, or improper use of guardianship or power of attorney.

MALE VICTIMIZATION

Males experience and describe the experience of intimate partner violence differently than do women, and the notion about the differences is not well understood by the medical community. Men tend to deny victimization for the same reasons women deny the occurrence, but with an additional burden that includes threats to reveal sexuality to family or friends. In one study, 50% had experienced partner abuse within the last year, and over 23% had experienced poly-victimizations over a 6-year period.

While intimate partner violence is more prevalent than rape, all men are potential victims of sexual violence as demonstrated in the study about incarcerated and community male victims. About 3% of American men (2.78 million men) have experienced rape at some time in their lives, where 1 in 10 reporting victims in 2003 were male. As with other types of victimization of children, 71% of the male victims were under 18 years of age. Male victims of rape in the community experience more weapon usage, whereas victims in the prison experience multiple assailants. Prison is a particularly vulnerable place for males, with over 420,000 males raped each year while incarcerated. Perpetrators of this type of crime consider the penetration of another indiscriminately, and many offenders were reported to have multiple types of victims over the course of their criminal sexual pursuits.

Male rape victims react to rape similarly to women in that there is predictable psychological trauma associated with rape, including depression, anger and guilt, self-blame, and sexual dysfunction. Flashbacks may feed mental health pathology, resulting in suicide ideation and attempts. This has lead to the belief that gay and heterosexual men respond to rape differently in that

> gay men have difficulties in their sexual and emotional relationships with other men and think that the assault occurred because they are gay, whereas straight men often begin to question their sexual identity and are more disturbed by the sexual aspect of the assault than the violence involved. (Brochman, 1991)

Questions about sexuality in the heterosexual male is complicated and a source of confusion and stress to the male victim when ejaculation is part of the rape experience. Given that the research is aging and the focus on violence against women is institutionalized and well funded, the topic of rape of males remains a taboo subject that is not currently a priority in most communities. Men should, however, continue to seek care through the local rape crisis centers as policy and legislative stakeholders push to ensure equal and competent care of the male rape victim.

Also within the typology of violence is **self-directed violence.** Self-directed violence refers to violence in which the perpetrator and the victim are the same individual and is subdivided into self-abuse and suicide (see Chapter 10 for more information).

THREE LEVELS OF PREVENTION

Primary prevention is action taken to prevent the development of a disease or injury. Most population-based health promotion activities are prevention activities directed toward at-risk populations, and the outcomes are measured by improvement of identified and targeted elements in health behaviors through evidence-based measures. The role and activity are distinct and should not be confused. Confusion about primary care providers (e.g., internist or family practice health-care providers) and primary prevention occurs because the primary health-care provider role will implement all primary, secondary, and tertiary prevention activities by providing health promotion, disease or injury identification, and/or restorative care.

Primary care delivery of prevention activities includes scientific-based health promotion. Health promotion is the evidence-based change in population activities and individual lifestyles that are believed to assist populations to reach and maintain optimal health. The World Health Organization defines it as the process of enabling populations to increase control over and improve their health by avoiding disease and injury.

Health promotion is a coordinated community action in which governments and communities partner to implement healthy lifestyle plans. These plans are specific to a community in that they account for social, cultural, and economic systems unique to the community. Groups involved include government, social and economic sectors, nongovernmental and voluntary organizations, local industry, local authorities, and media. Mediation between differing interests rest on the subject matter expertise of health-care professionals and the social groups demanding change.

Interpersonal violence, and in particular, intimate partner violence (IPV), were initially seen as distinct issues: husbands beating their wives versus child abuse versus gang violence versus bullying versus gang rape, etc. The ACE study exposed the interconnectedness of all types of violence and the health outcomes that rob families of their loved ones through early death. For some vulnerable populations, violence is a continuum that begins at conception and ends with death (see Fig. 8.1) and could also be defined as family violence. Health promotion aims to use evidence-based activities to interrupt the addition of episodes of violence experienced by individuals, groups, and communities, thereby improving the likelihood of individuals reaching a healthy old age.

Public health nursing competencies address the domains and performance measures necessary for primary prevention activities. Examples of health promotion activities include legislative and funding changes that are based in policy generated between the social activist, the subject matter expert, and the researcher in the specific area of violence. Taking it to the organizational level where policies and procedures are generated, the worker can never identify the effects of violence if the organization fails to implement legislation or policy. The spectrum of prevention in sexual assault is directed toward norm change and includes six levels:

- Strengthening an individual's knowledge and skills, for example, providing multiple skill sessions to high school students related to sexual violence
- Promoting community education, for example, fostering media coverage of IPV with focus on solutions and awarding good media coverage
- Educating providers, for example, training Little League coaches to recognize bad behavior that diminishes another and correct it

- Fostering coalitions and networks, for example, bringing stakeholders together in collaboration
- Changing organizational practices, for example, implementing physical changes in the environment that diminishes opportunity for crime
- Influencing policies and legislation that support health community norms and a violence-free society, for example, promoting and informing full implementation of Title IX

Secondary prevention activities encompass activities directed toward early disease detection, thereby increasing opportunities for comprehensive interventions to prevent progression of the disease or injury and emergence of other symptoms. Secondary prevention occurs during primary care encounters in clinic settings when a health-care provider identifies disease and prescribes medication. This occurs because patients go to their primary care providers when they are in need of immunizations (primary prevention), are sick or are injured (secondary prevention), or need continual stabilization for illness or injury (tertiary prevention). Confusion about the primary care role occurs because the primary health-care provider role implements all levels of prevention, including primary, secondary, and tertiary prevention activities in the community. In secondary prevention, however, the role of primary care provider is limited to identification of disease and injury.

Tertiary prevention reduces the negative impact of an already established disease or injury by restoring function and reducing disease- or injury-related complications. In health-care delivery, this health-care provider works with those incarcerated, institutionalized or homebound, or in need of reconstructive care. These health-care providers are specialized in their field and work to maintain or improve the outcome disease or injury. A plastic surgeon who repairs facial injury following a domestic assault would be considered a tertiary provider, as there is stabilization and even reversal of the effects of injury present.

Common Codes

CSA—Child Sexual Assault
CPA—Child Physical Assault
DFSA—Drug Facilitated Sexual Assault
IPV—Intimate Partner Violence; or
IPV—Interpersonal Violence
PA—Physical Assault
SA—Sexual Assault

Case Study

THREE LEVELS OF PREVENTION

An occupational health nurse for a tire company in the Midwest demonstrates primary, secondary, and tertiary prevention as part of her scope of work for all employees. An example of primary prevention shows the occupational health nurse providing annual health examinations that include screening for immunizations, safety-related work issues and initiatives, as well as violence prevention resources and information.

Jackie, a 23-year-old employee, sees the nurse for her annual health check, and the nurse observes that she has an old bruise over her left eye that she received in an argument with her significant other. This is not the first time there has been physical injury in this relationship. Secondary prevention is illustrated here with the nurse caring for Jackie's left eye bruise and discussing follow-up as well as referrals to assist the employee. The nurse will see her in 3 to 4 weeks in a follow-up appointment.

At the 4-week follow-up appointment, Jackie discloses that she is feeling depressed and has missed 3 days of work this past month. This example of tertiary prevention will show the nurse working with Jackie on addressing the depression to prevent further sequelae by providing referrals to a health-care provider for follow-up as well. The client now has health issues from the violence that are affecting work and the quality of her life.

REGULATORY CONSIDERATIONS

Occupational Safety and Health Act and Workplace Violence

There are currently no specific government standards for workplace violence. However, the Occupational Safety and Health Act (OSHA) (1970) highlights the *Federal Register's* rules, proposed rules, and notices, and includes standard interpretations, for example, official letters of interpretation of the standards related to workplace violence.

> Section 5(a)(1) of the Occupational Safety and Health Act, often referred to as the General Duty Clause, requires employers to "furnish to each of his employees employment and a place of employment which are free from recognized hazards that are causing or are likely to cause death or serious physical harm to his employees.
>
> Section 5(a)(2) requires employers to "comply with occupational safety and health standards promulgated under this Act." (U.S. Department of Labor, 2007).

In 2002, OSHA defined workplace violence as

> . . . violence or the threat of violence against workers. It can occur at or outside the workplace and can range from threats and verbal abuse to physical assaults and homicide, one of the leading causes of job-related deaths. (U. S. Department of Labor, 2007).

Section 5(a)(2) requires employers to "comply with occupational safety and health standards promulgated under this Act." Violence remains a growing concern for employers and employees nationwide.

Health Insurance Portability and Accountability Act

The Health Insurance Portability and Accountability Act of 1996 (HIPAA; 45 CFR §§ 160–164) establishes national standards that protect the privacy of an individual's medical record and other personal health information. Importantly, the rules apply to health plans, health-care clearinghouses, and providers that conduct health-care transactions electronically. The law requires safeguards to protect the privacy of personal health information and sets the limits on disclosure of information without the patient's authorization. Ultimately, HIPAA gives control over the medical record to the patient. In addition, patients have a right to examine, obtain a copy of, and request corrections in their health record.

While HIPAA provides broad protections from unauthorized disclosure of patient health information, it does not inhibit the following:

- Disclosures of health information for public health prevention, surveillance, criminal investigation, and intervention activities
- Reporting of child abuse and neglect
- Protections for child victim health information (but disclosures can still be made with victim's consent or where necessary to prevent serious harm to that victim or other potential child victims)
- Courts, law enforcement agencies, and those determining the cause of child deaths from accessing relevant health information

- Protection of child victim health information to prevent its disclosure to parents or other adult representatives when disclosure would be contrary to the child's best interests.

Other organizations exempt from HIPAA may include:

- State agencies, such as child protective service agencies
- Law enforcement agencies
- Municipal offices

Emergency Medical Treatment and Active Labor Act (EMTALA)

The Emergency Medical Treatment and Active Labor Act (EMTALA) was passed as part of the Consolidated Omnibus Budget Reconciliation Act of 1986 (COBRA). The federal statutory and regulatory legislation consists of laws passed by Congress and regulations adopted by the Centers for Medicare and Medicaid Services (CMS) enforced by Department of Health and Human Service.

EMTALA governs when and how a patient may be (1) refused treatment or (2) transferred from one hospital to another when she or he is in an unstable medical condition. EMTALA applies to most hospitals with few exceptions. EMTALA was passed to prevent discrimination toward those who could not afford to pay for medical care in a hospital. Therefore, any person who goes to an emergency department seeking medical care must be provided with an appropriate medical screening examination (MSE) to determine if, in fact, the person is in need of emergency medical care (EMC). If the person's condition is unstable, the hospital is obliged to provide the patient with treatment until he or she is stabilized.

If the patient is stable and does not have an emergency condition, there is no obligation to treat the patient in the hospital. Interpretive Guidelines §489.24(c) for EMTALA state that if the MSE reveals the condition is not an emergency, the hospital may have procedures that allow for a qualified medical provider (QMP) to conduct a specific MSE if the examination is within the scope of practice for the QMP. The hospital's obligation under EMTALA ends at the completion of the MSE, and hospitals are not obligated to provide services beyond those needed to determine there is no emergent condition.

There are exemptions from EMTALA, and they are complex. It is in the hospital's best interest to probe in cases in which patients present to the ED and do not appear to have a EMC to determine the extent of the EMTALA obligation. The circumstances surrounding why a request is being made would confirm if the hospital in fact has an EMTALA obligation.

When services are requested for a nonmedical condition (e.g., immunization, allergy shot, or flu shot) or when evidence of a crime has occurred and the patient is considered "walking-well" (e.g., sexual assault/abuse or blood alcohol), the hospital is not obligated to provide a MSE under EMTALA. However, if the individual brought in by police was injured or may have sustained significant injury and presents to the ED, a MSE would be warranted to determine if a need for EMC exists.

When law enforcement officials request hospital emergency personnel to provide clearance for incarceration, the hospital has an EMTALA obligation to provide a MSE to determine if an EMC exists. If no EMC is present, the hospital has met its EMTALA obligation and no further actions are necessary for EMTALA compliance.

When audited, EMTALA surveyors will evaluate each case on its own merit when patients request service for non-EMC following crimes, for example, evidence collection in criminal justice proceedings. In the patient without injury following sexual assault and abuse cases and some domestic violence cases, many hospitals have existing protocols that allow triage to the Sexual Assault Nurse Examiner (SANE), Sexual Assault Forensic Nurse Examiner (SAFE), Sexual Assault Response Team (SART), or Domestic and Other Violence Emergencies (DOVE) programs if there is no EMC. This is especially true when specialized knowledge, skills, and abilities related to forensic care are needed to evaluate and document the effects of the crime.

The Joint Commission for Accreditation on Healthcare Organization (JCAHO/The Joint Commission)

The Joint Commission standards for accreditation determine a health-care organization's level of performance in specific areas by evaluating the observable. The Joint Commission standards present the minimum performance expectations for actions that affect the quality of care of patients in the institution that is seeking accreditation. These standards are developed in consultation with health-care experts, providers, measurement experts, purchasers, and consumers, and they are usually updated every 2 years.

In 2004, the Joint Commission introduced a new standard for hospitals' response to IPV, neglect, and exploitation. The elements of the standard include development or adoption of criteria for identifying victims and education of staff about identification, referral, community resources, and mandatory reporting laws and compliance. The Joint Commission also requires emergency and ambulatory care facilities to have established policies for identifying and assessing possible victims of rape and other sexual molestation and requires staff to be trained on these policies. As part of the assessment process, The Joint Commission requires these facilities to define their responsibilities related to the collection and preservation of evidentiary materials. Sexual assault examiner programs are helping many health-care facilities carry out these requirements for victim populations, both IPV and sexual assault and abuse.

Mandatory Reporting

There are a variety of mandatory reporting statutes in all states and territories in the United States for a variety of crimes, with one major exception. Every state requires all citizens to be mandatory reporters if child abuse and elder abuse is suspected. However, states vary in their laws regarding reporting of other types of crimes. The National District Attorneys Association and the American Prosecutors Research Institute address issues affecting the prosecution of crime, in particular violence against women.

Nurse Practice Acts

Nurse practice acts are legislation that governs the practice of nursing in a state or territory. Each legislation and regulation is unique, but they all have a common theme, that is, to protect the life, health, property, and public welfare of the people of that state from the unauthorized, unqualified, and improper delivery of services by individuals in the practice of nursing.

In recent years, environmental changes in the health-care delivery system, technological advances, and changes in the expectations of the health-care consumer have necessitated revisions in the way nursing is regulated to ensure the protection of the public. A number of potential regulatory models were proposed, and in 1999 the National Council of State Boards of Nursing (NCSBN) created a new regulatory model for the profession of nursing called the mutual recognition model. Public health programs, as well as health-care and legal systems, are being evaluated, and changes to support evidence-based practice are emerging to support the forensic nursing role at all levels and in all settings.

OVERARCHING CONTEXTUAL ISSUES

People are part of a community that includes family, neighbors, and organizations that function to provide services. How people connect to their community is directly related to the cultural acceptance of the behavior in the family and in their wider community. Therefore,

forensic nurses have a responsibility to assess the patient within the patient's cultural context, not the environment of the nurse. The patients' experiences may include previous victimizations and the normal responses to the abnormal events in their lives. These responses may include self-medication (addictions) for emotional or physical pain, behavioral choices that are high risk for early death, and attention seeking (e.g., teen pregnancy, child abuse, early sexual debut with multiple sex partners, prostitution, smoking, obesity, or domestic violence). Additionally, those with life-style vulnerabilities or vulnerabilities that create dependency (e.g., intellectual, physical, mental health diagnoses) are at higher risk than are those without the vulnerabilities noted here.

With the advent of significant technological advances, virtual violence using technology as a tool, much like a robber would use a gun, results in another vulnerable group—unsupervised adolescents. Dating violence has been recognized for its impact on adolescent development; however, virtual violence has resulted in new crimes such as cyberbullying and sex-texting. Persons who stalk others are using technology to increase control and fear as a method of intimidation. Virtual violence not only includes cyberbullying and stalking, but also unwanted sexual solicitation; sex-texting; graphic violence in videos, games, music and lyrics; phasing; sex that focuses on controlling, sadism, masochism, incest, and devaluating women; and preoccupation with the occult songs about sadism, trafficking, and human sacrifice, and the apparent enactment of the rituals in concerts. When caring for patients who are vulnerable and at risk for violence in its many forms, crisis intervention, with acceptance of the patient's choices, knowledge of available resources, and teaching safety planning, are nursing skills that empower and protect individuals and families from further harm (Box 8.3).

EVIDENCE-BASED CARE FOR RESPONDERS

Responders to traumatic situations are at risk of developing changes in psychological and biological indices. These changes can result in health-care providers experiencing a variety of symptoms that can impact the quality of their work and the safety of their patients. These reactions have garnered a variety of different names that address the vicarious trauma or compassion fatigue often experienced by caregivers of forensic patients. Diagnoses include acute stress disorder (ASD), secondary traumatic stress (STS),

Box 8.3   Common Case Presentations of Interpersonal Violence Across the Life Span

Typical Childhood Case Histories

1. 3-year-old female whose mother verbalizes suspicion about the boyfriend (intimate partner violence–IPV)
2. 6-year-old child with bruises on arms (IPV)
3. 9-year-old child with depression and suicide attempt (IPV, CSA, CPA, neglect)
4. Family of children in custody for abandonment (IPV)
5. 11-year-old female with poor attendance in school with failing grades (CSA)

Typical Adolescent Case Histories

1. 13-year-old female caught with street drugs (IPV)
2. 13-year-old male is bullying victim (interpersonal violence)
3. 14-year-old pregnant teen (IPV, rape)
4. 14-year-old gang initiation ("sexed in" or "beaten in")
5. 16-year-old teen with black eye (gay, bullying, IPV)
6. 16-year-old teen sex-texting (dating, acquaintance)
7. 16-year-old runaway (trafficking, IPV)
8. 17-year-old teen with sexually transmitted infections

Typical Adult Presentation

1. Drug-facilitated sexual assault
2. Dating violence
3. Drug use
4. Gang rape
5. False allegation
6. Stalking
7. Strangulation
8. Stranger–homicide
9. IPV rape
10. Workplace violence

Typical Older or Vulnerable Person Presentation

1. Nonreporting generational view
2. Child abuse survivor and offender (gender roles)
3. Comorbidities (mental health and dementia)
4. Early dementia, consent, and self-neglect
5. Institutional abuse
6. Caregiver abuse (financial, physical, isolation)

---

posttraumatic stress disorder (PTSD), burnout, vicarious trauma (VT), and compassion fatigue (CF). While similar, they have unique characteristics that differentiate them, such as (1) a time frame, where persistent symptoms of ASD and PTSD differ in the length of time present; (2) the location of the trauma, where burnout and CF are similar in that they occur in the workplace; or (3) the type of trauma, where workplace burnout is related to physical and mental exhaustion from job stresses and CF is secondary to the vicarious experiences seen, heard, or identified with regarding the patient who is traumatized.

Vicarious trauma occurs when individuals are exposed to graphic and/or traumatic material, as told by patients, that results in changes in the nurses' view of the world and of themselves (Box 8.4).

Compassion fatigue describes emotional, physical, social, and spiritual exhaustion that overtakes a person and "causes a pervasive decline in his/her desire, ability, and energy to feel and care for others" (Box 8.5). Compassion fatigue is secondary traumatic stress syndrome, secondary victimization, secondary survival, emotional contagion, countertransference, or provider fatigue. Although it is similar, CF is not PTSD or burnout.

Burnout is a "subtle process in which an individual is gradually caught in a state of mental fatigue and is completely empty and drained of all energy." Burnout is associated with the workplace and occurs when forensic nurses take multiple shifts or double shifts with

Box 8.4   Case Example 1

The divorced nurse has evaluated hundreds of child sexual assault victims at the clinic for years. She has been exposed to secondary traumatic stress through the forensic medical histories of her child patients. She no longer dates or hires male babysitters for her children. She is experiencing vicarious trauma (VT).

Box 8.5   Case Example 2

The nurse has volunteered at the rape crisis center for years. She has been exposed to secondary trauma through the histories given to her by the patients. Lately she has been very tired and has taken several days off by calling in sick because she could not get out of bed to go perform her volunteer work. She is experiencing compassion fatigue syndrome.

turnarounds over a short period of time without a substantial break. Mental fatigue is dangerous for the patient and the nurse, and although regulated for resident physicians, maximum hours and scheduling are not regulated for nurses (Box 8.6).

Box 8.6   Case Example 3

The occupational health nurse has burnout. She has completed her fourth 16-hour day this week in a flu immunization clinic at the factory. This is a typical work week for her. She is exhausted, and in the last hours of the fourth day does not ask an employee about allergies before giving the immunization. The employee has a reaction and is taken to the hospital. This error is due to the mental fatigue in burnout.

In acute stress disorder, the person has been exposed to a traumatic event in which the person experienced, witnessed, or was confronted with an event that involved actual or threatened death or serious injury. The response has been reported to be intense fear, helplessness, or horror. The person may experience dissociative symptoms that include numbing, detachment, or absence of emotional responsiveness.

This person may not be aware of his or her surroundings and report being in a "daze." This can include a derealization or depersonalization with dissociative amnesia and an inability to recall important aspects of the trauma. The person reexperiences recurrent images and thoughts in dreams, illusions, and flashbacks that are stimulated by noise, odors, or visual cues. Reliving the experience causes distress and results in avoidance of the stimuli to the arousal when recalling the traumatic event. The expected anxiety symptoms of ASD will prevent restful sleep and increase irritability and poor concentration. The person may become hypervigilant, have an exaggerated startle response, and kinetic restlessness. These symptoms will result in disruption of routine social and occupation tasks and activities where the person's impairment may result in avoidance of significant actions necessary for seeking assistance. The ASD may last up to 4 weeks after the traumatic event and is not related to existing medical or psychological diagnoses (Box 8.8.).

Box 8.7   Case Example 4

An 8-year-old child was injured in a crash that resulted in hospitalization. The child cried frequently, and when he returned to school, he could not read at the same level, was irritable, and couldn't concentrate on his schoolwork. This reaction is expected and a result of acute stress reaction.

PTSD is a psychiatric diagnosis that occurs at least 4 weeks after and as a result of surviving a significant trauma. In WWI, it was known as "shell shock." It is also known as combat fatigue, combat neurosis, and war neurosis. Patients who experience an acute traumatic reaction may experience continuous emotional and physical symptoms long after the trauma. Typical events that may result in PTSD include rape, severe child abuse, war, crashes, or natural disasters. To date, there is no known intervention or medication that prevents PTSD (Box 8.8).

NURSING IMPLICATIONS

Program Response

One emerging specialty in nursing is the health-care response to the offenders and victims of violence in health-care systems. Included in the specialty is the evaluation of the systems themselves (Box 8-9).

The *Forensic Nursing Scope and Standards of Practice* define the forensic nursing role as nursing practice that intersects with the legal system in all nursing settings worldwide. Public health programs as well as health-care and legal systems are being evaluated, and changes to support evidence-based practice are emerging to support the forensic nursing role at all levels and in all settings. In particular, evidence reveals that forensic nurses are in the best position to provide direct care to patients who find themselves with injury related to violence, whether offender or victim. In addition, forensic nurses are developing systems that respond to and interface with the legal and public health systems nationally, resulting in significant inroads made in the care of patients whose lives intersect with the legal system. However, barriers exist in the health-care system that impact forensic nursing patients who are "never-served," and some easily identified barriers include health-care provider educational and psychomotor skill deficits.

Box 8.8   Case Example 5

The occupational nurse is walking through the factory to see some of the employees who are late for their annual health checkup. She is standing next to a rig that gives way, with large tires falling from the ledge and hitting an employee and grazing her. One year later she is again in the same area of the rig and tires and begins to feel anxious and hyperventilates. She is experiencing physiological reactions characteristic of PTSD, which is related to her trauma last year.

Box 8.9   Health-Care Provider Reporting Needs

- The Joint Commission Guidelines for reporting violent incidents
- Standard operating procedures for reporting to law enforcement or the state's human services department
- Membership on SART with community agencies, such as members of the legal community, including law enforcement and prosecution, community programs with legal advocates, state protective services for adults or children, forensic nurses and physicians, administrators of community stakeholder agencies, or citizen groups
- Decision tree for health-care provider who is likely the first responder in an emergency department
- Educational programs for team members that address standards of practice and guidelines for education that include team building for patient-centered care, addressing the biological, psychological, and social needs of victims of violence
- Quality control and improvement process to address the needs of the distinct disciplines within the team, which should include experts from the unique disciplines

As the evidence base increases, one first step in health care is to ensure that the victim and offender are recognized when they present with intentional or unintentional injury. Recognition will ensure that the patient who is in need of the complex interactions from a highly skilled forensic nurse is served in the emerging health-care system. Built on the Memphis sexual assault response model, evolutionary growth has resulted in a national model that exists in Duluth, Gwinnett County, Georgia. It combines forensic nursing, advocacy, and statewide educational programs to respond to victims of family violence, intimate partner/domestic violence, child maltreatment, sexual assault, and abuse across the life span, as well as collaborates with the local legal, educational, and health-care systems. They do this by providing statewide educational programs with national and local speakers to address the unique needs in Georgia, the military, and the federal jurisdictions. They also respond to all offenders when there is a search warrant and will travel to local emergency departments to provide specialized medical forensic services to those unable to leave the hospital environment due to urgent medical or health-care needs. There are other models that exist; however, in the economic downturn, agencies are evaluating their expenditures and eliminating duplication. This summative process requires collaborative effort with common goals of efficiency with enhanced victim-centered outcomes.

The result of formative and summative evaluation is that forensic nursing programs in the same geographic areas are combining and expanding services to meet the comprehensive needs of the citizenry. When community programs segregate populations of victims, inefficiencies and duplication of efforts occur. In particular, when programs are legislated or population needs are not addressed (e.g., older and vulnerable person abuse, neglect and exploitation, and domestic violence or adolescent and child abuse), community programs become self-promoting and may not consider the expensive outcomes of running more than one program. Legislated programs are another barrier because legislation restricts funding for specific services or funding streams for programs, patient type (e.g., limited to rape only), or forensic nursing practice. Existing and future programs should address these and other important issues to ensure care is patient-centered or victim-centered.

Response to Clients

Identification of victims of violence has improved with screening tools developed for use in the emergency departments with all adult female patients who may have been subjected to domestic violence (Box 8.10). A recent published evaluation of the effectiveness of these screening tools has identified a lack of impact. However, these population-based evaluations cannot predict the individual benefit to a victim or offender as awareness is raised with each inquiry, and some recently have been found to be predictive.

Selected IPV Screening Tools

IPV screening tools include the following.

- HITS (Hurt, Insulted, Threatened, and Screamed) is a four-item scale with 5 points for each item. Sensitivity

Box 8.10   Health Professionals Actions With Victimized Patients

- Identify the abuse and implement ADPIE.
- Validate the patient's experience by saying, "I am sorry this has happened to you."
- Assess the patient and patient's safety upon the leaving the health-care arena.
- Document in both written and photographic form.
- Refer to stakeholder organizations providing the variety of services to wrap around the health-care role.
- File reports.

(Data taken from Houry, D., Sachs, C. J., Feldhaus, C. J., & Linden, K. (2002). Violence inflicted injuries: Reporting laws in the fifty states. *Annals of Emergency Medicine, 39*(1), 56-60.)

is 96% and specificity is 91%, using a cutoff of 10.5 as indicative of abuse. Its internal consistency, using Cronbach's alpha, is 0.80. The HITS historical development and tool are found at http://www.orchd.com/CommunityViolence/DomesticScreenTool.pdf

- CTS (Conflict Tactics Scale) is considered the gold standard for detection, but it is not practical for community clinical practice because it is time-consuming, with 19 items on a 7-point scale. Results of HITS and CTS were correlated ($r = 0.85$).
- PVS (Partner Violence Screen) has four questions and shows sensitivity of 71.4% and specificity of 84.4%. PVS had a higher sensitivity and specificity when compared to the ISA (see below) (64.5% and 80.3%) or CTS (71.4% and 84.4%).
- AAS (Abuse Assessment Screen) has three questions and is designed to address IPV in pregnancy. Women identified as abused on the AAS also scored significantly higher on the ISA, CTS, and DAS.
- ISA (Index of Spouse Abuse) is a standard for detection, but it is cumbersome and time-consuming for clinical practice. It has 30 items on a 5-point scale, with a score of greater than 19 being indicative of IPV. Modifications have been recommended to improve validity of the tool.
- DA (Danger Assessment) assesses the risk factors for lethal intimate partner violence. It has recently been revised to improve the likelihood of identification and now scores the level of risk.
- HARASS assesses the barriers faced by women trying to leave an abusive relationship.
- WAST (Women Abuse Screening Tool) is a short tool useful in community clinical practice.

Domestic homicide has been linked to positive scores on DA, AAS, and HARASS. With the new scoring system for the DA implying odds of lethality ($OR = 0.90$) when injury is identified related to IPV, the Danger Assessment should be used in every emergency department and community clinic.

Health-care providers have long avoided asking their patients questions related to violent crimes such as rape or child abuse. With the Joint Commission's newest recommendations, all emergency departments must have policies and procedures in place to respond to the effects of violence. For many, the discovery of a violent event, such as domestic violence, often meant that patients' needs would fall behind those with life-threatening injury or illness. Today, well-developed decision trees (e.g., algorithms) are used in communities nationwide. They all have similar structure and resemble the generic decision tree in Figure 8.5.

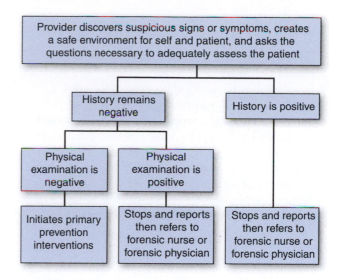

■ **FIGURE 8.5** Health-care provider decision tree.

Key Points

There are several key points for health-care providers to consider when responding to patients in clinical settings, including personal, patient care, and system response issues.

Accreditation

- All patients should be screened routinely.
- All professional schools, including medical, nursing, social work, and public health, should incorporate into the existing curricula issues covering violence and victimization.
- In accordance with the Joint Commission, hospitals should have established policies and procedures that address the safety of the health-care provider upon discovery of the effects of violence.
- There should be protocols for appropriate notification of staff as well as the safety and security for all during the initial discovery of violence.
- Legislation related to reporting violent crime should be incorporated in all policies and procedures with the recognition that states are different in the identification of age of consent for sexual activity and reproductive health.

EMTALA

- There should be a referral system in place that addresses the issues in EMTALA, and all personnel should know it and be able to provide the referrals easily.
- To decrease the risk to the facility, legal advice should validate efforts to protect the patient and providers, as well as the institution.

- Developing a process is part of the program development, occurring before forensic nursing programs are initiated.

Cultural Competence

- Health-care personnel and the staff of the agency should be culturally competent.
- Services augmenting patient communication should be available and planned for in any new program, including signing, translating, and conducting developmental assessments for consent in intellectually challenged individuals of all ages.
- Techniques for approaching the patient, as well as any evaluation, should be culturally sensitive and taught in educational programs.

Prevention

Today there are prevention programs that target youth by teaching them what families taught 100 years ago—rules related to dating. In addition, in enlightened communities these interventions have demonstrated a reduction of intimate partner dating violence as well as an increase in condom use.

Over the last 25 years, myriad agencies have developed programs that address aspects of intervention, each filling a niche when gaps were identified. No one agency can do it all. Coordinated community responses that pull together resources in the community are the latest evolutionary permutation of the first team response that took place in Memphis in 1974. Today, many programs used as referral sources incorporate the community team approach. One such program is the Sexual Assault Response Team (SART), which includes health-care (mental and physical), law enforcement (police departments and attorneys), and advocacy services to ensure that humane and patient-centered services are provided. A second example is the Child Advocacy Center (CAC) program, which focuses services on victims who are under 18 years old. Another service is the rape crisis centers, some of which include medical forensic services, counseling, and advocacy services, although some offer only one type of service. Domestic violence intervention (DVI) programs in communities may also offer legal and counseling services for families and individuals. There are also child protection investigation teams (CPIT) that review cases of suspected abuse and determine relevancy of information to be included and documented in the child welfare system. The team may include administrative personnel, case workers, and professionals from health care and law enforcement.

The approach to prevention or intervention cannot be resolved with one professional, one agency, or one intervention. An overall team approach with multiprofessional participants will ensure the best results of legal and patient outcomes, investigation, and recovery.

Interventions are inherent in the face-to-face communication with a client who is sitting in the office or examination room and includes making statements of fact to the traumatized client regarding what is the law and what is institution policy, explaining mandatory reporting, and providing validation that the client has experienced a negative life event or trauma that he or she did not deserve. Supportive statements should be repeated at every visit, and help should be given to a client to place the event aside so that it takes the role of an occurrence in the client's past life, but does not continue to replay in the client's mind and ruin or maintain its destruction of his or her future.

CONCLUSIONS

The forensic nursing specialty role is well developed in many areas and practice settings. There are commonalities between and among forensic nursing programs that service victims and the suspects. Many forensic nursing services that initially were for sexual assault of adults only are expanding to include victims and suspects of domestic violence, child abuse, and elder and vulnerable person assault, abuse, neglect, and exploitation. This maturation of the specialty practice has placed nurses in institutions (e.g., prisons and hospitals), nonprofits (e.g., advocacy and crisis centers), as well as in entrepreneurial settings (e.g., community settings). As a result, the nurse is sometimes co-opted by employers or response team members to take positions about forensic nursing practice that dictate and limit the forensic nursing role (e.g., to evidence collection only), rejecting the holistic practice of nursing and the added WHEEL of knowledge, skills, and abilities of forensic nurses. The limited view of nursing care of victims and offenders are myopic and based in part on limited beliefs that the nurse is there for courts only (law enforcement or prosecution) or to protect the patient from court outcomes (advocacy). Some forensic nurses may even adopt a police investigative role and deny they are practicing nursing altogether. Successful coordinated teams that address all aspects of criminal violence responses respect each team member's educational foundation, role on the team, and contributions to the outcomes of the collaboration, whether for the individual, the family, the community, or the society at large (Box 8.11).

Box 8.11   Emerging Pitfalls in Beliefs About Forensic Nursing Practice

"**I**'m here to collect evidence."

No, you practice as a registered nurse governed by legislation and regulation.

"No one asks for the photographs, so I don't release them."

OR

"I'll release the photographs that are representative of this case."

No, all records are released under HIPAA when requested by law enforcement.

"I can't testify for the defense."

OR

"I'm collecting evidence to get the bad guys."

Nursing care occurs in the course of performing health care, and that process is useful to the courts, but not necessarily to one legal position over another. Your nursing practice should be comprehensive, based on nursing theory and ADPIE process, unbiased, and culturally competent. The facts emerge from the documentation of the unbiased forensic nursing evaluation. The adversarial legal system will argue the merits of your evaluation under the legal rules, and if there is an element of bias, credibility of your practice and the practice of others in your organization will be questioned.

Forensic nurses who adopt the investigative role of law enforcement will run the risk of being labeled as biased for the prosecution and identified by the court as a testimonial witness, unable to testify about the patient's history of the event and the biological, psychological, sociological, and spiritual health risks, sequelae, and nursing interventions. Rulings that label forensic nurses as testimonial witnesses will increase if nurses do not understand and cannot explain that they are first registered nurses, legislated and regulated in the practice that inevitably leads to diagnosis and treatment of the health and medical concerns of the patient.

As forensic nurses head back to school in record numbers, they should be good consumers of the educational offerings from a variety of organizations and institutions. The differing offerings should be evaluated and respond to the need of the forensic nurse, whether continuing education for beginning practice in an area or certification or formal academic education that results in a degree. The nurse will need to decide if the degree is in nursing or one outside nursing and recognize the implication of each. In summary, each level of education will provide the information and training necessary to improve forensic nursing practice globally.

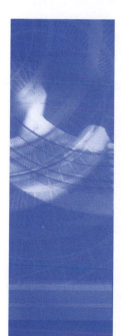

EVIDENCE-BASED PRACTICE

Reference Question: For women who are abused by their intimate partner, does the use of an advocacy (group social support) intervention prevent violence within 12 months of the intervention?

P = Women abused by intimate partner
I = Advocacy
C = Usual care
O = Prevent violence
T = 12 months

Database to Search: Cochrane Library

Search Terms: Because the Cochrane Library is a small database, doing a simple keyword search is usually sufficient. Searching for "intimate partner abuse" finds two reviews in Cochrane. One is appropriate for the question.

Selected References From Search:

1. Cook, R.J, Dickens, B.M. (2009). Dilemmas in intimate partner violence. *International Journal of Gynecology & Obstetrics, 106*(1):72-75.

(evidence-based practice box continued on page 134)

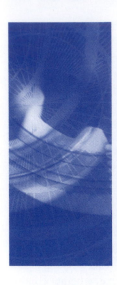

EVIDENCE-BASED PRACTICE (continued)

2. Ramsay, J., Carter, Y., Davidson, L., et al. (2009). Advocacy intervention to reduce or eliminate violence and promote the physical and psychosocial well-being of women who experience intimate partner abuse (Review). *The Cochrane Collaboration, 1*(3)1-23.

Questions Used to Discern Evidence:

Read the studies listed and answer the following questions:

1. What are the differences between the two studies in respect to design, methods, and results?
2. What are the similarities between the two studies in respect to the number of subjects, measures used, and interventions, if any?
3. What skills do you need to learn to work with women who survive intimate partner abuse?

REVIEW QUESTIONS

1. Compassion fatigue is described as:
   A. Following a witnessed traumatic event of actual or threatened death or serious injury
   B. Gradually becoming caught in a state of mental fatigue and drained of energy
   C. Emotional, physical, social, and spiritual exhaustion that leads to a pervasive decline in ability and energy to feel and care for others
   D. Feeling the trauma of another person and taking it on as one's own

2. The health-care provider's role in the recognition and response to violence is:
   A. Promoting community education on all levels
   B. Implementation of procedures and policy in identification and treatment of patients who have been abused
   C. Elimination of organizations in the community who deal with perpetrators
   D. Both B and C

3. The definition of community violence is:
   A. Exposure to acts of interpersonal violence committed by individuals who are not intimately related to the victim
   B. Exposure to acts of interpersonal violence committed by a relation
   C. Exposure to acts of violence across the life span by individuals known or related to the victim
   D. Exposure to acts of violence other than rape and sexual assault

4. Virtual violence has resulted in new crimes surfacing rapidly in communities. An example of virtual violence is:
   A. Bullying on the playground
   B. Stalking by using technology to track the victim
   C. Sexual stimulations of unwanted touching
   D. Consenting sex among underage adolescents

5. The spectrum of prevention in sexual assault described by Cohen includes levels such as:
   A. Fostering a cost-effective jail health system
   B. User-friendly treatment materials that are accessible by organizations that provide services for sexual assault patients
   C. Fostering networks and coalitions in the community
   D. Reporting violent events to law enforcement

6. An example of primary prevention in sexual assault care is:
   A. Providing emergency contraception to a patient who has been raped
   B. Collection of evidence for the patient who has been physically abused
   C. Maintaining the chain of custody
   D. Discussion of high-risk behavior reduction to a person one is standing next to in the grocery store checkout line

REVIEW QUESTIONS—cont'd

7. The Occupational Safety and Health Act, often referred to as the General Duty Clause, requires employers to:
   A. Furnish a place of employment that is free from recognized hazards that may cause death or serious harm
   B. Supply risk management-mandated payment and reporting of noncompliance with staffing mandates
   C. Provide bullet-resistant glass and walls in the emergency rooms
   D. Make referrals for coverage of sexual harassment counseling to reduce lawsuits

8. The Joint Commission states that hospitals will respond to patients who present for IPV, neglect, and exploitation. This might include:
   A. Demonstration of staffing flexibility based on level of care
   B. Cross-trained ED staff for collection of evidence based on DHS protocol
   C. Trained and educated ED staff on the identification of victims of violence
   D. Organizational policy for treatment of injury related to violence that is documented with concept maps and decision trees

9. A 29-year-old female enters a clinic complaining of abdominal pain, and assessment reveals multiple bruises in different stages of healing on her torso and breasts. The woman explains that she is clumsy and runs into objects a lot. The nurse examiner should:
   A. Obtain a full body MRI or X-rays
   B. Consider the diagnosis of a bleeding lesion from a concussion
   C. Gather more history, with specific questions about violence in her life
   D. Call and report potential violence to law enforcement

10. Cyberbullying includes:
   A. Sending or forwarding mean text messages
   B. Posting pictures with consent
   C. Encouraging people to share personal information
   D. Informing a person that you do not want them to e-mail you again

11. Many teens do not report dating violence because they are afraid to tell friends and family. Which of the following is correct regarding the occurrence?
   A. 72% of eighth and ninth graders report dating violent friends
   B. Adolescents rarely report verbal, physical, emotional, or sexual abuse from a partner
   C. About 50% of students nationwide report being physically hurt by a boyfriend or girlfriend in the past 12 months
   D. Most adolescents experience more violence in nondating and family relationships

References

Allen, J.P., Maisto, S.A., & Connors, G.J. (1995). Self-report screening tests for alcohol problems in primary care. *Archives of Internal Medicine, 155*(16):1726-1730.

American Nurses Association (ANA). (2009). *Forensic nursing: Scope and standards of practice*. Washington, DC: American Nurses Association.

American Psychological Association (APA). (2000). *Diagnostic and Statistical Manual of Mental Disorders* (4th ed.). Washington, DC: APA.

Anda, R.F., & Brown, D.W. (2007). Root causes and organic budgeting: Funding health from conception to the grave. (Commentary). *Pediatric Health, 1*(2):141-143.

Anda, R.F., Dong, M., Brown, D.W., Felitti, V.J., et al. (2009). The relationship of adverse childhood experiences to a history of premature death of family members. *BMC Public Health, 9*(106). Retrieved from http://www.biomedcentral.com/1471-2458/9/106. doi:10.1186/1471-2458-9-106

Anda, R.F., Felitti, V.J., Bremner, J.D., Walker, J.D., et al. (2006). The enduring effects of abuse and related adverse experiences in childhood: A convergence of evidence from neurobiology and epidemiology. *European Archilves of Psychiatry and Clinical Neuroscience, 256*(3):174-186.

Bair-Merritt, M.H., Blackstone, M., & Feudtner, C. (2006). Physical health outcomes of childhood exposure to intimate partner violence: a systematic review. *Pediatrics, 117*(2):e278-290.

Baird, K., & Kracen, A.C. (2006). Vicarious traumatization and secondary traumatic stress: A research synthesis. *Counselling Psychology Quarterly, 19*(2):181-188.

Bauer, N.S., Herrenkohl, T.I., Lozano, P., Rivara, F.P., Hill, K.G., & Hawkins, J.D. (2006). Childhood bullying involvement and exposure to intimate partner violence. *Pediatrics, 118*(2):e235-242.

Brochman, S. (1991). Silent victims: Bringing male rape out of the closet. *The Advocate, 582*:38-43.

Brown, J.B., Lent, B., Schmidt, G., & Sas, G. (2000). Application of the Woman Abuse Screening Tool (WAST) and WAST-short in the family practice setting. *Journal of Family Practice, 49*(10): 896-903.

Campbell, J., Webster, D.W., & Glass, N. (2009). The danger assessment: Validation of a lethality risk assessment instrument for intimate partner femicide. *Journal of Interpersonal Violence, 24*(4):653-674.

Campbell, J.C., Sharps, P.W., Sachs, C., & Yam, M.L. (2003). Medical lethality assessment and safety planning in domestic violence cases. *Clinics in Family Practice, 5*(1):101-112.

Center for Democracy & Technology. (2009). *Health privacy*. Retrieved January 16, 2010, from http://www.cdt.org/issue/health-privacy

Center on the Developing Child. (n.d.). *InBrief: The impact of early adversity on children's development*. Retrieved November 7, 2009, from http://developingchild.harvard.edu/library/briefs/inbrief_series/inbrief_the_impact_of_early_adversity/

Centers for Disease Control and Prevention. (2006). *Intimate partner violence: Fact sheet*. Retrieved August 16, 2009, from http://www.cdc.gov/violenceprevention/pdf/IPV_factsheet-a.pdf

Centers for Disease Control and Prevention. (2009). *Youth violence prevention scientific information: Definitions–definition of youth violence*. Retrieved September 30, 2009, from http://www.nccev.org/violence/community.html

Centers for Disease Control and Prevention. (2009). Definition of elder maltreatment. *Elder Maltreatment*. Retrieved August 16, 2009.

Centers for Disease Control and Prevention. (n.d.). *New technology and youth violence*. Retrieved November 7, 2009, from http://www.cdc.gov/ncipc/dvp/electronic_aggression.htm

Chasson, S., & Russell, A. (2002). Sexual assault: Clinical issues. Do SANE examinations satisfy the EMTALA requirement for "medical screening"? *Journal of Emergency Nursing, 28*(6):593-595.

Chiodo, D., Wolfe, D.A., Crooks, C., Hughes, R., & Jaffe, P. (2009). Impact of sexual harassment victimization by peers on subsequent adolescent victimization and adjustment: A longitudinal study. *Journal of Adolescent Health, 45*(3):246-252.

Cohen, L. (1999). The spectrum of prevention: Developing a comprehensive approach to injury prevention. *Injury Prevention, 5*:203-207.

Continuum of family violence. (n.d.). *Replace fear with hope*. Retrieved January 13, 2010, from http://www.mcleancountyil.gov/statesattorney/pdf/Continuum_Of_Family_Violence.pdf

Cook, S.L., Conrad, L., Bender, M., & Kaslow, N.J. (2003). The internal validity of the index of spouse abuse in African American women. *Violence and Victims, 18*(6):641-657.

Cyberbullying Research Center. (2009). Retrieved November 7, 2009, from http://www.cyberbullying.us/publications.php

Dahlberg, L.L., & Kruge, E.G. (2002). Violence: A global public health problem. In E.G. Krug, L.L. Dahlberg, J.A. Mercy, A.B. Zwi & R. Lazano (Eds.), *World report on violence and health*. Geneva: World Health Organization, pp. 1-22.

Davis, R., Parks, L.F., & Cohen, L. (2006). Sexual violence and the spectrum of prevention: Toward a community solution. Retrieved from http://www.nsvrc.org/sites/default/files/Publications_NSVRC_Booklets_Sexual-Violence-and-the-Spectrum-of-Prevention_Towards-a-Community-Solution.pdf

Department of Health and Human Services, Administration for Children and Families. (2006). *Child Maltreatment 2006*. Retrieved from http://www.acf.hhs.gov/programs/cb/pubs/cm06/cm06.pdf

DeSantis, L.A., & Lipson, J.G. (2007). Brief history of inclusion of content on culture in nursing education. *Journal of Transcultural Nursing, 18*(1):7S-9s.

Dominguez-Gomez, E., & Rutledge, D.N. (2009). Prevalence of secondary traumatic stress among emergency nurses. *Journal of Emergency Nursing, 35*(3):199-204.

Dube, S.R., Anda, R.F., Whitfield, C.L., Brown, D.W., Felitti, V.J., Dong, M., et al. (2005). Long term consequences of childhood sexual abuse by gender of victim. *American Journal of Preventive Medicine, 28*:430-438.

Duhart, D.T. (2001). Violence in the workplace, 1993-99. *Bureau of Justice Statistics: Special Report, 12*. Retrieved from http://bjs.ojp.usdoj.gov/content/pub/pdf/vw99.pdf

Durose, M.R. (2005). *Family violence statistics: Including statistics on strangers and acquaintances, 1t 31-32*. Bureau of Justice Statistics. Retrieved November 7, 2009, from http://www.abanet.org/domviol/statistics.html

Edwards, S., Dube, S.R., Felitti, V.J., & Anda, R.F. (2007). It's ok to ask about past abuse. (Commentary with discussion). *American Psychologist, 62*(4):327-332.

Federal Bureau of Investigation. (2004). *Crime in the United States 2004, uniform crime report*. Retrieved September 30, 2009, from http://www.fbi.gov/ucr/cius_04/documents/CIUS2004.pdf

Feldhaus, K.M., Koziol-McLain, J., Amsbury, H.L., Norton, I.M., Lowenstein, S.R., & Abbott, J.T. (1997). Accuracy of 3 brief screening questions for detecting partner violence in the emergency department. *Journal of American Medical Association, 277*(17): 1357-1361.

Felitti, V.J., Anda, R.F., Nordenberg, D., Williamson, D.F., Spitz, A.M., Edwards, V., et al. (1998). Relationship of childhood abuse and household dysfunction to many of the leading causes of death in adults. The Adverse Childhood Experiences (ACE) Study. (See comment). *American Journal of Preventive Medicine, 14*(4):245-258.

Finkelhor, D., Ormrod, R.K., & Turner, H.A. (2009). The developmental epidemiology of childhood victimization. *Journal of Interpersonal Violence, 24*(5):711-731.

Finkelhor, D., Turner, H., Ormrod, R., Hamby, S., & Kracke, K. (2009). Children's exposure to violence: A comprehensive national survey. *Juvenile Justice Bulletin, 12*. Retrieved from http://www.ncjrs.gov/pdffiles1/ojjdp/227744.pdf

Garcia-Moreno, C., Jansen, H., Ellsberg, & Heis, L. (2005). World Health Organization. *(WHO) multi-country study on women's health and domestic violence against women.* Retrieved November 7, 2009, from http://www.who.int/gender/violence/who_multicountry_study/en/

Gates, D.M., & Gillespie, G.L. (2008). Secondary Traumatic Stress in Nurses Who Care for Traumatized Women. *Journal of Obstetric, Gynecologic, & Neonatal Nursing, 37*(2), 243-249.

Glass, N., Perrin, N., Hanson, G., Bloom, T., Gardner, E., & Campbell, J.C. (2008). Risk for reassault in abusive female same-sex relationships. *American Journal of Public Health, 98*(6):1021-1027.

Groth, A.N., & Burgess, A.W. (1980). Male rape: Offenders and victims. *American Journal of Psychiatry, 137*(7):806-810.

Hillis, S.D., Anda, R.F., Dube, S.R., Felitti, V.J., Marchbanks, P.A., & Marks, J.S. (2004). The association between adverse childhood experiences and adolescent pregnancy, long-term psychosocial consequences, and fetal death. *Pediatrics, 113*(2):320-327.

Holden, G.W. (2003). Children exposed to domestic violence and child abuse: Terminology and taxonomy. *Clinical Child & Family Psychology Review, 6*(3):151-160.

Houry, D., Sachs, C.J., Feldhaus, C.J., & Linden, K. (2002). Violence inflicted injuries: Reporting laws in the fifty states. *Annals of Emergency Medicine, 39*(1):56-60.

Human Rights Watch. (n.d.). *No escape: Male rape in U.S. prisons.* Retrieved July 17, 2009, from http://www.hrw.org/legacy/reports/2001/prison/

International Association of Forensic Nurses. (2004). *Core competencies for advanced practice forensic nursing.* Retrieved June 11, 2008, from http://www.forensicnurse.org/associations/8556/files/APN%20Core%20Curriculum%20Document.pdf

International Labour Organisation. (2002). *A future without child labour.* Retrieved July 17, 2009, from http://www.ilo.org/wcmsp5/groups/public/—-dgreports/—-dcomm/—-publ/documents/publication/wcms_publ_9221124169_en.pdf

International Labour Organisation. (2007). *Towards the elimination of the worst forms of child labour (TECL): Note on the definition of 'child trafficking.'* Pretoria, South Africa: International Labour Organisation.

Isley, P. (1991). Adult male sexual assault in the community: A literature review and group treatment model. In A. Burgess (Ed.), *Rape and sexual assault III: A research handbook.* New York: Garland Publishing.

Kennedy, A.C., Bybee, D., Sullivan, C.M., & Greeson, M. (2009). The effects of community and family violence exposure on anxiety trajectories during middle childhood: The role of family social support as a moderator. *Journal of Clinical Child & Adolescent Psychology, 38*(3):365-379.

Kernic, M.A., Holt, V.L., Wolf, M.E., McKnight, B., Huebner, C.E., & Rivara, F.P. (2002). Academic and school health issues among children exposed to maternal intimate partner abuse. *Archives of Pediatrics & Adolescent Medicine, 156*(6):549-555.

Lawyers.com. (n.d.). *Criminal law: Crime definition FAQs.* Retrieved November 24, 2009, from http://criminal.lawyers.com/Criminal-Law-Crime-Definition-FAQs.html#8

Leeb, R.T., Paulozzi, L.J., Melanson, C., Simon, T.R., & Arias, I. (2008). *Child maltreatment surveillance: Uniform definitions for public health and recommended data elements.* Retrieved from http://www.cdc.gov/ncipc/dvp/CM_Surveillance.pdf.

Lefley, H.P., Scott, C.S., Llabre, M., & Hicks, D. (1993). Cultural beliefs about rape and victims' response in three ethnic groups. *American Journal of Orthopsychiatry, 63*(4):623-632.

Lipscomb, G.H., Muram, D., Speck, P.M., & Mercer, B.M. (1992). Male victims of sexual assault. *Journal of American Medical Association, 267*(22):3064-3066.

MacMillan, H.D., Wathen, C.N., Jamieson, E., Boyle, M.H., et al. (2009). Screening for intimate partner violence in health care settings: A randomized trial. *Journal of American Medical Association, 302*(5):493-501.

Mao, C. (2002). Teaching residents humanistic skills in a colposcopy clinic. *Academic Medicine, 77*(7):742.

Marshall, V.W., & Altpeter, M. (2005). Cultivating social work leadership in health promotion and aging: Strategies for active aging interventions. *Health & Social Work, 30*(2):135-144.

Maternal and Child Health Bureau. (2009). *Cyberbullying; Tolls and tips for prevention and intervention.* Retrieved November 7, 2009, from http://webcast.hrsa.gov/Postevents/archivedWebCastCaptionDefault.asp?aehid=1304

McCall, M.A., & Sorbie, J. (1994). Educating physicians about women's health. Survey of Canadian family medicine residency programs.(See comment). *Canadian Family Physician, 40*:900-905.

McFarlane, J., Campbell, J.C., Wilt, S., Sachs, C., Ulruch, Y., & Xu, X. (1999). Stalking and intimate partner femicide. *Homicide Studies, 3*(4):300-316.

McFarlane, J., Parker, B., Soeken, K., & Bullock, L. (1992). Assessing for abuse during pregnancy: Severity and frequency of injuries and associated entry into prenatal care. *Journal of American Medical Association, 267*(23):3176-3178.

McHolm, F. (2006). Rx for compassion fatigue. *Journal of Christian Nursing, 23*(4):12-21.

McKinney, C.M., Caetano, R., Ramisetty-Mikler, S., & Nelson, S. (2009). Childhood family violence and perpetration and victimization of intimate partner violence: Findings from a national population-based study of couples. *Annals of Epidemiology, 19*(1):25-32.

MedLaw.com. (n.d.). Interpretive guidelines. *EMTALA and Healthlaw Resources for Healthcare Professionals, Hospitals, and Their Attorneys.* Retrieved January 30, 2010, from http://www.medlaw.com/healthlaw/EMTALA/guidelines/interpretive-guidelines.shtml

Men's Advice Line. (n.d.). *Male victims of domestic violence: Our position.* Retrieved July 17, 2009, from http://www.mensadviceline.org.uk/pages/advice-frontline-workers.html

Mercy, J.A., Butchart, A., Farrington, D., & Cerda, M. (2002). Youth violence. *World report on violence and health.* Retrieved from http://www.who.int/violence_injury_prevention/violence/global_campaign/en/chap2.pdf

Mollica, R. F., & Son, L. (1989). Cultural dimensions in the evaluation and treatment of sexual trauma. An overview. *Psychiatric Clinics of North America, 12*(2):363-379.

Moracco, K., & Cole, T. (2009). Preventing intimate partner violence: Screening is not enough. *Journal of American Medical Association, 302*:568-570.

National Center for Children Exposed to Violence. (2006). *Community violence.* Retrieved September 30, 2009, from http://www.nccev.org/violence/community.html

National Institute of Occupational Safety and Health. (2009). Occupational violence. *NIOSH safety and health topic.* Retrieved October 30, 2009, from http://www.cdc.gov/niosh/topics/violence/

National Scientific Council on the Developing Child. (2005). *Excessive stress disrupts the architecture of the developing brain: Working paper No. 3.* Retrieved November 7, 2009 from http://developingchild.harvard.edu/library/reports_and_working_papers/working_papers/wp3/

National Youth Violence Prevention Resource Center. (2008). *Media violence facts and statistics: Prevalence of media violence.* Retrieved November 7, 2009, from http://www.safeyouth.org/scripts/faq/mediaviolstats.asp

Occupational Health and Safety Administration. (2007, July 20). *OSHA Standards. Workplace Violence.* Retrieved January 12, 2010, from http://www.osha.gov/SLTC/workplaceviolence/standards.html

Office on Violence Against Women. (2004). *A national protocol for sexual assault medical forensic examinations: Adults/adolescents.* Retrieved from DATE www.ncjrs.gov/pdffiles1/ovw/206554.pdf

Oppeal, S., Lamanna, B.F., & Glenn, L.L. (2006). Comparison of the dissemination and implementation of standardized public health nursing competencies in academic and practice settings. *Public Health Nursing, 23*(2):99-107.

Quad Council of Public Health Nursing Organizations. (2003). *Quad Council PHN competencies.* Retrieved January 10, 2010, from http://www.astdn.org/publication_quad_council_phn_competencies.htm

Rennison, C.M. (2002). *Rape and sexual assault: Reporting to police and medical attention, 1992-2000.*

Rennison, C.M. (2003). Intimate partner violence, 1993-2001. *Bureau of Justice Statistics Crime Data Brief,* (NCJ 197838). Retrieved from http://bjs.ojp.usdoj.gov/content/pub/pdf/ipv01.pdf

Rizzo, V.M., & Seidman, J. (2008). Health promotion & aging. *Council on Social Work Education.* Retrieved from http://www.cswe.org/File.aspx?id=24022

Runyan, D., Wattam, C., Ikeda, R., Hassan, F., & Ramiro, L. (2002). Child abuse and neglect by parents and caregivers. In E.G. Krug, L.L. Dahlberg, J.A. Mercy, A.B. Zwi & R. Lozano (Eds.), *World report on violence and health*, pp. 59-86. Geneva, Switzerland: World Health Organziation.

Schultz, P.N. (2002). *Rape in the context of intimate partner violence.* Unpublished Ph.D. Texas Woman's University, Houston, TX.

Self directed violence. (2002). In E.G. Krug, L.L. Dahlberg, J.A. Mercy, A.B. Zwi & R. Lozano (Eds.), *World Report on Violence and Health.* Geneva, Switzerland: World Health Organization.

Sheridan, D.J. (1998). *Measuring harassment of abused women: A nursing concern.* Unpublished Dissertation. Oregon Health Sciences University, Portland, OR.

Sherin, K.M., Sinacore, J.M., Li, X.Q., Zitter, R.E., & Shakil, A. (1998). HITS: A short domestic violence screening tool for use in a family practice setting. *Family Medicine, 30*(7):508-512.

Shonkoff, J.P., Boyce, W.T., & McEwen, B.S. (2009). Neuroscience, molecular biology, and the childhood roots of health disparities: Building a new framework for health promotion and disease prevention. *Journal of American Medical Association, 301*(21):2252-2259.

Shuey, K., & Hoaks, D. (1989). Brief: ADPIE—the game is on. ADPIE is an extension of the nursing process acronym, APIE (assessment, planning, implementation, and evaluation) to include "diagnosis". *Journal of Continuing Education in Nursing, 20*(4):184-185.

Speck, P.M. (2002). *Things you didn't learn in nursing school: Forensic nursing principles—WHEEL.* Paper presented at the Emergency Nurses Association.

Speck, P.M. (2005). *Program evaluation of current SANE services to victim populations in three cities.* Unpublished dissertation, University of Tennessee Health Science Center, Memphis, TN.

Speck, P.M., Connor, P.D., Hartig, M.T., Cunningham, P.D., & Fleming, B. (2008). Vulnerable populations: Drug court program clients. *Nursing Clinics of North America, 43*(3):477-489.

Speck, P.M., & Patton, S.B. (2010). Qualifications of the forensic nurse in sexual assault evaluation. In L.E. Ledray, A.W. Burgess & A.P. Giardino (Eds.), *Medical Response to Adult Sexual Assault.* St. Louis, MO: GW Medical Publishing.

Stewart, D.W. (2009). Casualties of war: Compassion fatigue and health care providers. *MEDSURG Nursing, 18*(2):91-94.

Tewksbury, R. (2007). Effects of sexual assaults on men: Physical, mental and sexual consequences. *International Journal of Men's Health, 6*(1):22-35.

The Adverse Childhood Experiences (ACE) Study. (n.d.). *Bridging the gap between childhood trauma and negative consequences later in life.* Retrieved January 29, 2010, from http://www.acestudy.org/index.html

The National Campaign to Prevent Teen and Unplanned Pregnancy. (n.d.). *Sex and tech: Results from a survey of teens and young adults.* Retrieved July 17, 2009, from http://www.thenationalcampaign.org/sextech/PDF/SexTech_Summary.pdf

Thoman, E. (n.d.). *Beyond blame: Media literacy as violence prevention.* Retrieved July 17, 2009, from http://www.medialit.org/reading_room/article93.html

Tjaden, P., & Thoennes, N. (1998). Stalking in America: Findings from the national violence against women survey. *National Institute of Justice Centers for Disease Control and Preventions Research in Brief.* Retrieved November 24, 2009, from http://www.ncjrs.gov/pdffiles/169592.pdf

Tjaden, P., & Thoennes, N. (2000a). *Extent, nature, and consequences of intimate partner violence.* Retrieved November 7, 2009, from http://www.ncjrs.gov/pdffiles1/nij/181867.pdf

Tjaden, P., & Thoennes, N. (2000b). *Full report of the prevalence, incidence, and consequences of violence against women.* Retrieved November 7, 2009, from http://www.ncjrs.gov/pdffiles1/nij/183781.pdf

Tjaden, P. & Thoennes, N. (2000c). *Full report of the prevalence, incidence, and consequences of violence against women: Findings from the national violence against women survey*. Vol. Report NCJ 183781. Washington, DC: National Institute of Justice.

Tjaden, P., & Thoennes, N. (2006). Extent, nature, and consequences of rape victimizaton: Findings from the national violence against women survey. *NIJ Special Report*, 46. Retrieved from http://www.ncjrs.gov/pdffiles1/nij/210346.pdf

The National Center for Victims of Crime. (2007). *Male rape*. Retrieved July 17, 2009, from http://www.ncvc.org/ncvc/main.aspx?dbName=DocumentViewer&DocumentID=32361

U.S. Department of Health and Human Services. Health information privacy. *Office for Civil Rights*. Retrieved January 15, 2010, from http://www.hhs.gov/ocr/privacy/

U.S. Department of Labor. (2007). *Workplace violence: OSHA standards*. Retrieved January 10, 2010, from http://www.osha.gov/SLTC/workplaceviolence/standards.html

United Nations Children's Fund. (2005). *The state of the world's children 2006: Excluded and invisible*. Retrieved July 17, 2009, from http://www.unicef.org/sowc06/pdfs/sowc06_fullreport.pdf

Violence Prevention Alliance. (2009). Definition and typology of violence. *Global Campaign for Violence Prevention*. Retrieved from http://www.who.int/violenceprevention/approach/definition/en/index.html

Violence Prevention Alliance. (2010). The ecological framework. *The VPA Approach* Retrieved November 11, 2009, from http://www.who.int/violenceprevention/approach/ecology/en/index.html

Walker, E.A., Gelfand, A., Katon, W.J., Koss, M.P., et al. (1999). Adult health status of women with histories of childhood abuse and neglect. (See comment). *American Journal of Medicine, 107*(4):332-339.

Walker, E.A., Unutzer, J., Rutter, C., Gelfand, A., Saunders, K., VonKorff, M., et al. (1999). Costs of health care use by women HMO members with a history of childhood abuse and neglect. *Archives of General Psychiatry, 56*(7):609-613.

Weiss, M.J., & Wagner, S.H. (1998). What explains the negative consequences of adverse childhood experiences on adult health? Insights from cognitive and neuroscience research. (Editorial). *American Journal of Preventive Medicine, 14*(4):356-360.

Williams-Evans, S.A., & Sheridan, D J. (2004). Exploring barriers to leaving violent intimate partner relationships. *Association of Black Nursing Faculty Journal, 15*(2):38-40.

World Health Organization. (2008). *The Ottawa charter for health promotion*. Retrieved December 20, 2010, from http://www.who.int/healthpromotion/conferences/previous/ottawa/en/

World Health Organization. (2010). Social determinants of health. *Social Determinants of Health*. Retrieved January 29, 2010, from http://www.who.int/social_determinants/en/

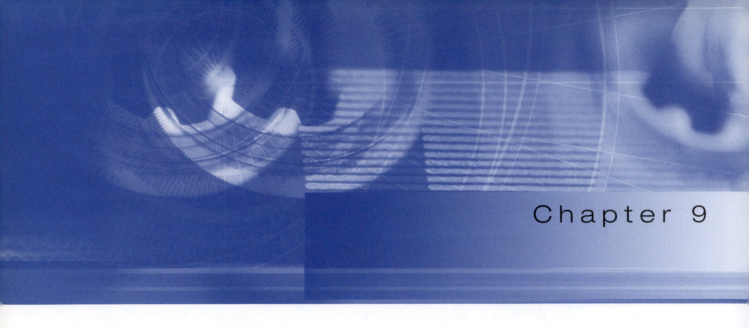

Chapter 9

Violence: Sexual Assault and the Forensic Nurse

Catherine J. Carter-Snell

" 'Normal' is just a setting on the dryer."
Barbara Johnson

Competencies

1. Discussing the available evidence underlying the effectiveness of SANEs.
2. Analyzing key elements of sexual assault care.
3. Assessing evidence in current or future sexual assault care practices.
4. Comparing and contrasting evidence collection in sexual assault of adolescents and adults.

Key Terms

Assessment
Evidence-based nursing practice
Interventions
Sexual assault
Sexual assault nurse examiners

INTRODUCTION

Sexual assault (SA) is an invasive and traumatic event for both men and women. Hundreds of thousands of people are victimized yearly in both the United States and Canada. The 2002 National Violence Against Women survey in the United States revealed that 17.6% of women (1 in 6) and 3.0% of men (1 in 33) had experienced a completed or attempted rape at some time in their life, with estimates of at least 876,064 SAs per year. The group at highest risk consists of women from 18 to 24 years of age. The most comprehensive Canadian survey of violence against women was conducted in 1993, in which 39% of women reported at least one SA since the age of 16 years. Subsequent General Social Surveys (GSS) consistently reveal that approximately 3% of Canadian women have been sexually assaulted within the preceding year. Based on 2006 census data, that means that at least 402,432 females age 15 or older have been sexually assaulted.

The personal and social impact of SA can be devastating. Short-term consequences include genital or nongenital injury, dissociation, acute stress disorder, and disruption of work and family life. Long-term consequences include chronic health disorders, post-traumatic stress disorder (PTSD), suicide, alcohol or drug dependency, and revictimization.

The purpose of this chapter is to discuss the services provided by Sexual Assault Nurse Examiners (SANEs) and many of their care elements. The focus is primarily on evidence related to SA of adolescents and adults.

CONSEQUENCES OF SA

The impact of SA on individuals, families, and health-care systems is significant. Long-term health-care costs for women after SA have been estimated to be in the billions of dollars in the United States and Canada.

Historically, the health services provided to sexually assaulted clients have been provided in busy emergency departments. Staff is often unfamiliar with care options or with evidence preservation or collection. Victims may be left waiting for significant periods until staff is available, often dehydrated and fatigued yet not being allowed to eat, drink, or void until after the examination. Care has been found to be incomplete or insensitive, especially for women of color, women who went to a Catholic hospital, women who were assaulted by someone they knew, women who had multiple forms of penetration, or women who presented in a less than sympathetic manner. Staff members have been found to negatively react to disclosures of SA

if not seeking that information. Negative reactions to disclosure have been associated with increased severity of PTSD symptoms. These gaps in care have been identified as secondary victimization, which has been associated with greater severity of PTSD symptoms and poor client outcomes.

Rates of PTSD are estimated to be between 47% and 55%, which is two to three times higher than for any other trauma. Data on male victims of SA also suggest extremely high rates of PTSD. Once disorders such as PTSD develop, they are difficult to treat, especially in women. Cognitive behavioral therapy (CBT) has been found to be one of the more helpful strategies. Unfortunately, CBT is not widely available to victims of SA or routinely part of subsidized counseling services provided to victims.

PTSD is also associated with high rates of depression and revictimization. Women who have been sexually assaulted have been shown to have significantly higher rates of substance abuse, sick time and health visits, and increased rates of suicide, especially if both PTSD and depression are present.

The gaps in comprehensive care and low rates of prosecution contributed to the development of the role of patient advocate in the United States in the 1970s, in which counselors pushed for improved legislation and standards of care for all SA victims. Soon after the advocate role began, Sexual Assault Nurse Examiners (SANEs) began to be trained. The first SANEs began to practice in 1977 in Minnesota, and slowly the role expanded across the United States. It is now estimated that there are thousands of sexual assault response teams (SARTs) across the United States. The SANE did not emerge in Canada until the mid-1990s, with the development of the first teams in Winnipeg, Vancouver, Edmonton, and Toronto. There are now SARTs in over half of the Canadian provinces, with more being planned.

EVIDENCE-BASED NURSING PRACTICE

The term "evidence-based" practice emerged initially in medicine to describe professional practice that relies on the integration of the best available evidence with professional expertise and client values. The "gold standard" of evidence in medicine and nursing is the randomized controlled trial (RCT). However, the RCT is not always the best method with which to gain understanding of nursing issues. Nursing is both an art and a science, combining caring and compassion with multiple forms of science and philosophy. **Evidence-based nursing practice** involves incorporating the best level of available evidence into care. Evidence includes research findings as well as factors such as clinical expertise, client preference, circumstances, and setting and resource constraints.

A hierarchy of sources of evidence has emerged (Fig. 9.1), which is usually illustrated in ascending order of quality or strength of evidence.

While there is considerable consistency among the hierarchies described in the literature, there is some movement between the placement of systematic reviews and qualitative research studies. Systematic reviews are more than a typical "literature review." They are rigorous reviews of the existing research on a particular topic involving extensive efforts to identify the research, documentation of the process, and specific guidelines for analysis. The Cochrane Collaboration Group is one of the leaders in setting standards for conducting and reporting systematic reviews, and it collects systematic reviews conducted by various research teams. Reviews are reported either descriptively or, where there are comparative quantitative data, in the form of meta-analyses. This type of review allows for pooling and synthesis of similar studies, strengthening the ability to detect the true magnitude of a difference if it exists.

Systematic reviews were originally intended to include only RCTs, but methods have been described for observational cohort studies, which are typical of most quantitative nursing research studies. Systematic reviews are also sometimes known as "metasyntheses." They have a lower status than quantitative systematic reviews. Standards for the conduct of qualitative systematic reviews/metasyntheses have been developed by groups such as the Cochrane Qualitative Methods Research Group and the Qualitative Metasynthesis Project researchers. There are also systematic reviews in which qualitative and quantitative research have been combined. In general, systematic reviews of any type are generally considered to provide higher levels of evidence than single studies, regardless of the type of research, as long as they are conducted properly and only similar studies and populations are pooled.

It should be noted that within each level of evidence there are also embedded levels and quality of evidence. For instance, a cohort study on risk factors for injury using multivariate analysis may provide a depth of data and relationships between risk factors that would not be captured by a cohort study in which rates of injury are reported for lists of single risk factors. A study involving complex multivariate methods, such as structural equation modeling or hierarchical linear modeling, also provides higher-level information due to its inherent management of error measurement and ability to detect interaction between factors. Flaws in research methods and conclusions also affect the strength of the evidence. Even higher levels of research methods are weakened if a sample does not represent typical SA populations, the methods used to examine the clients do not reflect recommended practices, or there are flaws in measurement.

Methods for measuring the quality of individual studies differ across the literature and the type of research. Quality measures typically examine factors related to the research design, the accuracy of measures, and the consistency of the findings and conclusions. There is little existing literature in which the quality of SA research has been quantified. One evaluation was conducted of the quality of the research used for a systematic review of risks for SA injuries. The research was examined using a validated tool for noncomparative observational research known as the MINORS scale, which assesses aspects of research design. A second tool was developed by the reviewer to include measures thought to affect quality or best practices of the studies, such as use of aids to visualization and specialized examiners, such as SANEs. The instrument was called the Sexual Assault Quality Score (SASQ). The MINORS score was quite low across the research and did not change appreciably among studies conducted prior

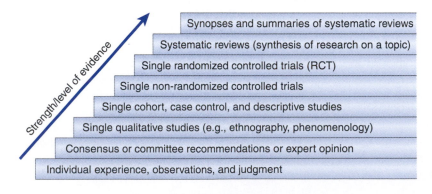

Strength/level of evidence

Synopses and summaries of systematic reviews

Systematic reviews (synthesis of research on a topic)

Single randomized controlled trials (RCT)

Single non-randomized controlled trials

Single cohort, case control, and descriptive studies

Single qualitative studies (e.g., ethnography, phenomenology)

Consensus or committee recommendations or expert opinion

Individual experience, observations, and judgment

■ **FIGURE 9.1** Levels of evidence.

to 2000 (mean = 58%; SD = 9) compared with those conducted between 2000 and 2006 (mean = 63%; SD = 10). In contrast, the mean SASQ score was 15% higher (mean = 66%; SD = 15) in studies conducted since 2000 compared with earlier time periods. Significantly fewer studies scored less than 60%, reflecting improvements in techniques and examiner skill. All of the research involved individual cohorts with mostly univariate or bivariate analyses. The results apply only to the quality of the studies in the review; however, it is anticipated that similar results will be found in other areas of SA study quality. The nature of the trauma and clients limits the ability to perform randomized controlled trials or more sophisticated designs. To strengthen the evidence we therefore have to explore methods such as multivariate analysis in single studies and systematic reviews of multiple studies related to the same topic.

This discussion will be used as the guideline with which to evaluate the level or strength of the evidence in the subsequent discussions.

SEXUAL ASSAULT NURSE EXAMINERS

Sexual Assault Nurse Examiners (SANEs) make up one of the largest subspecialties of forensic nurses found in either the International Association of Forensic Nurses (IAFN) or the Forensic Nurses' Society of Canada (FNSC). This area of forensic nursing was also the first to be formally certified as a specialty by the IAFN through an optional examination and recertification process. The first examinations were for sexual assault nurses caring for adults and adolescents (SANE-A) and were written by American SANEs in 2001. The first Canadian nurse (the author of this chapter) was certified in 2002. A certification process is now in place for SANEs for pediatric clients (SANE-P). The initials "SANE" can be used following a nurse's name only if the nurse has met the certification requirements of the IAFN or similar agency granting certification. Forensic nurses in Canada are now exploring specialty certification through the FNSC and the Canadian Nurses' Association. Many nurses in North America have received education in SA care, usually consistent with the IAFN curriculum requirements, but have not taken the IAFN examinations. These nurses may use "sexual assault nurse examiner" as a job description but cannot use the initials. In the SA literature, the term SANE is used often, but it is not clear if all nurses are certified. For the purposes of this chapter, all nurses providing care for SA clients will be referred to as SANEs, recognizing that only some may be certified.

Role of SANEs

The IAFN has described forensic nurses as integrating forensic knowledge into their existing biological, psychological, and social nursing knowledge while caring for victims of violence or trauma. SANEs, therefore, combine knowledge related to objective evidence collection and forensic examination with knowledge related to comprehensive health-care needs of clients who have been sexually assaulted.

The cost of health care is prohibitive for clients who do not report to police in the United States, leading to a trend to have private clinics or centers funded by government agencies. Surveys of SA programs in the United States indicate that the most specialized SA nursing programs are still based in health-care settings. The minority (10% to 40%) is located in community-funded facilities or with police services.

Despite the push to specialize and at least three decades of experience, a number of regions in the United States still provide nonspecialized care to sexually assaulted clients in emergency departments using staff unfamiliar with care options, although advocates are increasingly available to help clients understand their range of options in these settings. In the United States these advocates are also seen as important to ensure the client receives support without damaging the SANE's credibility as an unbiased witness in court. The standards and expectations for witness testimony are different in Canada. Provision of empathetic, compassionate care is recognized as part of nursing and therefore not seen as potentially biasing in the courts. In Canada all SA services are located in health-care centers, either emergency or stand-alone clinics. Unfortunately, specialized SA services are relatively new in Canada and are therefore found only in major urban centers.

A review of SA programs suggests that health-care–based programs receive more survivors than police-based programs. This is supported by victimization survey data in which almost three times as many Canadian women (30%) reported they sought health care after their SA, compared with the number who reported to police. Over half of respondents in a U.S. study reported seeking health care after their SA compared with 32% who reported to police. These findings have important implications for SANEs. We are more likely to interact with victims of SA. This may also be the victim's only interaction with the health-care system, as only a third of clients have been found to return for follow-up. Failure to provide comprehensive services when clients do decide to seek care may result in serious consequences for the client.

Health-seeking behaviors of SA clients also suggest important social policy actions for nurses. Clinical experience has shown that health services are often sought mainly to obtain prophylaxis for pregnancy and sexually transmitted infections, but on arriving, clients find even more options and services available to them. Women's groups have lobbied to make emergency contraception available on the shelves of many Canadian pharmacies to make it more readily available. The move may have unanticipated drawbacks, however. It may reduce the number of women seeking health care after an SA and reduce their awareness of both the risks and the services available. There is no requirement for pharmacists to provide information about local SA services or options. A Canadian study compared the volume of women accessing emergency contraception when only physicians could prescribe compared with the post-policy change in which pharmacists could dispense the contraception in one province. The number of women accessing emergency contraception more than doubled in the 5-year interval, more than accounted for by population growth. Over 55% were using it for unprotected intercourse, but it is unknown how many of these women were sexually assaulted. It is also unknown if any of these women then sought additional SA services. SANEs need to be aware of the potential impact of legislative changes such as this and work to find effective solutions to aid SA victims in locating and accessing care options after SA.

Models of Care

Most information regarding models of SANE care is anecdotal or descriptive in nature. Identification and description of such models are important for evaluating effectiveness of programs. A common theme in SA care is empowerment. Empowerment allows the client to regain control after an assault. A model of "empowering care" has been described in which SANEs provide health care, crisis support, and resources. Key components include treating all clients with dignity and respect regardless of circumstances, accepting the client as a person, believing the history of the assault, assisting clients in restoring control over their lives and making their own choices, and respecting their decisions. The client is offered a comprehensive range of services and may select those best suited to his or her unique needs. Services include an examination for physical or psychological consequences of the assault (e.g., injuries or acute stress), involvement of police and evidence collection, access to medications to prevent pregnancy and sexually transmitted infections,

crisis intervention, and referral to follow-up services aimed at reducing the health consequences of the assault. Effectiveness of SA services and nurses would therefore be measured on the range of services provided, client satisfaction, and client outcomes rather than on prosecution or forensic outcomes.

An empowerment model of care brings with it a need for the SANE to also advocate for the client's access to comprehensive health care, including the provision of sensitive, compassionate care. The ability of the SANE to advocate in this way can be a challenge; however, if a SANE is employed by the police or justice system, it may be seen as a bias. There are some potential benefits to working through a health-care or neutral agency. This care may not always result in involvement of police and evidence collection if it is not desired by the client. Reporting is not always a benefit to the client. There is some preliminary evidence in domestic violence situations that while reporting may produce positive feelings, there are negative consequences for the client if the case goes to court. Although a portion of sexually assaulted clients are also victims of partner violence, further research is required in this area before results can be applied.

Comprehensive or holistic models of care have emerged as a common framework for many SA services. The next step is to evaluate these models in terms of SANE effectiveness and impact on client outcomes.

Effectiveness of SANEs

A number of researchers have studied the effectiveness of SANEs using a variety of measures. Most studies are descriptive, using retrospective convenience or cohort samples and outcome measures established after the fact. Conclusions from these individual studies are therefore tentative until more rigorous research is conducted or findings are confirmed across multiple studies. The perceived effectiveness of a team is also affected by its mandate; is it health care or forensic in nature? For instance, a team that is based on a justice model may consider successful prosecution as a measure of success, whereas health models may not.

Comprehensive Care

The effectiveness of SANEs or use of comprehensive care principles in preventing long-term consequences is anticipated but has not yet been well established. Multiple areas of effectiveness were examined in a well-designed quasi-experimental study across disciplines, using both qualitative and quantitative methods to study sexually assaulted client services both before and after the introduction of a SA team. The SANEs provided more prophylaxis, and clients were found to accept more treatment, report to police more often, were more likely to consent to evidence collection, had twice as many referrals, and experienced shorter stays in the department. These findings were supported in other single cohort studies in other settings. SANEs spent less time than when physicians were involved and more consistently obtained consents and consent for evidence collection.

Client Well-Being

Programs that address clients' physical and emotional needs after the assault have been found to have positive outcomes on client well-being by numerous researchers. The positive impact of programs on post-assault well-being addresses clients' physical and emotional needs.

One of the first studies to research SANE effectiveness in psychological outcomes looked at client reports of their psychological outcomes after being seen by SANEs. The majority of the 52 clients assessed reported overwhelmingly positive psychological outcomes after care by SANEs, including feeling cared for, supported, informed, and not pressured to report. Earlier qualitative research with a small group of sexually assaulted clients cared for by SANEs also reported clients felt supported, in control, and having choices. Neither study included a group cared for by nonspecialized health professionals nor longitudinal examination of outcomes such as PTSD, but they do provide key directions for further investigation and practice.

Further areas for future research on well-being outcomes include the effectiveness of both comprehensive care and specific **interventions** on the rates of short and long-term client consequences. Examples of these include differences in dissociation, acute stress disorder or PTSD, substance abuse, revictimization, or chronic health problems with measures such as facilitating client control and choice, reframing, crisis intervention, use of positive acceptance, grounding techniques, referrals for follow-up, and screening for suicide risks.

LEGAL OUTCOMES

Quality of evidence collection may affect successful prosecution and client outcomes if clients wish to proceed with the legal system. SANEs were found to collect evidence more accurately compared with emergency nurses or physicians. There is some individual variation in what is collected between examiners, and the rationale was not always found to be consistent. While individualizing is deemed preferable to a standard method for all, the authors emphasized the need for improved information for examiners to guide their decisions.

Some teams routinely collect SA forensic samples on all clients to avoid burdening clients with decisions. Using the same or standard interventions for all may not be seen as helpful by all clients. When clients were asked to rate various aspects of their care as having a positive or negative impact, they rated the forensic examination as less positive. The authors speculated that it may be due to the more circumscribed and routine nature of the examination. The difficulties with the evidence kit collection are further highlighted in qualitative interviews of sexually assaulted women seen by a Canadian SANE team. The women revealed that the sexual assault examination kit (SAEK) was one of the more difficult experiences they encountered, along with blood-taking and the speculum examination. Despite the difficulty, some women also described the evidence collection as empowering. The impact of SAEK collection is unknown among male victims, children, and women from other settings. It is recommended SANEs have a better understanding of the adverse and beneficial effects for all clients before changing practices to routine standard sampling.

Laying of charges and convictions are somewhat tenuous measures of nurses' effectiveness. It has been shown that charges will be laid in only a small proportion of cases, fewer will proceed to court, and even fewer will result in conviction. This attrition has been termed a "funnel effect." A global review of medicolegal outcomes after SA revealed that evidence and injury were not relevant to the outcome in over half the cases proceeding to court. The reasons for this low response may be well beyond the actions or scope of the SANE practice. The research on SA legal outcomes with cohort groups typically suggests that charge laying and prosecution are more likely if the assailant was a stranger or intimate partner rather than a recent acquaintance, if the victim was younger than 18, or if a witness was present. The SANE role is more likely to impact evidence collection and injury documentation. The impact of these on legal outcomes is less clear. In two U.S. and one Canadian cohort study, prosecution was more likely if the victim sustained more severe injuries. In contrast, the collection of specimens and presence of injuries were not found to result in more charges being laid in two Canadian and one Danish study. Differences in these results exist due to comparisons between charge laying and prosecution outcomes due to attrition, the way injuries are documented or analyzed (number versus severity), and perhaps cross-border differences in police and prosecution of SA cases.

A review across multiple studies of SANE teams and practices, mainly in the United States, revealed that SANEs positively impact the legal process. Measures included the comprehensiveness of the evidence collected, documentation, and chain of custody.

Experience of Staff

Provision of specialized SA services offers another potential benefit with increased education levels of nurses and increased comfort or experience with sexually assaulted clients. An increased exposure to sexually assaulted clients and additional education requirements may contribute to the nurse's confidence in assessment, procedures, and recommendations for interventions. Experience has been described as necessary to be able to detect genital injuries with direct visualization. The role of experience is not consistently supported in the literature, however. Residents with more SA examination experience reported lower rates of genital injury than the less-experienced junior residents with the same training. Comparisons of injury rates were not conducted on the same clients, however, so it is unclear if junior residents were incorrectly naming a normal finding as an injury or if the injuries in the populations examined were significantly different between groups due to use of cohort samples. The number of SA cases seen was also not compared between the junior and senior residents. Increased levels of experience and exposure to more sexually assaulted clients may also have benefits in terms of prevention of vicarious violence (burnout). In a study of counselors of sexually assaulted clients, it was found that experience and seeing larger numbers of clients reduced the risk of vicarious violence.

Staff configurations also impact effectiveness through experience. Some teams provide SANE coverage primarily through on-call casual staff, while others have part-time or full-time rosters of SANEs. Staff turnover on SANE teams is relatively frequent, but there is no comparison as yet of turnover and burnout among regular staff compared with casual staff. A meta-analysis of burnout studies suggests that increased staff experience has a beneficial effect in preventing burnout. A study of female nurses found less burnout in older nurses, perhaps also reflecting experience. The "casualization" of nurses was identified in a qualitative study of mental health nurses, although this may reflect job insecurity versus experience. Anecdotally, our experience on one Canadian team has been high turnover when staff was exclusively casual (on call) because staff were not regularly seeing clients and were therefore uncomfortable with their skills working alone. Turnover rates and costs decreased significantly once there was a change to an almost exclusively regular part-time roster. Further research is required in this area with SANEs.

EPIDEMIOLOGIC ISSUES WITH SA

The quality of information in SA research is affected by the type of data collected and its source. This must be considered when interpreting the evidence. There is considerable variability in the SA data in particular as it relates to definitions of SA and rape, sources of data, and the breadth of data.

SA and Rape Terms

Clinically the terms "rape" and "sexual assault" are often used interchangeably. Legally, these terms have quite different meanings, both within the country and between countries. In many U.S. states and across Canada, the term "rape" was initially limited to acts of vaginal-penile penetration and usually required "completed" penetration (penetration of a certain amount into the vagina). Acts such as penetration with a foreign body, attempted assault, fondling, and oral copulation or acts against men were not included. In the early 1980s the Canadian Criminal Code experienced a series of major amendments. The category of "sexual assault" was added to include all prior acts (rape and sodomy) as well as any unwanted act of a sexual nature. The emphasis began to shift in the legislation from the victim to the offender. There was less emphasis on prior sexual activity and likelihood of consent; husbands could now be charged; males could be victims; and there were a number of other forms of contact included as SA beyond vaginal-penile penetration. The acts and charges were also subdivided into ascending levels of severity based on levels of injury and aggression. These changes led to a rise in reporting of SAs.

Parallel changes occurred with the U.S. Federal Code related to "sexual abuse" in 1986. The amendment resulted in more gender-neutral legislation, an offender versus victim focus, inclusion of a broader range of unwanted sexual activities, removal of the requirement of resistance, inclusion of assault while intoxicated, removal of spousal immunity, and expansion of laws to include offenses committed in federal prisons. There is also legislation in each U.S. state for rape, SA, or both, resulting in a fair amount of diversity across the states. Some states retained their original rape legislation and added laws for "sexual assault" to encompass the wider range of unwanted activities of a sexual nature, whereas others have expanded their definition of rape to include additional acts. The term "sexual assault" was chosen for use throughout this chapter due to its more inclusive nature in both types of acts and gender.

The diversity of definitions between countries and even within countries creates some challenges for nurses caring for clients after SA. To begin with, it is difficult to interpret statistics on SA or rape. Statistics on SA may vary widely if different definitions or laws are in place as they may differentially include various types of penetration, exclude incomplete penetration or touching, and include only one gender. This variability becomes more complex when looking at the source of the statistics. If the data are from police or legal sources, the data are likely to include only those reporting their assault to police. It is well recognized that this number can significantly underrepresent the actual number of assaults taking place.

Knowledge of the wording and implications of local SA legislation is vital not only for understanding rates of assault and injury, but also for clinical care of sexually assaulted clients. The national or state legislation usually has a different level of assault or different penalties for various acts. Most notably, fear for one's life, restraint, presence of a weapon, and extent of injury will impact the charges and sentencing. The SANE must be aware of local legislation when obtaining the history of the assault to recognize relevant statements. For example, if the client states "I thought I wouldn't get out of there alive" or "I thought he had a knife," those statements would be significant to document both due to the psychological impact on the client and for the type of charges considered.

SA Data Sources

The data on SA rates and trends are directly affected by the source of the data, the definition of SA acts, and the type of question asked. Sources of data are most typically either from police reports (e.g., FBI uniform crime report) or from victimization surveys. Data from police reports are likely to seriously underestimate the prevalence of SA. Only 38.3% of those who indicated they had been sexually assaulted had reported to the police. Even fewer reported to police in Canada, with only 10% of sexually assaulted respondents having reported to police in both the 1993 and 1999 surveys. In the 2004 GSS, only 8% of the sexually assaulted women surveyed had reported to police. Police data are therefore not representative of the majority of the SA population.

Difficulties with using data from the police or from counselors may exist both from the use of self-report data and potential differences in injuries between those reporting to police and those who do not. A systematic review was conducted of SA injury research in which women's risks for injury were examined. There were three studies reporting tenderness and pain in women with injuries. Tenderness was defined as an objective response to palpation

such as wincing, withdrawing, and moaning, whereas pain was stated subjectively by the client. Among the 1183 women with injuries included in the review, almost half had tenderness to palpation whereas only 18% reported pain. The nurse and client may not realize there are injuries without conducting a comprehensive physical examination that includes palpation. Lack of awareness of injuries may also influence client decisions to report to police.

In a systematic review of research on risks for injuries up to January 2007, there were three studies identified in which injury rates were compared between women who did and did not report to police. All women had a physical examination. Rates of "physical" or "nongenital" injury were almost twice as high among women who reported to police compared with those who did not report. There were limited numbers of participants available in the three studies, but the differences suggest the necessity for further exploration into potential differences with injury outcomes and in the context of the SAs. These must be considered prior to attempting to combine or compare findings from police settings with those from either clinical settings or victimization surveys.

The victimization survey has become the standard for determining SA rates. The SANE needs to understand the question asked in each survey, however, and its implications. For instance, in the GSS the question is whether respondents have been assaulted within the last 12 months. Frequency and severity are not included. The specificity of the definition of SA used by researchers or perceived by respondents will also affect the data. Respondents may consider only stranger assaults or completed vaginal penetration. Limitations of the victimization survey include the role of memory and self-report on factors such as severity, nature of events, and specific details, as well as injuries.

Breadth of SA Data

Much of the SA literature has focused on female adolescents and adults. This is understandable given the high rates of assault among the college-age population. Less is known, however, about the risk and rates of SA against other groups including males, gay or lesbian populations, the disabled, and various ethnic groups. It is estimated from male surveys of SA that at least 3% to 7% of men have been sexually assaulted at least once in adulthood. At least 61% of American men assaulted as adults had also been sexually assaulted in childhood. It is thought that men underreport their assaults and that one factor may be the limited number of services for male clients. Another barrier to reporting assault among college males in one survey was the fear of being labeled as gay despite being heterosexual.

Sexual minorities are at particular risk of SA and revictimization. Gay men and bisexual men were found to be particularly vulnerable to revictimization in two studies, compared with lesbians or heterosexual clients. More work is needed to understand the unique needs of these populations and types of services that will allow them to feel empowered after SA.

Most U.S. research reports on white, black, and Hispanic populations and Canadian SA research has demonstrated very little examination of racial differences in SA other than among aboriginal (native Canadian) populations. It has been identified that Native American populations face significantly higher risks of violence and severity of violence than do Caucasian groups. Aboriginals in the province of Alberta were found to have 6.75 times more visits to emergency departments for violence-related injuries than non-aboriginal clients, and females between 20 and 29 years old had the highest number of violence-related visits. Native American adolescents who had been sexually assaulted faced higher risk of PTSD than did non-Native American adolescents. Little work has been done to explore reasons underlying these risks. Further work is required in both Canada and the United States on this high-risk population and risk factors. More work is also required on SA among immigrant groups. Some immigrants may have experienced SA as a consequence of war, torture, or other forms of oppression and may continue to be at risk even after immigrating. Further information is required regarding types of barriers to accessing services, culturally sensitive strategies for interviewing and examination that minimize further trauma, and appropriate sources of support.

Any examination of the SA literature requires that the SANE be familiar with the population of interest and source of the data. This will aid in interpreting the implications and applicability of the results.

Assailant Types

It is well documented that the majority of women are assaulted by acquaintances, either recently met or known for some time. The bulk of the data we have on sexual offenders has been drawn from incarcerated sexual offenders or pedophiles, forming the basis of the FBI typology of assailants. These incarcerated assailants are usually strangers to the victim or are pedophiles and have been convicted for their crimes. More typically the victims we see have been assaulted by someone known to them, either a recent acquaintance or an intimate partner. Acquaintance assailants are less likely to get caught

or to be prosecuted or for their victim to even report the assault to police.

Another profile has been described of the "undetected serial acquaintance" assailant. In a study of 1882 college men, 120 committed acts that were legally considered rape but for which they were never prosecuted. Approximately 1225 acts of interpersonal violence were committed by the 120 men, including battery and child abuse as well as rape, with many men each committing multiple acts of rape (mean = 5.8). The acquaintance rapist is described as someone who does not acknowledge their actions as SA, who "grooms" their victims by using social graces and often alcohol to reduce their resistance, then "isolating" them from friends. Lisak describes the undetected rapist as someone who has more sexual encounters than usual. This profile has changed police interviewing, leading some investigators to interview prior dates of the accused and to have the victim conduct a pretext call with the offender, often yielding a description of what occurred.

Victim Risks

Nurses must clearly understand that the SA is due to the actions of the assailant, not of the victim. There are, however, factors that have been associated with increased likelihood that the assailant will be able to access the victim and complete the assault. One notable example is the use of alcohol or drugs affecting the client's perception of risk or ability to resist.

Prior SA, either as a child or a young adolescent, has been associated with significant risks for subsequent revictimization in adulthood. A study of a cross-section of women revealed that those who had histories of childhood or adolescent SA were almost six times more likely to experience another SA as adults compared with those without a history of assault. Women who were revictimized were significantly more likely to develop mental health problems such as PTSD and depression than women assaulted only in childhood or only in adulthood. The risk of revictimization was found to be accentuated by alcohol use in a prospective study of college-age women. Women who had been previously assaulted and who used moderate to high levels of alcohol were four to seven times more likely to be sexually assaulted in the 2 months following initial assessment and three to five times more likely to be assaulted within 6 months compared with those with no history of victimization. The presence of low self-esteem and high-risk sexual behaviors after childhood SA was associated with a greater risk of revictimization. This may be a factor in increasing their vulnerability, particularly in the face of acquaintance assailants who are seeking vulnerable victims. Further work is needed on the pathways through which prior assaults lead to revictimization before prevention efforts will be successful with either victims or offenders.

Many rape myths are used in court to defend the accused. There is little empirical evidence to support these myths, leading to many myths now being struck down in court decisions. Canadian examples of myths that were ruled out are related to women's behaviors, credibility, or emotions. Many rape myths have been struck down in Canadian courts in recent years as irrelevant, including the expectation that behaviors by the victim made her responsible, such as getting into a car with the accused, going into a bar (*R. v. Seaboyer*) or entering into a private space with the accused (*R. v. Ewanchuk*), wearing provocative clothing (*R. v. Ewanchuk*), or behaving or appearing provocatively (*R. v. Osolin, R. v. Seaboyer, and R. v. Ewanchuk*). Other discounted myths included accusations the women had decreased credibility and were inclined to lie (*R. v. Osolin, R. v. Seaboyer,* and *R. v. Ewanchuk*), or that they were less believable if they were not respectable (*R. v. Osolin*), or were on social assistance (*R v. Ewanchuk, R. v. Osolin*). Emotional myths struck down included expectations that "real victims" would get hysterical and not be "cool," or that nonconcurrent or delayed reporting suggested decreased credibility (*R. v. Osolin, R. v. Seaboyer*). SANE and SART members, including police and prosecutors, need to be aware of local or federal cases that challenge these myths. Education of the public and other health-care professionals is also required, as many of these myths are still upheld, particularly if a client returns with a subsequent SA.

Interaction of Factors

None of these statistics or risk factors can be analyzed in isolation. For instance, it has been suggested that reports to police have stabilized or decreased over time. At the same time, the rates of nonstranger assaults are high. National Victimization of Women 1995 data were further analyzed for reasons why women do not report to police, and it was found that women were less likely to report the SA if the assailant was known to them. The level of intimacy has implications for the force and types of contact experienced. The interaction of multiple factors such as these highlights the need for more sophisticated research designs in which the influence of variables on both outcomes and other variables is examined. This can be examined using techniques such as multiple regression, structural equation modeling, or hierarchical modeling.

ASSESSMENT TECHNIQUES

Timing of the Examination

Many clients present hours or even days after an SA, coming in after they have disclosed to family or friends or had time to consider the impact of the trauma. Those coming in more than 24 hours after the assault are generally considered to be delayed. Delays have been consistently associated with knowing the assailant. In one study they were also linked to having lost consciousness during the assault or being physically assaulted as well as sexually assaulted. While necessary for the client, the delays may impact the ability to retrieve evidence or observe injuries. It is common for many SA protocols to specify a limit of less than 72 hours post-assault in which to collect forensic evidence. There is limited evidence to support the use of 72 hours as an absolute cutoff in adults. The period of 24 hours or less has been shown to yield the most evidence from the body in children and young adolescents, and most of the evidence in children is on clothing and bedding rather than the victim. In adults the timing is affected by the type of sample. The vaginal pool was found most likely to contain semen evidence within the first 24 hours in adults and adolescents, whereas samples from the cervical os were more likely to be positive for longer periods of time after assault. This is because cervical mucus retains the sperm for longer. A study of a cohort of 86 women was conducted with 36 pairs of forensic samples obtained. Semen persisted for more than 72 hours in a small number of the cervical os samples.

Some types of biological evidence from adolescents and adults may be retrieved beyond 72 hours. The decision for a time limit should be based on the type of evidence to be collected, the circumstances, and knowledge of testing methods available. A summary of ranges of evidence recovery is shown in Table 9.1.

Consent

Consent of the client is required before a physical examination is performed, even if the client has reported to the police. The client needs to understand not only what can be offered and implications of interventions, but also the medical and legal implications of declining interventions. Victims cannot be forced to submit to a physical examination. There are different approaches to the client who is unconscious or who does not have capacity for consent at the time of the examination. There have been attempts by physicians to either deem it "medically necessary" or to obtain warrants for DNA sampling by police and courts. Obtaining DNA is never medically necessary, although it

TABLE 9.1 **Evidence Persistence**

Evidence Source	Retrieval Time Frames	References
Mouth	28–31 hours	Rogers, D., & Newton, M. (2006). Evidence-based forensic sampling—more questions than answers. *Journal of Clinical Forensic Medicine, 13*(4):162-163.
Saliva on skin	0–24 hours	Sweet, D., Lorente, J.A., Valenzuela, A., Lorente, M., & Villanueva, E. (1997). PCR-based DNA typing of saliva stains recovered from human skin. *Journal of Forensic Sciences, 42*(3):447-451.
Fingers on neck	10 days	Rutty, G.N. (2002). An investigation into the transference and survivability of human DNA following simulated manual strangulation with consideration of the problem of third party contamination. *International Journal of Legal Medicine, 116*(2):170-173.
Vagina	6 days 7 days <24 hours	Davies, A., & Wilson, E. (1974). The persistence of seminal constituents in the human vagina. *Forensic Science, 3*(1):45-55. Morgan, J.A. (2008). Comparison of cervical os versus vaginal evidentiary findings during sexual assault exam. *Journal of Emergency Nursing, 34*(2):102-105.
Cervix	>72 hours (up to 7–10 days)	Morgan, J.A. (2008). Comparison of cervical os versus vaginal evidentiary findings during sexual assault exam. *Journal of Emergency Nursing, 34*(2):102-105. Silverman, E.M., & Silverman, A.G. (1978). Persistence of spermatozoa in the lower genital tracts of women. *Journal of the American Medical Association, 240*(17):1857-1875. Morrison, A.I. (1972). Persistence of spermatozoa in the vagina and cervix. *British Journal of Venereal Diseases, 48*(2):141-143.
Anus	72 hours (longer if immobile)	Willott, G.M., & Allard, J.E. (1982). Spermatozoa—Their persistence after sexual intercourse. *Forensic Science International, 19*:135-154.

may aid in attempts to identify and/or prosecute the assailant. This topic is a focus of debate in both legal and health-care circles, particularly in Canada due to privacy of medical information and human rights legislation. Some areas have developed regional guidelines or legislation addressing evidence collection with unconscious clients. In the absence of such guidelines, it has been argued that nurses can be charged with battery or negligence if they provide health care without consent, although Lee argues that obtaining forensic evidence is technically not health care. The argument is posed that the victim may wake and feel violated or even be placed at more risk if an investigation has proceeded and he or she is not safe or prepared to proceed with an investigation. Obtaining evidence while the client is unconscious also violates the notion of empowerment, removing control and choice.

Evidence collection while the client is unconscious may be seen as a violation of the client's right to informed decision making, as outlined in the Canadian Nurses' code of ethics, in which the client is to be given choice. It is also potentially in violation of the American Nurses' code of ethics in which the nurse supports the client's right to self-determination. Legislation differs across the United States. In Maine, for instance, it is admissible for health professionals to collect forensic evidence from an unconscious victim if a "reasonable person" thinks there are exigent circumstances warranting collection of evidence. Multidisciplinary groups, including victims, victim advocates, police, health-care professionals, ethicists, and the legal community, are currently exploring legislation in some areas of Canada to draft legislation to deal with this issue. There is no research to date in which the impacts (positive or negative) for the unconscious client have been examined when evidence was obtained without consent. The SANE must be familiar with local legislation regarding consent and evidence collection.

Interviewing and Crisis Intervention

After assessing for immediate threats to the client's health or safety, the SANE conducts an interview to obtain the medical history and the history of the SA. One of the risks during collection of information about the SA is retraumatizing the client and potentially contributing to increased risks of arousal and dissociation during the visit or to their risk of PTSD in the long term. Crisis intervention is required throughout the acute post-assault phase, including the interview and examination, in an attempt to minimize the risks of long-term consequences.

Crisis Intervention

Crisis intervention techniques are woven into the interview and subsequent care. While it is recognized that acute interventions are required, the nature of these actions has changed over time. The traditional debriefing models of crisis intervention have now been found to be ineffective and potentially harmful in the acute post-trauma phase by increasing arousal and anxiety, even if clients reported subjectively feeling better after the interventions. It has been speculated that victims of trauma who are made to repeat their history of events before they are ready to do so face increased risks of PTSD. Thousands of PTSD therapists arrived in New York City after the destruction of the World Trade Center, assuming that early intervention would be effective in reducing risk of PTSD. Although many victims reported feeling the interventions were helpful, there was no evidence that the debriefing techniques used were helpful, and in fact they were thought to decrease victims' resiliency to cope with the event. It has been hypothesized that the added trauma was due to having victims relate their experiences too soon after the event and the single-session nature of the debriefing. This rationale also highlights the need to limit clients' retelling their assault history to multiple people during their visit. There has been no research showing the effectiveness of debriefing at any point after the assault in preventing long-term consequences such as PTSD.

An alternative strategy for crisis intervention has been developed, which is known as psychological first aid (PFA). Initially designed for use with disaster and terrorism operations, it has merit for use with any client experiencing assault or trauma. An added advantage is that it can be easily learned by professionals as well as families. PFA consists of a set of core actions that may be used while working with the client:

- Contacting and engaging using a compassionate, non-intrusive manner
- Providing safety and physical and emotional comfort
- Calming and stabilizing overwhelmed victims and providing support
- Gathering information about needs, concerns, and alternatives from the client perspective to tailor appropriate interventions

- Planning for and providing practical assistance in addressing needs
- Facilitating connection with social supports (formal or informal)
- Providing information on coping and stress reactions
- Linking with collaborative services for subsequent assistance

The type and number of actions are dependent on the status of the client, the situation, and the resources available. In most acute crisis situations, the health professionals must at least define the problem, ensure safety, and provide support. Specific interventions found to assist in providing PFA include promoting safety, promoting calming, promoting sense of self and community efficacy, promoting connectedness, and instilling hope.

The PFA model is relatively new, and there is little research evaluating its overall effectiveness. Each of the components of the model, however, has been linked to evidence of positive client outcomes. The initial contact is important in promoting trust and gaining disclosure. Use of negative responses to disclosure by health professionals has been linked to increased risks of PTSD. Negative social reactions and self-blame were the strongest correlates of PTSD symptoms in testing a multivariate model. Self-blame and guilt have been found to be higher in women assaulted by someone they know (confidence assault) and are linked to feeling they cannot trust or are not able to determine trustworthiness. In the same study, a stranger attack (blitz) was associated with greater feelings of an unsafe world and an inability to protect themselves. Promotion of safety can reduce biological stress reactions and reduce either type of distorted trauma thoughts, such as inability to trust or never feeling safe again. Other examples of distorted trauma thoughts include believing the assault was preventable, especially in hindsight; believing it is their fault and neglecting the combination of factors beyond their control that caused the event; and negatively evaluating the actions they did or didn't take. Self-blame and fear of future revictimization are both linked to poor psychological outcomes. Sustained or significant physical reactions to stress (e.g., cortisol and catecholamine release) have been associated with subsequent biological changes seen with PTSD and depression. The risk of PTSD is associated with the intensity of the acute reaction to the trauma. Reframing is a cognitive strategy that may be helpful even in acute stages to reduce distorted thoughts and perhaps encourage the client to consider more positive alternatives. For example, if they say they will never be safe again, ask if they feel safe now and identify what they will need to feel safe tonight when they go home. Dissociation is a symptom sometimes seen with acute stress after SA. Examples of dissociation include becoming detached or estranged, feeling like it is not really happening (derealization), out-of-body experiences, and flashbacks or reexperiencing. This peritraumatic dissociation may be an indicator of risk for subsequent development of acute stress disorder or PTSD and has been found to occur among sexually assaulted clients if they had experienced childhood SA or abuse as well.

The client is most likely to dissociate when experiencing stressful events after the assault. Examples may include having to retell the events or having blood taken or a speculum examination. They might suddenly switch from being conversational to staring into space, reflecting their distress. Grounding techniques during a dissociative episode will help to reduce distress. The SANE speaks to the client softly, not expecting answers, but encourages the client to think of the sounds, smells, and feelings in order to reengage the client in the present. Strategies to prevent such episodes can also be used, such as engaging the client in conversation, particularly during distressing aspects of the examination (e.g., blood-taking or the speculum examination). Both reframing and grounding may reduce stress, provide hope, and help calm the client.

Calming will control the trauma-related anxiety, reducing its potential generalization to other activities beyond the trauma. Anxiety is a key factor in development of PTSD and depression. Analysis of a theoretical model revealed that the presence of acute stress symptoms, the magnitude of the biological response, and hyperarousal were key risk factors in the development of PTSD and comorbid depression or anxiety disorders.

Gathering information about the client's needs allows for individualization and promotion of client control of recovery. Control over the immediate situation, such as the SANE examination, has been linked to improved adaptation to the stress. Provision of tangible assistance, such as giving medications and making referrals, combined with a positive response, has been found to be helpful in reducing distress.

Coping and self-efficacy is enhanced through reminding clients of previous positive efforts and coping and helping them identify current strategies. It may also include helping them reflect on realistic goals or expectations. If they have been previously assaulted, they may have preexisting health consequences (e.g., PTSD, substance abuse, depression). In these instances, their coping mechanisms may not be effective, and the SANE may have to help them identify short-term sources of support and coping that may help them. Use of support systems may be particularly helpful in their recovery.

Social support has been linked to better recovery from trauma, including SA. Supporting efforts to connect with significant support people is therefore important. If individuals have few social supports or are unlikely to use them, the importance of formal support services should be emphasized further.

Interviewing Techniques

The concepts of PFA can be incorporated into the interviewing process, which consists of a medical history and a history of the assault. It is important to let the client pace the timing of the examination. Key interviewing techniques include the use of open-ended questions and listening. Interviewing guidelines have been developed for children 3 to 13 years of age, known as the National Child Interviewing (NICHD) protocol. Analysis of the interview content obtained before and after the introduction of the protocol revealed that more open-ended questions and fewer suggested prompts or closed yes/no questions yielded more information in both English and French-Canadian populations. There is very little available research on forensic interviewing techniques and their effectiveness with adolescent or adult SA clients. Much of the interviewing literature has to do with police interviews, which have a different focus from the SANE history of the SA. Communication and interviewing concepts in the SANE literature are largely derived from anecdotal literature or borrowed from other fields such as counseling.

The purpose of the medical history is to identify conditions or factors that may increase a client's risk for infection or other health issues, identify potential risks to health during the examination, aid in explaining findings throughout the examination, and guide interventions and discharge decisions or teaching. Examples include factors that might prolong bleeding or cause easy bruising, conditions such as asthma or allergies that may alter care, and a history of depression. Prosecutors sometimes request that the breadth of the medical history be limited in order to keep that information out of court. If the information is required to make health-care decisions, it is strongly recommended that it continue to be collected. An example is a history of prior suicide or use of antidepressant medications, which could suggest increased risk of suicidal attempts after discharge or affect decisions to discharge.

The breadth of the history of the SA itself is varied across teams. The purposes of the SA history are to guide the physical examination, to identify risks for injury or health consequences, and to compare mechanisms of injury from the history with expected patterns of injury. Key areas of the interview include date and time of the assault to aid in injury interpretation and timing of tests;

consensual vaginal intercourse in the last week or anal/oral intercourse in the last 3 days, as this could alter DNA results; post-assault activities that may interfere with evidence preservation (e.g., bathing, voiding, eating or drinking); physical symptoms that may indicate drug-facilitated assault, medical stability, or alter risks for injury (e.g., unconsciousness during assault, loss of consciousness, pain or bleeding, vomiting, amnesia); conditions of the SA surroundings, as these may help interpret trace evidence or injuries (e.g., mud, patterned flooring, carpets, stick shift in car); methods used by the assailant, such as restraint, licking, ejaculation, attempted strangulation, threats or coercion, and use of a weapon; and any injuries that the client may have inflicted on the assailant. There is little information gathered related to the assailant other than that required to guide the examination and evidence collection. For instance, knowing the relationship of the assailant assists in determining risks for safety and reexposure as well as the likelihood that the client will know the assailant's habits and subsequent risks for infection. If trace fibers are found later, the examiner may then wish to ask about what the assailant was wearing or what types of fabrics and fibers were at the scene. Some teams invite the police into the SA interview to minimize retelling. The risk with this, however, is that the client may feel obliged to reveal confidential health information to which the police would not normally have access to address SANE information needs. This would be in violation of Canadian health information acts unless the clients know they have a right not to reveal this information.

Police and prosecutors sometimes recommend the SANE collect intensively detailed information about the assailant and circumstances of the assault. This may result in the client retelling the assault at least twice to the SANE and police, which is counterproductive to the principles of PFA. It is recognized that in acute stress the client may have incomplete recall, particularly immediately after the event. Survivors of traumatic events, including SA, recalled more information after being given time to reevaluate the events. When combat veterans with preexisting PTSD were put into stressful situations again, researchers found decreased blood flow to the prefrontal and temporal region (responsible for executive decision making, speech, and episodic memory) while there was increased blood flow to the amygdala (primitive center). These findings have not been replicated with SA victims, but many victims do have preexisting PTSD. It is possible that the details given to the SANE may contradict later statements given to police, that police hear information that appears "new," or that clients may become so stressed during the examination that they can't speak of the assault.

Any of these occurrences could ultimately harm the prosecution of the case. The SANE requires information about the event that will impact determination of health consequences and interpretation of findings. For instance, it is important to know if the assailant is known or unknown, if the client is safe or likely to see the assailant again, and what are the factors impacting the potential HIV risk.

Cognitive behavioral therapy has been recognized as one of the most helpful strategies for prevention or recovery from posttraumatic stress. Most work on CBT, however, involves interventions occurring more than 14 days after the trauma. Some strategies of cognitive behavioral therapy such as reframing and grounding have been used in acute settings, but there is very little research to show the effectiveness of using CBT immediately after the assault in preventing long-term consequences.

Indicators of Increased Risks

Some indicators that may be seen in the initial visit have been associated with increased risks of PTSD in various trauma populations. Some of these include the presence of dissociation in the acute stage, particularly if it persists. Other risk factors include a history of prior SA as a child or adolescent, presence of injury from the assault, the extent of shame and self-blame, and preexisting psychiatric disorders, such as depression or anxiety disorders. Knowledge of the role of these indicators in sexually assaulted clients may allow more effective preventative efforts. Survivors of SA were interviewed regarding factors that aided in their recovery. Helpful strategies included being made to feel safe and having SANEs avoid behaviors such as minimizing the trauma with comments about how lucky they are to have survived and controlling behaviors such as rushing clients through rather than allowing them to pace the examination. Another strategy is to limit the number of professionals interacting with clients to minimize the number of times they repeat the history, keeping the purpose and focus of the interview focused on information needed to guide the examination and assess health risks (as compared with police, who focus on information for the investigation and truth verification), and providing dedicated staff who have time to spend with clients.

PHYSICAL EXAMINATION

The format and extent of physical examinations vary across teams and their philosophy of care and setting. If a comprehensive approach is used, it is recommended that a systematic method of physical examination be used. One such method is the conduct of a primary, secondary, and focused survey. This method is based on examination of trauma patients in emergency departments and is well suited to SA clients, who have also been victims of trauma.

The primary examination is a brief 30- to 60-second assessment of the ABCDs (airway, breathing, circulation, and disability of the central nervous system). The goal is to identify immediate threats to life or limb in core systems. If there are threats, these have to be resolved before further assessments can be conducted. The secondary survey consists of exposing the client for physical examination and conducting a head to toe examination. This is also a brief examination to identify potential problems in body systems. In clients who are not emergent and who are not unconscious or intoxicated, this may consist of merely asking if there are any problems in a particular body system or may involve at least inspection and palpation of the system. A more in-depth assessment of a specific body system may then be conducted if problems are suspected or need to be ruled out. This latter examination is known as a focused assessment. An example of a focused **assessment** would be an examination for pupil reactivity and presence of hemotympanum, Battle's sign, raccoon eyes, or other signs of blunt trauma for a client who reports being struck in the head. Clearly, it may be seen that this method is applicable to sexually assaulted clients as long as the focus is on identifying physical or psychological effects of SA rather than identifying diseases.

The secondary survey should be conducted in ambient (room) lighting with both inspection and palpation from head to toe. Ideally, a second examination with inspection only would be conducted with either ultraviolet light or an alternate light source. There is no research available on the benefits or risks in conducting one before the other. Clinical observations suggest that the ultraviolet light examination may be best first, as it is intended to identify semen. In that way a semen stain can be identified before it is potentially disrupted with palpation during the secondary survey in normal light. There is no research, however, that has identified the impact of variations in the depth of the physical examination nor the effects of different orders of the examination. It is based on clinical experience.

Ultraviolet Lights and Alternate Light Sources

The terms "ultraviolet light" and "alternate light source" are sometimes used interchangeably in practice. There are differences between the two that have implications for practice. Ultraviolet lights come in short, medium, and long wavelengths. The traditional Wood's lamp used short to medium wavelengths, typically around 254 to 365 nm. Both short- and medium-wavelength ultraviolet lights are very sensitive to stains, but are very nonspecific, meaning most substances will fluoresce but not necessarily be semen. The high false-positive rate places an unnecessary load on the forensic laboratory, and it is recommended lights in these wavelengths not be used. There are also risks of burns and corneal damage due to exposure to these lights. Longer ultraviolet wavelengths are more effective for forensic purposes and less likely to be associated with burns. The term "alternate light source" was originally intended to refer to argon laser lights, but it is now also used to refer to lights with wavelengths higher than 400 nm (beyond the ultraviolet wavelength), such as the LED lights.

There are two types of light emitted when using ultraviolet or alternate lights. These are excitation light and emission light. The excitation light is not visible at ultraviolet wavelengths (less than 400 nm), making the emission light on the stain visible to the naked eye. The excitation light is visible at wavelengths greater than 400 nm and therefore obstructs the ability to see the stain in the emission light unless barrier goggles are used to filter out the excitation light. Semen stains are best seen at wavelengths of 400 nm or more, thus requiring barrier filter goggles. Most of the research on ultraviolet and alternate light sources have been conducted on fabric rather than skin. A limited number of small trials have been conducted using semen on skin. Three of these studies involved examining the fluorescence of multiple substances in addition to semen using ultraviolet and/or alternate light sources. One study used a single volunteer with multiple fluids randomly applied to numbered regions on the forearms, including two semen stains, urine, saliva, water-soluble lubricant, condom lubricant, powder, Polysporin, soap, and a blank control spot. Two separate pilot studies were conducted, first with 7 volunteer raters (including five SANEs) and then at another site with 27 volunteers (all nurses or police with SA teams). Raters used each of four different wavelengths of light (254 to 450 nm) in random order to assess the stains, blinded to which stains were semen. Almost all substances fluoresced with short and medium wavelengths, while only the semen stains showed with the 450-nm lights. In a second study, multiple fluids were applied on forearms of eight volunteers, this time from eight different sources, including semen, blood, and urine, as well as lubricants. Lights used ranged from 370 to 500 nm. Semen and urine fluoresced only faintly on five of eight stains and when using the higher wavelength lights. The fluorescence persisted in three of the five positive stains on the second day. A comparison of the same semen samples on fabric showed the stains were much more fluorescent and visible on the fabric than on the skin. Unfortunately, raters were not blinded to which stains were semen. A study of a Wood's lamp (365 nm) showed high specificity to semen (95%) but poor sensitivity.

The information on use of the light is mainly anecdotal, especially as it relates to where to hold the light in relation to the skin. Wawryk and Odell found the best results if they initially placed the light within approximately 1 in. (3 cm) of the skin to initiate the fluorescence, and then holding the light at approximately 8 in. (20 cm) from the skin to look for stains. Lincoln found that semen stains were best seen at closer ranges, such as 2 to 4 in. (5 to 10 cm) as compared with 8 in. (20 cm). The stain was also more visible if more semen was present (e.g., 10 µL). The anecdotal literature also contains differences in the color of stains to expect if semen is present. The wavelength of light is one reason for the variability in descriptions about semen stains in the descriptive literature. Wavelengths of 360 nm have been found to produce blue fluorescence, whereas wavelengths of 430 to 470 produce orange fluorescence. This corresponds with data from Carter-Snell and Solty's study. Raters described stains seen with wavelengths of less than 400 nm as blue or blue-green, whereas stains were described mostly as white, yellow, or orange when the viewer was wearing orange barrier goggles and using lights over 400 nm.

Long-wavelength lights may be useful for injury identification as well. Nongenital (body) injuries may not yet be visible if clients arrive within 24 to 48 hours of the assault. Lights of 450 nm or more have been reported to augment early injuries such as deep bruises and to reveal old injuries or bite marks not yet visible on the skin. The light is absorbed by hematological components in the injury, and the surrounding dermal tissue fluoresces, thereby augmenting the appearance of marks. The lights have also been helpful in identifying further detail on tattoos in postmortem examinations. Skin conditions such as vitiligo (uneven skin coloring), dry skin, or lesions such as acne scars have been seen clinically to fluoresce, but they are consistent with flaking or scars and unlike the smear or drip patterns typically seen with semen stains. Further work is needed in this area to determine the circumstances under which bruises or other blunt injuries appear under lights when not visible in ambient light.

Little is known about how long semen remains on skin in various body regions, the fluorescent properties of stains, and other factors affecting visibility. There is mention in the literature that semen may not fluoresce if too soon after the assault or too late, although these time frames are not specific. One study examined wet semen stains compared with dry semen stains and found that wet semen did not fluoresce on the skin. It is not known how long the stain would remain fluorescent or if this varied by body part or skin color. It is evident, however, that SANEs need to know what type of light they are using, what to expect if positive stains are present, and the strengths or limitations in viewing stains.

No studies have been reported in which the timing of the ultraviolet examination has been considered. It is unknown if semen stains will be disrupted if palpation occurs, although it would seem logical that they would. For this reason, some teams that use lights will conduct the ultraviolet light examination first, noting and swabbing any positive areas, followed by the inspection and palpation in ambient light.

The research evidence to date is limited by small sample size, although the results are largely consistent that long-wavelength lights are recommended if looking for semen. Concerns have been raised about the utility of ultraviolet lights on skin as semen is less visible on skin than on fabric. The implications are most important for a negative ultraviolet light result on skin. Positive fluorescence is more likely to be semen with higher wavelengths, but is not confirmatory. Negative fluorescence may still occur in areas where semen was ejaculated. A recommended practice is to swab areas in which there was suspected or reported ejaculation even if there is no fluorescence. It has been suggested, however, that the long-wavelength lights may still offer benefits to guide more effective swab collection from stains compared with blind swabs without the lights.

Direct Visualization of Genitals

Direct visualization of the genital region is performed using the naked eye and with a series of techniques including labial separation, labial traction, and eventually speculum insertion.

Legal concerns are sometimes raised that perhaps in the process of the examination injuries were caused by these techniques. An expert SANE and midwife anecdotally describes lacerations of the posterior fourchette if labial separation and traction are performed in lateral directions rather than downward and diagonally. Very little research has been done on the before and after effects of these procedures. A sample of 27 women was examined before and after speculum insertion using toluidine blue dye applied to the genital region. There were 18 women with genital injuries seen before the speculum insertion. One additional woman showed a labial abrasion after the speculum insertion. Although further research is required, it is generally recommended that the initial genital examination be conducted prior to speculum insertion.

Various client positions have been shown to reveal hymen injuries differentially. A group of 47 prepubertal and 74 pubertal girls who were suspected to have been sexually abused were studied using three different examination techniques. Supine labial separation, supine labial traction, and prone knee-chest positions were used to examine their hymens. Hymen injuries were not visible in all three methods for both groups of girls, although the prone knee-chest position showed the injuries most often, followed by supine labial traction, although each technique had strengths for showing injuries in specific areas. The results lend further support to earlier work recommending multimethod examination techniques for prepubertal girls. It is one of the first studies also recommending multimethod techniques for adolescents. The prone knee-chest position is not routinely used on adolescents nor has experience shown it is accepted readily by adolescents.

Assisted Visualization of Genitals

Genital injuries from SA are sometimes difficult to visualize, especially with limited experience in examining sexually assaulted clients. A few comparisons have been conducted using direct visualization (naked eye) and use of either toluidine dye or colposcopy with magnification.

Toluidine

Toluidine blue dye is a stain that is applied to epithelial regions (e.g., genitals, breast tissue), left to dry for approximately 60 seconds, and then wiped off with either water-soluble lubricant or 10% acetic acid. If epithelial cells are intact, the dye is wiped off with little or no residue remaining (no uptake). If the underlying nucleated cells are exposed, such as with a laceration or excoriation, the cells will take up the dye and a dark purple/blue stain will remain in the exposed area. The dye will not be taken up in areas of superficial injury, such as superficial abrasions or in older injuries that have begun to reepithelialize or form scar tissue. Toluidine application is not recommended for use on mucous membranes (inner vaginal walls), as it spreads easily and is difficult to remove, thus obscuring visualization of bruising. Use of toluidine dye has been found to increase rates of observed injury from 4% to 28% in adolescents and from 16.5% to 33% in pediatric cases. Rates increase from 16% with direct visualization to 40% in adult SA victims.

Colposcopy

The use of colposcopy has been described as the standard in the United States, and it has been included as part of the U.S. Department of Justice's national protocol for SA.

Colposcopy can be used both for visualization and for photodocumentation. Use of magnification with the colposcopy is optional. Use of magnification has been shown to increase the ability of practitioners to detect genital injuries. A systematic review of the literature was conducted relevant to use of colposcopy in SA and abuse examinations. In a study using either colposcopy or toluidine, the use of colposcopy revealed injuries in 85% of women, and 11% of these could not be seen without colposcopy. The toluidine was used for 765 cases and there were injuries identified in 75% of these. The authors did not describe any simultaneous comparison of toluidine and colposcopy within the same cases, however, and further information was unavailable. Numerous descriptive studies reported an increase in ability to detect genital injuries when the colposcope was used, both in adult and adolescent females. In contrast, colposcopy was found to have no advantage over visualization with the naked eye in children's examinations, perhaps as the majority of children subjected to sexual abuse will have no injuries present. The issue of magnification with the colposcope was not specifically addressed in Templeton's review.

In a systematic review of research on injuries and risks for injuries, it was noted that the use of toluidine and colposcopy with magnification was exclusively used in studies involving SANEs. Almost half of all studies involving SANEs included at least one aid to visualization. If colposcopy was used by physicians, magnification was not used. The rates of genital injury reported when examinations were conducted by nurse examiners were found to be three times higher in these studies than rates reported by either emergency physicians or physicians specially educated in SA.

The use of magnification with colposcopy is controversial among some SA practitioners. It has been suggested that if magnification is required to see injuries, they are not likely to be clinically significant. It may be argued that the presence of a break in skin integrity, microscopic or not, poses an increased risk for sexually transmitted infections. Another argument criticizing the use of magnification centers on the increased expectations by the courts that injury should be present, despite many women being uninjured.

Comparisons of Toluidine and Colposcopy

Colposcopy is expensive and not widely available. Making it a standard of care may pose the risk of SANE care being considered substandard if only toluidine is used. Only two studies have been identified to date in which toluidine and colposcopy have been compared in the same study. A total of 837 genital injuries were identified among 445 consecutive female SA clients ranging from

13 to 74 years old when examined by SANEs, each of whom had seen at least 200 cases. Only 63% of the injuries were identified with unassisted (direct) visualization. An additional 34% were identified with the use of toluidine dye. Only 3% more injuries were noted with colposcopy using 16 times magnification compared with toluidine, and most of these were redness or swelling. Only 1% of the injuries (3 of 837) were injuries other than redness or swelling that could not be detected by direct visualization or with toluidine application. Researchers concluded that when skilled examiners were available, the only additional benefit of the colposcopy over the other methods was photodocumentation. A second study on 120 volunteers after consensual intercourse found more tears were identified with toluidine than either direct visualization or colposcopy (p <0.5). One flaw in their methods, however, was the application of toluidine after the speculum insertion. It cannot be ruled out that the insertion may have added injury not previously present. There were, however, more injuries in the anal region seen with toluidine as well.

Without such comparisons it cannot be said that one method is better than the other. The issue again becomes one of clinical significance if either aid to visualization is used. The injuries seen in SA tend to sometimes be quite subtle. A review of the injury literature showed higher rates of injury seen with direct visualization (naked eye) in more recent years, and this was attributed to increased examiner knowledge and skill related to the appearance of injuries and what to expect. Experience is required to correctly identify injuries. If this is the case, then it could be argued that aids to visualization should be used to ensure all injuries are noted regardless of experience levels. Some teams have begun to indicate if injuries were seen with direct visualization, aids to visualization, or both. The legal significance of this information is also unknown.

Hymen Visualization

It is sometimes difficult to examine the hymen, particularly on women with redundant folds of hymen. One of the techniques suggested to help view the edges of the hymen is balloon visualization. This can be done with the use of a Foley catheter, such as a 14 Fr. catheter. The technique has also been used clinically for menarchal adolescents who have not had prior intercourse and/or tampon use if they refuse the speculum insertion or if it would be too traumatic for them. The balloon would allow the nurse to view the edges of the hymen without further traumatizing the client. If this technique is used in the latter instance, a "blind" swab of the end of the vagina/cervix

may also be desired for DNA retrieval. No research was located to indicate the effectiveness of blind swabs for DNA retrieval. It should also be noted that neither blind swabs nor balloon visualization would be recommended if the female is less than Tanner stage 3 (premenarchal), as the nonestrogenized hymen would be extremely sensitive.

Photographs

Photographs may be taken during the SA examination for either quality assurance and peer review or for legal purposes. The client must be involved in the decision to photograph and to provide consent to have them taken. Once taken, the defendant and the court have access to the photographs as well, and the client must be prepared for this. The use of photographs is not without its limitations. In some Canadian jurisdictions there has been reluctance to use photographs as even relatively large genital injuries are likely to be smaller in size than the jury might expect. There are fears the jury or judge may then reduce the perceived seriousness of the assault. In the United States, digital or colposcopic photographs are a routine part of the forensic examination for most teams. There are still concerns that have to be addressed, such as that photographs are too invasive and may offend.

Another concern with photographs is that they may yield less information and miss more injuries than if the clinician were able to manipulate the tissues. Findings such as redness and swelling were particularly difficult to assess by photographs when comparing inter-rater reliability.

INJURIES

There are a number of issues with the evidence as it relates to types, categories, severity, rates, and risks for injuries after SA. The definitions of injuries and types of injuries used as outcomes vary across the literature. These differences have an impact on severity, rates of injuries, and our understanding of risks for injuries. Injury has been defined as "damage to any part of the body due to mechanical force." At one end of the spectrum are those researchers who include redness and swelling as injuries along with other more traditional injuries, whereas those on the other end include only lacerations. Differences in types of injuries studied leads to variability in injury rates. An example is seen in Table 9.2. These data are the result of a preliminary analysis of the data used in an injury risk study. The rates of nongenital injury remain very high compared with genital injury, but both the mean number of injuries per client and the rate of injuries are quite a

TABLE 9.2 **Injury Rates by Injury Types (n-927)**

Injury Category	Description	All Injuries	All but Redness and Swelling	All but Redness, Swelling, and Tenderness
Nongenital	% Injured	91.3	90.3	86.4
	Mean no. Injuries	10.8	10.0	9.4
Genital	% Injured	75.8	62.2	57.1
	Mean no. Injuries	3.2	2.7	2.6

bit lower when redness and swelling are excluded from the injury count and even lower when tenderness is also removed.

Injury Definitions and Mnemonics

Mnemonics offer ways in which to organize thoughts or assessments to help remember key points or practices. The most familiar mnemonic for SA injuries is TEARS (tears, ecchymosis, abrasions, redness and swelling). This mnemonic has been extremely helpful in guiding nurses as to expected injuries. Unfortunately, this mnemonic is incomplete and mostly relevant to genital injuries only, potentially contributing to either incomplete examinations or documentation. There are a number of nongenital injuries that may be seen with SA that are not included. An additional problem is the definitions used. The "T" refers to tears, which are defined as "any breaks in tissue integrity, including fissures, cracks, lacerations, cuts, gashes or rips." The mechanism of injury for lacerations is significantly different for lacerations and cuts. Lacerations are tears or rips in the skin that are the result of blunt injury, and cuts (incised wounds) are from penetrating trauma. Putting the two terms together under the heading "tears" may contribute to further confusion between the mechanisms. There is no mention in the mnemonic of other forms of penetrating trauma, such as stabs or punctures. The remainder of the terms included in "tears" are findings that are not necessarily due to injuries, such as cracks or fissures. Anal fissures, for instance, are defined as tears of the skin that are most likely to occur from nontrauma mechanisms such as straining from stool, especially if the fissure is not on the midline region. The use of the term "ecchymosis" is seldom used as it is poorly defined and is more commonly associated with medical disorders such as bleeding disorders than with trauma. The mechanisms of injury in SA may include either blunt or penetrating forces, and they need to be included in injury mnemonics. Blunt force injuries include abrasions, contusions, lacerations, and fractures. Petechiae are usually characteristic of compression leading to rupture of venules. The one

exception is petechiae to the cervix, which are seen with blunt injury due to the rich capillary supply to the cervix. Penetrating injury typically results in incised wounds (also termed "cuts") or stab wounds. Stabs may be from knives or any other sharp object, such as flying debris or ice picks. Firearm injuries are a unique form of penetrating wound that may also contain abrasions, burns, and trace evidence such as clothing wads or gunpowder deposits. It may not always be known if firearms were the mechanism of injury, and the SANE may only be able to identify the wound as a stab type of penetrating wound rather a bullet wound.

An alternate injury mnemonic was developed to provide forensic nurses with a more comprehensive mnemonic to guide their physical examination and to assist with their documentation. This mnemonic (Table 9.3) was termed BALD STEP and has now been used across Canada as part of the revision of the Royal Canadian Mounted Police evidence kits. The BALD STEP mnemonic includes a broader range of injuries and physical findings typically seen in forensic physical examination. The mnemonic is also useful as a key for traumagrams to indicate findings more succinctly. The first two initials of each finding are indicated beside the body part, along with measurements, color, and any other key characteristics

TABLE 9.3 **BALD STEP Forensic Physical Findings Mnemonic**

BALD STEP Mnemonic for Physical Findings

B	Bruises (BR)	S	Stain (ST)
	Bite marks (BI)		Swelling (SW)
	Bleeding (BL)	T	Tenderness (TE)
	Burns (BU)		Trace evidence (TE)
A	Abrasions (AB)	E	Erythema (ER)
	Avulsions (AV)	P	Patterned injury (PA)
L	Lacerations (LA)		Petechiae (PT)
D	Deformities–acute (DE)		Penetrating (PE) +
			incised (I), chop (C)
			stab (S), gunshot(G),
			or puncture (P)

(e.g., PA, BR-round blue 3 cm to indicate a patterned bruise, which is round, blue, and 3 cm in diameter). The shape could then be drawn onto the traumagram or photographed.

Standard definitions are essential for both clinical care and legal testimony. It is strongly recommended that we use terminology consistent with forensic pathology and forensic emergency medicine. This is particularly important in areas in which another professional is expected to give expert testimony based on the SANE's documentation or if multidisciplinary research is considered. The descriptive literature contains many erroneous and inconsistent descriptions, including charts of aging of bruises. It is not possible to age a bruise because individuals progress differently through the color phases depending on factors such as their metabolism, medications, age, and general health. The only factor that may aid in aging a bruise is that the presence of yellow on the bruise has been found across the existing studies to indicate bruises are at least 24 hours old or more. Absence of yellow, however, does not mean it is less than 24 hours old.

Consistency of definitions and documentation of the range of nongenital and genital injuries seen will facilitate a more comprehensive understanding of patterns of injuries seen with various types of SA (e.g., stranger, nonstranger). A pattern of injury describes a collection of injury types and locations associated with various mechanisms of injury. This information is valuable in helping the nurse to assess if the history and findings are consistent and to guide the physical examination. For instance, if a client states she fell on a slippery (bald) step and slid down the stairs, the nurse would expect a pattern of injuries including friction abrasions to limbs in contact with the stairs and bruising at points of impact. It would be helpful to be able to describe patterns of genital and nongenital injury typically seen with SA under various circumstances and with different assailant types. It has been suggested that we expand the definition of pattern to include severity as well as prevalence, type, frequency, and location.

Severity of Injury

Definitions and classifications or rating scales for severity of injury are only minimally described in the SA literature. There has been some work done to validate the Injury Severity Score (ISS) and Abbreviated Injury Scale (AIS) with forensic clients. The difficulty with these scales is that they mainly rate threats to life and limb. Those types of injuries are relatively rare in SA. A mean of 6% of women (SD = 3, median = 4%) were admitted to the hospital as a result of their injuries from SA across studies reporting admission for injuries. The AIS and ISS

would suggest the remaining women were not severely injured. That raises the larger issue of clinical significance with SA injuries. Are the injuries found among sexually assaulted clients occurring in greater frequency? Are there more sites of injury or only specific sites involved? Are there complications involved with presence of nongenital or genital injuries?

Hospital admission or threat to life and limb may not be the best marker of severity of injury for sexually assaulted clients. Preliminary analysis on the data from a group of sexually assaulted women was conducted. Only 1.2% of 917 women were admitted to the hospital, and 82.8% were able to be discharged. The SANEs were in a position as consultants, coming into the emergency department to provide the SA care, then collaborating with the physician to either discharge clients or leave them in the emergency department for further medical care outside the scope of SA care. At least 1 of 6 women (16.3%) had to remain in the emergency department for further medical care, including intervention for suicidal ideation, fluid replacement, sutures, radiology, or treatment of other abnormalities discovered during the SANE's physical examination. Discussions of severity of injury require more in-depth analysis of the acute health-care needs of SA clients beyond admission and the long-term implications of these needs.

Types of Injury Outcomes

The type of injury outcome poses problems for analyzing evidence of injury and for reporting. The bulk of the SA literature reports only on either genital injuries or on physical injuries (which may or may not include genital injuries). Genital injuries are sometimes limited to vulvovaginal regions or may include anal regions, or are termed "anogenital." Physical injuries may be limited to nongenital body trauma or may include both nongenital and genital trauma. Very few studies separated their analyses into genital and nongenital injuries. The mechanism of injury is sometimes quite different for nongenital injuries than for genital injuries. Clients may sustain punches or blows to nongenital areas or sustain a penetrating injury, whereas injuries to the genital region are more typically from blunt mechanisms. Unless we examine both types of injury outcomes, we will not have a clear picture of how different risk factors contribute to either type of injury outcome or the patterns of injury to expect.

Rates of Injuries

Rates of injuries vary widely across the literature, even across studies using the same type of injury outcome. A review of the literature indicated that genital injuries seen with direct visualization were reported among 40% to 60% in research after 1995, compared with rates of 5% to 40% in the years preceding 1995. One of the reasons for this change may be examiner experience. In the systematic review of injury literature, there were significant differences found between rates of injury reported by emergency physicians and those reported by SANEs. The SANEs reported genital injury at rates more than three times higher than those reported by the emergency physicians. In contrast, the emergency physicians reported absence of any injury in twice as many women, and rates of nongenital injuries were almost three times higher for women examined by emergency physicians compared with women examined by SANEs. This may be partly explained by experience as to injury types and patterns seen most often by either group. SANEs would have more experience with the types and patterns of genital injury seen with SA. Emergency physicians are specialists in trauma medicine and would understandably be able to detect even early signs of trauma to nongenital areas. It was of note that none of the studies involving emergency physicians used aids to visualization, such as either toluidine dye or colposcopy with magnification, whereas these aids were used in almost all the SANE studies.

Risks of Injuries

There are many descriptive studies in which risk factors for injury have been examined. Most of these provide univariate frequencies of injuries based on presence or absence of various perceived risk factors, and the results vary across studies. Only a few multivariate studies are available in which risk factors are considered together in injury outcomes.

A structural equation model was developed to test a theory of the influence of various hypothesized risk factors and the pathways through which they led to either genital or nongenital injury. The model was tested on data from 485 sexually assaulted women who had both a physical and genital examination when seen by SANEs. The only direct influences on nongenital injury were physical resistance by the victim and use of physical aggression by the assailant. The hypothesized risk factors contributed indirectly by working through either aggression or resistance. The only direct influence on genital injury was completed penetration (anal, vaginal, or multiple sites). The association between genital and nongenital injury was found to be related to attempted penetration. Attempts at penetration were associated with increased victim resistance, and in turn increased assailant aggression, therefore contributing to increased nongenital injury.

Consensual Versus Nonconsensual Injury

Most of the injury literature involves cohort studies containing only sexually assaulted women or women after consensual sex. There have been only a few studies comparing injuries between consensual and nonconsensual populations in the same study. A preliminary meta-analysis of these studies revealed the following:

- Women with any genital injuries were 1 to 18 times more likely to be in the nonconsensual group, although high heterogeneity indicates need for further research.
- There were twice as many genital injuries in the nonconsensual group compared with the consensual group (mean = 2.1 vs. 1.1, $p = 0.03$), with only moderate heterogeneity.
- If women had two or more genital injuries, they were 19 times more likely to be in the nonconsensual group ($p = 0.0006$), with no heterogeneity.
- Abrasions to the labia minora were 4.2 times more likely in the nonconsensual group, with none being found in the consensual groups of women and significantly fewer present in consenting adolescents.

There were a number of methodological issues in the studies and considerable heterogeneity (variability) between study findings. Despite the limitations in all of these studies (e.g., small sample size, definitions of injuries), these findings lend support to the likelihood of more genital injuries in nonconsensual groups and differences in location of injuries. Further study is needed in this area to describe patterns of injury more fully.

One area of contention in court is the attempt to link the presence of injuries in nonconsensual intercourse to the lack of the normal human sexual response. This response involved lubrication and pelvic tilting to accommodate the insertion of the penis. Too many variables have yet to be explored, such as the role of fear on lubrication and vaginal responses, the effects in situations where sex may have begun consensually, and the presence of injuries with lubrication. A nurse's testimony in the United States was discounted based on this lack of evidence.

EVIDENCE PRESERVATION AND COLLECTION

One of the most fundamental aspects of evidence preservation and collection is the concept of chain of custody. This refers to ensuring that the evidence has not been contaminated or altered in any way between the time of collection and police receipt. Once the evidence is collected, it must be kept with the SANE at all times until handed over to police, and there should be documentation of anyone who has had contact with the evidence. The types of evidence collected will vary by police jurisdiction, forensic laboratory, and local practices. In Canada the Royal Canadian Mounted Police (RCMP) forensic laboratories process forensic kits for all but two provinces, regardless of whether they or other police forces authorize the kits. The current SA kit has been significantly revised based on the yield of evidence and quality of the samples received by the forensic laboratory.

Trace Evidence

Trace evidence such as glass, grass, or fibers may be on the client's body or clothing. Some protocols involve the use of a drop sheet. Staff may place a large piece of paper on top of a clean sheet or other clean item and have the client stand on the paper while they undress. The intent is to catch trace evidence falling from their clothing. In 2009 this practice was discontinued from the Canadian RCMP kits due to the low yield of trace evidence. It is still possible, however, to use the drop sheet for specific clients if trace evidence is visible and likely to be collected in this manner.

Trace evidence, such as hair and fibers, was found on either a child's clothing or bedding in 64% of cases seen. Adults may also have trace evidence on their clothing. Clothing that is likely to have trace evidence or DNA (e.g., semen) should be collected if the case is being reported to the police. Typically, the panties are collected from an adult or adolescent (or slacks if no panties are worn). Other items may also be collected if there is a history of ejaculation, saliva, or other body fluids being in contact with clothing over that area.

Other techniques include collecting the trace items with tweezers or tape and inserting it into an envelope. If the item can be scratched (e.g., bullet casing), metal instruments should be avoided.

DNA Reference

A sample of the client's DNA is required so the laboratory may differentiate the victim's DNA from the assailant's. Many of us recall having to pull hairs with the root intact from the victim's head and pubic area. Thanks to the evolution of improved DNA analysis this technique is no longer required. PCR technology for DNA replicates small samples of DNA millions of times. DNA can be identified from a very small blood stain, even just a few skin cells, compared with older methods requiring the size of a quarter. While this is now very helpful, it means

SANEs must be very careful to not contaminate samples with their own DNA. If blood cannot be obtained at all from the client, a buccal swab may be performed. This is a swab of the inside of the cheek to collect the client's epithelial cells. A buccal swab cannot be used for DNA reference if there has been oral sex without the use of a barrier device and probable ejaculation, which would cause DNA contamination. If neither blood nor a buccal swab can be obtained, then it may still be necessary to obtain plucked hairs.

One of the problems with traditional DNA collection is that samples of blood or saliva are wet. If not properly dried, the DNA is very susceptible to mold and degrading. An alternate technique has been identified in which hydrophilic adhesive tape is applied behind the person's ear. The DNA identification was 100% accurate. At this time, this is not a commonly used practice.

Body Stains

The general rule for obtaining swabs from the body is that dry stains are obtained with wet swabs and wet stains are obtained with dry swabs. If there is crusting of a dry stain, it may also be possible to scrape the excess material into a paper envelope. Water is usually used to moisten swabs. This is due to concerns that saline will crystallize on the slides in the laboratory. Swabs are taken of both visible stains and areas suspected to have had contact from ejaculation, biting, sucking, or licking. A number of clients do not know if these events occurred since alcohol is involved in many SAs. It would be reasonable to consider routinely swabbing the breasts of any client who was severely incapacitated or who does not know what type of contact occurred.

A double-swab technique is recommended for collection of evidence from bite marks. This technique was developed by a forensic odontologist and involves use of a moist swab over the bite mark followed immediately by a dry swab. The moisture is described as "wicking" the embedded assailant DNA upward to the surface, which is then captured by the dry swab. There is some initial evidence that this technique may be more effective on dry surfaces.

Internal Genital Samples

Internal forensic samples from female clients usually include vaginal wall swabs, cervical os swabs, and collection of vaginal fluid from the posterior fornix (also called a vaginal pool). The vaginal pool is collected by inserting 1 to 3 mL of fluid into the posterior fornix with a tube attached to a syringe or a long 14-gauge intravenous catheter, then it is aspirated out. Practices vary as to whether saline or water is used. The rationale for saline is to prevent the rupture of sperm seen when water is used. The counter argument is that the saline results in crystallization patterns on the slides when analyzed in the laboratory, so some protocols suggest use of small amounts of water instead. The practice of vaginal pool samples is no longer being used in some laboratories (e.g., RCMP laboratories) as they are not found to yield additional information that the cervical os swab did not already give. The likelihood of detecting semen evidence decreases in the vaginal pool after 24 hours, whereas semen may yield positive results days later. The cervical swabs are taken by swabbing over the cervix, since the cervical mucus is likely to trap any sperm.

Drug-Facilitated Sexual Assault

SA may be made easier or facilitated by the use of drugs or alcohol, either voluntarily or involuntarily. The true rates of drug-facilitated sexual assault (DFSA) or incapacitated sexual assaults are difficult to determine. Incapacitated SA was found to be more common on college campuses than in population samples based on a national survey. At least two thirds of the 300,000 college women estimated to be sexually assaulted in 1 year were either considered drug-facilitated (involuntary consumption) or incapacitated (voluntary). Incapacitated SA has been found to be more common than DFSAs in both the college population and in a large community sample.

One key factor in determining rates of DFSA is the delay in presenting for examination. Delays in presenting for examination contribute to difficulties in identifying offending agents. Drug metabolites clear the blood and urine within less than 12 hours for some of the drugs commonly thought to be seen in DFSA, such as flunitrazepam (Rohypnol) or gamma-hydroxybutyrate (GHB), and many others are cleared within 24 hours. The majority of clients do not come in until 12 to 24 hours after assault or even longer, well past this window of detection. The testing for some drugs such as flunitrazepam is not widely available; a benzodiazepine screen from a hospital or local laboratory may be negative, but it would not have been able to detect Rohypnol. Experiencing SA while incapacitated can be very traumatic for clients. The decreased memory and ability to reconstruct events can lead to long-term psychological sequelae.

Even if DFSA testing is available or performed early, it is often limited to those clients for whom there is a history suggestive of involuntary ingestion or symptoms suggesting DFSA. Common findings with DFSA include neurological effects (i.e., confusion, dizziness, drowsiness, impaired judgment, antegrade amnesia, loss of consciousness), lack of muscle control, reduced inhibitions, nausea, and cardiovascular effects such as hypotension and bradycardia. There are high rates of drug or alcohol involvement found in three U.S. studies. A large study was conducted of all samples ($n = 1179$) submitted from across the United States from SA teams whose clients were thought to have experienced DFSA. A total of 60% of samples were positive: alcohol (63%); marijuana (31%); cocaine (14%); benzodiazepines (14%); amphetamines (7%); GHB (7%); opiates (4%); other narcotics or barbiturates (2%). Two thirds of the samples were positive for drugs or alcohol in a similar study of samples submitted with suspected DFSA ($n = 2003$). Alcohol was present in 63% of the samples and marijuana in 30%. Only 3% were positive for Rohypnol or GHB. Both of these studies only involved samples in which DFSA was suspected. A subsequent study was conducted in which all sexually assaulted clients presenting to four different regions were approached for testing of their urine and hair (Juhascik et al. 2007). Alcohol or drugs were present in 43% ($n = 144$) of all assaulted clients. Alcohol was the most commonly reported or confirmed agent (43%), followed by marijuana (33%), cocaine (18%), opioids (7%), amphetamines (7%), and benzodiazepines (3%).

DFSA testing usually involves collection of urine and blood, ideally both at approximately the same time. Metabolites of drugs are recovered much later from urine than for the blood, and the differences between the blood and urine levels allow calculation of clearance as well as time frames and dose of the drug. Blood is collected in two gray-topped tubes containing sodium fluoride and potassium oxalate or lithium heparin, and they should be refrigerated. Urine samples should be collected in containers with an O-ring seal to prevent leakage, or may also be transferred into gray-topped tubes. At least two tubes of each fluid are required, but the exact amount of blood and urine may vary by forensic laboratory and its equipment. Some forensic laboratories are capable of testing hair, which retains evidence of drugs for much longer. Drugs usually take 4 to 6 weeks to show in the hair with new growth areas. Hair sampling may therefore be useful only in the immediate post-assault phase as a baseline for subsequent testing. Alternatively, it may be useful in cases in which the assault is reported later or where initial blood and urine samples were not available. Hair testing is not currently performed in Canadian forensic laboratories.

Given the suspected high rates of DFSA, involuntary or otherwise, one would anticipate that SANEs would routinely test all clients. This decision should take into consideration the client distress reported earlier in this chapter. The client who is fearful of needles may be able to be tested for sexually transmitted infections (STIs) with urine samples and vaginal swabs and have a buccal swab. Sampling of urine and hair may be an alternative, depending on laboratory practices and local protocols.

STI Testing and Prevention

The guidelines for treatment of sexually transmitted infections are developed nationally in both the United States and Canada. The 2009 recommendations are shown in Table 9.4.

Cefixime is the preferred medication, with good evidence for its effectiveness. It is no longer included in the CDC recommendations, however, due to problems with availability of cefixime in the United States. Note in Table 9.4 that Canada and the United States differ in their recommendations for metronidazole and hepatitis B immune globulin (HBIG) use. These recommendations may reflect differences in the risk of these disorders, population risk, and individual opinions in the value of the available evidence.

Prophylactic treatment for STIs is usually offered if the contact was within approximately 72 hours of the assault. Beyond that time testing is recommended, and clients are treated based on results rather than prophylactically. Testing prior to 48 hours post-assault is likely to provide a false negative result, so it is not usually required prior to prophylaxis. Some teams choose to perform baseline testing to identify preexisting STIs. This is to ensure that the prophylaxis is also effective for the existing STI and to facilitate contact tracing. This practice may be problematic in some regions due to potential for introducing prior sexual history into the court case. This risk will vary with case law and local legal practices and should be weighed against the health-care risks of untreated STIs. Note that STIs are reportable diseases, and local practices must be followed for reporting positive findings.

Follow-up testing is recommended in approximately 1 month for any client younger than 14 years old, for those who receive alternate rather than recommended treatments, and for those with risks of pharyngeal infection. Each of these factors are associated with decreased effectiveness of the drug regimen. For instance, children metabolize drugs differently, and the adult dose of recommended medications may be less effective in preventing STIs. There is insufficient evidence that pharyngeal gonorrhea is adequately treated by one-dose regimens of cefixime, although one small study has identified that cefixime

TABLE 9.4 STI Prophylaxis Guidelines

	Canada	United States
Chlamydia	▪ **Azithromycin*** 1 gm orally ×1 dose. (Alternate: Doxycycline 100 mg orally twice daily ×7 days.) If pregnant: Amoxicillin 500 mg three times daily ×7 days.** (May use azithromycin, but inform client that long-term fetal effects are unknown but not expected to be harmful.)	▪ **Azithromycin** 1 gm orally ×1 dose. (Alternate: Doxycycline 100 mg orally twice daily ×7 days.)
Gonorrhea	▪ **Cefixime*** 400 mg orally ×1 dose. (Contraindicated if allergy to cephalosporins or anaphylactic reaction to penicillins.) Alternate: Ceftriaxone 125 mg IM ×1 dose.	▪ **Ceftriaxone** 125 mg IM ×1 dose.
Trichomoniasis & Bacterial Vaginosis	▪ **Metronidazole*** 2 gm orally ×1 dose (only if test positive for trichomoniasis).	▪ **Metronidazole** 2 gm orally ×1 dose for all clients.
Hepatitis B (if not fully vaccinated)	▪ **Hepatitis B immune globulin (HBIG)** within 14 days of exposure. ▪ **Hepatitis B vaccine**, three-dose series (Oral-genital, oral-oral contact are not significant modes of transmission.)	▪ **Hepatitis B vaccine series** HBIG is given only if the assailant is known to be hepatitis B positive.

*These medications have been designated as having good evidence that treatment is effective and there has been at least one properly conducted RCT (Public Health Agency of Canada, 2008).
**There is fair evidence that these medications will be effective, and benefits outweigh risks.

effectively treated all but 1 of 45 patients with pharyngeal infections. The follow-up tests are recommended in approximately 1 month. Most testing is DNA based and will not be able to differentiate dead cells effectively treated by prophylaxis from live cells. Waiting approximately 1 month after medication will allow cells to clear from the system.

HIV Postexposure Prophylaxis

HIV postexposure prophylaxis (PEP) is much more controversial than prophylaxis for the other STIs. To begin with, the research on effectiveness of PEP has been taken mainly from cases in which health-care workers were exposed to potentially contaminated sharps. Therefore, the risks of PEP need to be weighed against the risks of acquiring HIV. Contacts that would be considered high risk include the following:

- Men who have sex with men
- Intravenous drug users
- History of incarceration
- Multiple assailants
- Use of sex trade workers
- Assailants from endemic areas (e.g., Africa)

Client risk factors for infection after exposure to known HIV sources are reported to be approximately 0.2% for receptive vaginal-penile intercourse and 0.3% for receptive anal intercourse. These risks increase for the client if there was no condom or the condom broke, there are open injuries present, or if there is a concurrent STI.

HIV PEP is usually recommended if vaginal or anal penetration has occurred, there was contact with secretions (e.g., no barrier protection), and the assailant is HIV positive or potentially high-risk status. The medication needs to be started as soon as possible within 72 hours of the contact. If providing PEP, it is recommended that clients receive a series of HIV tests to detect seroconversion and that they receive counseling. The counseling should address risk factors for HIV, side effects, and the follow-up protocols. The type and frequency of follow-up varies by region. It may be limited to an initial consultation and final follow-up visit or may be as often as weekly until the 28-day course of treatment is completed. It usually involves interaction with HIV/infectious diseases specialists. The HIV PEP is quite expensive, but in Canada it is paid for by the provincial governments under certain circumstances set out by the provinces. Clients are often given a 3- to 5-day supply to last them until they can attend a follow-up appointment with a specialist. Their treatment usually lasts at least 28 days. The regimens vary by province and state. In general, treatment consists of administration of antiretrovirals such as zidovudine (AZT) and lamivudine (3TC), which is widely available in a single tablet such as Combivir. Many protocols suggest the addition of a protease inhibitor such as a lopinavir/ritonavir combination (Kaletra) if the assailant is known to be HIV positive or high risk for HIV.

Despite the availability of national STI guidelines, the provincial or state guidelines and treatment choices vary widely between regions, teams, and even individuals making the decision to offer PEP. Arguments center on concerns about true level of risk of transmission, especially when assailant risk factors are unknown, when client compliance due to side effects is uncertain, and whether a client will develop treatment resistance to HIV if the client does not complete treatment and requires subsequent treatment.

Determination of assailant risk for HIV is difficult, particularly as most adolescents and adults have only recently met their assailants. A province-wide project was introduced in Ontario, Canada, to offer free HIV PEP to all high-risk and unknown-risk clients. As anticipated, the majority of clients (84.7%) did not know if the assailant had any risk factors for HIV. HIV PEP was accepted by 66.7% of those clients assaulted by high-risk assailants and 41.3% of those with unknown risk. Acceptance of PEP was more likely if they knew the assailant's HIV risk or status, had moderate to high anxiety levels about HIV, were assaulted by someone known less than 24 hours, were assaulted multiple times or by multiple assailants, or were younger than 18 or over 21 years old. Side effects were graded from level 1 (minor) to 4 (severe). Grade 2 to 4 side effects were reported by 77.1% of clients, with an average of three side effects per client. These included fatigue (58.5%), nausea (49.5%), diarrhea (27.5%), headache (20.7%), mood alterations (20.4%), and vomiting (16.4%). Vomiting was significantly associated with likelihood of not completing PEP. The full course of medication was completed by only 23.9% of the high-risk group and 33.2% of the unknown-risk group. Side effects were the top reason for not completing the medications within the first 2 weeks for 81.2% of clients. Other reasons for stopping medications included interference with daily activities (42%), inability to take time off for follow-up visits (21.7%), and believing the PEP was unnecessary (18.8%).

Follow-up testing for HIV antibody and antigen are usually recommended at 4 to 6 weeks, 3 months, and 6 months after exposure. Use of barrier devices should also be discussed for subsequent intercourse for the 6-month period until results are received if there has been potential for HIV exposure during the assault.

Emergency Contraception

Rates of pregnancy after SA are unknown. There are numerous methods for prevention of pregnancy after an SA, but the most commonly used method is the administration of levonorgestrel (Plan B). This is a progestin-only contraceptive that is given in a one-time dose of two pills. While most effective in the first few days after an assault, Plan B can be given up to 5 days later. Davidoff reviewed the research on reduction of pregnancy, finding it reduced risk by 59% to 94%, with the package insert claiming an 89% reduction. Plan B has been found to have fewer side effects such as nausea than the previously used Yuzpe method (combined dose of estrogen/progestin such as Ovral). The mechanisms of action for Plan B include preventing ovulation, especially if given before the luteinizing hormone surge in the cycle, and perhaps also by making ova resistant to fertilization if given after the surge. It has also been found to reduce sperm counts in the uterine cavity by alkalinizing the pH and to thicken cervical mucus. The research has established that there are no post-fertilization effects of Plan B.

The ethics of administering emergency contraception have been widely debated. The Roman Catholic church has allowed the use of Plan B since scientific evidence has established it works mainly through preventing ovulation rather than implantation. It is therefore not seen as abortion by some. Others may still choose to not give Plan B as it prevents pregnancy. If refusing to administer Plan B is a consideration for a SANE, then local and professional legislation and employer's position should be carefully examined before taking action. The client also has a right to treatment and should receive a referral to another center where she can obtain Plan B. A number of regions and countries such as Canada have now made Plan B available over the counter in pharmacies.

Referrals and Follow-Up

Clients should be advised when to return to the nearest emergency department or clinic, have self-care explained, and be instructed regarding health-care or counseling follow-up procedures. Clients need immediate medical help if they react to their antibiotics. Signs of immediate hypersensitivity/anaphylaxis should be discussed. Although there are fewer side effects with Plan B, it is still possible clients may have a deep vein thrombosis and embolism. Clients should be advised to seek immediate health care for symptoms such as sudden pain in the leg, abdomen, or chest.

Self-care is usually symptomatic. Injuries to the genital region heal within 3 to 5 days as it is a highly vascular region. Anecdotal evidence supports the use of warm baths, without irritating soaps, to increase blood supply to the area and theoretically speed healing. Nonsteroidal anti-inflammatory agents are helpful to manage inflammation and pain of soft tissue injuries. If there has been a head injury, clients may require further observation or admission and diagnostic imaging of the head or neck, particularly if there was a loss of consciousness or any other deficit. Clients who have had attempted or potential strangulation should also be observed or admitted, particularly if they lost consciousness during the strangulation, were incontinent, experienced any voice change, or had difficulty swallowing.

Follow-Up Visits

Some teams have been able to incorporate follow-up physical examinations into their protocols. These examinations have been reported anecdotally to be helpful in distinguishing subtle findings and ruling them out as injuries or by supporting identification of an injury. For instance, a mark may be present that appears to be a bruise, but if it is present 2 weeks later on follow-up examination, it is likely a normal finding.

TESTIMONY

Provision of fact-based or expert testimony regarding sexually assaulted clients is a relatively new experience for many nurses. Any SANE may be called to court as a fact witness to describe the actions taken during an examination and the findings. The prosecutor may be able to meet with the SANE prior to the court date to discuss the procedures and the type of questions that will be asked. The prosecutor must be careful during this meeting to not lead the SANE or tell the SANE what to say. The information provided during testimony should be concise, objective, and factual. Opinions and interpretations are to be avoided. There is an expectation that the nurse will be unbiased. The perception and definition of this is somewhat different in Canada compared with the United States. In the United States, it has resulted in the increased role of the advocate to ensure empathy and confidentiality with the client so that the nurse is unbiased. In Canada the courts generally recognize that compassion and empathy are part of the nursing function and that the SANE can still give unbiased testimony. The SANEs should, however, remember that their role is not to convict but rather to provide comprehensive care, including the objective observation of physical findings.

Expert witnesses are called to court to provide opinion on the findings. They may or may not have actually seen the client. Expert SANEs are typically asked to give opinion and/or explanation regarding human tissue (e.g., elasticity, resiliency to injury), anatomy, and possible causes of injuries if present or reasons why injuries may be absent. The requirements for qualifying a SANE as an expert witness are more stringent, particularly in some regions. The standard has generally been that if someone has more education and experience in a particular area than the average person he or she can be qualified as an expert by the judge in the case. This has been applied for experts in any area, ranging from plumbing to health care. In Canada the standards for qualifying a nurse as an expert in SA have become more stringent. A SANE was called to testify in one particular case, and when she admitted she was unaware of the research in a particular area her testimony as an expert was struck down. The result has been that only a few SANEs are now being presented for qualification as experts in court in some areas in an attempt to protect the SANE's reputation and credibility. These experts tend to be the nurse specialists or sexual assault researchers. Research is needed to compare and contrast the criteria for experts across the country and between nurses and physicians to better prepare SANEs for this area of practice.

Current Status of Evidence

We have seen throughout this review that the bulk of the evidence is clinical opinion, expert opinion, or nonexperimental research designs with cohort samples of sexually assaulted clients. Individual studies deal only with a limited concept, often in isolation. Only a limited number of multidimensional studies have been conducted to examine interactions between variables. Even fewer systematic reviews have been conducted across the existing studies, but the number is increasing each year.

Implementing Evidence-Based Sexual Assault Practice

The relatively short existence of specialized nurse examiners for SA clients poses challenges for evidence-based practice. The role has sometimes been interpreted differently, impacting the core knowledge and training required. Both the role and core knowledge needs must be clear before the existing evidence in those areas can be examined comprehensively. In addition, it takes time to build a body of research in a particular area and even longer to have enough studies on an individual topic to synthesize and summarize these for clinical implementation. As a result, some of the practices and beliefs held by sexual assault nurses may be founded on evidence of limited quality. It

is vital for nurses to have a solid understanding of the evidence underlying their practice, both for client outcomes as well as for legal outcomes and expert testimony. It is also important for our future care of sexually assaulted clients to recognize and develop areas for future research and understanding.

SANEs' knowledge of the current research is also relevant to their testimony in court and can affect case law. This was seen with the handling of expert witness testimony by SANEs in both the United States and Canada. Identifying higher quality evidence is only one step in implementing evidence-based practice. Efforts to implement change have not always been successful despite a variety of models available. A model has been proposed and tested in which three components have to be considered: context, facilitation, and evidence. Kitson found that lower levels in one aspect (e.g., context) may be compensated for by another (e.g., a strong facilitator or change agent) and that all three need to be considered for successful implementation of evidence-based practice.

CONCLUSIONS

Caring for the sexually assaulted person is challenging, and the context needs to be evaluated. The context is the setting in which the change is to take place. A context that will support change is one in which culture of the organization supports learning and continuing education, there are clear roles and effective teamwork, and there are measures of feedback on performance, such as peer review. We work in a setting involving multiple disciplines, particularly health care, social work, science, and justice. Each discipline offers a unique perspective and philosophy used in approaching sexually assaulted clients. Each discipline needs to have an understanding and respect for the differences in philosophy and approach to the clients. Multidisciplinary education is required for all team members. Expert opinion and research needs to be facilitated within this multidisciplinary context in order to effectively prevent SA or its consequences.

Facilitation describes the type of support available to help people in the change process. Successful facilitators demonstrate high respect, empathy, credibility, and authenticity; have clear authority and are accessible; are flexible and consistently supportive; and are present. The future of effective implementation of evidence-based practice is heavily reliant on strong facilitation by our leaders in SA care, research, and management. Advanced practice nurses and forensic nursing organizations are becoming increasingly active in lobbying governments and influential groups to help reduce risks of assault and improve care for SA victims. SANEs at all levels need to identify key facilitators in their region and work with them to resolve challenges in their community.

Evidence should be relatively strong to support the change, with high levels of consensus on the topic from experts and partnership with the client regarding the change. Research evidence in sexual assault nursing will rarely be at the level of true experimental designs in the hierarchy, due to the nature of our clients and their circumstances. Random assignment to assaulted and nonassaulted groups is clearly not possible. There is, however, substantial room to improve the designs of future research, such as including random selection of sexually assaulted clients and use of matched cohorts who have not been assaulted. Replication of individual research designs in different settings and with different clients is another way to strengthen the quality of the research. Sample size is often an issue in SA research; therefore, collaboration with other SA teams for multisite research is strongly encouraged. There is a move to more sophisticated forms of data analysis, such as multiple regression, structural equation modeling, and hierarchical modeling. These methods allow us to explore relationships between variables and to test theories and pathways as to how different outcomes develop. We are seeing more synthesis of research information on various topics in the form of literature reviews, and some of these follow the more rigorous guidelines of systematic reviews.

EVIDENCE-BASED PRACTICE

Reference Question: For women who are abused by their intimate partner, does the use of an advocacy (group social support) intervention prevent violence within 12 months of the intervention?

P = Women abused by intimate partner
I = Advocacy
C = Usual care
O = Prevent violence
T = 12 months

Database to Search: Cochrane Library

Search Terms: With the Cochrane Library being such a small database, doing a simple keyword search is usually sufficient. Searching for "intimate partner abuse" finds two reviews in Cochrane. One is appropriate for the question.

Selected References From Search:

1. Cook, R.J., & Dickens, B.M. (2009). Dilemmas in intimate partner violence. *International Journal of Gynecology and Obstetrics, 106*(1):72-75.
2. Ramsay, J., Carter, Y., Davidson, L., et al. (2009). Advocacy intervention to reduce or eliminate violence and promote the physical and psychosocial well-being of women who experience intimate partner abuse (review). *The Cochrane Collaboration, 1*(3):1-23.

Questions Used to Discern Evidence:

Read the studies listed and answer the following questions:

1. What are the differences between the two studies reviewed in the article in respect to design, methods, and results?
2. What are the similarities between the two studies reviewed in the article in respect to the number of subjects, measures used, and interventions, if any?
3. What skills do you need to learn to work with women who survive intimate partner abuse?

1. A common theme in sexual assault care is:
   A. Advocacy
   B. Empowerment
   C. Role modeling
   D. Telling their story

2. There are several kinds or types of assailants. Assailants who are less likely to get caught, be prosecuted, or for their victim even to report to police is the:
   A. Intimate partner assailant
   B. Family member assailant
   C. Stranger assailant
   D. Acquaintance assailant

3. Helpful strategies in the examination by SANEs of sexually assaulted clients include:
   A. Being made to feel safe
   B. Controlling client's response
   C. Maximizing the trauma
   D. Rushing the client through the examination

4. Reframing is a cognitive strategy that may be helpful even in acute stages to reduce distorted thoughts and perhaps encourage clients to consider more positive alternatives. An example of reframing is:
   A. If they say they feel extremely anxious, ask if they need an anti-anxiety medication.
   B. If they say their head hurts, ask if they have had bouts of headaches before.
   C. If they say they will never be safe again, ask if they feel safe now and identify what they will need to feel safe tonight when they go home.
   D. If they say the assailant will come back to hurt them badly next time, ask why they think this way.

5. There are two types of light emitted when using ultraviolet or alternate lights: excitation light and emission light. The excitation light is not visible at ultraviolet wavelengths (less than 400 nm), making the emission light directed on the stain:
   A. Invisible
   B. Visible to the naked eye
   C. Partially visible
   D. Movable

6. It is sometimes difficult to examine the hymen, particularly on women with redundant folds of hymen. One of the techniques suggested to help view the edges of the hymen is:
   A. Balloon visualization
   B. Toluidine visualization
   C. Colposcopic visualization
   D. Both D and C visualization

7. One of the most fundamental aspects of evidence preservation to ensure that the evidence has not been contaminated or altered in any way between the time of collection and police receipt is:
   A. Fully exposed photographs
   B. Grade of trace evidence
   C. Source of body stains
   D. Chain of custody

8. The general rule for obtaining stains from the body is by swabbing:
   A. Dry stains with dry swabs and wet stains with wet swabs
   B. Wet and dry stains with dry swabs
   C. Dry stains with wet swabs and wet stains with dry swabs
   D. Wet and dry stains with wet swabs

9. One key factor in determining rates of DFSA in sexual assault clients presenting in the emergency room is:
   A. Not consenting to prosecute the case
   B. Delays in presenting for examination
   C. Not consenting to inform family
   D. Asking for levonorgestrel (Plan B)

10. A model to implement change in the handling of expert testimony by SANEs in the United States and Canada, in which three components are considered, has been proposed and tested. The three components are:
    A. Context, facilitation, and evidence
    B. Context, victim risks, and interaction factors
    C. Evidence, outcomes, and SANE education
    D. Consent, timing, and evidence

References

Acierno, R., Resnick, H., Kilpatrick, D.G., Saunders, B., & Best, C.L. (1999). Risk factors for rape, physical assault, and posttraumatic stress disorder in women: Examination of differential multivariate relationships. *Journal of Anxiety Disorders, 13*(6):541-563.

Adams, J.A., Girardin, B., & Faugno, D. (2001). Adolescent sexual assault: Documentation of acute injuries using photo-colposcopy. *Journal of Pediatric and Adolescent Gynecology, 14*(4):175-180.

Adams, J.A., & Wells, R. (1993). Normal versus abnormal genital findings in children: How well do examiners agree? *Child Abuse & Neglect, 17*(5):663-675.

Ahrens, C.E., Cabral, G., & Abeling, S. (2009). Healing or hurtful: Sexual assault survivors' interpretations of social reactions from support providers. *Psychology of Women Quarterly, 33*(1):81-94.

Ahrens, C.E., Campbell, R., Ternier-Thames, N.K., Wasco, S.M., & Sefl, T. (2007). Deciding whom to tell: Expectations and outcomes of rape survivors' first disclosures. *Psychology of Women Quarterly, 31*(1):38-49.

Alberta Centre for Injury & Research. (2005). *Injury related health services use by First Nations in Alberta*. Hospital Admissions 200 & Emergency Department Visits, 2000. Retrieved August 5, 2007, from http://www.acicr.ualberta.ca/pages/documents/FirstNationsInjuriesHealthServiceUse.pdf

American College of Emergency. (2002). *Evaluation and management of the sexually assaulted or sexually abused patient*. Dallas, TX: American College of Emergency Physicians.

American Mental Health Counsellors Association. (2007). *Psychological first aid*. Retrieved June 5, 2009, from http://www.thefreelibrary.com/Psychological+first+aid-a0158907275

American Nurses Association. (2005). *Code of ethics for nurses with interpretive statements*. Retrieved August 21, 2008, from http://nursingworld/org/ethics/code/protected_nwcoe813.htm

Anderson, S., McClain, N., & Riviello, R.J. (2006). Genital findings of women after consensual and nonconsensual intercourse. *Journal of Forensic Nursing, 2*(2):59-65.

Andrews, B., Brewin, C.R., Rose, S., & Kirk, M. (2000). Predicting PTSD symptoms in victims of violent crime: The role of shame, anger, and childhood abuse. *Journal of Abnormal Psychology, 109*(1):69-73.

Archambault, J. (2005). *Time limits for conducting a forensic examination: Can biological evidence be recovered 24, 36, 48, 72, 84 or 96 hours following a sexual assault?* Retrieved from http://www.mysati.com/enews/May2005/practices_0505.htm

Baird, S., & Jenkins, S.R. (2003). Vicarious traumatization, secondary traumatic stress, and burnout in sexual assault and domestic violence agency staff. *Violence & Victims, 18*(1):71-86.

Balsam, K.F., Rothblum, E.D., & Beauchaine, T.P. (2005). Victimization over the life span: A comparison of lesbian, gay, bisexual, and heterosexual siblings. *Journal of Consulting & Clinical Psychology, 73*(3):477-487.

Bamberger, J.D., Waldo, C.R., Gerberding, L., & Katz, M.K. (1999). Postexposure prophylaxis for human immunodeficiency virus (HIV) infection following sexual assault. *The American Journal of Medicine, 106*:323-326.

Barsley, R.E., West, M.H., & Fair, J.A. (1990). Forensic photography: Ultraviolet imaging of wounds on skin. *American Journal of Forensic Medical Pathology, 11*(4):300-308.

Bays, J., Chewning, M., Keltner, L., Stewell, R., Steinberg, M., & Thomas, P. (1990). Changes in hymenal anatomy during examination of prepubertal girls for possible sexual abuse. *Adolescent Pediatric Gynecology, 3*:34-46.

Besant-Matthews, P.E., Lynch, V.A., & Duval, J.B. (2006). *Blunt and sharp injuries*, pp. 189-200. St. Louis, MO: Elsevier Mosby.

Birmes, P., Brunet, A., Carreras, J.L., Charlet, J.P., et al. (2003). The predictive power of peritraumatic dissociation and acute stress symptoms for posttraumatic stress symptoms: A three-month prospective study. *American Journal of Psychiatry, 160*(7):1337-1339.

Bisson, J.I., Shepherd, J.P., Joy, D., Probert, R., & Newcombe, R.G. (2004). Early cognitive-behavioural therapy for posttraumatic stress symptoms after physical injury. *British Journal of Psychiatry-Supplement. 184*:63-69.

Bowie, S.I., Silverman, D.C., Kalick, S.M., & Edbril, S.D. (1990). Blitz rape and confidence rape: Implications for clinical intervention. *American Journal of Psychotherapy, 44*(2):180-188.

Bownes, I.T., O'Gorman, E.C., & Sayers, A. (1991). Assault characteristics and posttraumatic stress disorder in rape victims. *Acta Psychiatrica Scandinavica, 83*(1):27-30.

Boyle, C., McCann, J., Miyamoto, S., & Rogers, K. (2008). Comparison of examination methods used in the evaluation of prepubertal and pubertal female genitalia: A descriptive study. *Child Abuse & Neglect, 32*(2):229-243.

Brennan, P.A. (2006). The medical and ethical aspects of photography in the sexual assault examination: Why does it offend? *Journal of Clinical Forensic Medicine, 13*(4): 194-202.

Breslau, N., Davis, G.C., Peterson, E.L., & Schultz, L. (1997). Psychiatric sequelae of posttraumatic stress disorder in women. *Archives of General Psychiatry, 54*:81-87.

Brewer, E.W., & Shapard, L. (2004). Employee burnout: A meta-analysis of the relationship between age or years of experience. *Human Resource Development Review, 3*(2):102-123.

Brewin, C.R., Andrews, B., & Valentien, J.D. (2000). Meta-analysis of risk factors for posttraumatic stress disorder in trauma-exposed adults. *Journal of Consulting and Clinical Psychology, 65*(5):748-767.

Britton, J.C., Phan K.L., Taylor S.F., Fig L.M., & Liberzon. I. (2005). Corticolimbic blood flow in posttraumatic stress disorder during script-driven imagery. *Biological Psychiatry, 57*(8):832-840.

Brymer, M., Jacobs, A., Layne, C., Pynoos, R., et al. (2006). *Psychological first aid (PFA) field operations guide* (2nd ed.). Retrieved June 10, 2009, from http://www.ncptsd.va.gov/ncmain/ncdocs/manuals/PFA_2ndEditionwithappendices.pdf

Burgess, A.W., Hazelwood, R.R., & Burgess, A.G. (2001). Classifying rape and sexual assault. In R.R. Hazelwood & A.W. Burgess (Eds.). *Practical aspects of rape investigation*, pp. 165-176. Boca Raton, FL: CRC Press.

Butterfield, M.I., Panzer, P.G., & Forneris, C.A. (1999). Victimization of women and its impact on assessment and treatment in the psychiatric emergency setting. *Psychiatric Clinics of North America, 22*(4):875-896.

Campbell, R. (2008). The psychological impact of rape victim's experiences with the legal, medical and mental health systems. *American Psychologist, 63*(8):702-717.

Campbell, R., Ahrens, C.E., Sefi, T., Wasco, S.M., & Barnes, H.E. (2001). Social reactions to rape victims: Healing and hurtful effects on psychological and physical health outcomes. *Violence & Victims, 16*(3):287-302.

Campbell, R., & Bybee, D. (1997). Emergency medical services for rape victims: Detecting the cracks in service delivery. *Womens Health, 3*(2):75-101.

Campbell, R., Patterson, D., Adams, A.E., Diegel, R., & Coats, S. (2008). A participatory evaluation project to measure SANE nursing practice and adult sexual assault patients' psychological well-being. *Journal of Forensic Nursing, 4*(1):19-28.

Campbell, R., Patterson, D., & Lichty, L.F. (2005). The effectiveness of sexual assault nurse examiner (SANE) programs. *Trauma, Violence & Abuse, 6*(4):313-329.

Campbell, R., & Raja, S. (1999). Secondary victimization of rape victims: Insights from mental health professionals who treat survivors of violence. *Violence & Victims, 14*(3):261-275.

Campbell, R., Sefi, T., Barnes, H.E., Ahrens, C.E., Wasco, S.M., & Zaragoza-Diesfeld, Y. (1999). Communiy services for rape survivors: Enhancing psychological well-being or increasing trauma? *Journal of Consulting and Clinical Psychology 67*(6):847-858.

Campbell, R., & Wasco, S.M. (2005). Understanding rape and sexual assault: Twenty years of progress and future directions. *Journal of Interpersonal Violence, 20*(1):127-131.

Canadian Nurses Association. (2002). Position statement: Evidence-based decison making and nursing practice. Retrieved March 22, 2007, from www.cna-nurses.ca/CNA/documents/pdf/publications/PS63_Evidence_based_Decision_making_Nursing_Practice_e.pdf

Canadian Nurses Association. (2008). Code of ethics for registered nurses. Retrieved August 22, 2008, from http://www.cna-aiic.ca/CNA/documents/pdf/publications/Code_of_Ethics_2008_e.pdf

Canaff, R. (2004). Limits and lessons: The expert medical opinion in adolescent sexual abuse cases. Retrieved July 15, 2008, from http://www.ndaa.org/publications/newsletters/update_volume_17_number_3_2004.html

Carter-Snell, C. (2003). *ACCN 4453: Emergency nursing of the acutely ill and injured Part A.* Calgary: Mount Royal College.

Carter-Snell, C. (2005). *Forensic Studies 4413: Sexual Assault Examination and Intervention.* Retrieved from http://wwwacad.mtroyal.ca/forensic

Carter-Snell, C., & Hegadoren, K. (2003). Gender and stress disorders. *Canadian Journal of Nursing Research, 35*(2): 34-55.

Carter-Snell, C., & Soltys, K. (2005). Forensic ultraviolet lights in clinical practice: Evidence for the evidence. *The Canadian Journal of Police & Security Services, 3*(2):90-96.

Carter-Snell, C.J. (2007). *Understanding women's risks for injury from sexual assault.* Edmonton: University of Alberta.

Centers for Disease Control. (2006). Sexually transmitted diseases guidelines 2006. Retrieved July 20, 2007, from http://www.cdc.gov/std/treatment/2006/sexual-assault.htm

Christian, C.W., Lavelle, J.M., De Jong, A.R., Loiselle, J., Brenner, L., & Joffe, M. (2000). Forensic evidence findings in prepubertal victims of sexual assault. *Pediatrics, 106*(1):100-105.

Christofides, N.J., Muirhead, D., Jewkes, R.K., Penn-Kekana, L., & Conco, D.N. (2006). Women's experiences of and preferences for services after rape in South Africa: Interview study. *British Medical Journal, 332*:209-213.

Ciancone, A.C., Wilson, C., Collette, R., & Gerson, L.W. (2000). Sexual assault nurse examiner programs in the United States. *Annals of Emergency Medicine, 35*(4):353-357.

Cochrane Collaboration (2009). The Cochrane Collaboration. Retrieved from http://www.cochrane.org/

Crandall, C.S., & Helitzer, D. (2003). Impact evaluation of a sexual assault nurse examiner program: National Institute of Justice.

Croxatto, H.B., Ortiz, M.E., & Muller, A.L. (2003). Mechanisms of action of emergency contraception. *Steroids, 68*(10-13): 1095-1098.

Cyr, M. & Lamb, M.E. (2009). Assessing the effectiveness of the NICHD investigative interview protocol when interviewing French-speaking alleged victims of child sexual abuse in Quebec. *Child Abuse & Neglect, 33*(5):257-268.

Dancu, C.V., Riggs, D.S., Hearst-Ikeda, D., Foa, E.B., & Shoyer, B.G. (1996). Dissociative experiences and post-traumatic stress disorder Among female victims of criminal assault and rape. *Journal of Traumatic Stress, 9*(2):253-267.

Davidoff, F., & Trussell, J. (2006). Plan B and the politics of doubt. *Journal of American Medical Association, 296*(14): 1775-1778.

Davies, A., & Wilson, E. (1974). The persistence of seminal constituents in the human vagina. *Forensic Science, 3*(1):45-55.

Del Bove, G., Stermac, L., & Bainbridge, D. (2005). Comparisons of sexual assault among older and younger women. *Journal of Elder Abuse & Neglect, 17*(3):1-18.

Derhammer, F., Lucente, V., Reed, J.F., & Young, M.J. (2000). Using a SANE interdisciplinary approach to care of sexual assault victims. *Joint Commission Journal on Quality Improvement, 26*(8):488-496.

Desai, S., Arias, I., & Thompson, M.P. (2002). Childhood victimization and subsequent adult revictimization assessed in a nationally-representative sample of women and men. *Violence and Victims, 17*:639-653.

Du Mont, J., Miller, K., & Myhr, T.L. (2003). The role of "real rape" and "real victim" stereotypes in the police reporting practices of sexually assaulted women. *Violence Against Women, 9*(4):466-486.

Du Mont, J., & Parnis, D. (2000). Sexual assault and legal resolution: Querying the medical collection of forensic evidence. *Medicine and Law, 19*(4):779-792.

Du Mont, J., & White, D. (2007). *The uses and impacts of medico-legal evidence in sexual assault cases: A global review.* Retrieved June 12, 2009, from http://www.svri.org/medico.pdf

Du Mont, J., White, D., & McGregor, M.J. (2008). Investigating the medical forensic examination from the perspectives of sexually assaulted women. *Social Science & Medicine* (in press.)

DuMont, J., Humphries, H., Leeke, T., Loutfy, M., Macdonald, S., & Myhr, T. (2005). A prospective cohort study of HIV-1 post-exposure prophylaxis in Ontario sexual assault victims/survivors.

Eckert, L.O., Sugar, N., & Fine, D. (2004). Factors impacting injury documentation after sexual assault: Role of examiner experience and gender. *American Journal of Obstetrics & Gynecology, 190*(6):1744-1746.

Elliott, D.M., Mok, D.S., & Briere, J. (2004). Adult sexual assault: Prevalence, symptomatology, and sex differences in the general population. *Journal of Traumatic Stress, 17*(3):203-211.

ElSohly, M.A., & Salamone, S.J. (1999). Prevalence of drugs used in cases of alleged sexual assault. *Journal of Analytical Toxicology, 23*(3):141-146.

Emergency Nurses Association (ENA). (2007). *Emergency nursing core curriculum*. St. Louis: Elsevier.

Ericksen, J., Dudley, C., McIntosh, G., Ritch, L., Shumay, S., & Simpson, M. (2002). Clients' experiences with a specialized sexual assault service. *Journal of Emergency Nursing, 28*(1):86-90.

Ernoehazy, W., & Murphy-Lavoie, H. (2008). *Sexual assault*. Retrieved June 4, 2009, from http://emedicine.medscape.com/article/806120-print

Estabrooks, C.A. (1999). Will evidence-based nursing practice make practice perfect? *Canadian Journal of Nursing Research, 30*(4):273-294.

Felson, R.B., Messner, S.F., Hoskin, A.W., & Deane, G. (2002). Reasons for reporting and not reporting domestic violence to the police. *Criminology, 40*(3):617-648.

Foa, E.B., & Riggs, D.S. (1995). Posttraumatic stress disorder following assault: Theoretical considerations and empirical findings. *Current Directions in Psychological Science, 4*(2):61-65.

Foa, E.B., & Street, G.P. (2001). Women and traumatic events. *Journal of Clinical Psychiatry, 62*(Suppl 17):29-34.

Frazier, P.A. (2003). Perceived control and distress following sexual assault: A longitudinal test of a new model. *Journal of Personality & Social Psychology, 84*(6):1257-1269.

Frazier, P.A., & Haney, B. (1996). Sexual assault cases in the legal system: Police, prosecutor, and victim perspectives. *Law and Human Behavior, 20*(6):607-628.

Friedman, Z., Kugel, C., Hiss, J., Marganit, B., Stein, M., & Shapira, S.C. (1996). The Abbreviated Injury Scale. A valuable tool for forensic documentation of trauma. *American Journal of Forensic Medicine & Pathology, 17*(3): 233-238.

Funk, M., & Schuppel, J. (2003). Strangulation injuries. *Wisconsin Medical Journal, 102*(3):41-45.

Gabby, T., Winkleby, M.A., Boyce, W.T., Fisher, D.L., Lancaster, A., & Sensabaugh, G.F. (1992). Sexual abuse of children. The detection of semen on skin. *American Journal of Diseases of Children, 146*(6):700-703.

Gemzell-Danielsson, K. & Marions, L. (2004). Mechanisms of action of mifepristone and levonorgestrel when used for emergency contraception. *Human Reproduction Update 10*:341-348.

Gidycz, C.A., & Koss, M.P. (1991). Predictors of long-term sexual assault trauma among a national sample of victimized college women. *Violence & Victims, 6*(3):175-190.

Gidycz, C.A., Loh, C., Lobo, T., Rich, C., Lynn, S.J., & Pashdag, J. (2007). Reciprocal relationships among alcohol use, risk perception, and sexual victimization: A prospective analysis. *Journal of American College Health, 56*(1): 5-14.

Girardin, B.W., Faugno, D.K., Seneski, P.C., Slaughter, L., & Whelan, M. (1997). *Color Atlas of Sexual Assault*. St. Louis: Mosby.

Gnanadesikan, M., Novins, D.K., & Beals, J. (2005). The relationship of gender and trauma characteristics to post-traumatic stress disorder in a community sample of traumatized northern plains American Indian adolescents and young adults. *Journal of Clinical Psychiatry, 66*(9):1176-1183.

Golden, G.S. (1994). Use of alternative light source illumination in bite mark photography. *Journal of Forensic Sciences, 39*(3):815-823.

Golding, J.M. (1999). Sexual-assault history and long term physical health problems: Evidence from clinical and population epidemiology. *Current Directions in Psychological Science, 8*(6):191-194.

Gray-Eurom, K., Seaberg, D.C., & Wears, R.L. (2002). The prosecution of sexual assault cases: Correlation with forensic evidence. *Annals of Emergency Medicine, 39*(1):39-46.

Greenspan, L., McLellan, B.A., & Greig, H. (1985). Abbreviated Injury Scale and Injury Severity Score: A scoring chart. *Journal of Trauma-Injury Infection & Critical Care, 25*(1):60-64.

Hapke, U., Schumann, A., Rumpf, H.J., John, U., & Meyer, C. (2006). Post-traumatic stress disorder: The role of trauma, pre-existing psychiatric disorders, and gender. *European Archives of Psychiatry & Clinical Neuroscience, 256*(5):299-306.

Haynes, B. (2007). Of studies, syntheses, synopses, summaries, and systems: the "5S" evolution of information services for evidence-based healthcare decisions. *Evidence-Based Nursing, 10*(1):6-7.

Heidt, J.M., Marx, B.P., & Gold, S.D. (2005). Sexual revictimization among sexual minorities: A preliminary study. *Journal of Traumatic Stress, 18*(5):533-540.

Herbert, C.P., Grams, G.D., & Berkowitz, J. (1992). Sexual assault tracking study: Who gets lost to follow-up? *Canadian Medical Association Journal, 147*(8):1177-1184.

Herman, J.L. (2003). The mental health of crime victims: Impact of legal intervention. *Journal of Traumatic Stress, 16*(2):159-166.

Higgins, J.P.T., Thompson, S.G., Deeks, J.J., & Altman, D.G. (2003). Measuring inconsistency in meta-analysis. *British Medical Journal, 327*:557-560.

Hilden, M., Schei, B., & Sidenius, K. (2005). Genitoanal injury in adult female victims of sexual assault. *Forensic Science International, 154*(2/3):200-205.

Hochmeister, M.N., Whelan, M., Borer, U.V., Gehrig, C., et al. (1997). Effects of toluidine blue and destaining reagents used in sexual assault examinations on the ability to obtain dna profiles from postcoital vaginal swabs. *Journal of Forensic Sciences, 42*(2):316-319.

Holmes, M.M., Resnick, H.S., & Frampton, D. (1998). Follow-up of sexual assault victims. *American Journal of Obstetrics and Gynecology, 179*(2):336-342.

House of Representatives (1986). Sexual abuse act of 1986.

Hutson, L.A. (2002). Development of sexual assault nurse examiner programs. *Nursing Clinics of North America, 37*(1):79-88.

Ingemann-Hansen, O. (2008). Legal aspects of sexual violence: Does forensic evidence make a difference? *Forensic Science International, 180*:98-104.

International Association of Forensic Nurses. (2006). What is forensic nursing? Retrieved July 7, 2008, from http://www.iafn.org/displaycommon.cfm?an=1&subarticlenbr=137

International Association of Forensic Nurses (IAFN). (2008). IAFN reaches new landmark goal with the first SANE-pediatric (SANE-P) certification examination. *On the Edge, 14*(2).

James, R.K. (2008). Crisis intervention strategies. *Basic crisis intervention skills*, pp. 37-74. Belmont, CA: Thomson.

Jaycox, L.H., Zoellner, L., & Foa, E.B. (2002). Cognitive-behavior therapy for PTSD in rape survivors. *Journal of Clinical Psychology, 58*(8):891-906.

Joanna Briggs Institute (n.d.). *Cochrane qualitative methods review group*. Retrieved June 7, 2009, from http://www.joannabriggs.edu.au/cqrmg/about.html

Johnson, H. (2006). *Measuring violence against women: Statistical trends 2006*. Ottawa: Statistics Canada.

Jones, J.S., Dunnuck, C., Rossman, L., Wynn, B.N., & Genco, M. (2003). Adolescent Foley catheter technique for visualizing hymenal injuries in adolescent sexual assault. *Academic Emergency Medicine, 10*(9):1001-1004.

Jones, J.S., Dunnuck, C., Rossman, L., Wynn, B.N., & Nelson-Horan, C. (2004). Significance of toluidine blue positive findings after speculum examination for sexual assault. *American Journal of Emergency Medicine, 22*(3): 201-203.

Jones, J.S., Rossman, L., Hartman, M., & Alexander, C.C. (2003). Anogenital injuries in adolescents after consensual sexual intercourse. *Academic Emergency Medicine, 10*(12):1378-1383.

Juhascik, M.P., Negrusz, A., Faugno, D., Ledray, L., et al. (2007). An estimate of the proportion of drug-facilitation of sexual assault in four U.S. localities. *Journal of Forensic Science, 52*(6):1396-1400.

Kilpatrick, D.G., Resnick, H.S., Ruggiero, K.J., Conoscenti, M.A., & McCauley, J. (2007). *Drug-facilitated, incapacitated, and forcible rape: A national study*. US Department of Justice.

Kimerling, R., Alvarez, J., Pavao, J., Kaminski, A., & Baumrind, N. (2007). Epidemiology and consequences of women's revictimization. *Womens Health Issues, 17*(2):101-106.

Kitson, A., Harvey, G., & McCormack, B. (1998). Enabling the implementation of evidence based practice: A conceptual framework. *Quality in Health Care, 7*:149-158.

Krinsley, K.E., Gallagher, J.G., Weathers, F.W., Kutter, C.J., & Kaloupek, D.G. (2003). Consistency of retrospective reporting about exposure to traumatic events. *Journal of Traumatic Stress, 16*(4):399-409.

Kubany, E.S. (n.d.). *Trauma related guilt*. Retrieved June 4, 2009, from http://www.cbt.ca/trauma-related_guilt.htm

Lamb, M.E., Orbach, Y., Hershkowitz, I., Esplin, P.W., & Horowitz, D. (2007). Structured forensic interview protocols improve the quality and informativeness of investigative interviews with children: A review of research using the NICHD investigative interview protocol. *Child Abuse & Neglect, 31*(11-12):1201-1232.

Larkin, H., Paolineti, L., Levitt, A., & Phelps, B. (1999). Determining a victim profile and the usefulness of colposcopy in sexual assault victims by a sexual assault victims by a sexual assault response team. *Academic Emergency Medicine, 6*(5):529.

LeBeau, M., Andollo, W., Hearn, W.L., Baselt, R., et al. (1999). Recommendations for toxicological investigations of drug-facilitated sexual assaults. *Journal of Forensic Sciences, 44*(1):227-230.

Ledray, L. (1999). *Sexual Assault Nurse Examiner (SANE) development and operation guide*.

Ledray, L., & Barry, L. (1998). SANE expert and factual testimony. *Journal of Emergency Nursing, 24*(3):284-287.

Ledray, L., Giardino, A.P., Datner, E.M., & Asher, J.B. (2003). *SANE-SART history and role development*. St. Louis: G.W. Medical Publishing, pp. 471-485.

Ledray, L., & Simmelink, K. (1997). Efficacy of SANE evidence collection: A Minnesota study. *Journal of Emergency Nursing, 23*(1):75-77.

Lee, P. (2001). *In the absence of consent: Sexual assault, unconsciousness and forensic evidence*. Vancouver, BC: British Columbia Centre of Excellence for Women's Health.

Li, R.C., & Harris, H.A. (2003). Using hydrophilic adhesive tape for collection of evidence for forensic DNA analysis. *Journal of Forensic Sciences, 48*(6):1318-1321.

Lincoln, C. (2001). Genital injury: Is it significant? A review of the literature. *Medicine, Science and the Law, 41*(3):206-216.

Lincoln, C.A., McBride, P.M., Turbett, G.R., Garbin, C.D., & MacDonald, E.J. (2006). The use of an alternative light source to detect semen in clinical forensic medical practice. *Journal of Clinical Forensic Medicine, 13*(4):215-218.

Lisak, D., & Miller, P.M. (2002). Repeat rape and multiple offending among undetected rapists. *Violence & Victims, 17*(1):73-84.

Lynnerup, N., Hjalgrim, H., & Eriksen, B. (1995). Routine use of ultraviolet light in medicolegal examinations to evaluate stains and skin trauma. *Medicine, Science and the Law, 35*(2):165-168.

MacKenzie, E.J., Shapiro, S., & Eastham, J.N. (1985). The Abbreviated Injury Scale and Injury Severity Score. Levels of inter- and intrarater reliability. *Medical Care, 23*(6): 823-835.

Marc, B. (2008). Current clinical aspects of drug-facilitated sexual assaults in sexually abused victims examined in a forensic emergency unit. *Therapeutic Drug Monitoring, 30*(2):218-224.

Marinelli, L., Green, W.M., & Panacek, E. (2008). What really glows: Analysis of the Wood's lamp in detecting semen and saliva on human skin. *Annals of Emergency Medicine, 52*(4):S171-S171.

Marshall, S., Bennett, A., & Fraval, H. (2001). Locating semen on skin using live fluorescence. Retrieved October 4, 2005.

Martin, N.C., Pirie, A.A., Ford, L.V., Callaghan, C.L., et al. (2006). The use of phosphate buffered saline for the recovery of cells and spermatozoa from swabs. *Science & Justice, 46*(3):179-184.

Martin, S.L., Young, S.K., Billings, D.L., & Bross, C.C. (2007). Health care-based interventions for women who have experienced sexual violence: A review of the literature. *Trauma Violence & Abuse, 8*(1):3-18.

McCall-Hosenfeld, J.S., Freund, K.M., & Liebschultz, J.M. (2009). Factors associated with sexual assault and time to presentation. *Preventative Medicine, 48*(6):593-595.

McCann, J., Voris, J., Simon, M., & Wells, R. (1990). Comparison of genital examination techniques in prepubertal girls. *Pediatrics, 85*(2):182-187.

McCauley, J., Gorman, R.L., & Guzinski, G. (1986). Toluidine blue in the detection of perineal lacerations in pediatric and adolescent sexual abuse victims. *Pediatrics, 78*(6): 1039-1044.

McFarlane, A. (2000). Posttraumatic stress disorder: A model of the longitudinal course and the role of risk factors. *The Journal of Clinical Psychiatry, 51*(Suppl): 15-20.

McFarlane, A.C. (1997). The prevalence and longitudinal course of PTSD. Implications for the neurobiological models of PTSD. *Annals of the New York Academy of Sciences, 821*:10-23.

McGregor, M.J., Du Mont, J., & Myhr, T.L. (2002). Sexual assault forensic medical examination: Is evidence related to successful prosecution? *Annals of Emergency Medicine, 39*(6):639-647.

McGregor, M.J., Le, G., Marion, S.A., & Wiebe, E. (1999). Examination for sexual assault: Is the documentation of physical injury associated with the laying of charges? A retrospective cohort study. *Canadian Medical Association Journal, 160*(11):1565-1569.

McMillan, A., & Young, A. (2007). The treatment of pharyngeal gonorrhea with a single oral dose of cefixime. *International Journal of STD & AIDS, 18*(4):253-254.

McNally, R.J. (2003). Progress and controversy in the study of posttraumatic stress disorder. *Annual Review of Psychology, 54*(1):229-253.

McNally, R.J., Bryant, R.A., & Ehlers, A. (2003). Does early psychological intervention promote recovery from posttraumatic stress. *Psychological Science in the Public Interest, 4*(2):45-80.

Meiser-Stedman, R., Yule, W., Smith, P., Glucksman, E., & Dalgleish, T. (2005). Acute stress disorder and posttraumatic stress disorder in children and adolescents involved in assaults or motor vehicle accidents. *American Journal of Psychiatry, 162*(7):1381-1383.

Millar, G., Stermac, L., & Addison, M. (2002). Immediate and delayed treatment seeking among adult sexual assault. *Women & Health, 35*(1):53-64.

Miller, T.R., Cohen, M.A., & Rossman, S.B. (1993). Victim costs of violent crime and resulting injuries. *Health Affairs, 12*(4):186-197.

Ministers, F.P.T. (2002). *Assessing violence against women: A statistical profile.* Retrieved April19, 2006, from http://www.swc-cfc.gc.ca/pubs/0662331664/index_e.html

Montori, V.M., Swiontkowski, M.F., & Cook, D.J. (2003). Methodologic issues in systematic reviews and meta-analyses. *Clinical Orthopedics & Related Research, 413*:43-54.

Morgan, J.A. (2008). Comparison of cervical os versus vaginal evidentiary findings during sexual assault exam. *Journal of Emergency Nursing, 34*(2):102-105.

Morrison, A.I. (1972). Persistence of spermatozoa in the vagina and cervix. *British Journal of Venereal Diseases, 48*(2): 141-143.

Muram, D., & Elias, S. (1989). Child sexual abuse-genital tract findings in prepubertal girls. *American Journal of Obstetrics and Gynecology, 160*:333-335.

N.A. (2000). *A history of Canadian sexual assault legislation: 1900-2000.* Retrieved April 12, 2009, from http://www.constancebackhouse.ca/fileadmin/website/citation.htm

Nash, K.R., & Sheridan, D.J. (2009). Can one accurately date a bruise? State of the science. *Journal of Forensic Nursing, 5*:31-37.

National Forensic Nursing. (2006). T-blue swabs. Retrieved September 12, 2007, from http://www.nfni.org/t-blueswabs.html

National Institute of Justice (2007). Rape and sexual violence. Retrieved from http://www.ojp.usdoj.gov/nij/topics/crime/rape-sexual-violence/welcome.htm

Nelson, D.G., & Santucci, K.A. (2002). An alternate light source to detect semen. *Academic Emergency Medicine, 9*(10):1045-1048.

Oquendo, M., Brent, D.A., Birmaher, B., Greenhill, L., et al. (2005). Posttraumatic stress disorder comorbid with major depression: Factors mediating the association with suicidal behavior. *American Journal of Psychiatry, 162*(3): 560-566.

Parnis, D., & Du Mont, J. (2003). Examining the standardized application of rape kits: An exploratory study of post-sexual assault professional practices. *Health Care for Women International, 23*(8):846-853.

Peress, D.A., Ward, M.F., Rudolph, G., Ayan, J., et al. (2007). Factors associated with prompt vs. delayed treatment-seeking among sexual assault victims (Abstract). *Annals of Emergency Medicine, 50*(3):S134.

Pierce-Weeks, J. (2008). The challenges forensic nurses face when their patient is comatose: Addressing the needs of our most vulnerable patient population. *Journal of Forensic Nursing, 4*:104-110.

Polit, D.F., & Hungler, C.T. (2008). *Nursing research: Generating and assessing evidence for nursing practice.*

Public Health Agency of Canada. (2008). Canadian guidelines on sexually transmitted infections. Ottawa: Queen's Printer.

Ramin, S.M., Satin, A.J., Stone, I.C., Jr., & Wendel, G.D. (1992). Sexual assault in postmenopausal women. *Obstetrics and Gynecology, 80*(5):860-864.

Royal Canadian Mounted Police. (2003). Ultraviolet light sources and their uses. Retrieved October, 2004, from http://www.rcmp.ca/firs/bulletins/ultraviolet_e.htm

Rennison, C.M. (2002). *Rape and sexual assault: Reporting to police and medical attention, 1992-2000.* No. NCJ 194530. Washington, DC: U.S. Department of Justice.

Rich, V.L., & Rich, A.R. (2007). Personality hardiness and burnout in female staff. *Journal of Nursing Scholarship, 19*(2):63-66.

Rogers, A.J., McIntyre, S.L., Bacon-Baguley, T., Rossman, L., & Jones, J. (2009). *The forensic rape examination: Is colposcopy really necessary?* Unpublished Presentation Abstract, International Association of Forensic Nurses.

Rogers, D., & Newton, M. (2006). Evidence-based forensic sampling: More questions than answers. *Journal of Clinical Forensic Medicine, 13*(4):162-163.

Rose, S., Bisson, J., & Wessely, S. (2003). A systematic review of single-session psychological interventions ('debriefing') following trauma. *Psychotherapy & Psychosomatic, 72*(4):176-184.

Royce, R.A., Sena, A., Cates, W., & Cohen, M.S. (1997). Sexual transmission of HIV. *New England Journal of Medicine, 336*:1072-1078.

Rutty, G.N. (2002). An investigation into the transference and survivability of human DNA following simulated manual strangulation with consideration of the problem of third party contamination. *International Journal of Legal Medicine, 116*(2):170-173.

Sable, M.R., Danis, F., Mauzy, D.L., & Gallagher, S.K. (2006). Barriers to reporting sexual assault for women and men: Perspectives of college students. *Journal of American College Health, 55*(3):157-162.

Sackett, D.L., Rosenberg, W.M.C., Gray, J.A., Haynes, R.B., & Richardson, W.S. (1996). Evidence based medicine: What it is and what it isn't. *British Medical Journal, 312*(7023): 71-72.

Sandelowski, M., & Barroso, J. (n.d.). *Qualitative metasynthesis project.* Retrieved June 8, 2009, from http://www.unc.edu/~msandelo/qmp/

Santucci, K.A., & Nelson, D.G. (1999). Wood's lamp utility in the identification of semen. *Pediatrics, 104*(6):1342-1345.

Saukko, P., & Knight, B. (2004). *Knight's forensic pathology.* London: Arnold.

Schei, B., Sidenius, K., Lundvall, L., & Ottesen, G.L. (2003). Adult victims of sexual assault: Acute medical response and police reporting among women consulting a center for victims of sexual assault. *Acta Obstetricia et Gynecologica Scandinavica, 82*(8):750-755.

Schwartz, R.H., Milteer, R., & LeBeau, M.A. (2001). Drug-facilitated sexual assault. *Southern Medical Journal, 93*(6):558-561.

Shanks, L., & Schull, M.J. (2000). Rape in war: The humanitarian response. *Canadian Medical Association Journal, 163*(9):1152-1156.

Sheridan, D.J., & Nash, K.R. (2007). Acute injury patterns of intimate partner violence victims. *Trauma Violence & Abuse, 8*(3):281-289.

Shin, L.M., McNally, R.J., & Kosslyn, S.M. (1999). Regional cerebral blood flow during script-driven imagery in childhood sexual abuse-related posttraumatic stress disorder: A PET investigation. *American Journal of Psychiatry, 156*:575-584.

Shin, L.M., Wright, C.I., Cannistraro, P.A., Wedig, M.M., et al. (2005). A functional magnetic resonance imaging study of amygdala and medial prefrontal cortex responses to overtly presented fearful faces in posttraumatic stress disorder. *Archives of General Psychiatry, 62*(3):273-281.

Sievers, V., Murphy, S., & Miller, J.J. (2003). Sexual assault evidence collection more accurate when completed by sexual assault nurse examiners: Colorado's experience. *Journal of Emergency Nursing, 29*(6):511-514.

Silverman, E.M., & Silverman, A.G. (1978). Persistence of spermatozoa in the lower genital tracts of women. *Journal of American Medical Association, 240*(17):1875-1857.

Slaughter, L. (2000). Involvement of drugs in sexual assault. *Journal of Reproductive Medicine, 45*(5):425-430.

Slaughter, L., Brown, C.R., Crowley, S., & Peck, R. (1997). Patterns of genital injury in female sexual assault victims. *American Journal of Obstetrics and Gynecology, 176*(3):609-616.

Slim, K., Nini, E., Forestier, D., Kwiatkowski, F., Panis, Y., & Chipponi, J. (2003). Methodological index for non-randomized studies (minors): Development and validation of a new instrument. *ANZ Journal of Surgery, 73*(9):712-716.

Sokol, T. (2008). Anal fissures. Retrieved August 18, 2008, from http://www.medicinenet.com/anal_fissure/article.htm

Sommers, M.S. (2007). Defining patterns of genital injury from sexual assault: A review. *Trauma Violence & Abuse, 8*(3):270-280.

Sommers, M.S., Shafer, J., Zink, T., Hutson, L., & Hillard, P. (2001). Injury patterns in women resulting from sexual assault. *Trauma Violence & Abuse, 2*:240-258.

Soon, J.A., Levine, M., Osmond, B.L., Ensom, M.H.H., & Fielding, D.W. (2005). Effects of making emergency contraception available without a physician's prescription: A population-based study. *Canadian Medical Journal, 172*(7):878-883.

Sorenson, S.B., Stein, J.A., Siegel, J.M., Golding, J., & Burnam, M. (1988). The prevalence of adult sexual assault. *Journal of Sex Research, 24*:101-112.

Speck, P.M. (2009). The alphabet soup of credentials and sorting it all out. *On the Edge.* Retrieved from http://www.iafn.org/displaycommon.cfm?an=1&subarticlenbr=334

State of Maine. (2007). 24 §2986. *Performing forensic examinations for alleged victims of gross sexual assault.* Retrieved August 21, 2008, from http://janus.state.me.us/legis/statutes/24/title24sec2986.pdf

StatsCan. (1993). *The Daily.* Ottawa: Statistics Canada.

StatsCan. (2008). 2006 Census Data Search. Retrieved August 24, 2008, from http://www12.statcan.ca/english/Search/secondary_search_index.cfm

Stein, M.B., Lang, A.J., Laffaye, C., Satz, L.E., Lenox, R.J., & Dresselhaus, T.R. (2004). Relationship of sexual assault history to somatic symptoms and health anxiety in women. *General Hospital Psychiatry, 26*(3):178-183.

Stermac, L., Del Bove, G., Brazeau, P., & Bainbridge, D. (2006). Patterns in sexual assault violence as a function of victim perpetrator degree of relatedness. *Journal of Aggression, Maltreatment & Trauma, 13*(1):41-58.

Stermac, L.E., Du Mont, J.A., & Kalemba, V. (1995). Comparison of sexual assaults by strangers and known assailants in an urban population of women. *Canadian Medical Association Journal, 153*(8):1089-1094.

Stermac, L.E., & Stirpe, T.S. (2002). Efficacy of a 2-year-old sexual assault nurse examiner program in a Canadian hospital. *Journal of Emergency Nursing, 28*(1):18-23.

Stoilovic, M. (1991). Detection of semen and blood stains using polilight as a light source. *Forensic Science International, 51*(2):289-296.

Sulmasy, D.P. (2006). Emergency contraception for women who have been raped: Must Catholics test for ovulation, or is testing for pregnancy morally sufficient? *Kennedy Institute of Ethics Journal, 16*(4):305-331.

Sweet, D., Lorente, J.A., Valenzuela, A., Lorente, M., & Villanueva, E. (1997). PCR-based DNA typing of saliva stains recovered from human skin. *Journal of Forensic Sciences, 42*(3):447-451.

Tang, K. (1998). Rape law reform in Canada: The successes and limitations of legislation. *International Journal of Offender Therapy and Comparative Criminology, 42*(3):258-270.

Taylor, B., & Barling, J. (2004). Identifying sources and effects of career fatigue and burnout for mental health nurses: A qualitative approach. *International Journal of Mental Health Nursing, 13*(2):117-125.

Templeton, D.J., & Williams, A. (2006). Current issues in the use of colposcopy for examination of sexual assault victims. *Sexual Health, 3*(1):5-10.

Tewkesbury, R. (2007). Effects of sexual assault on men: Physical, mental and sexual consequences. *International Journal of Men's Health.*

Thorne, S., Jensen, L., Kearney, M.H., Noblit, G., & Sandelowski, M. (2004). Qualitative metasynthesis: Reflections on methodological orientation and ideological agenda. *Qualitative Health Research, 14*(10):1342-1365.

Tjaden, P. (2009). A comment on White and Du Mont's visualizing sexual assault: An exploration of the use of optical technologies in the medico-legal contact. *Social Science & Medicine, 68*(9-11).

Tjaden, P., & Thoennes, N. (2002). Full report of the prevalence, incidence, and consequences of violence against women. Retrieved May 14, 2006, from http://www.ncjrs.gov/txtfiles1/nij/183781.txt

Ullman, S.E., & Filipas, H.H. (2001). Predictors of PTSD symptom severity and social reactions in sexual assault victims. *International Society for Traumatic Stress Studies, 14*(2):369-389.

Ullman, S.E., Townsend, S.M., Filipas, H.H., & Starzynski, L.L. (2007). Structural models of the relations of assault severity, social support, avoidance coping, self-blame and PTSD among sexual assault survivors. *Psychology of Women Quarterly, 31*(1):23-37.

U.S. Department of Energy. (2009). Human genome project information. Retrieved June 15, 2009, from http://www.ornl.gov/sci/techresources/Human_Genome/elsi/forensics.shtml

U.S. Department of Justice (USDOJ). (2004). *A national protocol for sexual assault medical forensic examinations.* No. NCJ 206554. Washington, DC: U.S. Department of Justice.

U.S. Department of Justice (USDOJ). (2005). *A national protocol for sexual assault medical forensic examinations.* No. NCJ 206554. Washington, DC: U.S. Department of Justice.

U.S. Department of Justice (USDOJ). (2006). *Criminal victimization in the United States.* Retrieved July 23, 2006, from http://www.ojp.usdoj.gov/bjs/cvict.htm

Van Bruggen, L.K., Runtz, M.G., & Kadlec, H. (2006). Sexual revictimization: The role of sexual self-esteem and dysfunctional sexual behaviors. *Child Maltreatment, 11*(2):131-145.

Virginia v. Johnston: Notice and motion IN LIMINE to exclude opinion testimony of Suzanne Brown as scientifically unreliable (2000).

Washburn, P. (2003). Why me? Addressing the spiritual and emotional trauma of sexual assault. *Topics in Emergency Medicine, 25*(3):236-241.

Wawryk, J., & Odell, M. (2005). Fluorescent identification of biological and other stains on skin by the use of alternative light sources. *Journal of Clinical Forensic Medicine, 12*(6):296-301.

Waxman, H. (2008). Drug adherence and resistance. *HIV/AIDS Today, 1*(17):1-2.

White, D., & Du Mont, J. (2009). Visualizing sexual assault: An exploration of technologies in the medico-legal context. *Social Science & Medicine, 68*:1-8.

Willott, G.M., & Allard, J.E. (1982). Spermatozoa: Their persistence after sexual intercourse. *Forensic Science International, 19*:135-154.

Woolley, B., Jones, J.S., Rossman, L., & Bush, C. (2007). Comparative analysis of incapacitated versus forcible sexual assault in a community-based population. *Annals of Emergency Medicine, 50*(3):s133-s134.

Wyatt, J.P., Beard, D., & Busuttil, A. (1998). Quantifying injury and predicting outcome after trauma. *Forensic Science International, 95*(1):57-66.

Yehuda, R. (2000). Biology of posttraumatic stress disorder. *Journal of Clinical Psychiatry, 61*(Suppl 17):41-46.

Yehuda, R. (2004). Risk and resilience in posttraumatic disorder. *Journal of Clinical Psychiatry, 65*(Suppl 1):29-36.

Zadunayski, A. (2006). *Expert medical evidence in the criminal justice system: The case for sexual assault nurse examiners.* Edmonton: Alberta Association of Sexual Assault Centres.

Zink, T., Fargo, J.D., Baker, R.B., Buschur, C., Fisher, B.S., & Sommers, M.S. (2008). Comparison of methods for identifying ano-genital injury after consensual intercourse. *The Journal of Emergency Medicine.* (in press.)

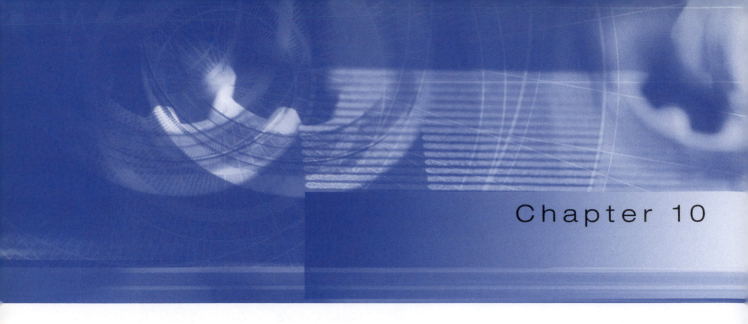

Chapter 10

SELF-DIRECTED VIOLENCE AND THE FORENSIC NURSE

Ann M. Mitchell, Irene Kane, Allyson Havill, and Christine Cassesse

"The test of friendship is assistance in adversity, and that too, unconditional assistance. Co-operation which needs consideration is a commercial contract and not friendship. Conditional co-operation is like adulterated cement which does not bind."

Mohandas Gandhi

Competencies

1. Defining self-injurious behavior.
2. Defining incidence of self-injurious behavior.
3. Identifying risk factors related to self-injurious behavior.
4. Identifying treatment options for self-injurious behavior.
5. Defining suicide attempt.
6. Identifying risk factors related to suicide.
7. Identifying protective factors related to suicide.
8. Conducting a suicide assessment.
9. Discussing components of a no-suicide contract.
10. Identifying evidence-based nursing interventions for the treatment of the patient with suicide ideation and/or a suicide attempt.
11. Describing protective and discharge planning factors to be taken into account at time of discharge.

Key Terms

Non-suicidal self-injurious behavior
Parasuicide
Self-injurious behavior
Suicide
Suicidal gesture
Suicidal ideation
Suicidal intent
Suicide attempt

INTRODUCTION

The forensic nurse employed in emergency, clinical, psychiatric mental health, or a correctional health-care setting may regularly encounter suicidal or self-injurious patients. Cognizance of the range of self-injurious behaviors and differentiation from suicide may be critical in assessment of living or deceased patients for the forensic nurse. **Suicide** is the ultimate act of self-destruction in which a person purposefully ends his or her own life. Even the most experienced forensic nurse may have difficulty assessing suicide and the range of self-injurious behaviors in a patient population. It is critical that the nursing assessment incorporate techniques to uncover the intention of behaviors and include close collaboration with caretakers, family, and friends, as well as the patients themselves.

SELF-INJURIOUS BEHAVIOR

Self-injurious behavior (SIB) is self-mutilating behavior, and it is an enigma even to those who study it. Part of the enigma is created by the lack of consensus over what actually constitutes SIB, what the intent of the behavior is, and who engages in SIB. Additionally, there is a lack of consensus regarding whether SIB exists as a separate diagnostic category or whether SIB is a symptom, transiently evident over many categories of psychopathology and as a marker of more severe pathology. There is evidence to support that SIB can occur in the absence of any DSM-IV–diagnosable psychopathology. Conversely, SIB has been noted to occur in a variety of DSM-IV diagnoses, including eating disorders, mood and anxiety disorders, bipolar disorders, psychotic disorders, and borderline personality disorder. Only borderline personality disorder includes SIB in its diagnostic criteria.

Incidence of Non-Suicidal Self-Injurious Behavior

Estimates of the incidence of SIBs vary widely because of the difficulty in finding consensus regarding the most accurate definition for it. The inclusion of behaviors that can be described as injurious but culturally acceptable (such as tattooing, piercing, and branding) in the definition of SIB is questioned by some researchers but accepted by others. Additionally, behaviors that are accepted in some cultures and communities as developmentally "normal" in adolescents are considered self-injurious by other cultures and communities. Behaviors such as jumping from heights, drug and alcohol use, and driving recklessly are accepted by some as self-injurious but refuted by others. Most researchers operationalize SIBs as being socially unacceptable and causing direct self-harm. **Parasuicide** is another term often used to define nonlethal but intentional self-harm.

The International Society for the Study of Self-Injury was founded in 2006, and it offers a unifying definition of **non-suicidal self-injurious behavior** (NSSI) as "the deliberate, self-inflicted destruction of body tissue without suicidal intent and for purposes not socially sanctioned."

Formation of a unified definition of SIB permits researchers and consumers to distinguish NSSI from culturally acceptable forms of display, behaviors such as drug overdose, and the SIBs engaged in by developmentally disabled or psychotic individuals. However, much research after 2006 continues to be inconsistent with the definition of SIBs, making generalizations difficult. The most current figures regarding SIBs place the incidence at somewhere between 7% and 30%.

Another dilemma in grasping the true scope of the problem relates to how the incidence of SIB is defined. Some researchers include a lifetime incidence of self-injury even if it occurred only once, whereas others look at self-injury within a given time frame or only in those who repeatedly self-injure. Importantly, one can make an argument for either approach. Some see one incident of self-injury as experimental and possibly caused by a contagion effect. Others see one episode of self-injury (or even sub-threshold self-injury) as being a mild form of a syndrome of emotional dysregulation that requires continuous monitoring and, perhaps, intervention. The extent of self-injury does appear to exist across a continuum, with sub-threshold, single-episode self-injury at one pole and addictive, repetitive self-injury at the other.

Another problem is apparent when comparing older research on SIBs (1980–1995) with more current offerings. Older research looks almost exclusively at clinical samples of individuals who self-injured. Because of the bias toward clinical samples, self-injurers were believed to be almost exclusively female, of low socioeconomic status, from a dysfunctional family, and to have borderline personality traits and evidence of a history of childhood trauma. Current research describes a fairly equal distribution of NSSI between males and females. Although there is some association with childhood trauma and family dysfunction, 50% of persons engaging in NSSI do not share this history. The incidence of NSSI in adolescents of high socioeconomic status equals the incidence in adolescents of low socioeconomic status. The association of borderline personality disorder is not generally applicable to adolescents engaging in NSSI. Considering these variations, this section describes the most common causes of SIBs, their differentiation from suicidal behaviors, and currently supported treatment for NSSI.

NSSI commonly includes cutting, branding, burning one's skin without suicidal intent, breaking bones, hitting, pinching, pulling out hair, punching walls, self-inflicting bruising through banging against objects, ingesting toxins, and interfering with wound healing. More subtle forms of self-injury, such as scratching, repetitive rubbing, and serious nail-biting, are considered sub-threshold NSSI and are often associated with anxiety, depression, and obsessive compulsive disorder.

NSSI has been postulated to begin in early to mid-adolescence, although reports of NSSI in childhood do exist. There is also some evidence to support NSSI's association with early-onset puberty. This association parallels findings of higher rates of other psychiatric and behavioral problems occurring earlier in life, including depression, anxiety, eating disorders, risky sexual behaviors, aggressive and antisocial behaviors, and substance abuse. NSSI peaks in late puberty and early adulthood, with up to one third of students at one university sample engaging in NSSI. NSSI in adulthood reduces to 4% in adult community samples, with the usual course of NSSI spanning a 5- to 10-year period. Although some studies have found a preponderance of white adolescents engaging in NSSI, other studies have found the incidence of NSSI in minority populations to be just as prevalent.

Traditionally, SIBs were strongly linked to suicidality, with adolescents and others being hospitalized for self-injury without other symptoms. Later research refuted the association of NSSI with suicidal thoughts, plans, or intent, except in those with other psychopathology. In fact, some researchers believe NSSI is engaged in at times by the adolescent as a failed form of suicide or homicide prevention. Adolescents believe they can avoid the permanent solution (suicide) by temporarily relieving their stress or emotional dysregulation. But in a large community sample of 7000 high school students, NSSI and suicidality could not be so neatly separated. While initially NSSI is distinct, with the adolescent strongly believing that he or she does not want to die, if the NSSI no longer works, the adolescent becomes increasingly vulnerable to other, more dangerous, solutions to emotional dysregulation, including suicide. Of the 17.5% of adolescents in this sample, 48% had some degree of suicidality associated with their behaviors. Additionally, there is a cohort of adolescents who vacillate between NSSI and **suicidal ideation,** which is defined as thoughts about killing oneself.

While studies from the 1980s and 1990s endorse a significant relationship between NSSI and attachment, childhood trauma, family composition, and abuse, later research describes a mild-to-moderate effect. There is some evidence that a critical parenting style, with subsequent alienation of the adolescent from his or her parents, may be associated with the onset and continuation of NSSI. Significant correlates for NSSI include emotional dysregulation, feelings of overwhelming stress with poor or maladaptive coping skills, and significant impulsivity. NSSI often occurs in adolescents searching for strategies for managing strong affective states for which other forms of emotional regulation have failed. Nock and Prinstein suggest that NSSI be classified as either automatic (for the self) or social (peer-influenced). In her seminal work, Dr. Nancy Heath endorses that adolescents engage in NSSI for control, crisis intervention, calming and comforting, communication, coping, chastisement, cleansing, conformation of existence, and creating comfortable numbness. Of these, she believes adolescents who engage in NSSI for cleansing, confirmation of their own existence, and creating comfortable numbness most seriously and repetitively self-injure.

Comorbid psychiatric disorders that might include NSSI allow further comprehension of the role of emotional dysregulation. Eating disorders and self-injury may be manifestations of the same underlying dysfunction, both representing a physical attack on the body to relieve overwhelming distress. Although research on the association between adolescent eating disorders and NSSI is scarce, one study focuses exclusively on it. This study suggests that underlying features are shared between the two disorders irrespective of gender, including the adolescents' greater dissatisfaction with their bodies, greater bulimic behavior, decreased feelings of self-efficacy, poorer affective awareness, greater distrust of others, increased difficulty with social relationships, and greater impulsivity. Additionally, there are addictive qualities to both NSSI and eating disorders allowing the behavior to reinforce itself over time.

Continuum of NSSI to Suicide

1. Normal thoughts
2. Passive death wish
3. Suicidal ideation
4. Suicidal ideation with plan
5. Suicidal intent
6. Suicidal gesture
7. Completed suicide

Adolescents with mood or anxiety disorders present in ways different from that of adults. Irritability, anger, impulsivity, and hyperarousal are typical of adolescents with an anxiety or mood disorder. These adolescents may have difficulty tolerating distress and do have poorer problem-solving skills. Nock's study of physical hyperreactivity as measured by skin conductance, distress tolerance, and problem-solving abilities supports the hypothesis that adolescents with NSSI share these traits with their peers suffering from mood and/or anxiety disorders, but that physical hyperreactivity was most associated with NSSI.

Adolescents who self-injure are difficult to identify in the clinical setting. Although adolescents may share their SIBs with their peers, they are reluctant to endorse SIBs to teachers, counselors, parents, and clinicians. And few teachers and counselors believe they have been adequately prepared for identification of/or intervention with a student who engages in NSSI. For parents, there is often a gradual understanding of the fact that their child engages in such behavior. Confronting the child may lead to denial that is later rebutted by an outside agency, such as the child's school. Often, parents react with a certain amount of ambivalence regarding obtaining professional help for their child, further delaying treatment. Parents often feel "pushed" to consider treatment after further deterioration of the child or increasing behavioral problems. The discovery of the child engaging in NSSI is often disorienting and confusing for the parent; however, inclusion of the parents in treatment has been seen positively by adolescents and parents alike.

Treatment of NSSI

Treatment of NSSI is focused on safety. Monitoring for suicidal risk should occur on a continuous basis, as well as identification of psychiatric comorbidities. Assessment should focus on what need the behavior fulfills in the adolescent's life, and treatment should assist the adolescent to develop healthy methods of responding to that need.

SIBs are believed to be related to serotonin, norepinephrine, and dopamine dysfunction, as well as to the dysregulation of opioid receptors, particularly the dynorphin receptors, directly reactive to dopamine dysregulation. The use of medication therapy, except in the context of treating an underlying psychiatric disorder, is not currently recommended. Significant comorbidity between NSSI and internalizing disorders, such as depression and anxiety, and externalizing disorders, such as conduct disorder and Tourette's syndrome, exists. Psychiatric evaluation and treatment should be considered. There is some anecdotal evidence for using naltrexone, an opioid receptor antagonist; however, no evidence has been developed to establish it as a standard treatment option.

Currently, the best-supported option for the treatment of SIB has been adapted from research regarding individuals with borderline personality disorder. A specific form of cognitive behavioral therapy, dialectical behavioral therapy (DBT), has been endorsed in randomized control trials. DBT uses both individual and group therapy to teach emotional regulation skills, interpersonal effectiveness, mindfulness, and self-management. But it has considerable clinical and financial drawbacks. Furthermore, few clinicians are trained or reimbursed to perform DBT with adolescents. There are other therapies for helping adolescents develop a mindful awareness of their symptoms, learn relaxation and distraction techniques, and develop a cohort of healthy peers with whom they can communicate. Adolescents must be encouraged to increase their affective language skills and improve their communication and problem-solving skills. Both family and group therapies have been supported as being helpful in this regard.

Even the most skilled and experienced forensic nurse may have difficulty assessing for SIBs in the adolescent, although it is critical that the nursing assessment incorporate techniques to uncover the intention of behaviors. Differentiating nonsuicidal from suicidal behaviors can have serious implications for the safety and protection of the adolescent. Understanding the triggers for SIB and suicide is essential in making a complete and accurate assessment. A **suicide attempt** that is motivated by a desire to end one's life should be differentiated from a **suicidal gesture,** which is an attempt that is planned to be discovered and is made for the purpose of influencing others.

EVIDENCE-BASED PRACTICE: ASSESSMENT OF THE SUICIDAL PATIENT

Safety Is the Priority

An emergency psychiatric suicide assessment begins with securing the patient's safety. The first step is to get

---

Forensic Nurse Alert: NSSI Assessment

Not all SIB relates to suicidality. However, a complete and thorough clinical assessment must be completed on all individuals.

the suicidal patient safely into an emergency department (ED) for a diagnostic evaluation to prevent an actual suicide attempt, which is SIB with a nonfatal outcome, accompanied by evidence that the person intended to die.

Once inside a protective environment, the patient's belongings and any potentially harmful objects are removed and stored to provide as safe an environment as possible. An evidence-based treatment plan must be developed. Decisions regarding patient care are based on a precise suicide risk assessment. The assessment must take into account all associated patient factors—environmental, genetic, medical, psychiatric—including forensic issues, to provide a full and complete picture of the patient and his or her lifestyle.

Forensic Nurse's Role

Forensic nurses are frequently in a key position to assess and intervene with suicidal patients. They may be among the first to come into contact with individuals having suicidal thoughts or exhibiting suicidal behaviors. Forensic nurses employed in inpatient care, outpatient care, and EDs need to be skilled in assessing the patient's suicidal potential. The investigation of injury, self-harm, potential of suicide, legal issues, and the protection of the patient and others are issues in which the nurse with forensic education and training may be instrumental as a consultant on the management team.

It is also essential that assessment skills be grounded in evidence-based practice. To this end, forensic nurses must be well-informed about suicide literature based on empirical data. In order to develop and establish comprehensive practice guidelines for suicide risk assessment, it is important to identify the risk factors associated with suicide, as well as to define the key elements of a suicide assessment interview.

SUICIDE RISK FACTORS

Patients who complete suicide often do not communicate their intent to do so during their final contact with a mental health professional. This presents an obvious challenge for nurses and others who are in the position of attempting to predict and prevent suicidal behaviors. Fortunately, there is significant empirical evidence that can provide a foundation for clinical decision making by the nurse. Suicide risk assessment is a systematic process in which the clinician uses specific data to formulate a clinical judgment that serves as the foundation for appropriate treatment and management.

In a comprehensive review of the suicide literature in the American Psychiatric Association's (APA's) *Practice Guidelines for the Treatment of Psychiatric Disorders Compendium,* the following empirically based risk factors were identified: demographic characteristics, the presence of psychiatric disorders, the presence of physical illnesses, family histories, and psychosocial issues.

Demographic Characteristics

Multiple demographic factors appear to be related to an increased risk of suicide, and they must be viewed within the context of other characteristics, such as age, gender, race, and marital status. According to the National Vital Statistics Report, suicide rates for adolescents, young adults, and the elderly are the highest among any other age groups. Men are four times more likely to die by suicide than women, and suicide rates for whites and Native Americans are twice as high as those for any other ethnic groups. In prospective studies of over 95,000 widowed persons, Kaprio and Koskenvuo and Luoma and Pearson found evidence to suggest that single people have double the suicide risk of those who are married; those who are divorced, separated, or widowed are four to five times

Case Study

CASE STUDY OF JEAN L.: A SUICIDE ATTEMPT

Jean L., a 28-year-old, married, white female, is escorted into a psychiatric emergency department (ED) by her husband and the local police, following medical clearance after an interrupted suicide attempt by taking an overdose of her Zoloft prescription. On the previous day, Jean had been remanded to a court appearance for payment of damages from her involvement in an alcohol-related altercation at a local bar. ED clinicians recognized Jean from a prior hospitalization 8 months earlier. Jean relates to the staff that she "has no reason to live—even my husband has given up on me." She sits slumped in the interview chair with a flat affect, arms dangling at her side, head slightly bent and moving back and forth, as she mumbles, "I can't do anything right. I hate my job. I am trying to have a decent marriage."

Case Study

CASE STUDY OF JEAN L.: A SUICIDE ATTEMPT (continued)

Her husband, who initiated the emergency commitment, is the primary source of information. Arriving home from work early, he found her in their bathroom, slumped over the toilet, her prescription bottle empty on the floor next to an empty bottle of wine. He is resolutely informing the ED nurse that he is "done with Jean and can't take it anymore."

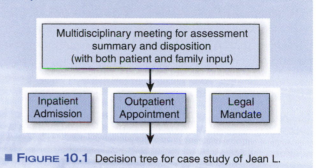

■ **FIGURE 10.1** Decision tree for case study of Jean L.

more likely to complete suicide. Further, data suggest that gays, lesbians, and bisexuals are more likely to attempt suicide than others.

Psychiatric Disorders and Physical Illnesses

Having been diagnosed with a psychiatric disorder is thought to be one of the strongest risk factors for suicide. More than 90% of completed suicides are by individuals who were diagnosed with one or more psychiatric disorders. Harris and Barraclough conducted a meta-analysis of 249 published studies and found that the psychiatric diagnoses associated with an increased risk of suicide include major depression, bipolar disorder, schizophrenia, anorexia nervosa, alcohol and other substance use disorders, and cluster B personality disorders (Box 10.1). The authors found clear indications that having a physical illness is associated with an increased risk for suicide. They

Box 10.1   Cluster B Personality Disorders

People with personality disorders often appear to be dramatic, emotional, or erratic. Cluster B personality disorders include the following:

- **Antisocial personality disorder**: a pattern of disregard for, and violation of, the rights of others
- **Borderline personality disorder**: a pattern of instability in interpersonal relationships, self-image, affect, and marked impulsivity
- **Histrionic personality disorder**: a pattern of excessive emotionality and attention-seeking behavior
- **Narcissistic personality disorder**: a pattern of grandiosity, need for admiration, and lack of empathy

(Adapted from DSM-IV-TR, 2004.)

found a number of studies supporting a link between suicidal behavior and AIDS, brain and spinal cord injuries, cancer, epilepsy, and Huntington's disease.

Psychosocial Issues

Certain psychological symptoms and clinical issues have been empirically linked to an increased risk of suicide. Hopelessness, a history of childhood physical and sexual abuse, absence of social support and religious beliefs, and a family history of suicide have been found to be associated with suicide rates.

There are empirical studies that examine the relationship between completed suicides and the existence of suicidal ideations, suicidal plans, and methods of suicide. In a 20-year prospective study, the presence of suicidal ideation was positively correlated to completed suicide. Kessler, Borges, and Walters found evidence that forming a suicide plan frequently came before a suicide attempt. But even without a plan, a suicidal person who acts impulsively may successfully complete suicide if there is a lethal means of suicide readily available. In a controlled study, Brent and others showed a positive relationship between the accessibility of firearms and the completion of suicide in adolescents. Therefore, it is essential to identify the accessibility of a lethal method for those who are at risk for suicide.

There are several scales and tools available to assist in the assessment of suicide risk, and some of these, as well as the Nurses' Global Assessment of Suicide Risk (NGASR) tool developed by Cutliffe and Barker, will be presented next.

Suicide Assessment Tools

The use of a tool to determine suicide risk is only one aspect of the broad assessment a nurse employs during the suicide risk review. Scales such as the Suicide Intent Scale, the Scale for Suicide Ideation (SSI), the NO HOPE Scale, the SAD PERSONS Scale, and the NGASR are a few examples of such tools (Box 10.2). Although currently no large-scale validation studies have been conducted on the NGASR, it provides a valuable support for nurses who are novices in such assessments.

Nurses' Global Assessment of Suicide Risk

The NGASR is a tool to determine (rates) risk factors that have been positively correlated with suicide risk. The NGASR was developed in a mental health facility in the United Kingdom, and it is an evidence-based suicide assessment tool that also helps nurses develop care interventions based on that risk. The clinical presentation of suicidal patients is quite varied and specific, so the NGASR is to be used *only as a guide* in the assessment of suicide risk.

The NGASR is composed of several sections and 15 identified risk factors (Box 10.3). Each factor is weighted as either 1 (less critical risk) or 3 (greater critical risk). The first factor is the level of hopelessness. Feelings of hopelessness are highly correlated with suicide risk and are determined by self-report and careful attention to verbalization and behavior suggesting hopelessness. In the case study, Jean L.'s perception that "even her husband has given up," is one such example. Second, one must assess for evidence of loss of interest and/or pleasure (for Jean L. this is evidenced by her statement, "I can't do anything right any more") and level of depression (for Jean L., her overdose and current verbal and nonverbal behaviors). Three additional high-risk factors to be observed include recent bereavement or relationship problems such as divorce, separation, or breakups (for example, Jean L.'s relationship with her husband); prior suicide attempts (i.e., Jean L.'s prescription overdose); and evidence of a plan (as demonstrated in Jean L.'s statement in the case box on page 184 to "figure out a way to choke myself"). At this point in the

---

Box 10.2 Suicide Assessment Measures

- Suicide Intent Scales
- Scale for Suicide Ideation
- NO HOPE Scale
- SAD PERSONS Scale
- Nurses' Global Assessment of Suicide Risk

There are numerous other suicide assessment measures for children and adolescents and for adults and older adults.

Box 10.3 NGASR Key Indicator Variables

- Feelings of hopelessness
- Depression/loss of interest or pleasure
- Evidence of suicide plan
- Recent bereavement or relationship breakdown or problems
- Prior suicide attempt
- Recent stressful life events
- Presence of persecutory voices or beliefs
- Withdrawal from interpersonal or social interactions
- Warning of suicidal intent
- Family history of serious psychiatric illness or suicide
- History of psychosis
- Widow or widower
- Socioeconomic stressors or deprivation
- Alcohol or substance misuse
- Presence of terminal illness

Additionally, presence of lethal means or weapons (Adapted from Cutcliffe & Barker, 2004.)

---

assessment, the score for Jean L. on these five factors is 15, the highest score that can be assigned using this tool.

The nurse continues with the assessment of recent stressful life events. The number and severity of a patient's stressors may deplete the person's resources and/or sources of support. Again in the example of Jean L., job difficulties, arrest, and perhaps financial worries must be considered. The assessment continues evaluating other key areas such as unhealthy interpersonal and social relationships, overall status in society, evidence of withdrawal, presence of hallucinations or delusions, and physical health status. A new diagnosis of a terminal illness may contribute to a patient's suicidal ideation and belief that the patient is taking control of an uncontrollable situation in his or her life.

The application of the NGASR in the case of Jean L. is evident. Upon completing the NGASR interview, the nurse determines the patient's total score and assigns the patient to one of four categories. The patient can be assigned a score from a very little, to intermediate, to high degree, or to an extremely high degree of suicide risk. Jean L.'s NGASR score is 22, putting her at a very high risk of suicide. How this information is applied by the nurse can be seen in the case example presented earlier. The nurse placed Jean L. on constant observation, and there has been no change since last night. With information gathered from the use of the NGASR, nursing interventions can be readily determined based upon risk, and secondly, the information provides an effective method of presenting assessment data to other team members.

Health professionals who use the NGASR report consistent satisfaction with the ability to identify critical suicide risk factors. The findings of an expert panel consisting of senior clinical nurses and psychiatrists concluded the tool has high face validity because it consists of well-established factors and that it has high contextual validity because there were no clear omissions in it.

In summary, the risk assessment score serves as a guide for the nurse to determine patient suicide risk, evaluate the level of nursing care to be employed with the assessed patient, and (as in the case of Jean L.) collaborate with the ED team to decide if further psychiatric consultation and/or treatment is necessary for the safety of the patient.

THE CLINICAL INTERVIEW

The clinical interview is the most important aspect of the suicide risk assessment. The *APA Practice Guidelines for the Treatment of Psychiatric Disorders Compendium* identifies guidelines and critical domains of the clinical interview for the nurse clinician. But it is the relationship of the clinician with the patient and the ability of the clinician to establish rapport and communicate empathy that provide the foundation for assessing the risk of suicide. The clinician will also want to ensure the patient's immediate safety.

The scope of the interview will vary depending upon the setting and the patient's ability and/or willingness to provide information. Additional sources of information may include previous contacts with the patient, as well as supporting information from other mental health professionals, medical records, and family members or others in the patient's support network.

The clinician must understand that simply asking patients about suicide will not necessarily mean that they will share accurate or complete information. Cultural, social, or religious beliefs about suicide may restrict a person's willingness to talk about the possibility of suicide, let alone the likelihood of acting on suicidal impulses.

ASSESSMENT OF LETHALITY

Because there is no single cause for suicide, no two suicides can be understood to result from exactly the same constellation of factors. Therefore, the effectiveness of measures designed to screen for suicide will depend upon the degree to which causal factors have been identified, the strengths of the causal relationships and suicide, and the prevalence of the causes in the specific population. The areas explained below have been identified in the *APA*

Practice Guidelines as key components of the suicide assessment interview.

Identify Specific Psychiatric Symptoms

The nurse identifies specific symptoms that are associated with an increased risk of suicide. Symptoms such as agitation, aggression, anhedonia, anxiety, depression, hopelessness, impulsivity, insomnia, and panic attacks have been correlated to an increased risk of suicide.

Assess Past Suicidal Behavior and Degree of Intent of Suicide Attempts

A history of past suicide attempts is one of the most important risk factors for predicting future suicide. Therefore, it is critical for the nurse to ask about past suicide attempts, including the context of the life stressors leading up to the attempt. Also, the patient's perception regarding how lethal the attempt was, as well as his or her level of ambivalence toward living, should also be explored. These factors will allow the nurse to document the degree of intent associated with past suicide attempts.

Review of Past Treatment History

A critical aspect of a suicide risk assessment is obtaining a review of the patient's treatment history. This can provide valuable information on comorbid diagnoses that may increase the patient's risk of suicide and may lead to information regarding suicidal ideation and past suicide attempts. It is useful to obtain a past medical history as well, as this may provide information about suicide attempts that were serious enough to require hospitalization and identify medical conditions that may be associated with an increased risk of suicide.

Identify Family History of Suicide, Mental Illness, and Dysfunction

Asking about family history is especially important when assessing for suicidal risk. Specifically, the nurse clinician should ask about suicide or suicide attempts in family members, as well as any psychiatric illness or hospitalizations. Also, the patient's childhood and current family situation should be discussed, including a history of family conflict, separation, forensic issues such as legal problems, substance abuse, domestic violence, and physical or sexual abuse.

Assess Current Psychosocial Issues and the Nature of the Present Crisis

Specifying the patient's current psychosocial issues is an important part of the suicide risk assessment to determine if there are acute or chronic psychosocial stressors, such as financial or legal problems, interpersonal conflicts or the loss of a significant relationship, an educational or professional failure such as the loss of a job, or problems with housing. It will also be helpful to gain an understanding of the patient's psychosocial situation to identify and mobilize social supports that have a protective function.

Identify Areas of Psychological Strength and Vulnerability

Psychological strengths and vulnerabilities include issues such as adaptive coping skills, personality traits, and cognitive styles. For instance, traits such as aggression, hopelessness, and impulsivity may be associated with an increased risk of suicide. Prevalence of the traits is also associated with individuals who exhibit cognitive rigidity characterized by polarized or constricted thinking. Another factor that may be a possible indicator of risk for suicide is perfectionist thinking, with a high expectation of the self.

Thoughts, Plans, and Behaviors

The nurse must inquire about the presence or absence of suicidal ideation. This is an essential aspect of the suicide risk assessment. Contrary to the idea that raising the topic of suicide may give the patient the idea to complete suicide, this is simply not the case. In reality, raising the issue of suicidal ideation may be a relief to patients as it allows them to talk about their feelings and to feel understood. When thoughts of suicide are raised by the patient, focusing on their nature, frequency, extent, and timing to understand the interpersonal, situational, and symptomatic context is critical.

Patients may deny having thoughts about suicide initially, so follow-up questions later in the interview are critical. The nurse may also need to ask follow-up questions even if at first the patient denies having thoughts about suicide. These may include asking about plans for the future or any recent self-harming behavior. Despite the best effort of the nurse, however, not all patients will admit to having suicidal ideation even when these thoughts are present. Depending on the individual situation, the nurse should talk to family members in order to learn whether they have observed any behaviors (such as the patient buying a gun) that may indicate the presence of suicidal ideation.

If the patient affirms the presence of suicidal ideation, the nurse then determines the presence of a specific plan for suicide and any movement by the patient toward carrying out such a plan. It is also important to question the patient about his or her perception of the lethality of the plan, as this may be as significant as the actual lethality involved in the plan itself. Any time there is suicidal ideation, the nurse should ask about the patient's access to firearms or other weapons. If the patient has such access, this should be discussed with the patient and a responsible family member for the purpose of making arrangements to restrict access. Finally, assessing suicidal intent and the lethality of a suicidal plan is crucial to minimizing the patient's risk of suicide. **Suicidal intent** is a subjective expectation and desire for a self-destructive act to end in death. Also included may be the personal verbal or nonverbal action that stops short of a direct self-harming act that suggests that a suicidal act or behavior might recur.

A plan that is not particularly lethal could still result in suicide if the patient has a strong level of intent and believes that the plan will result in death. Conversely, a patient with less suicidal intent could inadvertently succumb from carrying out a plan that he or she mistakenly believes is not fatal.

The completion of the clinical interview results in a multidisciplinary review that includes the forensic nurse's clinical assessment. Using patient Jean L., the multidisciplinary collaboration summary will be followed by an initial treatment plan based upon a clinically sound decision-making process.

THE DECISION TO HOSPITALIZE

The decision about whether or not to hospitalize a patient occurs once a clear picture of the situation has been established. All assessment factors must be pooled and taken into account to reach a satisfying and safe conclusion. Hospitalization will, in fact, occur when it is impossible to form or restore a treatment alliance between the clinician and the patient and if there is any question regarding the patient's ability to be safe.

The first determination of whether to hospitalize is the need for emergency stabilization. A behavioral emergency is an imminent risk that a patient will do something resulting in serious harm to self or others, while a behavioral crisis is a change in a patient's baseline functioning. Both can require hospitalization to help prevent further problems. A behavioral emergency almost always warrants a hospital admission, whereas a behavioral crisis might possibly be managed in an outpatient setting with increased visits or length of time.

A patient's baseline functioning is affected by both distal and proximal risk factors. Significant proximal risk factors may throw a vulnerable person into a behavioral emergency. These may include life events, an acute episode, stress, and alcohol or substance abuse. Changes in distal risk factors can also affect the patient's threshold for crisis by making them increasingly vulnerable to proximal risk factors.

The main goal of emergency intervention is resolving or reducing a crisis situation. Acute interventions need to occur next within the treatment continuum. Talking about suicide with the patient can be the most important and therapeutic issue. Unlike popular belief, talking about suicide does not "put the idea in the person's head." It is estimated that 65% to 85% of persons communicate about suicide before they attempt it. One of the most important ways to get patients to talk about their thoughts is to respect their autonomy by refraining from interrogating the patient. It is possible to maintain an "anti-suicide stance" while at the same time being able to listen to and empathize with the patient.

Determining the correct setting for care is the next step. The patient and, ideally, members of his or her support system should be involved in this process, if there are not legal issues precluding a mandate for inpatient treatment. The person must be asked if he or she would feel safe outside of the hospital or if the patient would act upon his or her suicidal feelings and thoughts once outside of the hospital. If the patient has a disturbance in his or her mental status, the nurse and other mental health professionals should never rely solely on the patient's word or validation of a no-suicide contract.

Furthermore, the commitment status of the patient must be established once the decision to hospitalize has been made. A voluntary commitment allows the patient to sign into a facility voluntarily. There is also an involuntary commitment, in which the patient must be suicidal, homicidal, or unable to care for self because of a mental disorder. (Box 10.4) A clinician must treat involuntary commitments carefully, because they may cause significant barriers between the patient and the clinician. However, a person who is involuntarily committed will have a legal hearing within some state-specific time frame to ensure that hospitalization is indeed necessary. If probable cause is not found, the patient may then be discharged. Once the decision for treatment setting and commitment status is finalized, the plan of care continues. For patient Jean L., this is to the inpatient setting.

EVIDENCE-BASED PRACTICE: PLANNING FOR THE SUICIDAL PATIENT

The Standards of Psychiatric and Mental Health Clinical Nursing Practice include Standard V (Planning),

Box 10.4   Against the Patient's Will

The psychiatric and suicide assessments may indicate the need for continued evaluation and treatment, which the patient may refuse. If the patient does not voluntarily elect to participate in the advised care plan developed to protect against a clear and present danger of self-harm, the multidisciplinary team may pursue involuntary treatment through a petition to the court for a legal commitment to treat. A decision to treat against the patient's will is a last resort to ensure patient safety and entails a legal process designed to protect the patient's constitutional rights and freedoms, while providing needed psychiatric treatment.

State laws detail the mental health procedures that authorize continued evaluation and care for the patient who is at risk for harm to self or others. Forensic nurses play a key role in providing comprehensive assessment data to distinguish not only a patient's risk for self-harm, but also the potential for violence toward others. If the patient is reporting homicidal ideation or an intentional desire to harm another, the forensic nurse is required to report any suspected violence, including physical (weapon threat, beating), sexual (forced sex, unwanted touching), or psychological (forcing another to perform degrading acts, controlling, or confining another individual).

which states that the nurse develops a plan of care that is discussed among the patient, nurse, family, and others to prescribe evidence-based interventions toward desired outcomes. The purpose of the plan is to guide interventions, document progress, and achieve desired patient outcomes. For the suicidal patient, this means planning interventions based on the risk factors identified.

For Jean L., an actively suicidal patient, the nurse provides for the first step, the patient's immediate safety. The multidisciplinary team has made the decision to hospitalize this patient. After the nurse mobilizes the resources necessary to provide a safe inpatient environment for the patient, the plan for achieving the goal of reducing the patient's risk of suicide is initiated. Because of the significant risk involved with the presence of a psychiatric disorder (i.e., mood disorder, schizophrenia, substance use disorder, etc.), one of the subsequent areas of focus for the nurse will be planning appropriate nursing interventions for any of the patient's assessed psychiatric disorder(s).

Planning interventions that include educating the patient about psychological factors such as coping skills and cognitive style are important to achieving desired outcomes. Inclusion of the patient's family, friends, and significant others may also help the nurse plan for meaningful interventions that target the patient's feelings of hopelessness and/or loneliness. Finally, collaboration and communication with other members of the health-care team and other mental health professionals are a critical part of the nurse's role. This assists the nurse in the process of collecting and sharing relevant information and data about the patient for the purpose of planning effective interventions resulting in successful patient outcomes.

EVIDENCE-BASED PRACTICE: INTERVENTIONS FOR THE SUICIDAL PATIENT

Astute assessment, diagnosis, and planning will lead to evidence-based practice interventions that will result in the sound management of the patient at risk for suicide. Once the nurse comprehensively reviews all assessment data for

No-Suicide Contract

No-suicide or no-harm contracts may be established between a patient and nurse in an attempt to guarantee that the patient will remain safe from self-harm for a specific period of time. During this period of time, if the patient feels unsafe, he or she will contract to get in touch with the patient's chosen or assigned clinician; if the patient is in an outpatient setting, go to an emergency room immediately, or if in an inpatient setting, seek out his or her inpatient nurse when these feelings are uncontrollable. Although these contracts may make the nurse feel safer, there is no solid evidence that those who contract for safety are less likely to commit suicide. Furthermore, when behavioral emergencies such as patient suicidal behaviors or suicide do occur, it may leave the clinician vulnerable to personal emotional distress. In a recent study done on patient's perceptions of no-suicide contracts, it was found that patients reported positive attitudes toward written no-suicide agreements, and there were no significant differences irrespective of these patients' age, gender, presence or absence of an Axis II diagnosis, or ratings of overall treatment helpfulness. However, prior experience with written agreements and recurring suicidality may lead multiple attempters to doubt the usefulness of this technique. Other research suggests that no-suicide or no-harm agreements are not an effective deterrent to self-harm. There must be continued and ongoing careful suicide risk assessments in lieu of relying too heavily on the no-suicide contract to protect the patient. Any contract against self-harm will only be as good as the underlying therapeutic alliance.

Case Study

CASE STUDY OF JEAN L.: IN PSYCHIATRIC TREATMENT

The multidisciplinary team gathers around the conference room table to listen to and discuss the morning report regarding their inpatient census. Lara, reporting senior psychiatric nurse, highlights an observational status change on one patient: "Night staff increased the observation status to constant observation on Jean L. During midevening checks, staff noted that Jean L. was sitting alone in a corner of the lounge and was not socializing even with her new friends, Anna and Riva. She seemed to be intensely preoccupied with her own thoughts, and when encouraged by Sam, the charge nurse, to talk about what was bothering her, she declined, stating, "Maybe later, I have to work on some stuff on my own." Staff attempted to engage her a second time when she returned to her room to rest on her bed, but she abruptly replied she "just needed to be alone for awhile." When the night staff made rounds at shift start, they noted that Jean L. was sitting cross-legged on her bed, head down, and hands twisting her top sheet like a rope. When approached, Jean L. looked up with a vacant stare, flat affect, and quietly asked, "What?" Jill, the night charge nurse, proceeded with a mental status exam. Jean ultimately shared that she "just wanted to be dead" and thought she could "figure out a way to choke myself." She was placed on constant observation and there have been no changes since last night. The staff is requesting immediate interventions but would also like to discuss all options since this hospital admission is similar to her last one.

suicide risk factors, completes additional inpatient assessment information as indicated, and reviews the multidisciplinary team plan of care, developing and implementing effective nursing interventions are the tasks at hand for short- and long-term risk management. Jean L. has numerous risk factors, including a diagnosis of major depression, alienation from others, unshakable difficulties resolving life issues (e.g., she hates her job and is experiencing marriage difficulties), irritability, a prior history of suicide attempts (including a previous hospitalization), and current suicidal ideation with imminent danger). Although these factors underscore the need for subsequent intensive nursing supervision, the management of patients identified at risk for suicide is individually determined based upon their psychological, social, historical, environmental, and ongoing clinical assessments.

A review of the literature indicates that precise guidelines for the management of the patient at risk for suicide are limited. However, recent research by Cutcliffe and others and Sun and others employing grounded theory methods offers suggestions for nursing care of the suicidal patient. The center of Cutcliffe's premise is a core variable defined as "reconnecting the patient with humanity." This core is described as a process composed of three stages whereby the nurse sets the stage for interaction interventions with empathic, nonbiased care that guides the suicidal patient toward attaining power over his or her suicidality, ultimately emerging with the confidence to live again. This is accomplished through (1) creating a warm, interpersonal setting; (2) offering security while exploring insight into suicidal beliefs; and (3) making sense of suicidal thoughts to reset goals and establish a hopeful future. A nursing care theory developed by Sun and others presents four categories for an action-interaction strategy, with the core category identified as a therapeutic relationship vested in safe, compassionate care. Performing holistic assessments (vigilant observations, skillful interviewing, noting suicide signals and cues), protecting the patient, providing basic mental and physical care, and employing compassionate, hope-inspiring advanced healing care are the four categories underpinning this core.

Larsson and colleagues suggest the implementation of the sympathy-acceptance-understanding-competence (SAUC) model based upon the work of Gustafsson as a tool to guide the care of the suicidal patient. In this model, the patient works toward the goal of successful self-relation (improved understanding of oneself) through an interactive communication process with the nurse. This phased relationship process, with the primary goal of the patient developing a revised self-relation, includes sympathy and concern related to anxious feelings (S), acceptance and respect with nonjudgment (A), understanding and support of the situation creating suicidal feelings (U), and competence and trust (C) that assist the patient to recognizing his or her health-inspiring self-resources.

Whether the focus is reconnecting the patient with humanity, using nursing actions and interactions to intervene to prevent suicide and promote healing, or developing a goal-directed revised self-relation, the key factor underpinning all three of these interventions within the nursing process is a compassionate, caring base. Therefore, the challenge at the outset of the nurse-suicidal patient relationship is to negotiate an evidence-based, mutually agreed upon, empathic, interventional strategy (see Table 10.1). The challenge of negotiating interventions is the initial tactical strategy employed in the plan of care for the nurse–suicidal inpatient relationship with Jean L.

TABLE 10.1   Patient Care Plan: Building an Evidence-Based Therapeutic Alliance

	Risk Factors	Nursing Actions	Evidence-Based Rationales	Outcome/Evaluation
Clinical Build an empathic therapeutic relationship (Cutcliffe et. al, 2007; Sun et. al, 2006; Larsson, et al, 2007).	Depressed mood, flat affect, irritability.	Convey attentive, supportive, and curiously interested reflections (Cutcliffe et al, 2007; Billings, 2004).	Authentic empathy increases patient trust, the hallmark of relation building and decreases loneliness pain (Billings, 2004).	Patient confides inner thoughts, suicidal ideations, and/or plans.
	Hopelessness.	Inspire hope through unconditional caring practices (Cutcliffe et al, 2007; Larsson et al, 2007).	Inspiring hope implicitly through unconditional acceptance, tolerance, and understanding improves patient self-view, decreasing risk for self-harm (Cutcliffe et al, 2007; Larsson et al, 2007).	Patient offers suggestions to resolve issues (job, divorce) that are contributing to sense of hopelessness.

(table continued on page 188)

TABLE 10.1 **Patient Care Plan: Building an Evidence-Based Therapeutic Alliance** (continued)

	Risk Factors	Nursing Actions	Evidence-Based Rationales	Outcome/Evaluation
	Suicidal thoughts and difficulty with impulse control.	Establish ongoing mini-assessments, vigilant observations and routines (including unit environmental safety checks); using empathic clinical curiosity and sensitivity to engage patient in self-support (Larsson, 2007; Sun et al, 2006; Varcarolis, 2004).	Increase nurse-patient alliance for safety, which contributes to reduced suicide risk (Larsson, 2007; Billings, 2004).	Patient shares desire to live concurrent with denying suicidal ideation.
Historical Establish the degree of suicide risk (Billings, 2004).	Prior suicide attempt.	Obtain vigilant and comprehensive assessment of past suicidal thoughts, plans, attempts, and recent related situations (Sun et al, 2006; Billings, 2004).	Reducing suicide risk through understanding past-present contributing factors is a crucial responsibility of the inpatient psychiatric nurse to promote patient protection as well as insight, knowing that the best predictor of suicidal behavior is a past history of a suicide attempt (Cutcliffe et al, 2007; Sun et al, 2006; Sher, 2004).	Patient shares circumstances surrounding previous and current history for self-harm thereby participating in self-understanding of contributing factors to decision-making actions.
Psychosocial Identify contributing stressors to current situation (Sun et al, 2006; Sanchez, 2001).	Lack of social support network (e.g., few friends).	Assist patient with identifying probable or possible supportive relationships and practice reviewing old and employing new but self-comfortable social methods (Larsson et al, 2007).	Reconnecting the person with humanity (second phase) involves assisting the patient with seeking novel, supportive relationships to strengthen positive life feelings (Cutcliffe et al, 2007).	Patient seeks new friendships on the inpatient unit to try out new social approaches and reports progress.
	Divorce and loss of significant relationship.	Review marital relationship demonstrating genuine concern coupled with seeking understanding of the patient's contributions to the marital history (Sun et al, 2006; Sanchez, 2001; Mann et al, 1999).	Causal conditions contributing to suicide risk identified by Sun and others (2006) include enduring painful experiences such as loss/abandonment through divorce. Understanding the influence of the experience upon suicidal ideation contributes to insight and relearning to live (third phase of reconnecting to humanity) (Cutcliffe et al, 2007).	Patient recognizes spouse and self-contributions to the ineffective marital relationship and identifies alternatives for future relationship success.

	Risk Factors	Nursing Actions	Evidence-Based Rationales	Outcome/Evaluation
Environmental Identify employment responsibilities and contributing performance factors.	Career dissatisfaction.	Identify patient's coping skills and factors contributing to job performance and satisfaction (Cutcliffe et al, 2007; Larsson et al, 2007; Sanchez, 2001).	Causal conditions contributing to suicide risk identified by Sun and others (2006) include stress and a history of trauma. Recognition of how the patient is contributing to job dissatisfaction or identifying factors within control may improve evaluation of employment status (Sanchez, 2001).	Patient identifies areas for current job self-improvement and/or opportunities for job change.

Additional common themes permeate the three theories and underscore the interventional guidelines or steps unique to each model. For example, ensuring safety and security for the patient, assisting the patient to gain insight into self-skills, and deriving patient goals vested in hope are recurrent themes. Using the unique theoretical approaches suggested, these themes are exemplified with Jean L.

Management of the suicidal inpatient requires the collaboration of the inpatient psychiatric team, which not only includes the psychiatric nurse, but also mental health professionals such as psychiatrists, social workers, and milieu therapists. Therefore, the Jean L. scenario reflects a multidisciplinary case review process that results in a comprehensive patient care plan incorporating evidence-based nursing interventions.

A focused, interventional care plan is critical to the nurse-inpatient relationship and the successful management of suicide risk. An intervention and treatment plan for Jean L. provides an example. It is also recommended that any nurse working with a suicidal patient periodically ask specific questions regarding what constitutes best practice in the management of the patient at risk for suicide. Stone recommends asking this question in the PICO format, where *P* is problem, *I* is intervention, *C* is comparison, and *O* is outcome (see Table 10.2). This affords the professional nurse a standard for ensuring the implementation of sound, evidence-based practice options.

TABLE 10.2   PICO: Evidence-Based Practice Options

Problem	
Intervention Search Terms: suicide, suicidal patient, patient at risk for self-harm, standard of practice, management of suicide, guidelines for the patient at risk for suicide, nursing (Cutcliffe et al, 2007; Sun et al, 2006; Larsson et al, 2007).	What is the standard of nursing practice for the management of the patient identified as at risk for suicide? The key factors underlying evidence-based practice are establishing a compassionate, safe, and caring base for nurse-patient interactions. From this foundation, keen interviewing skills provide intervention strategies from: 1. exploration of the factors of influence (psychological, social, historical, environmental, and clinical), and 2. identification of self and support resources to enable the patient to re-create expectations and opportunities for the future.
Comparison	Comparison and evaluation of three recommended interventional strategies using the AGREE (http://www.agreecollaboration.org/instrument) standardized evaluation tool encourage a knowledge-driven eclectic nursing approach to the care of the suicidal patient. The common themes (e.g., security, goals, future, hope, and resources) within the three theoretical frameworks allow the

(table continued on page 190)

TABLE 10.2   PICO: Evidence-Based Practice Options (continued)

	nurse to strategically individualize the unique steps recommended within each theory with a coherent and astute patient-focused plan of care.
Outcome	Following evidence-based recommendations, the nurse-patient relationship progresses through steps that promote patient trust, lead to the identification of coping skills and assets, and result in a sense of hope and a future focused on life versus death.

EVIDENCE-BASED PRACTICE: EVALUATION AND DISCHARGE PLANNING FOR THE SUICIDAL PATIENT

Generally, the inpatient care plan for the at-risk patient focuses on acute interventions that facilitate discharge and return to the community. When multidisciplinary assessment and collaborative evaluation indicate that the risk for suicide is eliminated, discharge may be imminent. However, previous research has identified that follow-up care for the suicidal patient is critical, given the risk for suicide (14% for men and 22% for women) following discharge.

The necessity for ongoing suicide risk assessment after discharge highlights the critical need for not only accurate, empathic assessment of suicide risk for inpatients prior to discharge, but also continuation of care in the outpatient setting. The brief, short-term treatment initiated on the inpatient unit is the start of the recovery process that must be maintained with qualified long-term clinical intervention. Postdischarge intervention includes the reassurance of continuity of care with the patient's outpatient clinician to ensure an uninterrupted care-planning process. Continuous care is a critical risk management factor.

Along with risk factors for suicide, protective factors will also be present (Box 10.5). These are factors that can help decrease the risk of suicide. When patients deny suicidal ideation or endorse suicidal ideation but state that they would not act on it, protective factors that may be operating as deterrents against suicide should be assessed by the forensic nurse.

CONCLUSIONS

In summary, there are some risk factors shared by both SIB and suicide. However, suicide and self-harmful behaviors are often unrelated. The astute forensic nurse must incorporate evidence-based assessments and diagnostic tools when differentiating self-harm and suicide. Diagnostic and

treatment plans should incorporate contemporary interventions backed by high-level evidence when available.

The effective assessment and management of the suicidal patient require a comprehensive and systematic approach by the forensic nurse. Sound clinical decision making predicated on an evidence-based theory of suicide assessment and intervention can be used to guide nursing practice with suicidal patients. A careful suicide assessment founded on a skillfully conducted clinical interview can be the foundation for the identification of risk factors and the planning of appropriate nursing interventions. Such a systematic theoretical and clinical approach can lead to successful outcomes for suicidal patients.

Box 10.5   Protective Factors

- **Stable social support system**: People in patients' social support systems may keep them company and talk with them and can serve to distract them from their feelings of self-worthlessness. Social isolation that often accompanies depression may also be decreased.
- **Availability and the ability to use adaptive coping skills**: Patients' abilities to problem-solve will enable them to find other, less self-destructive ways to deal with their feelings in order to alleviate the desperation and despair felt with depression and suicidal ideation.
- **Actively participating in one's treatment**: Being involved actively in treatment may serve to make it less intimidating for the patient to come forward and discuss uncomfortable or unwanted feelings with the treatment team.
- **Sense of hopefulness**: Allows patients to see the "light at the end of the tunnel" and helps to alleviate the impulse toward self-harm.
- **Spiritual inclinations**: Being afraid of suicide or death may help prevent patients from acting on impulsive ideas.
- **Pregnancy or having children under the age of 18 in the home**: Having children in the home may promote a sense of being needed in patients.

(Adapted from White, J. (2007). Suicide risk and protective factors for youth. *Crosscurrents, 10*(2):10.)

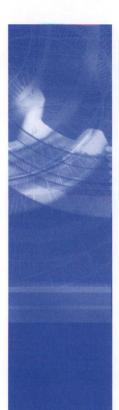

EVIDENCE-BASED PRACTICE

Reference Question: Does rape increase the likelihood of suicidal ideation and/or suicidal attempts in adult women?

Database(s) to Search: PubMed, PsychInfo

Search Strategy: Using the MeSH terms "Suicide," then "Rape," and joining them with "AND," works best. To find the more recent articles, simply limit the search to only those articles published in the last year.

Selected References From Search:

1. Belik, S.L., Stein, M.B., Asmundson, G.J., & Sareen, J. (2009). Relation between traumatic events and suicide attempts in Canadian military personnel. *Canadian Journal of Psychiatry, 54*(2):93-104.
2. Halligan, F.R. (2009). Youth and trauma: Terror, war, murder, incest, rape, and suicide. *Journal of Religion and Health, 48*(3):342-352.
3. Banks, L., Crandall, C., Sklar, D., & Bauer, M. (2008). A comparison of intimate partner homicide to intimate partner homicide-suicide: One hundred and twenty-four New Mexico cases. *Violence Against Women, 14*(9):1065-1078.

Questions Used to Discern Evidence:

Choose two studies among the studies listed, read about them, and answer the following questions:

1. What are the differences between the two studies in the design, methods, and results?
2. What are the similarities between the two studies in the number of subjects, measures used, and interventions, if any?
3. What skill do you need to learn to prepare for forensic nursing practice with this population?

REVIEW QUESTIONS

1. Which one of the following could be considered a culturally acceptable definition of SIB:
   A. Self-poisoning
   B. Superficial cutting
   C. Strangulation
   D. Tattooing

2. Persons who engage in SIBs:
   A. Are predominately female
   B. Are represented in every race and culture
   C. Have poor relationships with their parents
   D. Rarely have a DSM-IV-TR diagnosis

3. Therapeutic interventions that can be helpful in treating adolescents who engage in SIB include:
   A. Cognitive behavioral therapy
   B. Pharmacologic intervention
   C. Web-based therapy
   D. E-mail therapy

4. Parasuicide refers to which one of the following?
   A. A suicide attempt that is planned to be discovered and that is made for the purpose of influencing others
   B. The subjective expectation and desire for a self-destructive act to end in death
   C. A nonlethal but intentional self-harm
   D. SIB with a nonfatal outcome, accompanied by evidence that the person intended to die

5. The decision to treat a patient against his or her will may be a necessary last resort because it:
   A. Ensures patient will be safe from all harm
   B. Provides for necessary psychiatric treatment
   C. Bypasses the legal process to ensure patient's constitutional rights
   D. Bypasses the assessment process

(review questions continued on page 192)

6. One of the strongest risk factors for suicide found in over 90% of completed suicide cases is:
- **A.** Being middle-aged
- **B.** Being Caucasian
- **C.** Being a gun owner
- **D.** Being diagnosed with a psychiatric disorder

7. Which of the following provides the most important foundation for assessment of suicide?
- **A.** The use of suicide assessment scales
- **B.** The therapeutic relationship that the clinician is able to establish with the patient
- **C.** Assessment data from other health-care professionals
- **D.** Sound pharmacological management

8. Psychological traits associated with an increased risk of suicidal behavior include which one of the following?
- **A.** Hopelessness, polarized thinking
- **B.** Polarized thinking, parasuicidal behavior
- **C.** Hopelessness, sexual deviance
- **D.** Perfectionism, parasuicidal behavior

9. What does Cutliffe's premise of "reconnecting the suicidal patient with humanity" mean?
- **A.** A family meeting with a Bowen family therapist who specializes in reconnecting the suicidal patient back into the family system
- **B.** A discharge planning process whereby the patient actively participates in choosing his or her community residence and employment opportunities
- **C.** A staged process for nursing interventions with empathic, nonbiased care to guide the suicidal patient toward attaining power over suicidality and emerging with the confidence to live again
- **D.** A treatment plan focusing on involving the patient in community activities

10. The association between suicidal behaviors and SIBs:
- **A.** Is not well understood
- **B.** Has the common association of bipolar disorder
- **C.** SIB can be a strategy by the adolescent to prevent suicide
- **D.** Is the norm in 50% of adolescents and adults

References

Abou-Saleh, M.T. (1992). The management of patients at risk for suicide. *Journal of Psychopharmacology, 6*(2):304-311.

American Psychiatric Association. (2000). *Diagnostic and statistical manual of mental disorders-text revision.* (4th ed.). Washington, DC: American Psychiatric Association.

American Psychiatric Association. (2006). *Practice guidelines for the treatment of psychiatric disorders compendium.* Arlington, VA: American Psychiatric Association.

Anderson, R.N. (2001). Deaths: Leading causes for 1999. *National Vital Statistics Reports, 49*:11.

Antai-Ontong, D. (2008). *Psychiatric nursing: Biological and behavioral concepts* (2nd ed.). Clifton Park, NY: Delmar Learning.

Beck, A.T., Kovacs, M., & Weissman, A. (1979). Assessment of suicidal ideation: The scale for suicidal ideation. *Journal of Consulting and Clinical Psychology, 47*(2):343-352.

Beck, A.T., Schuyler, D., & Herman, J. (1974). Development of suicidal intent scales. In A.T. Beck, H. Resnick, & D. Lettieri (Eds.). *The prediction of suicide.* Oxford: Charles Press, pp. 45-69.

Billings, C.V. (2004). Psychiatric inpatient suicide. *Journal of the American Psychiatric Nurses Association, 10*(4):190-192.

Bostwick, J.M., & Rackley, S.J. (2007). Completed suicide in medical/surgical patients: Who is at risk? *Current Psychiatry Reports, 9*:242-246.

Brent, D., Oquendo, M., Birmaher, B., Greenhill, L., et al. (2002). Familial pathways to early onset suicide attempt: Risk for suicidal behavior in offspring of mood disordered suicide attempters. *Archives of General Psychiatry, 59*: 801-807.

Brent, D., Perper, J., Allman, C., Moritz, G., Wartella, M., & Zelenak, J. (1991). The presence and accessibility of firearms in the homes of adolescent suicides: A case control study. *Journal of American Medical Association, 266*:2989-2995.

Brown, G.K. (2002). *A review of suicide assessment measures for intervention research with adults and older adults.* Rockville, MD: National Institute of Mental Health.

Brown, G.K., Beck, A.T., Steer, R.A., & Grisham, J.R. (2000). Risk factors for suicide in psychiatric outpatients: A 20 year prospective study. *Journal of Consulting and Clinical Psychology, 68*:371-377.

Brown, L.K., Houck, C.D., Grossman, C.I., Lescano, C.M., & Frenkel, J.L., (2008). Frequency of adolescent self-cutting as a predictor of HIV risk. *Journal of Developmental and Behavioral Pediatrics, 29*(3):161-165.

Buzan, R.D., & Weissberg, M.P. (1992). Emergency medicine in review. *Journal of Emergency Medicine, 10*(3):335-343.

Centers for Disease Control and Prevention. (2000). Fatal injury data for 2000. Web-based injury statistics query and reporting system. Atlanta, GA: National Center for Injury Prevention and Control.

Cowman, S. (2007). Commentary on Sun, F.K., Long, A., Boore, J., & Lee-Ing, T. (2006). Patients and nurses' perceptions of ward environmental factors and support systems in the care of suicidal patients. *Journal of Clinical Nursing, 16*:805-806.

Croyle, K.L., & Waltz, J. (2007). Sub-clinical self-harm: Range of behaviors, extent, and associated characteristics. *American Journal of Orthopsychiatry, 77*(2):332-342.

Cutcliffe, J.R., & Barker, P. (2002). Considering the care of the suicidal client and the case for 'engagement and inspiring hope' or 'observations.' *Journal of Psychiatric and Mental Health Nursing, 9*:611-621.

Cutcliffe, J.R., & Barker, P. (2004). The Nurses' Global Assessment of Suicide Risk (NGASR): Developing a tool for clinical practice. *Journal of Psychiatric and Mental Health Nursing, 11*:393-400.

Cutcliffe, J.R., Stevenson, C., Jackson, S., & Smith, P. (2006). A modified grounded theory study of how psychiatric nurses work with suicidal people. *International Journal of Nursing Studies, 43*:791-802.

Cutcliffe, J.R., Stevenson, C., Jackson, S., & Smith, P. (2007). Reconnecting the person with humanity. *Crisis, 28*(2):207-210.

Davis, S.E., Williams, I.S., & Hays, L.W. (2002). Psychiatric inpatients' perceptions of written no-suicide agreements: An exploratory study. *Suicide and Life-Threatening Behavior, 32*(1):51-66.

Farrow, T.L., & O'Brien, A.J. (2003). No-suicide contracts and informed consent: An analysis of ethical issues. *Nursing Ethics, 10*(2):199-207.

French, L.A. (1985-86). Forensic suicides and attempted suicides. *Omega: Journal of Death and Dying, 16*(4):335-345.

Gustafsson, B. (2000). The SAUC model for confirming nursing, an action-theoretic approach to theory building and nursing practice. *Journal of Nursing Theory, 9*(1):6-21.

Harris, E.C., & Barraclough, B. (1997). Suicide as an outcome for mental disorders: A meta-analysis. *British Journal of Psychiatry, 170*:205-228.

Heath, N.L. (2009). Non-suicidal self-injury: The new challenge for counselors. Retrieved June 6, 2009, from http://www.education.mcgill.ca/healthresearchteam/images/CPA2009NSSIcounsellors.pdf

Henriksson, M.M., Aro, H.M., Marttunen, M.J., Heikkinen, M.E., et al. (1993). *American Journal of Psychiatry, 150*:935-940.

Horrigan, J.P., & Barnhill, L.J. (2000). Naltrexone treatment of self-injurious behavior. *Journal of the American Association of Child and Adolescent Psychiatry, 39*(9):1077-1078.

Hovey, J.D. (2000). Acculturative stress, depression, and suicidal ideation among Central American immigrants. *Suicide and Life-Threatening Behavior, 30*:125-139.

Kaprio, J., & Koskenvuo, R.M. (1987). Mortality after bereavement: A prospective study of 95,647 widowed persons. *American Journal of Public Health, 77*:283-287.

Kessler, R., Borges, G., & Walters, E. (1999). Prevalence of and risk factors for lifetime suicide attempts in the national co-morbidity survey. *Archives of General Psychiatry, 56*:617-626.

King, E.A., Baldwin, D.S., Sinclair, J.M., Baker, N.G., Campbell, M.J., & Thompson, C. (2001). The Wessex recent in-patient suicide study, 1: Case-control study of 234 recently discharged psychiatric patient suicides. *The British Journal of Psychiatry, 178*:531-536.

Kleespies, P.M., & Dettmer, E.L. (2000). The stress of patient emergencies for the clinician: Incidence, impact, and means of coping. *Journal of Clinical Psychology, 56*(10):1353-1369.

Kroll, J. Use on no-suicide contracts by psychiatrists in Minnesota. *American Journal of Psychiatry, 157*(10):1684-1686.

Larsson, P., Nilsson, S., Runeson, B., & Gustafsson, B. (2007). Psychiatric nursing care of suicidal patients described by the sympathy-acceptance-understanding-competence model for confirming nursing. *Archives of Psychiatric Nursing, 21*(4):222-232.

Luoma, J.B., & Pearson, J.L. (2002). Suicide and marital status in the United States, 1991-1996: Is widowhood a risk factor? *American Journal of Public Health, 92*:1518-1522.

Mann, J.J. (2002). A current perspective of suicide and attempted suicide. *Annals of Internal Medicine, 136*:302-311.

Mann, J.J., Waternaux, C., Haas, G.L., & Malone, K.M. (1999). Toward a clinical model of suicidal behavior in psychiatric patients. *American Journal of Psychiatry, 156*(2):181-189.

McGlothlin, J. (2008). *Developing clinical skills in suicide assessment, prevention, and treatment.* Alexandria, VA: American Counseling Association.

McKenzie, I., & Wurr, C. (2001). Early suicide following discharge from a psychiatric hospital. *Suicide and Life-Threatening Behavior, 31*(3):358-363.

McMyler, C., & Pryjmachuk, S. (2008). Do "no-suicide" contracts work? *Journal of Psychiatric and Mental Health Nursing, 15*:512-522.

Molnar, B.E., Berkman, L.F., & Buka, S.L. (2001). Psychopathology, childhood sexual abuse, and other childhood adversities: Relative links to suicidal behavior in the US. *Psychology and Medicine, 31*:965-977.

Nock, M.K., & Mendes, W.B. (2008). Physiological arousal, distress tolerance, and social problem-solving deficits among adolescent self-injurers. *Journal of Consulting and Clinical Psychology, 76*(1):28-38.

Nock, M.K., & Prinstein, M.J. (2004). A functional approach to the assessment of self-mutilative behavior. *Journal of Consulting and Clinical Psychology, 72*:885-890.

Nordentoft, M. (2007). Prevention of suicide and attempted suicide in Denmark: Epidemiological studies of suicide and intervention studies in selected risk groups. *Danish Medical Bulletin, 54*(4):306-369.

Odershaw, A., Richards, C., Simic, M., & Schmidt, U. (2008). Parents' perspective on adolescent self-harm: Qualitative study. *The British Journal of Psychiatry, 193*(10):140-144.

Omer, H., & Elitzur, A.C. (2001). What would you say to the person on the roof? A suicide prevention text. *Suicide and Life-Threatening Behavior, 31*(2):129-139.

Patterson, W.M., Dohn, H.H., Bird, J., & Patterson, G.A. (1983). Evaluation of suicidal patients: The SAD PERSONS Scale. *Psychosomatics, 24*(4):343-349.

Patton, G.C., Hemphill, S.A., Beyers, J.M., Bond, L., et al. (2007). Pubertal stage and deliberate self-harm in adolescents. *Journal of the American Academy of Child and Adolescent Psychiatry, 46*(4):508-514.

Paul, J.P., Cantania, J., Pollock, L., Moskowitz, J., et al. (2002). Suicide attempts among gay and bisexual men: Lifetime prevalence and antecedents. *American Journal of Public Health, 92*:1338-1345.

Peterson, J., Freedenthal, S., Sheldon, C., & Andersen, R. (2008). Non-suicidal self-injury in adolescents. Retrieved April 1, 2009, from http://www.psychiatrymmc.com/nonsuicidal-self-injury-in adolescents

Remifedi, G., French, S., Story, M., Resnick, M.D., & Blum, R. (1998). The relationship between suicide risk and sexual orientation: Results of a population-based study. *88*:57-60.

Ross, S., Heath, N.L., & Toste, J.R. (2009). Non-suicidal self-injury and eating pathology in high school students. *American Journal of Orthopsychiatry, 79*(1):83-92.

Roy, A. (2005). Relation of family history of suicide to suicide attempts in alcoholics. *American Journal of Psychiatry, 157*:2050-2051.

Sanchez, H.G. (2001). Risk factor model for suicide assessment and intervention. *Professional Psychology: Research and Practice, 32*(4):351-358.

Schmidt, H., & Ivanoff, A. (2007). Behavioral prescriptions for treating self-injurious and suicidal behaviors. In O.J. Rhienhaus & M. Piasecki, M. (Eds.). *Correctional psychiatry: Practice guidelines and strategies*. Dingston, NJ: Civic Research Institute, pp.1-23.

Sharma, V., Persad, E., & Kueneman, K. (1998). A closer look at inpatient suicide. *Journal of Affective Disorders, 47*:123-129.

Shea, S.C. (1999). *The practical art of suicide assessment. A guide for mental health professionals and substance abuse counselors*. Indianapolis: John Wiley & Sons.

Sher, L. (2004). Preventing suicide. *Quality Journal of Medicine, 97*:677-680.

Simon, R.I. (2008). Naked suicide. *Journal of the American Academy of Psychiatry and the Law, 36*(2):240-245.

Simon, R.I. (2000). Taking the "sue" out of suicide: A forensic psychiatrist's perspective. *Psychiatric Annals, 30*(6):399-407.

Simon, R.I., & Hales, R. (2006). *American psychiatric publishing textbook of suicide assessment and management*. Washington, DC: American Psychiatric Publishing.

Springhouse. (1998). Standards of psychiatric and mental health clinical nursing practice. In *Springhouse review for psychiatric and mental health nursing certification* (3rd ed.). Baltimore, MD: Lippincott, Williams & Wilkins, pp. 399-407.

Stone, P.W. (2002). Popping the (PICO) question in research and evidence-based practice. *Applied Nursing Research, 16*(20):197-198.

Sun, F.K., Long, A., Boore, J., & Tsao, L.I. (2005). Nursing people who are suicidal on psychiatric wards in Taiwan: Action/interaction strategies. *Journal of Psychiatric and Mental Health Nursing, 12*:275-282.

Sun, F.K., Long, A., Boore, J., & Tsao, L.I. (2006). A theory for the nursing care of patients at risk of suicide. *Journal of Advanced Nursing, 53*(6):680-690.

Sun, F.K., Long, A., Boore, J., & Tsao, L.I. (2006). Patients' and nurses' perceptions of ward environmental factors and support systems in the care of suicidal patients. *Journal of Clinical Nursing, 15*:83-92.

Szanto, K., Gildengerrs, A., Mulsant, B.H., Brown, G., Alexopoulos, G.S., & Reynolds, C.F. (2002). Identification of suicide ideation and prevention of suicidal behavior in the elderly. *Drugs & Aging, 19*(1):11-24.

Tsai, S., Kuo, C., Chen, C., & Lee, C. (2002). Risk factors for completed suicide in bipolar disorder. *Journal of Clinical Psychiatry, 63*:469-476.

Tueth, M.J. (1995). Management of behavioral emergencies. *American Journal of Behavioral Medicine, 13*(3):344-350.

Varcarolis, E.M. (2003). *Foundations of psychiatric-mental health nursing*. New York: W.B. Saunders.

Varcarolis, E.M. (2000). Psychiatric emergencies and forensic issues: Suicide behaviors. In E.M. Varcarolis (Ed.), *Manual of Psychiatric Nursing Care Plans*. New York: W.B. Saunders, pp. 446-456.

White, J. (2007). Suicide risk and protective factors for youth. *Crosscurrents, 10*(2):10.

Winchel, R.M., & Stanley, M. (1991). Self-injurious behavior: A review of the behavior and biology of self-mutilation. *American Journal of Psychiatry, 148*(3):306-317.

Wood, A., Trainor, G., Rothwell, J., Moore, A., & Harrington, R. (2001). Randomized trial of group therapy for repeated deliberate self-harm in adolescents. *Journal of the American Academy of Child and Adolescent Psychiatry, 46*(11): 1246-1253.

Yates, T.M., Tracy, A.J., & Luthar, S.S. (2008). Non-suicidal self-injury among "privileged" youths: Longitudinal and cross-sectional approaches to developmental process. *Journal of Counseling and Clinical Psychology, 76*(1): 52-62.

Yufit, R.I., & Lester, D. (2005). *Assessment, treatment, and prevention of suicidal behavior*. Hoboken, NJ: John Wiley & Sons.

Yurkovich, E., & Smyer, T. (2000). Health maintenance behaviors of individuals with severe and persistent mental illness in a state prison. *Journal of Psychosocial Nursing, 38*(6):26-29.

Zlotnick, C., Donaldson, D., Spirito, A., & Pearlestein, T. (1997). Affect regulation and suicide attempts in adolescent inpatients. *Journal of the American Academy of Child and Adolescent Psychiatry, 36*(6):793-798.

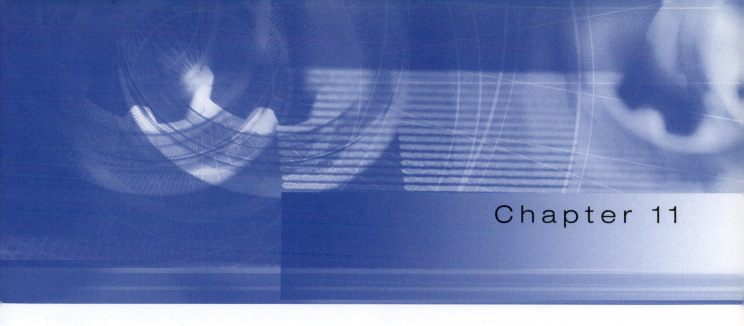

Chapter 11

Death Investigation and the Forensic Nurse

Stacey Lasseter Mitchell

"In three words I can sum up everything I've learned about life: it goes on."
Robert Frost

Competencies

1. Describing forensic nursing concepts and roles.
2. Describing death investigation systems.
3. Defining cause, manner, and mechanisms of death.
4. Verifying the significance of relationships with multidisciplinary team members.
5. Defining local/regional regulations and laws that govern practice.
6. Exploring community education and prevention opportunities.
7. Explaining the ethical and professional codes of conduct.
8. Describing the process of various death scene investigations.

Key Terms

Assessment
Cause of death
Coroner
Death scene investigation
Diagnosis
Evaluation
Forensic nurse death investigator
Implementation
Manner of death
Mechanism of death
Nurse coroner
Planning

INTRODUCTION

Care of the patient does not cease with the patient's death; it ends with the certification of the cause and manner of death. How and why a death occurred is important to many, such as individual families and those in legal systems and public health. Law enforcement investigates, and the courts will prosecute those responsible for intentional deaths. Public health officials track the incidence and prevalence of injury and disease processes that affect populations.

An attending or family physician or the medical examiner/coroner in the jurisdiction in which the person died is able to certify the cause and manner of death. The forensic nurse can play an important role in this process by conducting a thorough death investigation. The information gathered will affect the determination of cause and manner of death. Therefore, it is essential the forensic nurse develop an understanding of the medicolegal death investigation system and the death investigation process.

The **forensic nurse death investigator** (FNDI) and/or **nurse coroner** role is a subspecialty within the practice of forensic nursing. FNDIs may be employed in a medical examiner's office as nurse investigators to conduct the medicolegal death investigation, elected as coroners, or appointed as deputy coroners. Medical examiner or coroner law, as well as state nurse practice acts, will define the practice arena of the FNDI and nurse coroner. This chapter will discuss death investigator systems, the role of the FNDI/nurse coroner, and aspects of the death investigation.

DEATH INVESTIGATION SYSTEMS IN THE UNITED STATES

The United States has three types of death investigation systems: medical examiner, coroner, and mixed system. The oldest system is the coroner system, which traces its roots back to the English coroner or "crowner" system, initiated over 600 years ago. This was an appointed position. The coroner conducted inquests on bodies or assessed wounds of an individual, recorded the accusation, and if the injuries were likely to be intentional, arrested the accused. The coroner could conduct an independent investigation or be directed by a judge. Prior to the 12th century, the coroner also collected taxes in the name of the king. As time passed, the coroner's authority became limited to only conducting the death investigation. With their migration to America, the colonists brought with them the coroner system. Today, in states where the coroner system remains, the coroner is an elected position. In 1877 Massachusetts adopted a statewide system and replaced the coroner with a physician called a

"medical examiner." The physicians could be from any specialty, whether obstetrics, surgery, or family practice. It was not until 1918 in New York City that the first true medical examiner system was established, with the medical examiner having experience in forensic pathology.

Today, the death investigation system in the United States consists of both medical examiners and coroners. There are jurisdictions that are strictly coroner systems. Others are staffed by medical examiners. In a few states, there is a mixture of coroners and medical examiners. Currently, 12 states continue with established coroner systems, 22 use medical examiners, and 16 are mixed.

A **coroner** is an elected official who does not necessarily possess a medical degree. For those who are physicians, the specialty area is not delineated. For example, the coroner may be a family practice physician who performs the legal duties of the coroner in addition to treating private patients. In some jurisdictions, the sheriff may also be the coroner, thus having no medical background at all. In that situation, a pathologist is hired to perform the autopsy examination, but it is the responsibility of the coroner to determine the cause and manner of death and to complete the death certificate.

The coroner has the authority to hold an inquest or an official inquiry into the death. The information gathered during the investigation is presented in a courtroom setting. A judicial figure presides over the inquest with attorneys representing all interested parties. The outcome is documented in the public record, which is available to the community. This may, in turn, lead to other legal inquiries, either criminal or civil.

Medical Examiner

In contrast, a medical examiner does not have the ability to convene an inquest unless directed by law. However, the decision to conduct an autopsy examination is at the discretion of the medical examiner. A medical examiner is a licensed physician who in many cases is a board-certified forensic pathologist. The local government appoints the chief medical examiner to investigate and determine the cause and manner of death, especially deaths that are due to unnatural causes. Certain aspects of the death investigation, including the autopsy examination, postmortem laboratory testing, and examination of the decedent at the scene, are supervised by the medical examiner.

Forensic Pathologists

The forensic pathologist is a licensed physician who conducts the autopsy examination. Training includes a residency in pathology, which encompasses anatomic and/or clinical pathology. Anatomic pathology involves studying techniques, assessing organs and tissues to diagnose diseases, and evaluating cells to determine various benign and malignant conditions. Clinical pathology requires that the physician be familiar with the various laboratory tests that are routinely ordered. These involve hematology, toxicology, immunology, chemistry, and microbiology.

After completing a residency program, the physician takes part in a 1-year fellowship in forensic pathology. This fellowship is an intensive study in conducting medicolegal autopsies, interpreting laboratory reports, determining cause and manner of death, and testifying in court. The pathologist is then eligible to apply to sit for the board examination. With successful completion, the pathologist becomes a board-certified forensic pathologist.

Role of the Medical Examiner/Coroner

No matter the title, the roles of medical examiner and coroner are essentially the same. Both the medical examiner and coroner are responsible for the outcome of the medicolegal death investigation. Each state has legislation that outlines the types of deaths that are reportable to the medical examiner or coroner. Unnatural deaths and deaths due to trauma require extensive investigation into the circumstances, mechanism of injury, and any medical history or treatment that was rendered. The legal system may also investigate, and the findings may lead to criminal or civil proceedings. Nevertheless, state law identifies the specific responsibilities of the medical examiner/coroner.

The main duty of the medical examiner or coroner is to determine the cause and manner of death. **Cause of death** simply stated, is the medical finding of the reasons for death. It is the process that documents the sequence of events that result in death. **Manner of death** refers to the classification of the circumstances in which the death occurred. The categories of manners of death include homicide, suicide, natural, accident, and undetermined. To determine cause and manner of death, a scene investigation and laboratory studies must be conducted. The autopsy examination alone is not the sole source of information, but it is considered to be the ultimate peer review and the reference standard for postmortem evaluation to detect causes of death and traumatic injuries. Autopsies are very time-consuming and labor-intensive. Additional studies such as toxicology testing and histological review may be required. Evidence is collected and preserved as well.

Clinical autopsies are reported to be declining in number in many countries and in different types of institutions, and they require permission from the family of the deceased. However, the results of an autopsy may reveal the greatest quality of knowledge and surprising multiple coexisting medical conditions, as well as abuse and neglect. Forensic autopsies may be ordered by a legal authority. In some institutions, the declining number of autopsies has led to comparison of other methods used to evaluate the deceased.

One systematic review, using EMBASE and MEDLINE databases, assessed autopsy findings versus postmortem computed tomography (PMCT) in determining cause of death and identification of specific injuries in trauma victims. Outcomes were reported as percentage of agreement on causes of death and amount of injuries detected. Fifteen studies evaluated 244 deceased persons. The percentage of agreement in the comparisons ranged from 46% to 100%. The range of injuries detected ranged from 53% to 100%. Therefore, the researchers concluded that the evidence is inconsistent as to whether PMCT is reliable as an alternative to traditional methods of autopsy. Although PMCT is promising and able to detect injuries that may be overlooked with an autopsy, it is critical to conduct larger prospective studies before accepting PMCT as a valid alternative in determining cause of death.

Depending on state statute, additional responsibilities of the medical examiner/coroner can include identification of an unknown decedent. Methods used may be both scientific and nonscientific. Scientific methods include fingerprint identification, the use of dental records, and DNA comparison. Nonscientific means often augment the scientific methods. Descriptions of tattoos, scars, and other marks are useful. Visual identification is subjective and unreliable, but it is used very often. Once the decedent is identified, the medical examiner/coroner is responsible for notifying the next of kin.

Providing courtroom testimony is another duty of the medical examiner/coroner. The cause and manner of death are discussed, and details of the autopsy findings are provided to the court and juries. The medical examiner/coroner is the expert in terms of injury and how it occurs. Cause of injury related to the death is often the crux of the courtroom testimony. In addition, questions about possible alternatives of the scenario leading to death may be explored in court with the defense and prosecution challenging one another's witnesses and the evidence that is presented. The testimony is objective in nature and based upon research and accepted scientific practices. The use of high-level evidence is critical and should be familiar to the testifying witness.

THE ROLE OF THE FORENSIC NURSE

Forensic nurses must follow the nursing practice act for their individual state and work with multidisciplinary professionals in the field of death investigation.

Forensic nurses were first recognized as a beneficial resource to the medical examiner in Canada in 1975. John Butt, MD, chief medical examiner in Alberta, Canada, established a program using forensic nurses as medicolegal death investigators. Their nursing education, particularly that of disease processes, pharmacology, and ability to communicate effectively with families, was determined to be essential to the death investigation.

Since the 1970s, nurses have worked sporadically in medical examiners' offices as death investigators. As innovative as the role is, nurses often are unable to incorporate their nursing abilities to their fullest. Tradition shows that medicolegal death investigators were often former law enforcement officers. The idea of a forensic nurse or other health-care provider in this role is foreign and very nontraditional at best. The FNDI, although not officially defined as such, is a registered nurse who applies the nursing process, nursing knowledge and experience, and principles of forensic science to the medicolegal death investigation. This is a nontraditional role for nursing as well as for the medicolegal death investigation teams. It is one role that is not commonly thought of as being useful to the medical examiner or coroner. For many nurses, it is also considered an odd match because the "patient" is deceased and no longer in need of nursing care (Box 11.1).

However, the forensic nurse is an ideal complement to the medical examiner/coroner. Forensic nurses have a unique knowledge base that includes nursing science, forensic science, and criminal justice. The forensic nurse is able to conduct a more thorough *medical* investigation of the death. Questions are formulated based on medical knowledge. For example, the nurse is able to identify prescription medications at a scene and inventory them, thus distinguishing a potential overdose from a natural death.

The nursing skill sets of clinical care, family interaction and communication, and critical thinking are essential for the FNDI. Essential nursing skills allow the nurse to efficiently assess a scene and family interactions and to effectively communicate with all family members. One skill the nurse must develop is an understanding of the grief reaction, and more commonly courses addressing the human responses to death and trauma are being incorporated into nursing and health-professional education. An understanding of human responses to death and trauma is incorporated into forensic nursing practice and facilitates a rapid establishment of a rapport with the grieving family. The forensic nurse anticipates the family reaction and provides support while obtaining necessary information for the death investigation.

Patient education is another skill set the nurse translates to the death investigation process. In the death investigation, the forensic nurse explains cause and manner of death to the decedent's loved ones. For example, in a natural death from atherosclerotic cardiovascular disease, the forensic nurse will both explain the disease process to the spouse and take the opportunity to educate the spouse about a healthy lifestyle of diet and exercise.

Another benefit of using forensic nurses in the death investigation is the nurse's ability to analyze and summarize health records. Information gleaned by the forensic nurse assists the medical examiner/coroner in determining the need for any additional testing or specialty consultations that may be required to accurately identify the cause and manner of death. The forensic nurse reviews the medical record to discover the decedent's medical, social, and surgical history and to summarize the course of care. This relevant information is provided to the medical examiner/coroner so that the cause and manner of death determination may be expedited.

As an investigator, the nurse incorporates concepts of forensic science and forensic pathology. The technical aspects of crime scene investigation are protocol driven and easily learned. However, an overall evaluation of the decedent as related to the scene requires experience and medical knowledge. The nurse must be able to identify medications and reconcile them to disease processes to develop the "picture" of the decedent, his or her lifestyle and habits, and a possible cause of death. As an example, copious amounts of blood present at a scene do not necessarily mean a violent death. In fact, if the decedent has a history of chronic alcohol use as evidenced by findings of numerous beer or liquor bottles, the death could be due to exsanguination resulting from esophageal varices. The contributions of the forensic nurse to the death investigation are substantial and allow the pathologist access to a more thorough investigation.

Nurses with a mental health background and education may develop expertise in the psychological reasons

---

Box 11.1 Role of the Forensic Nurse in the Death Investigation

- Responds to the scene and conducts the investigation
- Obtains death reports per state statutes
- Provides case management to pathologists
- Interacts with and educates family members
- Notifies next of kin of the death
- Identifies decedents
- Provides community education
- Conducts research
- Develops and implements prevention strategies

leading to death. With sufficient knowledge and practice, forensic nurse investigators can focus on the deceased's life and emotional state leading up to death. A thorough examination of the deceased's psychological behavior can help determine the mode of death, which refers to the actual circumstances that led to the death, and determine if a death was intentional or accidental. According to Scott and colleagues, up to 20% of cases reviewed by the coroner/medical examiner are unclear as to the mode of death. The psychological autopsy can help to determine the reasons or events preceding death that may have prompted a suicidal action. Where did they do it? What was the reason? Why do it at a particular place or time?

For example, autoerotic asphyxia, the practice of seeking heightened sexual pleasure by inducing cerebral hypoxia, may indeed appear to be a suicide. But a skilled FNDI can interview friends and family to determine the person's intentions and actions, which, when combined with the death scene characteristics, can lead to a clear picture of the decedent's intentions at the time of death.

The statutory duties of the FNDI include conducting the death investigation either by responding to the scene or by obtaining information during a telephone interview, notifying next of kin that the death has occurred, and identifying the unknown. Other responsibilities such as case management, education of the community and family members, research and development, and implementation of prevention strategies may be incorporated into the role as well.

One excellent example of the application of forensic knowledge to clinical practice is reported by a European study that found in a systematic review of the literature that the incidence of sudden death documented in young men and women was of cardiac origin. The sudden cardiac death (SCD) incidence was 2.86 (per 100,000 person-years, males) and 1.24 (per 100,000 person-years, females). The primary cause was treatable cardiac disease, for which prevention strategies for young people instituted by nurses in a variety of clinical settings can help to avoid such deaths. Interventions in the primary care clinical settings can be developed directly for the living based on postmortem investigative information.

Guidelines for autopsy following SCD were developed by Basso and colleagues and may allow for a uniform method of investigating one of the leading modes of death in Europe and the United States. Current methods of death certification do not include categories of SCD. A protocol for cardiac assessment includes delineation of steps to be taken for heart examination, histology, and molecular sampling. Such a protocol, it is claimed, may allow for meaningful comparisons among communities

and countries as well as trends in disease patterns that result in death. As with protocols in all types of death, the nurse investigator may not perform the physical autopsy procedures. The communication with and explanations to the family members and gathering of the clinical information prior to the autopsy are crucial roles for a nurse.

Nursing expertise is beneficial to law enforcement officers in distinguishing between a natural death and a traumatic death. The child's death investigation is a unique area, and the final outcome and report may be within the forensic nurse's expertise. Using established protocols, the forensic nurse may respond directly to the hospital where the infant or child was pronounced dead and speak with the treating physician and family members to obtain the medical history and a description of the terminal events. Along with investigating officers, the nurse responds to the location where the incident occurred to conduct the scene assessment. If the incident occurred at the residence, the nurse obtains the social assessment of the family and location and documents the following:

- General area of the residence
- Condition of the interior of the home (cleanliness, lighting, and necessary facilities)
- Amount of food and items needed to care for the infant or child
- Any insect or rodent activity
- Any foul odors
- Any indication of alcohol or tobacco use inside or outside of the home
- Any other children in the home and their health status

The residential and social assessment, along with information about family behavior patterns, are crucial for the pathologist to be able to determine the overall status of the infant or child in relation to the autopsy findings. Classifying the cause and manner of death may be difficult or impossible without a thorough investigation, especially in cases where sudden infant death (SIDS), "bed sharing," or neglect may be issues. Adams, Good, and DeFranco cite a number of key recommendations for practice and family education that are based on the triple-risk model for which SIDS is the common pathway (Table 11.1).

The forensic nurse is able to obtain patient information and observe behaviors and family interactions when working with families in the clinical arena that will naturally benefit the investigation. This knowledge base and ability of a nurse assist law enforcement in understanding current medical issues that impact the child and in developing follow-up questions to determine if findings are consistent with the reported circumstances of death.

TABLE 11.1   **Clinical Recommendations for SIDS Based on Evidence**

Recommendation	Level of Evidence	References and Type
Place infant on back for sleeping	A	Five consistent high-quality studies
Firm sleeping surface, no soft bedding	C	Seven references: consensus, disease-oriented evidence, usual practice, expert opinion, case series
No overheating	C	Seven references: consensus, disease-oriented evidence, usual practice, expert opinion, case series
Smoke-free pregnancy, infant environment	C	Nine references: consensus, disease-oriented evidence, usual practice, expert opinion, case series
Separate crib, no co-bedding	C	Eight references: consensus, disease-oriented evidence, usual practice, expert opinion, case series
Offer pacifier	C	Four references: consensus, disease-oriented evidence, usual practice, expert opinion, case series

Adapted from Adams, Good, DeFranco, 2009.

Often diagnosed as SIDS, inflicted neurotrauma may be revealed only with an ocular autopsy. Guidelines for ocular autopsy are based on practice standards that have demonstrated the value of the examination in children who may have suffered from inflicted neurotrauma. Comparison studies with fatally abused children have revealed that ocular hemorrhages are far more common in neurotrauma than in other types of traumatic head injuries. Furthermore, optic nerve and orbital findings are significantly more common in abusive trauma. A rigorous best-practice protocol developed by Gilleland and colleagues specifically documents steps to be taken to standardize the ocular autopsy examination and to report clearly all the details of the examination. Removal of the eyes for examination deviates from some protocols, and examiners must be aware of the legislation in every jurisdiction. However, it may be worth pursuing, particularly in cases of children with head trauma. The forensic nurse's communication ability with families and legal authorities when there is a deviation from protocol may be critical. Communication with families and authorities is recommended, so that further comparisons will facilitate uniform descriptions of findings and pursuit of all potentially useful findings to be considered prior to the diagnosis.

Advances in the FNDI Role

There are areas in the United States where forensic nurses have accomplished a great deal of progress in the death investigation arena. In Charleston County, South Carolina, a nurse was elected as the coroner. Several of the deputy coroners are nurses as well. While they are known as "nurse coroners," their practice is not solely outlined by the state nurse practice act, but also by coroner law. Coroner law delineates their practice and provides much latitude in terms of the death investigation. This means that death investigation is the primary duty. However,

nursing skills and the many years of providing health care to families for a variety of health conditions are beneficial to the death investigation process. Nursing knowledge may be successfully integrated into the practice of death investigation, especially when interacting with family members.

In contrast, the forensic nurses at the Harris County Medical Examiner's Office in Houston, Texas, have a different type of practice. While still governed by the Texas nurse practice act and medical examiner law, the nurses have been able to incorporate the nursing process when investigating each case, with each family interaction, and when educating the public. For example, after the autopsy examination is completed, families are contacted by the nurses and the cause and manner of death are discussed. The nurses incorporate aspects of case management into the daily operations of the office. The pathologists are assigned nurses who assist with gathering additional information about the case, obtaining necessary police reports and medical records, and organizing multidisciplinary meetings to review difficult cases. Other states that use FNDIs as coroners and for a variety of responsibilities related to death investigation are Oregon, Louisiana, New Jersey, Pennsylvania, Wisconsin, and Maryland.

The implications for forensic nurses practicing in the death investigation arena are substantial. Interactions with families may be improved. The standard of death investigation may be elevated. However, there is limited evidence-based research regarding improved outcomes for families and the results of investigations. There are scant publications on nurses practicing in death investigation as a subspecialty of forensic nursing. Most information is delivered in lectures, as anecdotes, and through experience. The definition and description of the role of the forensic nurse death investigation must be clarified and clinical questions formulated for research projects. At present, lower levels of evidence include little more than case studies.

Research of the highest level, such as systematic reviews and comparison research, are conducted on the work done in medical examiner/coroner settings, such as that done by Scholing et al (2009), and best practices are developed to improve practice. However, there is little research being conducted by and about forensic nurses and their role and responsibilities as they pertain to how the nursing process impacts specific outcomes in death investigation. There are distinct differences and limitations for a nurse in this area of practice, depending on the system in which he or she practices.

Death Investigation and the Nursing Process

The death investigation not only includes collecting evidence and taking photographs of the scene, but it also involves conducting a thorough assessment of the decedent and the scene. To accomplish this in a systematic fashion, the nursing process should be used. The nursing process contains five important steps that are incorporated into the death investigation. Each will be discussed here in relation to the investigation process.

Assessment includes photographic and written documentation, according to agency protocol. In this step, data are collected and analyzed. The FNDI obtains initial information from law enforcement, family members, and others who are present at the death scene. This information encompasses the following:

- Demographics of the decedent
- Next of kin information
- Who found the decedent
- How was the decedent found
- Physical, mental health, medical, and social history
- Circumstances of death

Physical assessment of the deceased person is conducted as well. The nurse compares subjective information obtained from family members and treating physicians to the objective data collected (Lynch, 2006). The physical assessment findings confirm disease processes and identify mechanisms of injury and death.

Various protocols, depending on the suspected cause of death, may be followed and relate specifically to the physical autopsy findings. One example is the list of clinical information in the sudden cardiac death autopsy guidelines developed by Basso and colleagues (2007). Beyond routine medical history, questions related to details of cardiac symptoms, EKG results, etc., would be included.

Diagnosis results when the nurse identifies the diseases and health conditions of the deceased. Death does not preclude the nurse from diagnosing the patient. In fact, the diagnoses will help determine the route of a death investigation and subsequent information gathering that may be required for the forensic pathologist to determine the cause and manner of death. A diagnosis can be applied to the family members as well. The most common diagnosis that can be related to the family is grief. This leads the forensic nurse to the next step in the nursing process.

Planning is the nursing process stage at which the nurse sets goals and plans interventions that will achieve the desired patient outcomes. Further investigation strategies are planned, such as interviews with individuals and laboratory and other diagnostic tests that may be conducted to confirm findings and answer new questions. Appointments are set up for multidisciplinary team meetings to discuss difficult case findings.

Implementation requires use of good communication skills, which are essential during this phase. Interventions designed to attain the set goals are implemented. The forensic nurse continues the investigation by obtaining additional information, records, or photographs as required by the pathologist. Family and survivor needs are assessed, and referrals for counseling or support groups are made if they are not available on site.

Evaluation is the final phase of the nursing process, but it is actually an ongoing or developing phase of the nursing process. Goals are reviewed and interventions are examined to identify needed changes. Processes may not have elicited the desired results. Laboratories may have returned laboratory testing results more slowly than needed for a specific investigation. A specific witness interviewed may need to be reinterviewed for further information. Confirmation of laboratory and historical information may be necessary. After a process is complete, the nursing process may initiate again until all the questions can be answered. In the death investigation, the forensic nurse analyzes the investigation and documentation itself as well as the quality of the data obtained from all the investigatory processes. Laboratory studies are interpreted, and medical records are assessed. Further discussion with other investigating agencies will determine additional interventions. Generally, all goals are considered met when the pathologist ascertains the cause and manner of death and closes the case.

Statutes, administrative rules, and performance standards outline the duties of the forensic nurse who is either appointed or elected to the position. Even though forensic nursing practice is guided by policies, protocols, rules, and standards, the FNDI primarily acts as a nurse. The application and integration of the nursing process into the death investigation practice is essential.

THE DEATH INVESTIGATION

The death investigation is a systematic process in which information is gathered to determine the cause and manner of death. The cause of death is the injury or disease process that ultimately results in death. Examples of cause of death are atherosclerotic cardiovascular disease, gunshot wound of the head, or stab wound of the chest. This differs from the **mechanism of death,** which is defined as the physiological disturbance that is incompatible with life. The mechanism of death is *initiated* by the cause of death. For example, the stab wound to the chest (cause of death) that punctures the heart starts the hemorrhage that results in shock (mechanism of death) and the ultimate demise of the individual. Other mechanisms of death include cardiac arrest and sepsis. After determining what caused the individual to die, the pathologist must classify the manner of death. Manner of death is the categorization or legal classification of the death (Box 11.2).

The nurse is responsible for determining medical examiner/coroner jurisdiction when cases are reported. It is imperative the nurse be able to discern between each of these concepts. By knowing which questions to ask, the nurse will be able to obtain enough answers to satisfactorily identify a possible cause and manner of death and determine if this is a case requiring further investigation.

Components of the Death Investigation

The death investigation is a multidisciplinary effort. While the medical examiner/coroner conducts an investigation separate from law enforcement, much of the same information is shared by both. The pathologist will use information from the nurse investigator's written report, the scene investigation, and the autopsy examination to determine the cause and manner of death, which is the ultimate goal of the death investigation process.

Box 11.2   Manner of Death

Manner of death is the legal classification of death.

- Homicide
- Suicide
- Accident
- Natural
- Undetermined

Data from Spitz, W.U. (1993). *Spitz and fisher's medical legal investigation of death.* (3rd ed.). Springfield, IL: Charles C. Thomas.

Written Report

The investigative report is a written document outlining all the information from the investigation. The report is generated from information gathered from either a telephone interview or the scene investigation. It should be thorough and written in a timely manner. As additional information becomes available, the report should be updated so that those involved with the case will have access to the most current data.

The forensic nurse must ascertain certain information about the decedent to include in the report. Such data include demographics of the decedent and next of kin, when the decedent was last known to be alive and who saw him or her, how the next of kin was notified, date and time of death (if pronounced in a hospital, otherwise it will be known as a "found" time), how the decedent was identified, his or her medical history and name of personal physician, and decedent's social history. A narrative description of the scene should be included in the report as well. The nurse investigator objectively outlines all observations made at the scene. In the event of a death occurring at a hospital in which the nurse did not respond, the narrative report describes succinctly what was reported by staff as being the decedent's terminal events. The narrative section of the report should answer the questions Who? What? When? Where? Why? and How?

Death Scene Investigation

The forensic nurse investigator will respond to the death scene as part of the ongoing investigation. While documenting the scene during the **death scene investigation,** the nurse will study the surroundings. The circumstances of death are compared to the scene observations.

Through observations of surroundings and interviews with family members, friends, and acquaintances, the nurse is able to develop an understanding of the decedent, how the individual lived, and how he or she died. The information gained from responding to the scene will assist the pathologist in correlating injuries and determining the cause and manner of death.

Recording the observations from the scene of the death may be documented in several ways. A written description of the scene should objectively illustrate what the nurse has observed. Diagrams are often beneficial and will show the position of the decedent in relation to the rest of the surroundings, entrances, windows, weapons, blood stains, etc. Measurements of objects should be taken and noted on diagrams, and their locations should be sketched as accurately as possible. Lined graph paper is very useful for this task. Items that are recovered by law enforcement should be included. For example, the nurse responds to a scene where a suicide has been reported to have occurred.

The diagram should show where the weapon used is located in relation to the decedent. The measurements are to be noted as well. The scene should also be photographed. The photographs should lead the investigator from the farthest point, such as outside the door of the room, to inside the door, to views of each side of the room, and finally to the location of the decedent's body. They should also be taken from various angles, which will show all aspects of the scene. Close-up photographs of the decedent can focus on additional physical findings.

While at the scene, the nurse should look for any medications, drug paraphernalia, and items that may assist with identification of the decedent. Medications and drug paraphernalia present will guide the pathologist in ordering specific laboratory studies. The nurse will also have the opportunity to conduct a preliminary physical assessment on the decedent and speak with family members, friends, or acquaintances if present.

The Autopsy Examination

The autopsy, touted as the ultimate peer review, is the highest standard of postmortem examination, and it is essentially a laboratory test. Also known as "necropsy" or "postmortem examination," it involves a complete dissection of all organs in an effort to identify the cause and manner of death. Valuable information is provided to the pathologist about natural disease processes. Evidence such as bullets may be collected during the examination. Injuries are also photographed, diagrammed, and documented. In addition, the physical body art and piercings should be noted in writing and with images.

The examination begins with an external physical examination, a detailed visual inspection of the decedent. Clothing remains on the decedent and is photographed. It is then removed, and all aspects of the decedent are documented on diagrams, photographed, and the findings are dictated by the pathologist and transcribed. Beginning from the head and working toward the feet, the pathologist describes all aspects of the decedent from hair color and length to the condition of the toenails.

After this portion is completed, a Y-shaped incision is made to expose the organs of the chest and abdomen. The pathologist removes each organ, weighs it, and examines it. The cranial vault is opened, and the brain is removed and assessed. Injuries are examined, and wound tracks are identified. The pathologist is also able to determine if wounds were inflicted antemortem or postmortem (before or after death). Samples are collected for toxicological studies and other laboratory testing.

Not all autopsy examinations are performed by forensic pathologists in an effort to identify wounds and determine cause and manner of death. A clinical autopsy or hospital autopsy is completed by an anatomical/clinical pathologist, often at the request of family members or treating physicians to identify disease processes or the usefulness of a particular course of therapy. Permission must be obtained from the family. In contrast, the forensic autopsy is conducted to identify trauma, collect evidence, and determine cause and manner of death. The authority to conduct these autopsies is given by the state, and family permission is not necessary. Legal authority and family permission may precede the examination, but currently there are few standards or guidelines in Europe or the United States for conduction of additional testing, such as genetic testing, on cadaveric material. Special consent from the deceased prior to death, from an appropriate relative, or by power of attorney may need to be obtained.

The forensic pathologist may not perform an autopsy examination on all cases. An external examination may be completed in cases that are natural in nature for which there is no suspicion of foul play. This type of evaluation consists of a physical assessment, review of medical records, and review of the investigation. The pathologist will then determine the *most likely cause of death* based on all information gathered.

There is a global trend toward reduction in performance of the time-consuming autopsy examinations. Information about causes of death in all populations is critical to assessing health trends and planning prevention and health services. A verbal autopsy is frequently used in mid- to lower-income countries in which robust medical examiner or coroner systems do not exist due to organizational and economic constraints and other factors. In the language of nursing, the verbal autopsy is history related to the chief complaint, which is death in these cases. Verbal autopsy, as defined by the World Health Organization, is a method used to determine and document cause of death from data collected about the symptoms and signs of illness and the events that preceded death. One research study examined the implementation of a standardized verbal autopsy (VA) training program among physicians, nurses, and lay community workers in various communities. Knowledge required to classify perinatal causes of death was significantly improved in all groups. While not used in forensic autopsy, the training study tested by Engmann's team developed and standardized a verbal autopsy tool and training program to evaluate the use of the model in assisting physicians to document prenatal cause of death. The physicians and nurses had a comparable increase in knowledge after the training. The lay workers' knowledge scores improved significantly as well, but were lower than physicians' scores. The study determined that with appropriate training in verbal autopsy techniques the cognitive and applied knowledge needed to determine cause of death is similar for a variety of workers. This study suggests that there is a useful role for appropriately trained individuals to improve accuracy of documentation of perinatal cause of death in remote and rural areas. Perinatal deaths are the leading cause of death globally in children under 14 years old.

A review of 102 verbal autopsy research studies was conducted by Joshi, Kengne, and Neal and determined that there is no evidence that the design recommendations developed in the early 1990s for such studies had been uniformly applied. Seven key methodological indicators were recommended for research to evaluate the effectiveness of verbal autopsies. It is recommended that a combined questionnaire be used by a trained interviewer and a suitable respondent in a reasonable-recall period of time. Predefined algorithms are assigned, and an option for assigning multiple causes of death should be included. Follow-up validations studies should be conducted as well. Despite the need for such mortality surveillance in resource-poor countries, the ability to measure the effectiveness of the verbal autopsy cannot be verified completely when studies are not optimally designed to demonstrate improved outcomes. Trained forensic nurse involvement at all levels could have a significant impact on verbal autopsy training and research. Similar research is also severely limited on the effectiveness of FNDIs. Comparison studies between nurses and other professional death investigators would be very informative.

The nursing role may be to provide information to the physician performing the autopsy. The nurse may examine parts of the body, particularly if evidence of sexual assault is required, and participate in developing the physical findings. Communicating the autopsy results to the deceased's family members may be one of the most important roles for the forensic nurse working in death investigation. Keys and colleagues conducted retrospective telephone surveys with families whose family members had an autopsy; 32% of the relatives indicated that they were not adequately informed of the results. Results varied, but 54% of respondents were involved in a discussion of the results with a medical professional. More than half of the respondents wanted a copy, and two thirds of the families were satisfied with the explanations they received. Dissatisfaction was related to the unfamiliar medical terminology used. When family understanding was compared with autopsy reports, only 65% had an accurate knowledge of the findings. Over 90% of families believed the autopsy was useful for families. While there is an important need for families to know results, the purpose and findings may be best communicated in person and not over the phone or in a letter. Nurses have good communication skills, and the ability to explain medical results and findings to laypersons is an advantage of having nurses involved in informing the families of autopsy results.

Forensic Nurse Responsibilities Regarding the Death Investigation

Identifying Medical Examiner/Coroner Jurisdiction

State statutes outline which types of deaths are reportable to the medical examiner/coroner. It is the responsibility of the nurse to be thoroughly familiar with them (Box 11.3).

Whether the forensic nurse is notified of a death by law enforcement or a hospital, the nurse must gather enough information to determine if the death falls under the jurisdiction of the medical examiner or coroner. Certain questions, such as ascertaining the location of the decedent, any injuries identified, and the condition of the decedent's body must be asked. These answers will assist with determining jurisdiction. If the death does not fall under the state criteria, then the case is released for the primary care physician to complete the death certificate. However, if the nurse investigator establishes jurisdiction, a scene response must be decided. Agency protocols will delineate which types of deaths warrant an investigative scene response.

Box 11.3 Types of Reportable Deaths

The following are types of deaths that are reportable to the medical examiner/coroner. However, the nurse must be familiar with the particular state's statutes.

- Homicides
- Suicides
- Deaths of inmates in public institutions
- Poisonings or overdoses
- Unusual or suspicious circumstances
- Accidents (motor vehicle crashes, falls, etc.)
- Hyperthermia/hypothermia
- No physician to sign the death certificate
- Officer-involved deaths
- Neglect
- Burns/charred bodies
- Infants/children
- Maternal deaths
- Deaths occurring while at work

Data from Clark, S.C., Ernst, M.F., Haglund, W.D., & Jentzen, J.M. (1996). *Medicolegal Death Investigator.* Big Rapids, MI: Occupational Research and Assessment, Inc.
Descheneaux, K. (1991). Death investigations: How you can help. *Nursing,* 21(9):52-55.

Scene Investigation

It is commonly understood that the death scene belongs to the investigating law enforcement agency and the body belongs to the medical examiner/coroner. Therefore, the nurse must ask permission before entering the scene. Upon arrival, the nurse identifies the law enforcement officer who is in charge. The detective will walk the nurse through the scene, identifying key evidence and findings. Information sharing is common during this phase. The nurse will obtain demographics on the decedent and next of kin and a history of the events leading up to the death.

Next, the nurse will document the scene with photographs, diagrams, and notes. The photographs may be obtained with a 35-mm or digital camera, whichever is admissible in that particular jurisdiction. Then the nurse will identify any medications, noting the type, prescription, and number remaining in the bottle. Drug paraphernalia should be photographed. In the event of a homicide or forced entry to a residence, photographs of the door jams and locks should be taken. Special care should be taken for deaths of vulnerable populations such as the disabled, infants, and elders. Food, water, and the status of heating and cooling systems should be documented in addition to the general condition of the residence. While such findings may appear to be inconsequential, upon review of all the documentation and consultation with the investigatory team further exploration of the scene or questioning of key people often results.

As the law enforcement officer walks the forensic nurse through the scene, important aspects are pointed out and photographed to support nursing observation, to document, and to inform the pathologist. It may impact the determination of the cause and manner of death.

A preliminary physical examination of the decedent is conducted. Finally, family members will be interviewed for medical and social history and any knowledge of the circumstances of death. Vast information is gained from observation of the scene and from family demeanor, communication, interactions, and behaviors.

Physical Examination

The physical examination is a major part of the death investigation process. The nurse will document injuries or the lack thereof along with the condition of the decedent's body. Often a nurse's knowledge of signs and symptoms of disease pathology or specific medical conditions provides unique information on the deceased. Postmortem changes will allow time of death to be estimated and will further impact the law enforcement investigation. The types of injuries noted will allow the pathologist to match potential weapons that may be the cause.

The nurse should begin at the head and work toward the feet when conducting the physical assessment. Just like performing the physical examination on a living person, the nurse must assess each part thoroughly, documenting all findings. The head should be palpated for any trauma. Ligature marks may be mimicked by folds of skin. Petechial hemorrhaging may be difficult to recognize by the untrained eye, after postmortem changes, or on darker skin. Arms and hands are evaluated for defensive wounds and other injuries. Soot from firearms or various other organic elements or liquids may be viewed on the hands. Therefore, the hands must be placed in paper bags in all gunshot cases (homicides or suicides) or when there are findings. Wounds to the chest, abdomen, and back are noted, as well as findings on the legs and feet.

Identification of Wounds

Documentation of the physical examination necessitates that the nurse identify wounds by their appropriate names. Some injuries are due to blunt forces. They include abrasions, lacerations, avulsions, and contusions. An abrasion is a scraping away of the superficial layers of skin and is commonly called a "scratch." A laceration is a tear in the tissue that is caused by shearing or crushing forces. The edges are usually irregular with abraded edges and occur over bony prominences. Inside the wound, tissue bridging (threadlike strands of tissue that were not totally transected when the injury occurred) may be evident. An avulsion is a type of laceration in which the force that strikes the body at an angle causes the skin to be pushed or ripped off the bone. Often the direction the skin is pushed is clear evidence of the direction of force. Contusions are also known as bruises, and they may result from a blow or squeezing of the tissue. Blood vessels are crushed, and hemorrhage occurs under the skin. The skin is not broken, and the bleeding remains under the skin surface. Several blunt force injuries may appear in the same area, such as bruising beneath an abrasion that ends in an avulsion.

Injuries caused by sharp forces are known as cuts and stab wounds. The instrument is sharp enough to divide the tissue as it penetrates. A cut or incised wound is longer than it is deep and occurs when the sharp object is drawn over the skin. The edges are smooth. Tissue bridges are not evident in this type of wound. A stab wound differs from a cut in that a stab wound is deeper than it is long. According to DiMaio, the most common instrument used to create this type of wound is a knife. Stab wounds may also be caused by ice picks, pens, pencils, scissors, or broken glass.

Injuries from firearms are another type of wound that the forensic nurse will encounter. Firearm injuries may be caused by handguns, shotguns, and rifles. Each has a distinctive pattern, and the nurse must be knowledgeable about each and ensure the correct documentation.

Penetrating or perforating gunshot wounds are caused by handguns, either revolvers or semiautomatic guns. In a penetrating wound, the bullet enters but does not exit. The bullet enters and exits in a perforating wound. Wounds will look different based upon the range of the muzzle to the target. Entrance wounds are often mistaken for exit wounds by clinicians. The wound must be closely assessed to discern between the two. Entrance wounds characteristically have abrasions around the margins. This is a rare finding in exit wounds unless the decedent was leaning against a wall or hard floor or had an object pressed firmly against the body when being shot. Soot from the discharge of the weapon can be seen inside the wound when it is a contact wound. An imprint of the gun's muzzle may also be identified around the wound. In intermediate-range gunshot wounds occurring when the gun is held away from the body, burning gunpowder will sear the skin. The phenomenon is known as stippling or powder tattooing, and it gives rise to the punctuate abrasions that cannot be wiped off the body. Exit wounds are typically irregular in shape.

Shotguns and rifles cause extensive damage to the decedent's body. Shotgun shells contain a lead shot, pellets, and a wad (a filler in the shell). The farther away the shooter is from the decedent, the wider the pattern of disbursement of the pellets. Rifles are high-velocity weapons resulting in exit wounds that are devastating and characteristically larger than the entrance wounds.

A thorough study of gunshot wounds is beyond the scope of this chapter. Variations in range will affect the wound's presentation. In addition, gunshot wounds have been mistaken for other types of wounds until the autopsy examination. Therefore, the nurse should seek other avenues for gaining this knowledge base.

Postmortem Changes

As part of the physical examination, the nurse must identify any changes associated with death. These assist with estimating the time of death. The media provides a false impression that investigators are able to precisely pinpoint an individual's time of death. Only an estimation in hours, days, weeks, or months can be given and is based upon findings observed at the scene, such as algor mortis, rigor mortis, livor mortis, and decomposition.

Algor mortis is the progressive cooling of the body until it reaches ambient temperature after death. The body cools at a rate of 2° to 2.5°F per hour during the first hours after death and then slows to 1.5°F per hour for the next 12 hours. The decrease in temperature varies depending on the environment. The cooler the ambient temperature,

---

Box 11.4 Postmortem Changes

- Algor mortis
- Rigor mortis
- Livor mortis
- Decomposition

Data from DiMaio, V.J., & DiMaio, D. (2001). *Forensic pathology.* (2nd ed.). Boca Raton: CRC Press.

---

the quicker the temperature will decrease. A death that occurs midwinter in the Alaskan wilderness could result in a quickly frozen decedent who may remain preserved for months. If the environment is hot, the body will not cool as fast. This also holds true for the individual who is septic or perhaps running and collapses. The body temperature will lower more slowly.

It is difficult to pinpoint a time of death that is solely based on body temperature. There are several equations that are used, but they are based on a "normal temperature" at death.

Time of death = 37°C – Rectal Temperature (°C) + 3

or

Time of death = 98.6°F – Rectal Temperature (°F) / 1.5

Normal temperature is based on 98.6°F at death, which does not always occur. Therefore, these equations should be used with caution.

Rigor mortis is the progressive stiffening of the body after death. It results in the loss of adenosine triphosphate (ATP) in the muscle cells. Rigor develops and disappears at the same rate. However, it is more apparent in the smaller muscles first. Rigor mortis appears about 2 to 4 hours after death and is fully developed in 6 to 12 hours. The nurse must remember that the environmental temperature will affect the rate at which rigor mortis develops. As the decedent decomposes, the rigor will dissipate.

The reddish purple discoloration that is commonly found on dependent areas of the body is known as "livor mortis." The blood settles in the dilated and toneless capillaries of the decedent. Areas of the body that are resting against a surface when death occurs will be pale in color compared to nondependent areas of the body. Livor is usually evident 30 minutes to 2 hours after death. Between 8 and 12 hours, the lividity becomes "fixed." This means that if the nurse presses on an area of discoloration it will not blanch. If the nurse investigator notes that lividity is not present on a dependent area of the body, then it should be assumed that the body was moved some time after death.

Decomposition is the disintegration of body tissues after death. It involves the process of autolysis and putrefaction. Autolysis is the breakdown of the organs by the intracellular enzyme. Heat will accelerate this process; in contrast, the cold delays it. Putrefaction is the breakdown of the body due to bacteria, which is primarily dependent on the temperature of the environment. Decomposition begins with a greenish discoloration in the lower abdomen that is evident between 24 to 36 hours after death. Next, the head, neck, and shoulders become green and bloated. Marbling of the skin, the hemolysis of the blood in the vessels, becomes visible. Then there is generalized bloating and skin slippage. The entire body is a green-black color. Decomposition or purge fluid will drain from the body. This is often mistaken for blood. Insect activity is another marker used in documenting the presence of decomposition.

In dry climates, the body will dehydrate quickly, and the result is mummification. The skin will have a brown to black leathery appearance, and the organs will continue to decompose, often reduced to putty-like consistency.

Obtaining Medical and Social History

As part of the assessment process, the nurse must obtain a medical and social history of the decedent. Scene observations and speaking with the decedent's family and friends are key sources of information. Medications are inventoried and correlated with the history and any physician records. Discharge summaries from previous admissions are sufficient for establishing the medical history. The nurse should obtain information about primary care physicians, past surgical history, current list of medical diagnoses, and medications along with any history of smoking, alcohol, or drug use. The pathologist will use all of this information when reviewing the case and determining cause and manner of death. The medical and social history may be used when the pathologist is deciding whether to conduct an autopsy examination or an external examination only.

Identification of the Decedent

Another responsibility of the FNDI is to ensure the positive identification of the decedent. This is a priority for the nurse and should begin upon arrival at the scene. In the event the decedent's identity is unknown, aspects such as height, weight, hair color, eye color, and the presence of scars, marks, and tattoos are documented as quickly as possible so that inquiries from the community can be compared. A decedent's identification may be made by visual or scientific means (Box 11.5).

A visual identification may be sufficient in cases where the decedent died in a hospital and family members had visited or in cases where there is no head trauma or facial injury. The only caveat with a visual identification

Box 11.5   Scientific Identification

Scientific identification is accomplished through:

- Fingerprint comparison
- Dental record and radiograph comparison
- DNA testing of a blood relative
- Radiographs of healed fractures, prosthesis, or unique bone formations

is that they are subjective and often unreliable due to the fact that many people bear a close resemblance to others.

When there are multiple fatalities or severe head trauma rendering the decedent unviewable, the decedent must be identified by scientific means.

Scientific identification includes fingerprints, dental records, and DNA testing. Fingerprints are the most commonly used method. Fingerprints are unique to each individual, even identical twins. They may be compared to prints on file with local, state, and federal law enforcement agencies. When there are no fingerprints on file, then the nurse needs to ascertain from the family the whereabouts of any dental records. Once these records and any radiographs are obtained, a forensic odontologist is consulted. This forensic dentist compares postmortem dental radiographs to the antemortem records. Size and shape of teeth and dental restoration are used in the comparison evaluation.

In the event the decedent is too young to have dental records on file, then DNA testing will be necessary. DNA characteristics are passed from one generation to the next. Identification is made from antemortem samples taken from closely related family members and compared to tissue or blood samples obtained during the postmortem examination.

Scars, marks, and tattoos are often used to correlate any scientific measures that are used. Some medical examiner/coroner offices will use radiographs of joint replacements, healed fractures, and spine disorders to identify individuals. Identification means will be outlined by an agency's protocols.

Notification of Next of Kin

After the decedent's identification has been confirmed, the next of kin must be identified. It is imperative this be done in a timely manner. In jurisdictions where the medical examiner/coroner is mandated to notify next of kin, this duty may befall the forensic nurse investigator.

The death of a loved one is one of the greatest stresses a family can encounter. Therefore, any notification must be done quickly and compassionately. The nurse must not use words like "passed away" or "moved on to a better life." This leaves room for misinterpretation on the part of the family. The next of kin should be told their loved one has died. The word "died" is used. This term is generally understood by all.

All efforts should be made to notify the next of kin in person. The nurse makes a request for a law enforcement officer to accompany him or her when making the notification. If a telephone notification is found to be necessary, the nurse should ascertain if the family member is alone and should never inform a family member who is alone about the death. Coworkers, supervisors, friends, or clergy can assist with the notification process.

Documentation

When documenting injuries or the scene, the forensic nurse must describe the wounds as to their location, size, depth, color, and any other observations in the narrative report. The nurse's report should be clear and concise and should contain all relevant information that pertains to the case. Scene observations should be as detailed as possible. The nurse should document findings in a systematic manner so that information flows in a logical order.

Diagrams are often helpful when depicting large numbers of injuries. However, depending on protocol, the nurse may not be required to complete a diagram because the forensic pathologist will document all wounds during the autopsy. If policies permit the nurse to document all injuries on diagrams at the scene, discrepancies between the nurse's diagram and the pathologist's diagrams may be brought up in court. Each must be prepared to provide an explanation for discrepancies. Often, injuries may be unintentionally overlooked due to clothing, large amounts of blood, or other debris inhibiting the assessment.

When responding to a scene, a major responsibility of the forensic nurse is to document the site and the decedent. The forensic nurse at the scene is the eyes of the pathologist. This is best accomplished through the use of photography. Evidence is recorded in its original location. The photographs show position of the decedent, weapons, forced entry, if a struggle occurred, and the lifestyle of the decedent. The pathologist refers to the photographs when determining cause and manner of death. Injuries and injury tracks may be challenging to the pathologist, and photodocumentation of the scene and decedent may clear up any questions. The photographs of the scene and the decedent should include overall, orientation, and close-up images. The overall photograph shows the entire scene and provides a first-hand representation of the nurse's observations. Precise measurements of the scene and location of the body are included in written documentation. The nurse

will photograph the exterior of buildings and street signs. This puts the scene into perspective, especially for those who do not respond to the scene. The orientation photograph brings the area of interest closer. For example, the photographer may show an area of injury in relation to other parts of the body. The close-up photograph zooms in on the area of interest. For example, the nurse may want to show soot in a gunshot wound, so the injury must be magnified or a photograph is taken as closely as possible.

Documentation is extremely important in the death investigation. Details of the incident, scene findings, and wounds are preserved through the use of narrative description, diagrams, and photographs. There is only one opportunity to document and record the scene and the decedent as initially found.

Courtroom Testimony

There are times when the forensic nurse will be required to testify in court. Testimony about the contents of the written report may be needed to corroborate other aspects of the case. Therefore, it is necessary to ensure all observations are objectively documented.

When subpoenaed, the nurse should immediately contact the sender of the subpoena. The case should be discussed. The nurse will go over the case prior to any testimony. The report, photographs, and diagrams made will all be reviewed. The nurse should testify truthfully when answering all questions about the case.

EVIDENCE-BASED PRACTICE

Clinical questions specific to the nursing actions in death investigations remain undeveloped and unstudied. The evidence collection may have been practiced for years and make it to court, but it is not solidly tested with science. Nursing actions and interventions for assessment and diagnosis remain in need of verification with research studies. Responsibilities inherent in the role, as in all nursing roles, can be documented and assessed for impact and effectiveness of outcomes. Outcomes for the forensic nurse in death investigations may be unique, as they will not improve health outcomes or quality of life for the deceased. Outcomes may be related to competencies, behaviors, and techniques used, and the family and community outcomes are related to responses to nursing actions.

In addition to the fact that other sciences will impact on forensic nursing science and evidence for best practice, Farid opines that forensic science informs understanding of health-care issues. Specifically reporting on pressure ulcers, Farid notes that written documentation, admission, and progressive images for documentation may eliminate questions.

Processes such as the stages of decaying tissue and development of wounds may be enhanced by studying autopsies and pathology findings. Forensic findings inform clinical practice as well. Advances in the theoretical knowledge and temporal frames of reference for staging of pressure ulcers can benefit from understanding the dynamics of tissue death and the progress of decomposition variations in different climates and parts of the body. Although pressure management may benefit from alternating patient positions, the ability to document alterations in tissue perfusion and when tissue integrity is diminished can help to lock in times when tissue damage initiated and reduce lawsuits due to more accurate documentation.

Clinical practice benefits from forensic practice in other ways as well. Epidemiological findings from studies of hospital deaths from trauma and the impact of illegal or violent acts in communities inform scientists about patterns of mortality and its causes, which will lead to innovative strategies for prevention and interventions with the living, will help to focus resources in different communities to address prevalent issues, and will improve outcomes with the living and the deceased.

The novelty of the role of nurse as death investigator is decreasing as the benefits of having nurses in the role are being demonstrated by growing opportunity in many state coroner and medical examiner offices. The development and refinement of the role will solidify nursing clinical questions from which evidence of best nursing practice will emerge as the inevitable next step.

CONCLUSIONS

This chapter describes many aspects of the death investigation and evidence developed on processes and practices, but there are abundant individual nuances that exist in each state and country. The forensic nurse plays an important role in the process, bringing forth the nursing knowledge that can be applied to its fullest. The forensic nurse has an understanding of disease processes and its effects on the human body. Family interaction, behavior observation, and teaching are core functions of nursing professionals, and these skills transfer readily to the death investigation. Families, public servants, and the public at large want to understand how their loved one died. The nurse is able to explain complicated medical terminology and be the liaison between the pathologist and the community.

Forensic principles of evidence collection are easily taught. They are applied in conjunction with the nursing process in the death investigation. The nurse assists in establishing such things as the estimated time of death, the number and type of trauma present, medical history, and the circumstances of the death through thorough written, diagrammatic, and photographic documentation. These written and photographic aids will enable the nurse to refresh his or her memory when testifying to any observation in court. The FNDI is the perfect complement to the medical examiner or coroner.

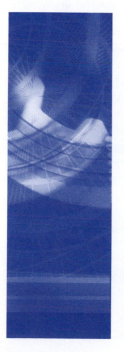

EVIDENCE-BASED PRACTICE

Reference Question: Do forensic nurses have a role in death investigations?

Database(s) to Search: PubMed, LexisNexis®

Search Strategy: "Forensic Nursing" should be used as a MeSH term and then "cause of death" as MeSH. Other terms related to "death" or "investigation" or "crime" may be helpful in locating more articles.

Selected References From Search:

1. Ciesiolka, S., Risse, M., Busch, B., & Verhoff, M.A. (2008). Philemon and Baucis death? Two cases of double deaths of married couples. *Forensic Science International, 176*(2-3):e7-10.
2. Gabriel, L.S. (2009). Patterns of injury in nonaccidental childhood fatalities. *Journal of Forensic Nursing, 5*(1):18-25.
3. Karger, B., Fracasso, T., & Pfeiffer, H. (2008). Fatalities related to medical restraint devices—Asphyxia is a common finding. *Forensic Science International, 178*(2-3): 178-184.
4. Hallady, J. (July 17, 2009). Nurses add detective work to their job skills: Program trains them to spot, collect evidence. *USA Today,* News: 3A.

(evidence-based practice continued on page 210)

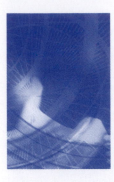

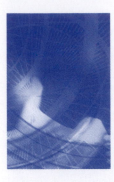*EVIDENCE-BASED PRACTICE* (continued)

Questions Used to Discern Evidence:

Choose two studies among the studies listed, read about them, and answer the following questions:

1. What are the differences between the two studies in the design, methods, and results?
2. What are the similarities between the two studies in the number of subjects, measures used, and interventions, if any?
3. What competencies do you need to acquire as a forensic nurse in death investigation?

REVIEW QUESTIONS

1. Which one of the following statements is true regarding death investigation in the United States?
   A. The medical examiner system is the oldest and most reliable.
   B. The coroner system originated in England, but was brought to this continent with the migration of the colonists.
   C. Forensic nurses can be elected to the office of Medical Examiner.
   D. The elected coroner is not allowed to sign the death certificate, only the physician is authorized to do so.

2. Manner of death refers to the classification of circumstances in which a death occurred. One example is:
   A. Gunshot wound
   B. Botched surgery
   C. Homicide
   D. Diagnosis of asthma

3. Extensive investigation may be required in a trauma or unnatural death based on:
   A. Circumstances of death and mechanism of injury
   B. Various circumstances, depending on medical examiner or coroner system
   C. Patient identification and insurance
   D. Absence of a qualified nurse investigator

4. Cause of death may include:
   A. Eye witness accounts
   B. Homicide
   C. Suicide
   D. Gunshot wound

5. Which one of the following is true regarding the forensic postmortem or autopsy examination?
   A. It is performed on all deceased persons.
   B. It can only be performed by the pathologist.
   C. Authority to perform is given by the family.
   D. Authority to perform is given by the state.

6. Nursing skills that may enhance outcomes in the death investigation role include:
   A. Nursing diagnoses and treatment plans
   B. Communication skills and critical thinking
   C. Knowledge of surgery techniques
   D. Nursing assessment knowledge

7. Which one of the following is a manner of death (MOD) that is consistent with the cause of death (COD)?
   A. COD: Cocaine toxicity; MOD: Overdose
   B. COD: Gunshot wound of the abdomen; MOD: Exsanguination
   C. COD: Hanging; MOD: Suicide
   D. COD: Exsanguination; MOD: Wrongful medication dosage

8. In the coroner system the following is true:
   A. Autopsies are done by the coroner.
   B. The coroner is always elected.
   C. The coroner is a physician, but not forensically trained.
   D. It is the system used in more than half of the states.

REVIEW QUESTIONS—cont'd

9. The medical examiner system:
   A. Uses only a medically trained forensic pathologist
   B. Uses a licensed physician
   C. Always convenes the inquest following a death
   D. Uses a licensed attorney

10. Deaths that are reportable to the coroner/medical examiner include:
   A. Inmates in public institutions
   B. Undiagnosed cancer patients
   C. Heart attacks
   D. All deaths in an ambulance

References

American Nurses Association (ANA). (2004). *Nursing scope and standards of practice.* Washington, DC: The American Nurses Association.

Basso, C., Burke, M., Fornes, P., et al. (2007). Guidelines for autopsy investigation of sudden cardiac death. *Virchows Archives, 452*:11-18.

Berman, A., Snider, S.J., Kozier, B., & Erb, G. (2008). *Fundamentals of nursing: Concepts, process, and practice.* (8th ed.). Upper Saddle River, NJ: Pearson Prentice-Hall.

Bowers, C.M. (2004). *Forensic dental evidence.* San Diego: Elsevier.

Clark, S.C., Ernst, M.F., Haglund, W.D., & Jentzen, J.M. (1996). *Medicolegal death investigator.* Big Rapids, MI: Occupational Research and Assessment, Inc.

Cohen, J.I. (2004). The forensic pathologist. Retrieved August 21, 2005, from: http://www.forensiconline.com/generallink.htm#a8

Descheneaux, K. (1991). Death investigations: How you can help. *Nursing, 21*(9):52-55.

DiMaio, V.J. (1999). *Gunshot wounds.* (2nd ed.). Boca Raton, CRC Press.

DiMaio, V.J., & DiMaio, D. (2001). *Forensic pathology.* (2nd ed.). Boca Raton: CRC Press.

Elger, B.S., Hofner, M.C., & Mangin, P. (2009). Research involving biological material from forensic autopsies: Legal and ethical issues. *Pathobiology, 76*(1):1-10.

Eliopulos, L.N. (1993). *Death investigator's handbook.* Boulder, CO: Paladin Press.

Hanzlick, R. (2007). *Death investigation: Systems and procedures.* Boca Raton: CRC Press.

Hanzlick, R., & Combs, D. (1998). Medical examiner and coroner systems: History and trends. *Journal American Medical Association, 279*(11):870-874.

Keys, E., Brownlee, C., Ruff, M., Baxter, C., Steele, L., & Green, F. (2008). How well do we communicate autopsy findings to next of kin? *Archives of Pathology Laboratory Medicine, 132*:66-71.

Knight, L.D., & Collins, K.A. (2005). A 25 year retrospective review of deaths due to pediatric neglect. *American Journal of Forensic Medicine and Pathology, 26*(3):221-228.

Knight, L.D., Hunsaker, D.M., & Corey, T.S. (2005). Cosleeping and sudden unexpected infant deaths in Kentucky. *American Journal of Forensic Medicine and Pathology, 26*(1):28-32.

Libow, L.S., & Neufeld, R.R. (2008). The autopsy and the elderly patient in the hospital and the nursing home: Enhancing the quality of life. *Geriatrics, 63*(12):14-28.

Lynch, V.A. (2006). *Forensic nursing.* St. Louis: Elsevier.

Mitchell, S. (2006). Integrating forensic nursing at the Harris County Medical Examiner's Office. National Association of Medical Examiners Scientific Meeting. Platform presentation. San Antonio, TX.

Pattison, N. (2008). Caring for patients after death. *Nursing Standard, 22*(51):49-56.

Ransom, D. (2003). Death investigation. In J. Payne-James, A. Busuttil, & W. Smock (Eds.). *Forensic medicine: Clinical and pathological aspects.* San Francisco: Greenwich Medical Media.

Saferstein, R. (2004). *Criminalistics.* (8th ed.). Upper Saddle River, NJ: Pearson Prentice Hall.

Scholing, M., Saltzherr, T., Fung Kon Jin, P., Ponsen, et al. (2009). The value of postmortem computed tomography as an alternative for autopsy in trauma victims: A systematic review. *European Radiology, 19*:2333-2341.

Scott, C., Swartz, E., & Warburton, K. (2006). The psychological autopsy: Solving the mysteries of death. *Psychiatric Clinics of North America, 29*:805-822.

Spitz, W.U. (1993). *Spitz and Fisher's Medicolegal investigation of death.* (3rd ed.). Springfield, IL: Charles C. Thomas.

Texas Code of Criminal Procedure. Chap. 49, Art. 49.25, Medical examiners. Retrieved February 4, 2009, from http://law.justia.com/texas/codes/cr/001.00.000049.00.html

The American Heritage Dictionary of the English Language, (4th ed.). Retrieved August 21, 2005, from Answers.com web site at http://www.answers.com/topic/coroner-1

N.A. (2005). The history of fingerprints. Why fingerprint identification? Retrieved October 2, 2005, from http://onin.com/fp/fphistory.html

Vaartjes, I., Henrix, A., Hertogh, E., Grabbee, D., et al. (2009). Sudden death in persons younger than 40 years of aged: Incidence and causes. *European Journal of Cardiology Prevention and Rehabilitation, 19*:592-596.

Vessier-Batchen, M. (2003). Forensic nurse death investigators. *The Web Mystery Magazine.* Retrieved September 12, 2005, from www.lifeloom.com

World Health Organization. United Nation's Children's Fund. (1994). Measurement of overall and cause specific mortality in infants and children: Memorandum from a WHO/UNICEF meeting. *Bulletin of the World Health Organization,* PMID: 7955018, 72:707-713.

Zercie, K.B., & Penders, P. (2006). Concepts of photography in forensic nursing. In R.M. Hammer, B. Moynihan, & E.M. Pagliaro (Eds.). *Forensic nursing: A handbook for practice.* Sudbury, MA: Jones and Bartlett.

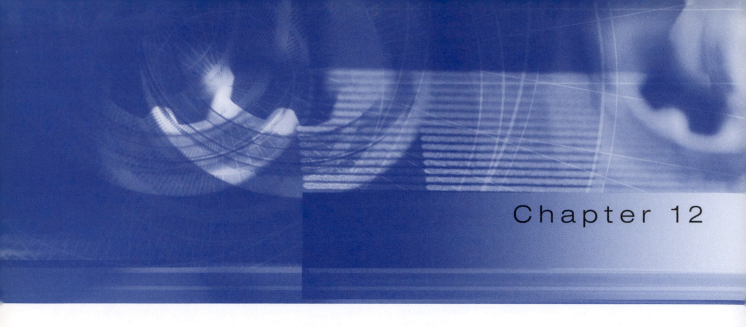

Chapter 12

Evidence: Collection, Preservation, Databases, and Cold Cases

Elaine M. Pagliaro

"We all participate in weaving the social fabric; we should therefore all participate in patching the fabric when it develops holes."

Anne C. Weisberg

Competencies

1. Understanding the role of evidence in the justice system.
2. Recognizing the types of physical evidence.
3. Determining the appropriate steps to take to preserve the physical and legal integrity of evidence.
4. Knowing how to preserve DNA evidence to avoid contamination and degradation of biological samples.
5. Understanding the various types of DNA analysis and the application of each to various types of physical evidence.
6. Recognizing the role of DNA analysis in the identification of suspects in unsolved cases.
7. Reiterating appropriate evidence guidelines for postconviction DNA testing.
8. Understanding the legal and ethical requirements for appropriate handling of evidence.

Key Terms

Biological evidence
Chain of custody
CODIS
Cold case
Contamination
DNA
DNA database
Documentation
Evidence integrity
Locard's Principle of Exchange
Mitochondrial DNA
Physical evidence
Polymerase chain reaction
Scientific evidence
Relevant evidence
Trace evidence

INTRODUCTION

Evidence gathered at a crime scene, from a victim, or from an alleged perpetrator must be collected and preserved properly for it to be admissible in a criminal proceeding. Forensic nurses must be aware of and follow strict guidelines throughout the evidence collection process. These guidelines include:

1. Ensuring that proper documentation is made prior to handling evidence
2. Maintaining the chain of custody or paper trail of how and by whom the evidence was handled
3. Applying appropriate analysis methods
4. Upholding legal and ethical standards
5. Preserving evidence properly so that it is usable in the future

The advent of DNA testing has revolutionized forensic analysis of biological evidence and greatly affected criminal proceedings. Various methods of DNA analysis, typing, and interpretation are discussed in this chapter.

In 1990, the FBI Laboratory developed the Combined DNA Index System (CODIS). This program provides software that enables federal, state, and local forensic laboratories to exchange and compare DNA profiles electronically. This tool has been instrumental in assisting law enforcement personnel to identify perpetrators by enabling them to submit a DNA profile from an evidence sample for comparison against profiles from convicted offenders currently in the CODIS database.

In addition to identifying a particular person as the perpetrator of a crime, DNA evidence has also been used by The Innocence Project to clear those who have been wrongly convicted.

The forensic nurse can play an important role in the collection, processing, analysis, and preservation of evidence.

Case Study

THE FORENSIC NURSE AND MOTOR VEHICLE ACCIDENT VICTIM

On a cold afternoon in October, two hunters discovered a partially clad young woman at the edge of the woods near a dirt road. She appeared to have been dumped in the area where she was found. She was severely injured and unconscious. The victim was immediately rushed to the hospital, where it was determined that she had multiple blunt force trauma consistent with motor vehicle impact. Her remaining clothing was removed in the emergency department (ED) during the initial examination. Because of the patient's condition, an ED employee with forensic nursing training collected the woman's clothing according to protocols appropriate for trace evidence preservation. The nurse had a discussion with her supervisor as to whether samples should be taken in the event that the woman was a victim of sexual assault; because of the need for immediate surgery, these samples were not collected. However, the nurse did retain the sheet that was under the woman while she was in the ED.

When the victim became conscious a few days later, she disclosed to medical personnel that she had been riding her bicycle on a deserted road when she heard a vehicle approaching from behind. She remembered little after that and had no explanation for her condition when she was found. At that time the patient consented to the release of evidence and agreed to speak with law enforcement.

The clothing and the sheet from the ED were sent to the laboratory. A search of the victim's shirt revealed rust, small fragments of automotive paint, and several black carpet-type fibers. The paint was determined to be similar to that used on Jeep-type vehicles in the late 1980s; the presence of rust on the sample with small pieces of the same paint adhered to the metal further supported the conclusion that the woman was hit by an older vehicle. Police began searching for owners of a Jeep who lived in the area where the woman was traveling when she was hit. Four such persons were identified.

The laboratory also found a small semen stain on the sheet that had been under the victim. DNA analysis and subsequent search of the evidence sperm-fraction profile against the state and national DNA databases did not reveal a suspect. The four persons who owned Jeeps were asked to supply buccal swabs for DNA comparison. Two of these men did provide DNA samples and were eliminated. One of the other persons drank a soda when the police questioned him. His soda can was swabbed and the DNA profile matched the semen from the sheet. A search warrant resulted in location of the suspect's Jeep with apparent recent damage. A sneaker matching the one the victim had on in the ED was found stuffed under the seat.

Because hospital personnel were aware of proper evidence collection procedures and the value of such evidence in forensic science investigation, the victim was able to see the man whose vehicle hit her, who sexually assaulted her, and who left her to die in a deserted wood brought to justice.

NATURE AND IMPORTANCE OF EVIDENCE

Legal Requirements for Evidence

As the above case study shows, awareness of the nature and importance of evidence in legal cases is among the most valuable forensic knowledge a nurse can have. Evidence is what attorneys use to "prove" their cases. Evidence is much more than either physical or eyewitness evidence. In court **relevant evidence** is anything that "makes the existence of any fact that is of consequence to the determination of the legal action more or less probable." Thus, evidence can be documents, medical observations, witness or suspect statements, patient statements, physical evidence, patterns, photographs, medical records, sounds, or anything else that can be shown to be related to a significant point in the legal case. The possibilities are almost endless. Clearly, relevant evidence is critical for proper investigation of an incident and, if collected and documented properly, any subsequent legal proceedings.

Just because evidence has been used in an investigation and is relevant to a case, however, does not mean that the attorney will be allowed to present that evidence in court. This is especially true when physical evidence is analyzed. Evidence must also be reliable for it to be used in trial or some other administrative hearing. Unless evidence can be relied on without significant questions, that evidence will never be heard by the trier of fact. Standards have been established in common law to assist the court in determining if expert testimony and evidence are reliable. These standards have been codified in both the *Federal Rules of Evidence* (2007) and the evidence codes of individual states. Several safeguards are in place in the legal system and forensic community to ensure the reliability of other types of evidence. For example, the rules against allowing hearsay, by definition unreliable in most circumstances, prevent statements made by others not present in the court to be related by another witness. Exceptions to the hearsay rules do exist, however, including statements made by patients to medical workers during treatment. These statements are considered more reliable because of the circumstances under which the information is conveyed. The court believes that a patient being questioned as part of a medical examination is going to tell the truth so he or she can obtain the best and most appropriate medical care. It is this exception that allows statements made by victims of sexual assault to be related by the Sexual Assault Nurse Examiner/Sexual Assault Forensic Examiner (SANE/SAFE) when testifying at a criminal trial. Other rules that ensure reliability of evidence require authentication of a document or photograph by an individual who can attest to its origins and that it is unaltered.

For any item of evidence that is going to be introduced at trial, an appropriate chain of custody for that physical evidence must be shown. The investigator must be able to account for the location and possession of evidence from the time it is identified until it is presented in the court. A detailed discussion of chain of custody requirements for physical evidence is provided in this chapter.

Investigators, medical practitioners, risk management consultants, and many others who often find themselves dealing with evidence are well trained in identifying relevant evidence and maintaining its integrity and reliability.

Classification of Physical Evidence

During the past few years, numerous television shows and movies about forensic science and crime scene investigation have become very popular. These television shows deal with the identification and analysis of what is referred to as physical or scientific evidence. Research has shown that there is a significant effect on the actions of jury members when they are exposed to stories about physical evidence and its potential to include or exclude a suspect (Tyler, 2006). **Physical evidence** is defined as material of a tangible or observable nature that may provide a fact relevant to the truth of what occurred or clarify a point at issue. **Scientific evidence,** which is physical evidence materials to which analytical procedures and the scientific method are applied to obtain facts, has become a critical part of many legal proceedings.

Some criminal and civil trials today will not proceed unless there is a presentation of physical or scientific evidence and the results of analysis of that evidence. As author Katherine Ramsland (2006) notes: "Through a proliferation of forensic television programs, the mass media has offered the public an education of sorts about forensic science and investigation, with a threefold effect. Until recently, a key issue in the legal process has been how to translate scientific testimony to laypeople on a jury, but these television shows have made potential jurors somewhat savvier about scientific methods and evidence. As a result, they often expect it and even look for better results than can be produced or techniques that may not exist. Thus, they may translate testimony from imperfect or technologically unsophisticated investigations into reasonable doubt and decline to convict."

Because of the expectations these programs have created, if no significant physical or medical evidence exists in a case, attorneys will often call experts to testify about reasons why there might not be such evidence. Common situations include the absence of semen and DNA or physical injuries in a sexual assault case.

In the early 20th century, a French criminologist, Edmond Locard, held that any time two objects come in contact with each other there is a mutual exchange of materials. **Locard's Principle of Exchange** became the basis of modern scientific investigation in criminal and civil cases. The transfer of materials between objects and the persistence of trace and transfer evidence on items continue to generate research studies. The proper identification, collection, and evaluation of transfer evidence are critical for justice to be served.

Physical evidence may be classified in many different ways. Classification schemes may be based on the nature or composition of the evidence, the analysis conducted on the evidence, or the type of incident investigated. Grouping evidence according to its nature may assist in determining its origin. Pattern evidence requires an answer to the question "What object or action created the pattern?" Types of evidence analysis include DNA analysis, firearms testing, fingerprint comparison, and tool marks. Classification by this method can be useful when considering the value of the evidence, but it may result in loss of evidence that can be subject to more than one type of testing. It is also useful to consider the nature of the incident when identifying and analyzing evidence. Incidents such as accidents, arson, medical malpractice, and sexual assault, for example, each have a different basis and set of factors that must be excluded or proved by evidence. Because classifying evidence by the type of incident or event concentrates on the legal or medical requirement that must be met, this helps the practitioner weigh the significance of each piece of evidence as it is identified and determine the scope of the incident. In addition, classifying by event relies on previous experience and national standards to assist practitioners when they evaluate patients, victims, injuries, or scenes.

COLLECTION AND PRESERVATION OF EVIDENCE

No matter what classification method is used to aid in the identification of evidence or the potential impact of an analysis, that evidence will be of little help in case evaluation if it is not properly collected and preserved. As the following case example shows, the importance of using appropriate procedures when handling evidence cannot be overstated.

Evidence that is well maintained can provide conclusive results even decades after collection. If, however, a sample is not properly packaged and maintained, the value of that evidence could be lost forever. In fact, if evidence is improperly handled, **contamination** can occur that alters the evidence to the extent that analyses could provide false associations or exclusions. This is particularly true in the collection and preservation of biological evidence. The discriminating power of DNA analysis and its potential to exonerate those who are falsely charged or convicted have been well publicized. The potential to identify suspects in crimes from biological evidence through use of DNA databases is unequaled. However, if evidence does not meet the scientific and

Case Study

VALUE OF FORENSIC EVIDENCE IN DEATH OF A STUDENT

A local university student was walking back to her dormitory from the student union late one Saturday night. While crossing the street to the main campus, she was struck by a motor vehicle. The car did not stop. Witnesses attempted to help the student and called 911. Within minutes the student was rushed to the university hospital, where she received emergency treatment. Her outer clothing was removed for medical procedures. One of the nurses on duty collected and packaged each item of clothing in clean paper as it was removed. That evidence was secured in a filing cabinet designated for such purposes until picked up by campus police. The student did not recover from her injuries. Although there were several witnesses, none could describe in any detail the vehicle that struck the student. Each item of clothing was examined at the laboratory, and each revealed different information that was useful in identifying the type of vehicle: paint smears on the victim's pants were analyzed and compared to the national paint database; possible make and model numbers were supplied to the police. A piece of broken plastic, less than ½ inch in size was found in the folds of her jacket. When the suspected SUV was located in the garage of the owner, that piece was subsequently physically fitted to a broken headlight structure on the vehicle. Rubber and other materials located on her shoes provided additional circumstantial evidence in the case. These items of evidence provided sufficient proof that the SUV located in another state was the vehicle involved in the hit and run accident. Because the evidence was collected quickly and appropriately and was secured until collected, there was no challenge to the physical evidence that linked the SUV to the crime. The driver of the SUV subsequently pled guilty to vehicular manslaughter.

legal requirements for proper collection and preservation, the value of that evidence is quickly lost.

Evidence Collection Guidelines

Nursing today involves interaction with numerous representatives of the law enforcement and justice systems. The background that nursing provides in critical thinking provides a good basis for the proper handling of evidence. The following discussion provides some general guidelines for the collection and preservation of various types of physical evidence.

By keeping in mind that the evidence must be "reliable" and its integrity must be without question, some common errors in collection and packaging can be avoided. **Evidence integrity** is usually shown in courts and other legal proceedings by providing proof of how the evidence was collected and that the evidence has not been altered. A chain of custody for each item of evidence is one way that this proof is shown. Forms and labels are commercially available to assist in the collection of complete chain of custody information.

Chain of Custody

The **chain of custody** usually begins when a practitioner locates or obtains physical evidence. That evidence must be properly documented as to how and where it is located prior to its collection. Any documentation of an item of evidence should begin with a description of the item, the date and time it was recovered, and from where it was recovered. The case or identification number must be noted as well as the number for the item itself. The initials or signature of the practitioner collecting the evidence should also appear. In some instances, such as standardized sexual assault evidence kits, recording the identification information is a simple process: the medical professional simply supplies the "chain" information in the appropriate locations on preprinted forms or packages. However, such standardized packages are not required for evidence to be documented properly.

Any subsequent transfer of that evidence item, such as from a SANE or a forensic nurse to a police officer, must also be documented. This paper trail that follows the transfer of evidence will provide a clear history as to how the evidence was handled and by whom. When documenting, it is best that the practioner include more rather than less information, as it may be important at a later time in the investigation. Because most evidence will be evaluated or presented in a legal proceeding some time after collection, the failure to note appropriate details could result in difficulties during testimony. The medical witness may not remember sufficient details of the procedures or item to be able to offer complete and accurate testimony. Improperly documented evidence or chain of custody could also result in a judge ruling that a piece of evidence is inadmissible during court proceedings.

Documentation of Evidence

If physical evidence, such as body fluid stains or trace evidence, is identified at a scene or during the examination of a patient, that evidence should be thoroughly documented prior to collection. There are many methods of **documentation** available, including notes, photographs, sketches and diagrams, and video or audio recording. Each method has advantages and should be employed as seems appropriate to the practitioner and the situation. As with other aspects of nursing, thorough and extensive notes are the foundation of good evidence documentation. These notes can provide the practitioner with important information after evidence collection. Notes also provide the link to other evidence documentation methods and key documents, such as chain of custody. In the collection of evidence from victims of abuse, for example, diagrams noting the location of injuries should accompany descriptive notes of any injuries noted.

Photographs of those injuries should also be taken at the time of examination. Whenever photographs are taken, an appropriate scale should be included to document the size and appearance of those injury patterns. Afterward, photographs should be taken without a scale. Attention to the curvature and shadows that may result from the location of those patterns is important. The "rule of three" is often used when photographing evidence (Zercie & Penders, 2006). This rule states that, at a minimum, evidence should be photographed (1) from an overall, (2) middle distance, and (3) close-up view to provide the context and detail necessary for good documentation. Additional photographs should be taken as needed to ensure proper representation of the injury. Such documentation is extremely important for reference at a later date. Proper photographic documentation has proven invaluable in assessing cases that have come up for postconviction review.

In clinical environments, it is important to have policies in place regarding use of photography to document injuries relating to trauma as well as domestic violence, sexual assault, or any means of abuse. These guidelines should include recommendations as to when photographs are indicated and what should be done with those photographs after they are taken. Improper storage of photographs that document physical injuries could result in that evidence being excluded during trial.

COLLECTION AND PACKAGING OF EVIDENCE

In general, physical evidence should be packaged to prevent alteration of the evidence or deleterious change. No matter when or how the evidence is collected, the evidence seal is one of the most important ways to demonstrate the integrity of the physical evidence. Use of a tamper-evident seal—a seal that will be broken whenever a package has been opened—assures the court and all who handle the evidence that it has not been handled or altered unknowingly. To further demonstrate the integrity of the seal, the individual who packages the evidence will initial, and often date, the evidence seal. Anyone who subsequently opens the package should do the same in an area away from the evidence seal. After laboratory analysis, for example, the scientist will place a new tamper-evident seal over the opening that was made in the package. Thus, when the evidence is used in court, there is a visible history of how many times, if at all, a package was opened and by whom.

The following guidelines for the packaging of commonly encountered physical evidence provide the general principles for handling various classes of evidence. More detailed suggestions are presented for the preservation and collection of biological evidence because of its great potential for individualizing evidence (linking to a particular person) and because it may be a source of contention in court proceedings. In general, common sense and an awareness of potential evidence in various nursing environments will prevent compromising physical evidence in most situations. The practitioner may rely on training and experience to determine what to collect, how it should be collected, and how much to collect. It is essential for the forensic nurse to be familiar with collection and packaging guidelines specific to the jurisdiction where the evidence will be tested.

Clothing

Each item should be collected separately and placed into a separate paper bag to avoid cross-contamination. If articles of clothing are wet, they should be air-dried on or over clean paper to collect trace materials before packaging. If this is not possible, articles may be put *temporarily* into separate plastic bags to avoid leakage or cross-contamination. Then, as soon as possible, the items must be opened one at a time in a place where they can be dried without the possibility of cross-contamination, such as in a drying room or evidence-drying cabinet. If evidence is not stored separately or dried appropriately, evidence can be transferred from one item to another. McNally and colleagues looked at physical evidence of various types submitted to a forensic laboratory and the results obtained from the analysis of biological stains on these items. They found if clothing is not completely dry prior to packaging, bacterial or mold growth, contamination, and breakdown of biological evidence often results. Even if the DNA actually remains unaffected, the improper packaging of wet evidence may raise questions in the mind of the trier of fact as to the reliability of any DNA profiles obtained from that evidence.

Any patterns on the clothing, including stains, transfer patterns, holes, or other damage, must be carefully noted at the time of collection. Practitioners should make every effort to preserve these patterns when packaging the evidence so that forensic specialists can examine the evidence at a later date. Clean paper placed on clothing that has bloodstain or semen patterns, for example, prior to folding it may prevent transfer of the body fluid to other portions of the garment or smudging of the pattern. Schwoeble found that the method of packaging and preserving clothing, such as keeping the items flat and wrapped in clean butcher-type waxed paper, limits the loss of gunshot particles and the alteration of gunshot residue patterns. A frequent mistake made by first responders and hospital personnel is to cut through the patient's clothing at the site of bullet holes, stab wounds, or tears in the fabric made by a penetrating object. When damage patterns are altered by subsequent actions by medical personnel, forensic laboratory examiners are often limited in their ability to interpret the patterns due to the evidence alteration. While it may be necessary to cut through clothing for proper medical treatment, defects in the clothing should be left intact whenever possible. Loss of evidence or alteration of body fluid patterns can often occur when clothing is removed from a patient in the emergency department. Hairs, fibers, body fluids, and other trace materials can sometimes be lost or gained when clothing is discarded on the floor during medical procedures. Chewning and colleagues (2009) conducted a controlled study of the persistence of fiber evidence, noting that even in that controlled situation, fibers were lost and transferred to other surfaces during packaging and handling. Thus, careful handling of items by the practitioner can help ensure the integrity of the physical evidence before it is examined in a laboratory by a forensic scientist.

Footwear

Footwear should be packaged separately from the clothing and each shoe packaged individually. Soil or other trace materials may collect within the grooves and ridges of the soles of shoes and may be linked to a source at a scene or from a vehicle. For example, a minute piece of metal found in the sole of a work boot collected from a suspect was found to match a piece of a broken lamp at the scene of an assault and removed from the victim's head wound. If footwear is placed with the other clothing, this same evidence could transfer to the other items in the package; such contamination of physical evidence could be detrimental to subsequent inquiries. Important evidence that may be gained from footwear also includes footwear sole patterns, stains, and evidence of blood spatter. In cases where footwear prints or shoe impressions are noted, these should be photographed with a scale for comparison to collected footwear.

Hairs, Fibers, and Other Trace Evidence

Hair and fiber evidence are among the most common forms of **trace evidence** encountered in case investigations. Often, the value of the hairs or fibers is unknown until samples are also collected from known parties and the various locations related to the incident. When handling trace evidence of unknown origin, it is important to package each questioned item (item of unknown origin) separately. Hairs may have root tissue that can provide information as to whether the hair was forcibly removed and on which standard DNA analysis can be conducted. Consequently, each hair should be placed on a separate sheet of paper, which is folded and placed in an envelope. This method prevents cross-contamination, damage to the hair, and potential loss. (A similar method should be employed for individual fibers that are collected.)

Hairs or fibers found on a victim's body are best preserved by carefully removing them. When appropriate, hair and fiber evidence may be collected by area, for example, the patient's right hand, or by pubic combing, although the occurrence of hair transfer in some types of cases may be very low. As early as 1998, Exline and colleagues demonstrated in a controlled study with heterosexual volunteers the low incidence of pubic hair transfers during intercourse, with only about 17% of the pairs showing some exchange. These researchers also noted that hairs were transferred more often to the male partner.

Hair and fiber evidence should *not* be removed from an article of clothing unless there is concern about damage or loss because the location of that trace on an item may have significance in a case investigation. In general, clothing that contains trace materials should be carefully folded and placed in a clean paper bag or in paper wrapping. If there is a concern that folding the item will redistribute the trace evidence, then the item should be wrapped flat in paper.

Biological Stains or Deposits

This category of evidence includes a large number of materials that can be found in several forms. The most commonly encountered types of **biological evidence** include blood, semen, saliva, tissue, and unprocessed plant materials. The method of choice for the collection and preservation of biological evidence primarily depends on the physical state of the evidence (wet, moist, or dry), the substrate on which the evidence is deposited, and the types of analyses that will be conducted. Since DNA analysis is the focus of many inquiries involving biological evidence, the forensic nurse must ensure that the biological evidence is not subject to alteration, degradation, or deterioration during collection, storage, or laboratory analysis. Extensive guidelines for the collection and preservation of biological evidence have been published. These recommendations are based on reviews of techniques employed by scientists in various jurisdictions, validation studies, analyses conducted by the authors and their coworkers, the results of screening tests, the quantity and quality of DNA obtained from the samples, and the potential for loss or contamination. Specific evidence collection guidelines, techniques, and choice of collection products vary somewhat among jurisdictions, depending on the experiences of medical personnel and laboratory analytical protocols. For example, Osborn and Neff (1989) and Gaensslen and Lee (2002) all found that whether hair was collected, or how it was collected, in sexual assault cases depended on the analytical capabilities of the local forensic science laboratory.

The following is a summary of the most commonly employed techniques for biological evidence.

Dried or semidried secretions on hard surfaces should be swabbed with a sterile cotton swab moistened with sterile water or saline. A minimum of liquid should be used to wet the swab to prevent dilution of the sample. Samples should not be scraped for collection purposes due to the risk of loss and contamination by small flakes of biological material. Multiple swabs should be avoided when small stain areas are being collected because this divides available material rather than concentrating the DNA on one swab. When feasible, swabs should be air-dried before packaging. Techniques for air-drying samples include drying swabs in a rack before inserting them into paper envelopes, using swab dryers to facilitate the drying process, and using commercially available tubes that cover the swab while allowing airflow. Caution should be used to avoid cross-contamination from other specimens in the dryer or the swab rack. Any drying apparatus must be cleaned with diluted bleach, treated with commercial DNA decontamination spray, or irradiated with UV light before and after each use to avoid contamination. Also, a dryer that has fans but no filters may introduce foreign airborne particles or bacteria onto the collected sample. One should also take care where the dryer is used because indoor environmental dust particles often contain skin cells. Toothman and colleagues obtained human DNA in 97% of environmental dust swabs tested, and most significantly, more than 60% of these samples yielded DNA alleles above the minimum limit of detection. Based on these results, the introduction of dust onto a case swab could potentially add alleles to DNA profiles and produce erroneous results.

Specially designed swab collection kits that allow collecting and subsequent drying of swabs within a container that allows airflow are commercially available. These kits allow collection and drying without the risk of contamination that may be present in a swab rack or dryer. Studies have shown that the swab dries within 3 to 5 hours in these boxes, with 100% of the samples yielding accurate screening tests and DNA profiles. Heat lamps or hair dryers should *never* be used to dry biological samples; researchers have known for years that heat degrades enzymes used for screening biological materials and breaks down DNA.

Liquid biological samples on hard surfaces, such as glass, tile, counters, and painted walls, may be collected in a sterile tube and refrigerated until submitted for analysis. If blood is collected, the tube should contain ethylene diamine tetracetic acid (EDTA) as a preservative. Tubes should not contain saline or other liquid that will dilute the sample. Liquid should not be frozen, since multiple freeze-thaw cycles degrade the sample and may make DNA results inconclusive. If the evidence cannot be brought to the laboratory in a timely manner, the liquid biological sample should be absorbed onto sterile swabs and air-dried.

Biological stains on absorbent surfaces, such as clothing, upholstery, carpets, etc., are best collected as a whole whenever possible. Warren (1991) studied several methods of collecting bloodstains from various surfaces and confirmed that direct removal of a stain on an absorbent surface yields the most conclusive results. If the item on which the stain has been deposited is large, the sample should be cut out and packaged in a clean, properly labeled envelope. There is no need to collect an unstained portion of the substrate unless required to do so by the local testing laboratory. Packaging must ensure that no transfer to other stain areas occurs; thus, individual stains from the same item should be packaged separately.

Tissue from wounds, at scenes or from medical procedures, should be packaged in clean, sterile glass or plastic containers. No liquid of any type should be added to these tissues. It is important not to add preservative to the tissue if it is collected as part of a medical procedure, for example, the product of conception from abortion or other surgically removed material. Some preservatives, such as formaldehyde substitutes and alcohol, may denature the DNA in the sample making the tissue unsuitable for some analytical procedures.

Firearms, Bullets, and Projectiles

Firearms and projectiles may contain various types of physical evidence, such as fibers, hairs, blood, and tissue. In the case of projectiles, they also may contain individual markings that allow for comparison to known firearms. Therefore, packaging of these objects must prevent the loss of trace amounts of materials and alteration of the individual characteristics. Firearms should be secured to prevent movement and should be made "safe" whenever possible before they are handled and packaged. Firearms should never be packaged in a paper envelope. Other than to ensure safety, firearms should be handled as little as possible and only while wearing gloves. Weapons are often swabbed for "touch" DNA, that is, for the DNA profile of the person(s) who handled the weapon. Thus, excessive handling of weapons could add biological material to the item or remove fingerprints and other evidence. Projectiles, fragments, and other small materials should be packaged in clean, paper druggist folds or gauze before sealing them in a clean envelope. The surface of the object should be protected from rubbing against hard surfaces or other objects to preserve evidence integrity.

Sharps

Sharp objects, such as needles, razor blades, glass fragments, or knives need to be secured in such a way that prevents injury to others and that preserves trace evidence on the item. Knives, for example, should be tied into cardboard holders or placed into specially designed sharps containers and be secured in cardboard boxes of the appropriate size. Specimen containers may be used to secure needles, razor blades, or pieces of broken glass.

Chemicals and Drugs

In cases of suspected poisoning, use of controlled substances, or effects from prescription medications, the collection of appropriate evidence and documentation is extremely important for treatment of the patient who presents at a medical facility or during a death investigation. At all times, the practitioner should ensure that all evidence is handled appropriately so that fingerprints, which may be important for linkage, or other evidence is not destroyed. If controlled substances are suspected, those drugs and associated materials should be noted to assist the toxicologist in the analysis of autopsy samples. In cases of suspected poisoning or prescription drug overdose, it is important for the medical team or forensic death investigator to obtain a social and medical history of the deceased. The practitioner should also take an inventory of prescription medications found at the scene or on the patient. Notes associated with the medications should include the following information, when available:

- Name of the patient
- Name of the medication
- Dosage
- Number dispensed
- Date filled
- Quantity of medication remaining in the container(s)
- Physician's name
- Pharmacy that dispensed the order

This information can be helpful when determining appropriate treatment for a surviving patient or can assist the forensic pathologist or death investigator during an autopsy. In addition, a medication record may be important when determining the cause of death. As with other evidence, any medications found at a scene should be photographed in place prior to complete inventory of the materials. Packaging should be appropriate for the type of container, such as paper or plastic bags, and a tamper-evident seal is necessary.

If poison is suspected, the investigator should look for possible sources of the chemical substance. Poisons can be introduced into the body by several methods. Thus, the critical thinking skills of the practitioner are extremely important when assessing the potential poisons in the environment and the possible method used to introduce the toxin to the body. In some cases, such as when Munchausen syndrome by proxy is suspected, Artingstall reported that poisonous agents used by perpetrators in the cases she reviewed often were readily available materials in the home or hospital room. In several reported cases, household cleaners, alcohols, and construction materials were found in appropriate locations in the suspect's home or workplace and were not initially considered as potential causes of the symptoms in the juvenile patients.

Legal Considerations for Evidence Collection and Documentation

Typically, biological standard materials, including blood or buccal swabs and hairs, are required during investigations. These materials are used for comparison to samples of unknown origin in criminal, accident, and paternity investigations. In cases of sexual assault, for example, the sexual assault evidence collection kit provides an appropriate means of collecting these samples as required by each jurisdiction to conduct forensic analysis and comparison. These "known" samples are requested from the victim, who has consented to the collection after appropriate explanation and counseling. Most jurisdictions provide for a signed consent during the sexual assault examination, which ensures the patient is aware of the purpose of the samples and her or his right to refuse to have the samples collected. This is especially important when collecting blood or urine in cases of suspected drug-facilitated sexual assault. Since testing at a forensic laboratory will show the presence of any drug present, even in small quantities or if taken willingly by the patient, it is important that the consent make clear the nature of the tests and, again, the patient's right to refuse the collection.

Known samples for comparison to evidence may also be requested from the suspected perpetrator by law enforcement. While a suspect can consent to this collection, consent should be obtained in written form. It is often necessary for law enforcement to obtain a search warrant from a judge to obtain samples from a suspect. The warrant process protects the suspect's constitutional rights and can assist in maintaining the proper chain of evidence. Some states may require a special warrant if clothing or other possessions of a suspect are to be collected and tested at a laboratory. In *all* instances, if the forensic nurse practitioner is asked by law enforcement to collect samples from an individual, a copy of the written consent or the signed search warrant should be made available to the nurse before the collection begins. It is a good practice to place a copy of the consent or warrant in the case file. Similar practices should be followed if samples are being collected at the request of the defense. Any practitioner who is likely to receive requests for the collection of known samples should consult with the local bar association and become familiar with the legal requirements for collecting evidentiary samples from suspects and victims.

Whenever documentation associated with evidence collection from victims or suspects is completed, the practitioner should consider issues of confidentiality as outlined by the Health Insurance Portability and Accountability Act (HIPAA) Section 160.103-191. Law enforcement officers will often request information related to these examinations; questions about HIPPA requirements could cause difficulty for health-care workers in these circumstances. In general, any person or institution that has physical control of health information must follow the HIPAA guidelines as they pertain to privacy and security. HIPAA sets guidelines for the use of forms for the release of medical information. Most health-care facilities will have established policies and procedures for implementing such forms. In addition, standard forms may be developed by other practitioners that could be used by the health-care professional. The standard consent forms included with many sexual assault evidence collection kits, for example, make it clear that the examination records and evidence may be provided to members of the criminal justice system for legal purposes. This statement, along with appropriate counseling and reporting of the assault to the police, may meet the standards necessary to release the appropriate materials in a victim's medical file. In addition, most law enforcement personnel will obtain a separate, appropriate written consent or search warrant to obtain the medical information that will be used as evidence in a case investigation.

Medical diagrams, notes, and photographic images are increasingly important as documentation and as evidence in legal proceedings. Policies and procedures regarding security of images, whether in hard copy or in digital form, must be implemented so that the privacy and confidentially of the patient is ensured. Specific reference to documentation should be included in any authorization for the release of this type of information. Each practitioner should be familiar with the procedures of the health-care facility in which the practitioner works regarding consent and the release of medical records.

DNA EVIDENCE

DNA has become a primary method employed in the fields of forensic science, forensic medicine, anthropology, botany, and paternity testing. The strength of DNA as evidence is based on its stability combined with the sensitivity and discriminating power of DNA analytical techniques. While only about 40% of forensic cases contain biological materials suitable for DNA analysis, for those cases using DNA testing the possibility of solving them greatly increases (U.S. DOJ, 2006).

Case Study

VALUE OF DNA EVIDENCE IN A SERIES OF CASES

In 1990, a woman was found unconscious and badly injured behind a local fitness center. She was partially clothed and had several bruises, stab wounds, and a bite mark on her shoulder. When she was taken to the hospital for medical assistance, a sex crimes evidence kit was collected, which included swabs of the bite mark; vaginal, oral, and anal samples; and pubic combings. Fibers and vegetation were noted on the victim's back and collected by medical personnel. After she regained consciousness, the woman reported that she had been abducted by a man who drove a dark-colored van. She could not describe the man, who initially wore a ski mask.

DNA analysis had recently been initiated in several laboratories in the country. Extracts of the bite mark swabs yielded insufficient DNA for the DNA restriction fragment length polymorphism (RFLP) testing of the time. While the anal swab demonstrated the presence of semen, the DNA obtained from the sample was degraded and was also unsuitable for DNA analysis. Because there was no named suspect in the case, little forensic comparisons could be done to identify a perpetrator.

In 1998, two homicides of women occurred in the same city. Semen was identified in samples taken from the victims at autopsy. DNA analysis was conducted, and the DNA profiles obtained from semen taken from both women were identical. Because there was no known suspect, the male DNA profile was searched against the DNA database. No match was obtained in 1998. Around this time, the samples in the 1992 case were retested using the latest DNA technology. The profiles from the bite mark also matched the profiles from the homicide victims. In addition, trace materials collected from the homicide victims were found to contain fibers that were microscopically and instrumentally similar to the fibers from the back of the woman who was kidnapped. This additional physical evidence provided additional support that the women were all transported in the same vehicle.

In 2005, a "hit" was reported between the unknown profiles and a convicted offender sample from Georgia. Investigation by local police showed that the offender had lived in the state at the time of the two murders and when the kidnapping-assault occurred in 1992. The defendant initially claimed that the bite mark was not inflicted as a result of the incident. Because evidence was properly collected and maintained, DNA was available for Y-short tandem repeats (STR) DNA testing on the anal swab. This Y-DNA profile also matched the profile of the defendant. While not as conclusive as standard STR typing, this result provided sufficient evidence to convince the defendant to agree to a plea bargain. He is now serving two consecutive life sentences, plus 25 years.

As shown by this case study, the advent of DNA testing has revolutionized forensic analysis of biological evidence. DNA technology was first applied to casework in the United Kingdom in 1985 to settle immigration issues. At that time, Dr. Alec Jeffries also used his newly developed DNA "fingerprinting" procedures during the investigation of a double rape-homicide case. In late 1986, DNA was accepted in a United States court in a paternity suit in the case *Pennsylvania v. Pestinikas* (1992). Once DNA was used for paternity testing, for which tubes of fresh blood could usually be obtained, paternity determination became much more straightforward, less time-consuming, and more discriminating than the previously applied serum protein testing. A few years later, in 1989, the FBI began accepting DNA cases and training other forensic laboratories in this new genetic testing method. By the mid-1990s, DNA analysis was widespread and accepted in courts throughout the United States.

When DNA fingerprinting* was first employed in casework, Adams and his colleagues reported that DNA of good quality, that is, not degraded, was necessary to obtain conclusive, discriminating results. In addition, the analytical method used at the time, RFLP, required relatively large quantities of DNA. Thus, some biological materials still were not suitable for DNA profiling. Semen stains the size of a dime or whole vaginal swabs were often required to get a DNA profile that could be compared to a suspect in a case. During the past decade, more sensitive and discriminating polymerase chain reaction (PCR) typing methods, the offender **DNA database,** and significant federal and state funding have greatly enhanced DNA typing in forensic casework.

From the time it was first used in U.S. courts, forensic DNA analysis has been vigorously challenged during many trials and hearings. The quality and quantity of DNA samples from criminal cases greatly vary. In addition, the proper collection and preservation of samples is critical for proper analysis and interpretation of DNA results and to prevent contamination. The majority of the challenges to admissibility of DNA evidence in today's courts usually are based on questions about the statistical significance of a "match" or the handling of evidence samples in specific cases. Thus, it is important for the practitioner to be aware of the implications of proper evidence collection and storage, particularly when DNA evidence is involved.

---

*DNA fingerprinting, while often used as a common term for DNA analysis, refers to the procedures developed by Dr. Alec Jeffreys and is licensed by Orchid Cellmark Corp.

DNA Structure and Genetics

DNA is the genetic or hereditary material in living cells. DNA is a polymer, with its individual building block called a "nucleotide." Each nucleotide consists of a sugar (deoxyribose), a phosphate group, and a nitrogenous base. There are four bases—adenine (A), guanine (G), cytosine (C), and thymine (T)—that are used to classify each nucleotide. The DNA polymer contains two long strands of DNA bound together by hydrogen bonds between complementary bases (adenine always pairs with guanine, thymine with cytosine). Because of this complementary bonding, the DNA molecule twists to form a double helix.

Most of the DNA in a cell is located in the nucleus and arranged into structures called chromosomes. In humans, there are 23 pairs of chromosomes. One-half the chromosome pair is inherited maternally; the other is derived from the father. While more than 98% of the human genome is the same among individuals (Lander, et al., 2001), there is considerable genetic variation of "noncoding" regions (not genes) of the DNA. It is these areas of the non-coding regions, commonly called "junk DNA," that are used in forensic DNA typing systems.

Most of the DNA in a cell is the nucleus, but DNA is also found in the mitochondria, in which are plentiful in the cytoplasm of cells. Mitochondria are maternally inherited; hence, all siblings within the maternal line will have the same **mitochondrial DNA** (mtDNA). During the past few years, scientists have applied mtDNA analysis to forensic samples. Because of the great number of mitochondria in a cell and their relative stability, mtDNA testing is successful in samples that are unsuitable for standard forensic DNA typing. These materials include hair shafts, old bones, and degraded samples. Melton (2005) conducted a retrospective review of the results of analysis of 691 casework hairs. She found that over 90% of samples of these hair shafts yielded partial or complete mtDNA profiles.

Biological Methods Employed Prior to DNA Analysis

Throughout most of the latter half of the 20th century, application of basic serological techniques, such as ABO blood typing, was essential to analyze biological evidence (Gaensslen, 1983). Today, serological analysis is generally limited to identifying the type of biological evidence present in a sample. This limited biochemical testing, however, is often necessary to prove the elements of crimes such as sexual assault. In addition, knowing the source of the DNA is often required for a complete and proper interpretation of the DNA results. For example, if a body fluid is identified on the skin of a victim when a SANE nurse uses an alternate/blue light, whether that sample is human and if it is saliva or semen will determine how it is extracted and its potential significance. After the type of biological material is identified, the evidence is individualized, that is, linked to (or excluded from) a particular person by DNA typing.

The process of examining items for the presence of biological evidence begins with recognizing and identifying materials for further testing. A critical step in this process occurs even before the evidence is submitted to the laboratory. The proper recognition of potential evidence and appropriate collection and packaging procedures by the practitioner can ensure the biological sample does not become degraded or destroyed. At the laboratory, various screening tests determine if a stain could be blood, saliva, semen, etc. Evidence screening saves considerable time and money by eliminating those stains that are not consistent with the body fluid of interest. The acid phosphatase (AP) test, for example, is a well-known screening test for seminal fluid. This test is only preliminary, however, and a confirmatory test must be performed to state that semen is indeed present. Researchers who tested common household products and other biological samples found that other substances also contain detectable amounts of AP and may give positive results when forensic samples are screened for this component. For example, in 1949 Kaye noted low, but detectable, reactions of the AP test with a number of body fluids (urine, serum, perspiration, feces); food products (milk, mushrooms, cauliflower); and other chemicals (alkaloids, albumins, choline).

Confirmatory tests conclusively demonstrate the presence of a particular body fluid. In most cases, trained laboratory personnel should conduct confirmatory tests. However, within some jurisdictions, SANEs have developed protocols with laboratory and criminal justice personnel to conduct microscopic identifications of spermatozoa. If the medical professional is going to be involved in the confirmation of a body fluid sample, procedures should be implemented only after consultation and cooperation with other forensic professionals and prosecutors. Unless confirmatory testing will consume the specimen, only after a sample has been identified will DNA individualize the body fluid.

Reddish-brown stains that may be blood are also screened prior to DNA typing. Most screening tests for blood are based on the property of the heme component of hemoglobin to catalyze the release of oxygen from peroxides. Various chemicals, such as o-tolidine, phenolphthalein (Kastle-Mayer), and tetramethylbenzidine, applied to the test sample will then change color when oxidized. These tests are extremely sensitive, and reactions with other chemical substances may result in so-called false positives. Thus, a positive reaction with any of these reagents indicates that the sample *could* be blood but should never be considered conclusive for the presence of blood.

As with body fluids, a confirmatory test is required to show that a specimen is, in fact, blood and not some other material. At one time microcrystal tests were used to confirm the presence of blood, but they do not indicate the species of origin: hence, a positive crystal test would be obtained from both human and animal blood. Except when non-human blood is suspected, the confirmatory test of choice in forensic cases will also determine if the blood is human.

The presence of *human* blood can be determined using any immunological method that tests for human hemoglobin. Rapid immunoassay using manufactured test strips is a one-step procedure and the preferred method in forensic laboratories today, since it consumes a small amount of sample and is extremely sensitive. Validation studies using commercially available test cards found a lower detectable limit of 0.07 μg/mL (Johnson, et al., 2003). These tests were also found to be highly specific and unaffected by a variety of common contaminants. However, if a sample is too small to conduct a confirmatory test prior to DNA analysis, the actual source of a human DNA profile obtained from a sample cannot conclusively be attributed to blood.

Semen is the body fluid most often identified and analyzed in the forensic laboratory. Statistics clearly show that sexual assaults constitute the largest percentage of cases involving interpersonal violence in which DNA is tested. As stated above, the common screening method for semen is the AP test. AP is usually present in high levels in semen, but it can also be found in other substances such as plant matter. The presence of semen must be confirmed by identifying spermatozoa microscopically or by detecting the human seminal protein p30, also called prostatic specific antigen (PSA). Positive detection of PSA by rapid immunoassay requires as little as 4 μg of that protein (Hochmeister, et al., 1999). PSA was detected by these researchers in samples up to 30 years old, including stains on clothing and vaginal swabs from sex crimes kits. This sensitivity could have significant implications for the confirmation of semen in samples from victims of sexual assault collected after 72 hours or that were diluted during the assault or prior to collection. Some practitioners have suggested that these tests be conducted by health-care professionals during medical and evidence examination procedures. However, this practice should be avoided because PSA testing has been shown to be affected by certain conditions, such as pH and high concentrations of semen; it may consume significant amounts of sample needed for DNA analysis; and it may raise issues of evidence contamination. In some laboratories, the identification of male DNA (Y chromosome DNA, or Y-DNA) is considered sufficient to confirm contact in sexual assault cases. These scientists do not look for sperm or p30 (PSA), and they proceed with DNA profiling after the Y-DNA has been identified.

Other enzyme, biochemical, and immunochromatographic tests may be conducted to identify biological substances such as saliva, urine, gastric fluid, and fecal matter. Microscopic examination may also be used for analysis of biological evidence. For example, hairs are examined microscopically, compared to reference samples from the victim and suspect(s), and checked for the presence of hair root material.

After biological evidence has been characterized, DNA analysis may be conducted on that sample. If the incident involves crimes against or injury to persons, the laboratory may require a known sample from those person(s) for comparison to any DNA profiles developed from the evidence specimen.

Forensic DNA Typing

In addition to sample quality and quantity, sample "purity" is also a major factor affecting DNA analysis. Sample mixtures may present problems when interpreting data. Certain biological samples, such as the vaginal swab from a sexual assault victim, are by their nature mixtures of victim and perpetrator cells. While procedures exist to separate sperm from epithelial cells in the DNA extraction process, scientists have shown that this separation is not always effective or complete (Ladd, et al., 2006). Mixtures may also be found in other types of samples that contain biological materials from two or more persons. Often, the analyst may be able to tell from the results if there is a major contributor and minor contributor(s) in these DNA mixtures. If both contributors are present in approximately equal amounts, the DNA profile from each source can readily be detected. However, with mixture ratios such as 25:1 or 50:1, the quantity of the major DNA specimen prevents the detection of the minor source. This situation has occurred with some vaginal swab samples

for which small numbers of spermatozoa have been detected. In cases in which semen is positively identified but no spermatozoa are present, standard DNA tests will detect only the victim's DNA profile.

DNA Typing Methods

DNA typing methods are based on two variations: sequence variation, which results from single base changes in the DNA molecule, and length differences, which are produced by a variation in the number of repeats in a row (in tandem) of a particular portion of the DNA sequence. It has been found that many regions, or loci, of the cell's DNA contain sets of nucleotides that are repeated; the number of repeated units at some loci can vary from person to person. DNA tests that detect such length differences are currently the most common type of variation studied in forensic nuclear DNA analysis.

The most common method used to detect variations in the DNA molecule employs a procedure called **polymerase chain reaction** (PCR). In PCR, small segments of DNA are copied, resulting in enough of the desired portion of the DNA to detect the variation present. At the end of the amplification process, more than one million times the amount of target DNA is in the sample (NIJ, 2005). Because of its speed and accuracy, PCR has become the method of choice not only in forensic science, but also in biological research and diagnosis.

The first PCR tests in widespread forensic use were commercially available as DQA1 and Polymarker (PM), which detected sequence variations as colored dots on a nylon strip. Another early PCR test identified length variations at D1S80 using gel electrophoresis to separate fragments of different length. These PCR procedures were highly sensitive, but they did not have the discriminating power that was seen in the more involved DNA fingerprinting method (RFLP analysis). However, when degraded or small amounts of DNA were present, these tests provided results for samples that were unsuitable for RFLP testing. Some cases for which these less discriminating tests were performed have been highly scrutinized during postconviction appeals. The DQA1, PM, and D1S80 tests are no longer used in forensic casework.

The standard DNA typing method employed by the forensic community today amplifies and detects the STRs in the DNA molecule (Butler, 2006). Various loci of the DNA molecule have been shown to exhibit variation in the number of repeated core elements they may contain. Like other PCR methods, STR typing is very sensitive. Current techniques allow for testing multiple loci (more than 16) in one tube at the same time, producing this powerful information using a minimum of sample and time. Because variations at multiple loci are tested for each sample, STRs have great discriminating power.

STR typing can also be focused on the Y chromosome. This is an important forensic development because it provides the possibility of obtaining a DNA profile in samples that have a low concentration of male versus female cells. In some cases, as described previously, only the female profile can be detected using standard STR systems. This is usually due to a large amount of female cells compared to cells of male origin, as when a vasectomized or otherwise aspermic/low sperm sample is encountered. By targeting only the Y chromosome during the amplification process, the female cells will not amplify, since they have only X chromosomes. The sensitivity of this test has proven valuable in the analysis of sexual assault evidence, particularly when spermatozoa are not identified in the specimen. Research has shown that DNA ratios of 1:500, male to female, readily produce reliable Y-STR profiles (Parson, 2003). Analytical schemes can be applied using Y-STR testing resulting in reliable profiles from postcoital samples collected at least 5 days after intercourse (Hall and Ballantyne, 2007). In addition, Y-STR typing may assist in evaluation of mixtures by providing information regarding the number of male contributors.

Y chromosomes are inherited through the paternal line, and all males within a family bloodline will have identical Y-STR profiles. Y-STR DNA testing is not as discriminating as standard STR analysis. Use of this method is increasing within the forensic community, and statistical data for various populations are readily shared among practitioners. In 2008, a comprehensive reference database of U.S. Y-STR profiles was compiled. These data, consisting of more than 13,000 sample profiles, were made available online as a searchable listing for use by practitioners.

Testing of single base differences, a procedure called SNP (single nucleotide polymorphism) determination, has been developed for use with forensic samples in recent years, especially when highly degraded samples are tested. Determination of SNPs is now a commonly used research tool for determining the genetic basis of disease and physiological conditions. These tests currently are not part of the routine forensic testing conducted in most public laboratories. They have been researched and validated by some laboratories and are available as additional tools when routine testing does not yield conclusive results. For example, SNP analysis played a major role in the successful identification of a portion of the remains collected after the destruction of the World Trade Center on September 11, 2001.

As stated previously, mitochondrial DNA analysis has recently been added to the battery of forensic tests employed in the analysis of biological specimens. Typically, mtDNA typing involves PCR amplification followed by determination of the actual base sequence of the amplified DNA. With the development of instrumental techniques for the determination of the DNA sequence, this procedure became more feasible as a forensic tool in cases where no other DNA results are possible. MtDNA analysis of hairs, for example, has provided an additional objective test that can be applied to hairs that could previously be compared only microscopically.

Mitochondrial DNA analysis was first introduced in a U.S. criminal trial in the summer of 1996 (*State of Tennesee v. Ware*, 1999). Since then, several state and local laboratories have incorporated mtDNA testing into their routine procedures. In 2003, the FBI established four regional mtDNA laboratories in association with state laboratories. This made mitochondrial DNA testing more readily available for use by all states. The analysis of unknown skeletal remains and associated samples for missing persons is now a major focus of the FBI mtDNA initiative. These data have been combined with mtDNA sequences developed by other laboratories to establish the Missing Persons mtDNA Database.

INTERPRETATION OF DNA RESULTS

When DNA analysis is conducted in a forensic setting, the goal usually is to compare DNA profiles obtained from evidence to DNA profiles developed from known samples—victim, suspect, or other named source—and to determine if that named person could be the source of the evidentiary DNA profile. Ultimately, there are only three basic interpretations that are possible:

- **Inclusion:** DNA detected from a known source "K" is present in the evidentiary sample, "Q." Therefore, person "K" could be the source of the DNA evidence. A statistical interpretation of this probability must be provided, based on the occurrence of each marker detected in the sample when compared to a database of known origin.
- **Exclusion:** DNA markers from the known source "K" are not present in the evidence or questioned sample. Therefore, person "K" could not be the source of the DNA profile developed from the evidence.
- **Inconclusive:** No conclusion can be made as to a possible source of the DNA evidence. Results, if any, are obtained, cannot be interpreted.

When the comparison results in an inclusion or DNA "match," the scientist must report the statistical significance of the match—how common or rare the evidentiary profile is. This typically involves calculating what is termed the random match probability, which is the expected frequency of individuals in the general population who could be the source of the DNA obtained from the evidence. The calculation is based on the number of times a particular allele has been demonstrated in a tested population. Depending on the type of DNA testing conducted, the frequency of occurrence in the population can be an extremely small number, for example one in millions. This statistic must then be weighed by the jury, along with other important facts relating to how the evidence may have been produced. It is important to keep in mind that whether a DNA sample can be obtained from a specimen, as well as the evaluation of the significance of any DNA profile obtained, will vary from case to case.

Low Copy Number DNA Testing

As the sensitivity of DNA testing increases and techniques to detect DNA present in extremely small quantities (low copy DNA) are applied to evidence, the interpretation of these data becomes more critical. Unfortunately, the increased PCR amplification necessary to develop profiles from low copy DNA (LCN) also results in amplification of background DNA contamination that may have been left by those who handled the object and not from those persons who were involved with the crime. The time at which biological material was deposited and whether more than one person contributed the DNA detected by these LCN methods must be considered. Valuable information may be gained from LCN techniques, however, because profiles can be obtained from fingerprints and from surfaces that may retain skin cells. Recognition of evidence, proper evidence handling, and appropriate documentation become even more critical if the significance of small quantities of DNA and the resulting profiles are going to be meaningfully interpreted.

Determination of guilt or innocence is the responsibility of the trier of fact and should never be the concern or focus of the forensic nurse. Unfortunately, the popular media may have contributed to false expectations and impressions of the general public as to the occurrence and significance of DNA in criminal and civil cases today. It seems that *every* criminal case on television involves a DNA match with the suspect—who then confesses and is quickly convicted. In fact, DNA profiles are developed in less than 50% of the cases submitted to forensic laboratories, and many of those DNA profiles match the victim or are not scientifically significant in a case. Jury members may expect DNA and other scientific evidence to be presented during a trial; if no such evidence is forthcoming, some jurors have been reluctant to find guilt beyond a reasonable doubt.

CONVICTED OFFENDER DATABASES

In 1990, the FBI Laboratory began a program called the Combined DNA Index System (**CODIS**). This program provided software that enabled federal, state, and local laboratories to exchange and compare DNA profiles electronically. Within a very short time, most states had passed laws that required certain convicted offenders to provide biological samples for DNA analysis and the creation of DNA data banks against which profiles from cases with no suspect could be compared. With the formation of the CODIS network, a revolution in forensic science occurred.

CODIS uses two main indices: a Forensic Index and the Offender Index. The Forensic Index contains DNA profiles from crime scene evidence. The Offender Index contains DNA profiles of individuals who have been convicted of various offenses defined by state and/or federal law. CODIS software enables Local DNA Index System (LDIS) laboratories to feed DNA data electronically to a designated State DNA Index System (SDIS) laboratory. Local laboratories cannot upload DNA profiles directly into the National DNA Index System (NDIS). Instead, each state's CODIS laboratory has an administrator who is responsible for maintaining the data and information in SDIS. The state laboratory then inputs data into NDIS, which also receives DNA profiles analyzed by the FBI Laboratory. NDIS became fully operational in October 1998. As of October 2007, NDIS contained more than 5 million DNA offender profiles and 200,000 sample profiles in the Forensic Index.

NDIS is administered and overseen by the FBI. As such, the FBI must ensure the quality of the profiles that are in NDIS. In addition, the privacy and security of the system must be maintained. The exchange of information within this secure CODIS system is controlled by and strictly limited to law enforcement. Quality and uniformity of data are also ensured by the DNA Advisory Board (DAB). The DAB continues to develop and revise recommended guidelines for quality assurance within forensic biology and DNA testing. These recommendations are published as *Standards for Forensic DNA Testing Labs* and *Standards for Convicted Offender Labs,* issued by the director of the FBI. States that participate in the national database verify in writing that the laboratory submitting DNA profiles to NDIS is in compliance with the published quality assurance standards. In addition, each CODIS-participating laboratory is subject to biannual external audits to confirm that quality procedures are being followed.

When a DNA profile from an evidence sample is submitted to the Forensic Index, that evidence profile is searched against the other profiles within the index. The evidence profile is also searched against the Offender Index. If CODIS software finds the same DNA profile in the Forensic or Offender Index, it identifies the two profiles as a "match," which is commonly called a "hit" by practitioners. After CODIS software produces a hit, qualified laboratory personnel analyze the DNA samples again to either confirm or refute the match. This confirmation is done to ensure that no problems or errors occurred that could have resulted in an incorrect DNA match. The verified DNA hit provides sufficient evidence to law enforcement to focus on a suspect in a previously unsolved case. Usually, law enforcement will then obtain a second sample from the offender by search warrant and test the new sample to compare the results with the evidentiary samples. Sometimes there is a hit between profiles in the Forensic Index with no corresponding association with an offender sample. Forensic Index hits provide valuable information to investigators by linking cases (even across jurisdictional lines) that previously were not known to be associated and by identifying serial cases. Thus, by comparing cases, additional investigative leads may be developed that could solve these cases, even if the perpetrator is not initially identified. As shown in the case study on page 228, "**cold cases**" continue to be solved with this technology.

Today, every state in the United States has a convicted offender law in place that requires persons convicted of violent crime to provide samples for inclusion in the DNA database. Variations of this law also allow the collection of samples from felons convicted of property crimes, such as burglary. The addition of large numbers of profiles to the DNA database has increased the efficacy of this forensic tool. Because of the effectiveness of DNA databases, some states are now passing laws requiring that biological samples be collected from arrestees in felony cases. Virginia began collecting DNA from individuals upon arrest for certain crimes in 2003. Between January 2003 and June 2006, the Virginia Department of Forensic Science reported 288 matches with arrestee samples that have aided investigations. Because of this reported success, by January 2008, 11 states had followed suit, with arrestee bills being proposed in many other legislatures. While the collection of DNA samples from arrestees has proven to be controversial, states that have incorporated arrestee profiles into their databases have reported a significant increase in the number of hits against no-suspect cases.

As the offender/arrestee databases increase in size, new evidence-based issues arise. For example, should "familial searches" be allowed? In some cases, a search of the offender database does not result in an exact match, but candidates with many alleles that match may indicate that a close relative of the registered offender is likely the donor of the unknown DNA profile. This would provide an investigative tool for law enforcement. Detractors have questioned the value of this practice in light of the possible violation of the constitutional rights of family members.

DNA and The Innocence Project

The power of DNA profiling to identify the perpetrator in a case was clear from the first use of the databank. Equally important is the ability of DNA to *exclude* individuals who have not contributed the biological sample, even if only a small amount of sample is present. Until DNA testing was routine, conventional serological testing, such as ABO and enzyme typing, was employed. This testing provided some ability to characterize the specimen. However, the discriminating power of these methods was vastly inferior to that of DNA analysis. For example, the least common blood type, AB, can only provide a random match probability of 1 in 25 (4%). By combing blood typing with additional markers found in the blood, the analyst might have been able to reach a somewhat better discrimination, but far less than that of current DNA technology. In addition, traditional serological techniques were unable to separate potential sources of the genetic markers in body fluid mixtures because those markers were found in the liquid portions of the sample. Thus, a vaginal swab from a sex crimes kit might yield results, but whether the blood group substances were from the male perpetrator, the female victim, or a consensual partner could not be determined. Certain procedures called differential extractions allow the DNA scientist to separate the sperm DNA and epithelial cell DNA, in effect eliminating any contribution from the victim when interpreting the offender's DNA profile.

Studies have shown that when DNA testing was conducted on samples where traditional serology included a suspect, the suspect was eliminated as a contributor to the DNA profile in up to 25% of those cases (Ladd, et al., 1996). Recognizing this power of DNA to exclude those who are falsely accused in criminal cases, attorneys sought to provide for DNA testing in postconviction appeals.

In 1992, attorneys Barry Scheck and Peter Neufeld started the Innocence Project at Yeshiva University in New York. Their efforts resulted in the first exoneration by DNA. Since that time, there have been over 215 postconviction exonerations. The Innocence Project is a group of

Case Study

DNA AS PROOF OF INNOCENCE

In the early 1990s a series of robberies and rapes occurred in the city of Chicago, Illinois. These crimes occurred about one block from each other and were initially considered two of a series of crimes that law enforcement believed were committed by the same person: John Willis was arrested for two of these crimes.

The first case occurred in a beauty parlor. The victim in that case was attacked and orally assaulted. After the attack, she spat onto a toilet paper wrapper that was later recovered by police. As the case went to trial in 1991, testing was performed on the wrapper at the Chicago Police Department's Serology Unit. Human semen was detected on the wrapper; however, conventional serological testing for ABO blood group substances was reported as inconclusive. The scientist reported that, based on her findings, she could not exclude Mr. Willis as the contributor of the semen. At the time, the actual test results were never supplied to the defense for review.

In 1992, Mr. Willis was convicted of this crime but continued to maintain his innocence. In 1994, another man, Dennis McGruder, was arrested for a 1992 rape and robbery that displayed a modus operandi similar to that of the assailant in Willis's case. Willis's appeal based on this evidence, however, was denied.

Willis was convicted of a second, similar crime in 1993. Although DNA testing was available to the prosecution, this testing was not conducted at the time of trial and the defense did not have access to the evidence. In spite of the fact that Mr. Willis claimed that McGruder admitted his guilt in the two crimes attributed to Mr. Willis, this evidence also was not allowed at trial.

Eventually, during the appeal process, the laboratory notes of the scientist were released and reviewed by other experts. It was clear that Mr. Willis's blood type, B, was not detected in the semen stain from the toilet wrapper. Information of this apparent exclusion had not been released prior to Mr. Willis's trial. As a result, the defense was provided with the remaining evidence, and DNA analysis exculpated Willis. In fact, the DNA profile developed from the sperm portion of the wrapper stain implicated Dennis McGruder. In 1999, John Willis was released from prison after spending 7 years incarcerated for crimes he did not commit.

programs in various jurisdictions that has the purpose of exonerating persons falsely convicted of serious crimes. These exonerations are achieved primarily through the implementation of DNA analysis on biological samples from the cases. DNA evidence has been used to reverse convictions based primarily on eyewitness misidentifications, false statements, suspected coerced confessions, and faulty or intentionally fraudulent forensic testing. Statistics maintained by the Innocence Project through March 2008 demonstrate the importance of this effort:

- Sixteen people were sitting on death row at the time they were exonerated by DNA testing.
- Over 70% of those exonerated were members of minority groups.
- Exonerations have been achieved in 31 states and the District of Columbia.
- The average time served by persons exonerated is 12 years.
- In more than 37% of the cases in which there were exonerations, the actual perpetrator was identified by the DNA profile developed from remaining evidence.

As new and more sensitive DNA methodologies are developed, it is expected that exonerations will continue

in the near future. It is also hoped that, as DNA testing is conducted by qualified scientists in more cases prior to adjudication, such injustice will occur infrequently in the future. Because of the clear impact that the Innocence Project has had on achieving justice for these more than 215 individuals, many states have now passed postconviction testing statutes. Postconviction laws focus on protecting the rights of the convicted in situations similar to those in which others were exonerated by DNA. The statutes usually allow convicted offenders to file a motion that DNA analysis be conducted on samples that were not tested for trial. As such, they also contain provisions that require law enforcement, laboratories, and the courts to maintain critical evidence for the length of a felon's sentence. Routinely, every item of evidence or every specimen from that evidence may not be tested in a particular case prior to trial; scientists will often test only those samples that appear to be significant to the case. Additional specimens may seem redundant, not as critical, or unsuitable for current technologies. For example, if a trail of bloodstains is found at a scene, the laboratory may test some of those stains along the entire trail, considering that the pattern indicates a single blood source. It should be noted that this practice also maintains the remainder of the samples for the opposition to test if they so desire. Postconviction DNA testing statutes provide the convicted felon access to those additional samples, even if there was no initial request by the defense to conduct DNA testing on the evidence. Access to future DNA testing by convicted offenders is particularly important because of the rapid development of forensic DNA methodologies.

FUTURE CONSIDERATIONS

Recently, the use of ethnic or race-specific DNA markers has been reported. By studying a set of DNA single nucleotide polymorphisms (SNPs), the DNAPrint Genomics Inc. laboratory was able to assess the "biogeographical ancestry" of a perpetrator in a 10-year-old sexual assault-murder case. Since the first widely publicized case of this kind in 2003, there has been much interest in biogeographical DNA testing by citizens and law enforcement alike. In fact, any individual may contact DNAPrint Genomics and similar companies for an ethnic ancestry assessment. This type of application of DNA typing clearly has its detractors among some scientists, privacy advocates, civil libertarians, and others. They argue that there is great potential for abuse of this technology in the form of racial profiling. Other scientists have been concentrating their efforts on pigmentation and eye color genes as sources for investigative leads, believing that such a focus would provide less divisive and inflammatory data.

Research has also been carried out in the area of non-human DNA. Cases have been reported in which DNA profiling of animal hairs and plant materials was used to link the suspect with the crime. However, some courts have rejected the use of this testing during trial because of the lack of appropriate databases or the inability to determine the significance of a match. Even in jurisdictions in which animal data are not admitted in court, these non-human DNA tests may provide valuable information to investigators.

Developments in the methods used by forensic laboratories have increased the efficiency and efficacy of DNA testing. Application of robotics to DNA analysis has greatly increased the productivity of DNA laboratories, especially when handling offender samples. In addition, automated testing reduces the possible sources of human error in various stages of the testing process. Portable DNA analysis instrumentation is being tested that could make preliminary results available at the scene, reducing the time required to provide investigative leads to the police or to conduct preliminary screening of multiple stains to identify biological specimens of greatest probative value. Questions about the potential for evidence contamination, consumption of samples, and affordability will need to be addressed if the portable DNA laboratory is adopted by the forensic scientific community.

ETHICAL ISSUES ASSOCIATED WITH EVIDENCE AND TESTING

While technological advancements in evidence processing are important, the most important issues raised concerning forensic DNA analysis or use of databases involve ethics. Numerous instances of forensic misconduct or failure to follow established guidelines have been fodder for the media. These instances of falsified evidence or other intentional acts are actually relatively uncommon. However, while most analysts are ethical and proceed according to established procedures, some critics have noted that unconscious bias or the association of laboratories with law enforcement agencies may taint the testing and interpretation of DNA evidence. Such bias has no place in the identification, collection, or interpretation of evidence.

Efforts to impose individual certification and facility accreditation are attempts at self-policing that have been successful to varying degrees. Quality control programs, including individual certification, are effective ways to monitor the technical or medical skills of individuals and the techniques employed at a facility. Unfortunately, these evaluation methods do not address the mental and emotional status of the forensic professional.

CONCLUSIONS

Forensic nurses play a vital role in the collection, analysis, interpretation, and preservation of evidence. Upholding scientific, legal, and ethical standards ensures that the probative value of evidence is not lost.

It is most important that the forensic nurse maintain independence and impartiality within the adversarial legal system. Forensic nurses must attempt to separate themselves from the personal nature of an incident, while at the same time providing compassionate care for a patient. In fact, by applying their critical thinking skills in a dispassionate and professional manner, forensic nurses can identify the best evidence, protect its integrity, and testify most effectively. Because physical evidence is so highly valued at this time in the justice system, the objective professionalism necessary to assess evidence is in itself among the best ways to serve the victim of a crime or an accident, as well the victim's family.

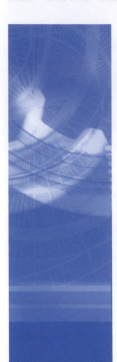

EVIDENCE-BASED PRACTICE

Reference Question: Do partial DNA matches call into question the validity of random match probability calculations?

Database(s) to Search: PubMed

Search Strategy: CODIS is unique and relatively new, so simply searching CODIS will be a good enough search term.

Selected References From Search:

1. Budowle, B., Baechtel, F.S., & Chakraborty, R. (2009). Partial matches in heterogeneous offender databases do not call into question the validity of random match probability calculations. *International Journal of Legal Medicine, 123*(1):59-63.
2. Liu, P., Yeung, S.H., Crenshaw, K.A., Crouse, C.A., et al. (2008). Real-time forensic DNA analysis at a crime scene using a portable microchip analyzer. *Forensic Science International Genetics, 2*(4):301-309.
3. Reid, T.M., Baird, M.L., Reid, J.P., Lee, S.C., et al. (2008). Use of sibling pairs to determine the familial searching efficiency of forensic databases. *Forensic Science International Genetics, 2*(4):340-342.
4. Riccardi, L.N., Melean, N.G., Rada, G., Tirado, N., et al. (2009). Genetic profiling of Bolivian population using 15 STR markers of forensic importance. *Legal Medicine (Tokyo) 11*(3):149-151.

Questions Used to Discern Evidence:

Choose two studies among the studies listed, read about them, and answer the following questions:

1. What are the differences between the two studies in the design, methods, and results?
2. What are the similarities between the two studies in the number of subjects, measures used, and interventions, if any?

REVIEW QUESTIONS

1. Television shows about forensic science and crime scene investigation have made it more difficult to prosecute cases with little physical evidence.
   A. True.
   B. False.

2. Which is *not* a method of classification of physical evidence?
   A. The nature of the incident.
   B. The type of analysis to be conducted.
   C. The cost of the type of analysis to be used.
   D. The type of the incident being investigated.

3. Recording the transfer of evidence from one person to the next is called:
   A. Evidence tracking.
   B. Material witness.
   C. Documentation log.
   D. Chain of custody.

4. Types of evidence generally allowed in court include all of the following *except*:
   A. Hearsay.
   B. Photographs.
   C. Video recordings.
   D. Documents.

REVIEW QUESTIONS—cont'd

5. It is not necessary to make notes, photographs, or diagrams of evidence prior to its forensic analysis.
A. True.
B. False.

6. When photographing evidence, it is best to use the "rule of three," which does *not* include photographing the sample:
A. In its entirety.
B. Close-up.
C. With an appropriate scale.
D. From a middle distance.

7. What provides a visible history of how many times a package of evidence has been opened and by whom?
A. Chain of custody.
B. Tamper-evident seal.
C. Evidence log.
D. Documentation notes.

8. The most common forms of trace evidence collected from crime scenes include:
A. Shoe print patterns.
B. Semen and body fluids.
C. Bullets and projectiles.
D. Hair and fibers.

9. The screening test for the presence of seminal fluid is:
A. Acid phosphatase (AP).
B. Phenolphthalein.
C. Polymerase chain reaction (PCR).
D. Short tandem repeats (STRs).

10. The Offender Index of CODIS contains:
A. DNS samples from crime scenes.
B. A list of cases that have been solved using DNA.
C. DNA profiles of convicted individuals.
D. Samples of DNA from cold case files.

References

Artingstall, K. (1999). *Practical aspects of Munchasen by proxy and Munchasen syndrome investigation.* Boca Raton, FL: CRC Press, pp. 156-157.

Biesecker, L.G., Bailey-Wilson, J., Ballantyne, J. et al. (2005). DNA identifications after the 9/11 World Trade Center attack. *Science, 310*:1122-1123.

Budowle, B., & van Daal, A. (2008). Forensically relevant SNP classes. *Biotechniques, 44*(5):603-610.

Bull, Morgan, Sagovsky, and Hughes, 2006

Butler, J. (2005). *Forensic DNA typing.* Burlington, MA: Elsevier Academic Press.

Cather, K. (2004). The C.S.I. effect: Fake TV and its impact on jurors in criminal cases. *Prosecutor*, Mar/Apr.

Chewning, D., Deaver, K., & Christensen A. (2008). The persistence of fibers on ski masks during transport and processing. *Forensic Science Communications, 7*(10):3. Retrieved April 19, 2009, from www.fbi.gov/hq/lab/fsc/backissu/july2008/research/2008_06_research01.htm

Committee on DNA Technology in Forensic Science, National Research Council. (1996). *The Evaluation of Forensic DNA Evidence.* Washington, DC: National Academy Press.

Conners, E., Lundgregan, T., Miller N., et al. (1996) *Convicted by juries, exonerated by science: Case studies in the use of DNA evidence to establish innocence after trial.* NCJ 161258. Washington, DC: U.S. Department of Justice, National Institute of Justice.

Cushwa, W.T., & Medrano, J.F. (1993). Effects of blood storage time and temperature on DNA yield and quantity. *Biotechniques, 14*(2):204-207.

Daniel, O. (2008). The stability of acid phosphatase in blood and other fluids. *British Journal of Urology*, 26(2):153-159.

Daubert v. Merrell Dow Pharmeceuticals, Inc. 509 US 579 (1993).

Exline, D., Smith, F., & Drexler, S. (1998). Frequency of pubic hair transfers during sexual intercourse. *Journal of Forensic Science, 43*(3):505-508.

Fatolitis, L., & Ballantyne, J. (2008). The US Y-STR Database. *Profiles in DNA, 11*(1):13-14.

Federal Bureau of Investigation (FBI). CODIS report. Retrieved December 20, 2007, from www.fbi.gov/hq/lab/codis

Federal Bureau of Investigation (FBI). (2007). *CODIS annual report.* Washington, DC: Federal Bureau of Investigation, U.S. Department of Justice. Retrieved December 21, 2007, from www.dna.gov

Federal Bureau of Investigation (FBI). (2007). *Standards for convicted offender labs.* Washington, DC: Federal Bureau of Investigation, U.S. Department of Justice.

Federal Bureau of Investigation (FBI). (2007). *Standards for forensic DNA testing labs.* Washington, DC: Federal Bureau of Investigation, U.S. Department of Justice.

Federal Rules of Evidence. (2007). Washington, DC: U.S. Government Printing Office.

Gaensslen, R.E. (1983). *Sourcebook in forensic serology, immunology and biochemistry.* Washington, DC: U.S. Government Printing Office.

Gaensslen, R.E., & Lee, H.C. *Sexual assault evidence: National assessment and guidelines.* Revised report compiled under Department of Justice grant 92-IJ-CX-0041. Retrieved May 10, 2009, from www.ncjrs.gov/pdffiles/nij/grants/191837.pdf

Gilbert, J.N. (2007). *Criminal investigation.* (7th ed.). New York: Pearson-Prentice Hall, p. 91.

Gramlich, J. (2006). States collecting DNA from arrestees. Stateline.org. Retrieved January 23, 2008, from www.stateline.org

Hall, A., & J. Ballantyne. (2003). Novel Y-STR typing strategies reveal the genetic profile of the semen donor in extended interval post coital cervicovaginal samples. *Forensic Science International, 136:*58-72.

Hochmeister, M.N., Budowle, B., Rudin, O., et al. (1999). Evaluation of prostate specific antigen (PSA) membrane tests for the forensic identification of semen. *Journal of Forensic Sciences, 44:*1057-1062.

Hochmeister, M., Eisenberg, A., Rudin, O., et al. (2001). A simple foldable cardboard box for the drying and storage of biological material recovered on cotton swabs. *Promega, 3:*21.

Johnston, S., Newman, J., & Frappier, R. (2003). Validation study of ABAcard® Hematrace® test for the forensic identification of human blood. *Journal of the Canadian Society of Forensic Science, 36*(3):173-184.

Kaye, S. (1949). Acid phosphatase test for identification of seminal stains. *Journal of Laboratory and Clinical Medicine, 34*(5):728-732.

Kumho Tire Company Ltd. V. Carmichael, 526 US 137 (1999) DC.

Ladd, C., Carita, E., Pagliaro, E., Garvin, A., & Lee, H. (2006). *Development of a high- throughput method to isolate sperm DNA in sexual assault cases.* Report of grant 2003-IJ-CX-K013. Retrieved March 10, 2009, from www.ncjrs.gov/pdffiles1/nij/grants/215339.pdf

Ladd, C., Messina, D., Reho, J., et al. (1996). Comparison of ABO typing and DNA analysis results in evidentiary and known samples. Unpublished data.

Lahiri, D., & Schnabel, B. (1993). DNA isolation by a rapid method from human blood samples: Effects of MgCl2, EDTA, storage time and temperature on DNA yield and quality. *Biochemical Genetics, 3*(7-8): 321-328.

Lander, E., Linton, L.M., & Birren, B. (2001). Initial sequencing and analysis of the human genome. *Nature, 409:*860-921.

Lee, H.C., Gaensslen, R.E., Bigbee, D., et al. (1992). *Guidelines for the collection and preservation of DNA evidence.* Washington, DC.: Federal Bureau of Investigation, U.S. Department of Justice.

Lee, H., & Ladd, C. (2006). The use of biological evidence and DNA databanks. In R. Hammer, B. Moynihan, & E. Pagliaro, (eds.). *Forensic nursing: A handbook for practice.* Sudbury, MA: Jones & Bartlett.

Lee, H., Palmbach, T., & Miller, M. (2001) *Henry Lee's crime scene handbook.* New York: Academic Press.

McNally, L., Shaler, R.C., Baurd, M., et al. (1989). Effects of environment and substrata on deoxyribonucleic acid (DNA): The use of casework samples from New York City. *Journal of Forensic Science, 34*(5):1070-1077.

Melton, T., Dimick, G., Higgins, B., et al. (2005). Forensic mitochondrial DNA analysis of 691 casework hairs. *Journal of Forensic Sciences, 50*(1):73-80.

National Conference of State Legislatures. (2008). State laws on DNA data banks—Qualifying offenses, others who must provide sample. Retrieved February 3, 2008, from http://www.ncsl.org/programs/cj/dnadatabanks.htm

National Institute of Justice. (2006). *Proceedings of the 2006 DNA grantees meeting.* Washington, DC: Department of Justice, Office of Justice Programs.

Osborn, M., & Neff, J. (1989). Patient care guidelines: Evidentiary examination in sexual assault. *Journal of Emergency Nursing, 15:*3.

Pagliaro, E. (2008). Personal communication, October, 2008.

Parson, W., Niederstatter, H., Brandstatter, A., et al. (2003). Improved specificity of Y-STR typing in DNA mixture samples. *International Journal of Legal Medicine, 117*(2):109-114.

Pennsylvania v. Pestinikas (1992. 617 A. 2d 1339 (Pa. Super)).

Peterson, J. (2005). *Census of publicly funded forensic crime laboratories, 2002.* Washington, DC: Department of Justice, National Institute of Justice. NCJ207205. Retrieved April 5, 2008, from www.usdoj.gov/publications

Ramsland, K. (2006). *The C.S.I. effect.* New York: Berkley Publishing Group, p. 91.

Reuters News Service. (2008). *DNA Print genomics helps Boulder police solve 10-year-old rape/murder case using cutting edge DNA technology.* January 30, 2008. Retrieved from http://www.reuters.com/article/pressRelease/idUS145130+30-Jan-2008+MW20080130

Schwoeble, A.J. (1999). GSR persistence on clothing. Oral presentation at the 26th annual meeting of the Mid-Atlantic Association of Forensic Scientists. Ocean City, MD, April 21–23, 1999.

State of Tennesee v. Ware (1999) WL233592 (Tenn. Crim. App.).

State v. Bogan.(1995). 183 Ariz. 506, 905 P.2d 515 (Ariz.App. Div. 1, Apr 11, 1995) (NO. 1CA-CR93-0453).

The Innocence Project. (2008). Retrieved March 21, 2008, from www.innoncenceproject.org

Thompson, W.C. (2006). Tarnish on the "gold standard": Understanding recent problems in forensic DNA testing. *The Champion, 1-2:*14-20.

Toothman, C., Kester, K., Champagne, J., Cruz, T., Street, W., & Brown, B. (2008). Characterization of human DNA in environmental samples. *Forensic Science International, 178*(1):7-15.

Tyler, T. (2006). Viewing CSI and the threshold of guilt. *Yale Law Journal, 115:*1050.

U.S. Congress, Office of Technology Assessment. (1990). *Genetic witness: Forensic uses of DNA tests.* OTA-BA-438. Washington, DC: Government Printing Office.

U.S. Department of Health and Human Services. (2003). HIPAA Section 160.103. Washington, DC: Government Printing Office.

U.S. Department of Health and Human Services, Health Insurance Portability and Accountability Act (HIPAA). (2003). Section 160.103-191. Washington, DC: Government Printing Office.

U.S. Department of Justice. (2006). *Principles of forensic DNA for officers of the court.* Washington, DC: National Institute of Justice.

United States v. Iron Shell, 633F.2d 77 (1980) *cert denied*, 450 US 1001 (1981).

Warren, J. (1991). Optimal medium for the transfer of crime scene stains for DNA analysis. Louisiana Association of Forensic Scientists Annual Meeting, October, 1991.

Washington v. Tuilefano & Lealuaialii. (1998). Superior Court of Washington for King County, No. 97-1-01391-3SEA & 96-1-08245-9SEA, 1/5/98.

Washington v. Tuilefano & Lealuaialii (2003). Court of Appeals, Division 1. 10/13/2003.

Wulff, P.H. (2006). Low copy number DNA: Reality vs. jury expectations. *Silent Witness Newsletter, 10*(3). Retrieved April 13, 2008, from www.ndaa.org/publications/newsletters/silent witness

Zercie, K., & Penders, P. (2006). Forensic photography. In R. Hammer, B. Moynihan, & E. Pagliaro (Eds.), *Forensic nursing: A handbook for practice*. Peabody, MA: Jones & Bartlett.

three

FORENSIC NURSING IN
SPECIAL AREAS OF PRACTICE

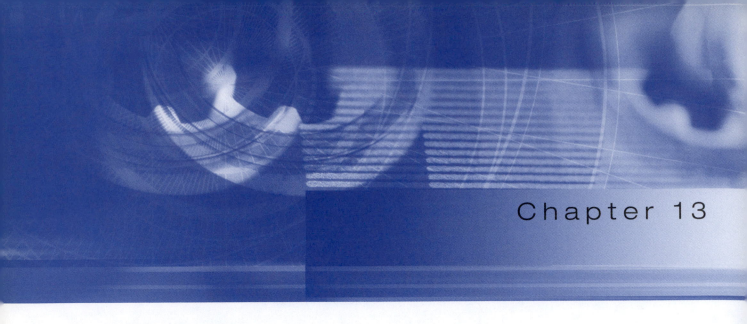

Chapter 13

FORENSIC PSYCHIATRIC MENTAL HEALTH NURSING

Mary Muscari, Alison Cole, and Daniele Wilcox

"A bend in the road is not the end of the road . . . unless you fail to make the turn."

Anonymous

Competencies

1. Describing the role of the forensic psychiatric mental health nurse.
2. Differentiating between therapeutic and forensic roles.
3. Discussing principles of collaboration and consultation.
4. Identifying the factors warranted to perform civil competency evaluations.
5. Critiquing the differences between competency to proceed and insanity in criminal cases.
6. Defining criteria used to perform sex offender assessments.

Key Terms

Actuarial risk assessment
Actus reus
Ad litem guardian
Civil competency
Collateral information
Competency to proceed
Conservator
Criminal responsibility
Dynamic risk factors
Guilty but mentally ill (GBMI)
Mens rea
Mental disease or defect
Mental state at the time of the offense (MSO)
Not guilty by reason of insanity (NGRI)
Pathway to offending
Power of attorney
Static risk factors

INTRODUCTION

Forensic Psychiatric Nursing

A subspecialty of forensic nursing is forensic psychiatric mental health nursing. This subspecialty has been defined as the psychiatric nursing assessment, evaluation, and treatment of individuals pending or following a criminal hearing or trial. The nurse focuses on the offender's thinking prior to and during the commission of a crime. Nurses also work as caregivers in forensic settings, forensic examiners, competency therapists, and consultants to law enforcement or attorneys. Psychiatric nursing is the core of practice, but the relationship between the nurse and client is markedly different from that in traditional psychiatric nursing. For example, evidence collection is a function of forensic nurses; thus, forensic psychiatric mental health nurses may participate in evidence collection to determine competency or to determine if a sex offender meets criteria to be deemed a sexually violent predator.

Forensic psychiatric mental health nurses also work with clients involved in civil law. Using Mason's definition in the context of the International Association of Forensic Nurses (IAFN) definition of forensic nursing, forensic psychiatric mental health nursing can be viewed as the application of psychiatric nursing science to public or legal proceedings. The application of the forensic aspects of mental health care are combined with the bio-psycho-social education of the registered nurse in the scientific assessment and treatment of persons with mental health problems who become involved with the legal system (Mason, 2002).

Forensic psychiatric mental health nurses may be generalist nurses who have a basic-level diploma, associate degree, or baccalaureate degree, or they may be an advanced practice nurse (APN), such as a clinical nurse specialist or nurse practitioner. Generalists typically provide direct care to offenders within a correctional or psychiatric setting, with the incarcerated or committed person as the client.

The APN typically acts as a forensic examiner, often hired by legal professionals to work indirectly with offenders to evaluate them or persons involved in civil matters, such as custody disputes and competency issues. The nursing roles, for the most part, are very different from the normal, routine expectations. They vary by place of employment and job requirements, and they are also being continually developed, expanded, and refined by nurses (Box 13.1 and 13.2.).

The APN's role as a forensic mental health professional may overlap with role responsibilities provided by psychiatrists and psychologists. "Correctional nursing," at times a term used interchangeably with forensic psychiatric

Box 13.1 Responsibilities and Functions of Forensic Psychiatric Mental Health Nurses

- Maintaining a nonjudgmental and professional attitude.
- Developing and sustaining knowledge of psychiatric mental health nursing principles.
- Developing and sustaining knowledge of psychiatric criminal and/or civil justice principles.
- Collaborating with members of the interdisciplinary team.
- Working in a secure environment.
- Serving as expert witness.
- Acting as consultant.

Box 13.2 Roles of Forensic Psychiatric Mental Health Nurses

- Correctional mental health nursing
- Criminal and civil competence
- Criminal responsibility
- Jury selection
- Risk and recidivism assessments
- Sex offender assessment
- Workplace violence
- Hostage negotiating
- Criminal profiling
- Disaster response
- Child custody evaluations
- Involuntary treatment
- Consultant

nursing, generally refers to nurses who provide nursing care for incarcerated individuals for a range of health-care problems.

THE DISTINCTIONS BETWEEN THERAPEUTIC AND FORENSIC ROLES

Interactions with the legal system can be challenging. Both the therapeutic and forensic roles require knowledge of psychiatric nursing principles and skills. However, there are distinct differences in the nature of the nurse-client relationship, the collection of historical data, and issues of confidentiality.

The therapeutic relationship is the core of psychiatric nursing treatment and is consistently focused on the client's needs. The nurse facilitates the client's ability to communicate distressing thoughts and feelings, helps with their activities of daily living, helps clients examine self-defeating behaviors and test alternatives, and promotes self-care and independence. The nurse generally listens to clients with empathy and in a nonjudgmental manner.

In contrast, the forensic psychiatric nurse, typically an APN, must remain unbiased, objective, and void of emotional attachment to the client. The manner in which the nurse gathers the information is methodical and purposeful, particularly as it relates to psycho-legal issues of the specific case.

Both therapeutic and forensic roles for nurses require the collection of historical data for assessment. In the therapeutic role, nurses obtain histories to better understand the client's intra- and interpersonal dynamics to make nursing diagnoses and develop treatment plans. In the forensic role, nurses commonly obtain collateral information regarding the psychological function of the person they evaluate. **Collateral information** may include medical, mental health, and school and work records, as well as juvenile, criminal, corrections, probation, and parole records (Box 13.3). The forensic nurse may interview others, such as a therapist, victim, or corrections officer. Interviews with the offender may not take place, if defense counsel asserts the offender's Fifth Amendment right against self-incrimination. Collateral data may be warranted to develop a benchmark against which to compare the consistency and/or discrepancy of the offender's account of the event.

Confidentiality Issues

Confidentiality is an important right of psychiatric clients. Privacy is protected, along with the confidentiality of treatment. Psychiatric nurses must obtain their client's permission to share information with persons not directly involved in the client's care. Confidentiality also applies to the offender's medical records, which should be read only by those directly involved in treatment or in monitoring the offender's care. Thus, clients must give written authorization to allow others to read their medical records. However, the forensic psychiatric mental health nurse may face dilemmas related to confidentiality.

According to the American Academy of Psychiatry and the Law (AAPL, 1995), practitioners should respect the client's right to privacy and confidentiality when performing forensic evaluations. Confidentiality should be maintained to the extent possible, given the legal context. Attention should be paid to the client's understanding of medical confidentiality. The forensic evaluation, however, requires that the client and collateral sources be informed of reasonably anticipated limitations on confidentiality.

Clients, third parties, and other appropriate individuals should be given notice of reasonably anticipated limitations on confidentiality. Professionals should indicate for whom they are conducting an examination and what they will do with the information.

Ethics guidelines may also be applied to forensic psychiatric APNs. Forensic psychiatric mental health nurses should inform the client or person they are evaluating that they are not their "nurse." The person being evaluated may develop the belief that there is a treatment relationship. The nurse is obligated to advise the client that this is not the case.

When the person being evaluated is incarcerated or on probation, parole, or conditional release, the nurse should be clear about confidentiality limitations and should ensure that these limitations are communicated to the person. The nurse should be familiar with institutional policies regarding confidentiality. If no policy exists, the nurse should attempt to clarify these matters with authorities and develop policies addressing confidentiality. Forensic psychiatric mental health nurses must also take precautions to ensure that confidential information is not released purposefully or inadvertently to unauthorized persons.

ISSUES RELEVANT TO FORENSIC PSYCHIATRIC NURSING

Forensic psychiatric mental health nurses face a number of issues because they are now able to treat clients that were solely the domain of psychiatrists and psychologists in the recent past. The forensic psychiatric mental health nurse collaborates with psychiatrists and psychologists and other professionals in their work with mentally ill offenders and with cases involving risk assessment and competency.

Box 13.3 Examples of Collateral Sources of Information

- Police reports
- Prison records
- Probation records
- Juvenile records
- Court records and/or transcripts
- Court orders
- Child protective records
- RAP (record of arrest and prosecution) sheet (criminal record)
- Child support records
- Prothonotary records (may show record of protective orders)

Traditionally, forensic psychiatric mental health nurses provide comprehensive care to mentally ill offenders, their families, and their communities by integrating nursing philosophy and practice within a social context that includes the criminal justice system. More than half of all prison and jail inmates had a mental health problem in 2005, which amounts to 705,600 inmates in state prisons, 78,800 in federal prisons, and 479,900 in local jails. Prison and jail inmates with psychiatric problems differ little from other psychiatric clients. They are principally disabled and distressed persons with multiple dysfunctions in need of a variety of therapeutic services. There are two critical features that differentiate forensic psychiatric clients. First, their problems are typically noticed only when they affect others. Second, the services they require are located at the shifting intersection of the criminal justice and mental health systems. Additionally, mentally ill offenders may be unwilling partners in their treatment.

Forensic psychiatric mental health nursing practice is affected by a set of issues outside the typical definition of nursing: the consideration of illness, treatment, crime, custody, and possibly punishment. Practice may take place in jails, penitentiaries, juvenile facilities, and community settings or in health-care facilities, such as psychiatric hospitals for those labeled "criminally insane." The dilemma in the nurse's role between custody and care is a significant quandary and is often simply stated, rather than described and discussed. Mason and Mercer state that the issue of custody versus care has stagnated, whereas Peternelj-Taylor and Johnson note that the principles of containment and care can coexist. Burrow and Nolan state that psychiatry is part of the regulatory structure of society, and psychiatric nurses are well versed in the task of combining treatment goals with those of detention and control. The custody versus care issue is critical to the practice of forensic psychiatric nursing, and it is equally important to correctional health nursing. Current descriptive and evidence-based literature has only minimally addressed issues and challenges at the most superficial level in the expanding role of the forensic psychiatric mental health nurse.

As a subspecialty of forensic nursing, forensic psychiatric mental health nursing challenges the notion that forensic mental health is the domain of psychiatrists and psychologists alone. Yet, the opportunity to be recognized as a psychiatric expert in federal immigration and naturalization court (INS) and offering testimony concerning petitioners for political asylum status may exist for few APNs or doctorally prepared nurses. Also, Shelton and Cashen describe the role of forensic psychiatric nurses working with juvenile delinquents. Forensic psychiatric nurses in juvenile settings work with patients who are characterized by higher degrees of social dislocation, abuse, mental illness, school failure, chronic physical health problems, and poverty than the general population. Forensic psychiatric mental health nurses function in and beyond prison walls, providing expert testimony and working with such issues as civil and criminal competency, risk assessment, and the evaluation of sex offenders for matters such as predatory status and civil commitment.

Another key issue for forensic psychiatric mental health nurses working with offenders is the association between substance abuse and criminal offending. Substance abuse is associated with numerous crimes as well as recidivism. Incarcerated criminals are more likely to reoffend after release if their substance abuse issue is not addressed before and after release. Furthermore, the combined issues of substance abuse, mental illness, and homelessness are associated with incarceration. The clinical and behavioral characteristics associated with homelessness and incarceration were assessed in individuals who entered the San Francisco County Jail system during the first 6 months of 2000 ($n = 12,934$) by McNeil, Binder, and Robinson. Research results reported that 16% of the inmates were homeless and 18% had a diagnosis of a mental disorder. Thirty percent of the homeless inmates had a diagnosis of a mental disorder during one or more episodes and 78% of the homeless inmates with a severe mental disorder had co-occurring substance-related disorders. Multiple regression analyses showed that inmates who were homeless with co-occurring severe mental disorders and substance-related disorders were jailed longer than other inmates who had been charged with similar crimes. The researchers concluded that homeless persons with mental illness, although representing a small portion of the total population, accounted for a substantial proportion of incarcerated persons in this setting. The increased duration of incarceration for the homeless persons with comorbid severe mental illness and substance abuse suggested that jails are de facto assuming responsibility for a population that needs a multiservice system approach to care.

COLLABORATION AND CONSULTING

Principles of Collaboration

Forensic psychiatric mental health nurses may work in collaboration with or as a consultant to other disciplines. Collaboration is a structured practice whereby two or more persons work together toward a common goal. It is both process and outcome oriented, with shared interests or conflicts that are addressed by key stakeholders. The stakeholders are those parties who are directly influenced by the actions taken to solve a complex problem. As such, the collaborative process is a synthesis of varied perspectives, and consequently, the collaborative outcome results from the development of integrative solutions that go beyond a single vision. Gardner presents 10 competencies for collaborative partnerships (Box 13.4).

Collaboration is a complex process that requires intentional knowledge sharing, joint responsibility, and mutual respect. Forensic psychiatric mental health nurses work in collaboration with other mental health professionals, law enforcement, and legal professionals.

Forensic Nursing Collaboration

It is critical that forensic psychiatric mental health nurses understand the educational and practice standards for collaborating professionals: forensic psychiatrists, psychologists

---

Box 13.4 Ten Competencies for Collaborative Partnerships

1. Know thyself. A prerequisite to trusting oneself and others is knowing one's own mental model (biases, values, and goals).
2. Learn to value and manage diversity. Differences are critical assets for effective collaborative processes and outcomes.
3. Develop constructive conflict-resolution skills. During collaboration, conflict is viewed as a natural opportunity to deepen understanding and agreement.
4. Use personal power to create win–win situations. Sharing power and the recognition of one's own power base are parts of effective collaboration.
5. Master interpersonal and process skills. Competence, cooperation, and flexibility are frequently identified attributes important to effective collaborative practice.
6. Recognize collaboration as a journey. Effective collaboration skills and knowledge take time and practice, and appreciative inquiry and knowledge of group process are all lifelong learning skills.
7. Leverage all multidisciplinary forums. Presence in team forums can provide an opportunity to assess how and when to offer collaborative communications for partnership building.
8. Appreciate that collaboration can occur spontaneously. Collaboration can happen spontaneously if the right factors are in place.
9. Balance autonomy and unity. Learn from your collaborative successes and failures and be willing to seek feedback and admit mistakes.
10. Remember that collaboration is not required for all decisions. Collaboration is not a universal remedy, nor is it warranted in all situations.

---

and social workers, and law enforcement professionals. The AAPL defines forensic psychiatry as a subspecialty of psychiatry that applies scientific and clinical expertise to legal issues in legal contexts embracing civil, criminal, correctional, or legislative matters. The AAPL further notes that forensic psychiatry should be practiced according to guidelines and ethical principles put forth by the profession of psychiatry. Forensic psychiatric fellows spend 1 year after their residency on developing their skills to deal with the civil and criminal legal system. They must become experts in the evaluation of competency, insanity, and provision of court testimony. Participation in clinical experiences with clients in jails and prisons is the core element of training.

Forensic psychiatric mental health nurses should also understand the roles of law enforcement and the legal professionals. Nurses must be well versed in the three phases of the criminal procedure: pretrial, trial, and posttrial. It is within these phases of criminal procedure that many forensic psychiatric mental health nurses function. For example, the nurse may be called to perform a competency assessment pretrial, supply an insanity evaluation during the trial, or collaborate on sentencing or treatment issues posttrial.

Principles of Consultation

Consultants are hired to give professional advice or services. Consulting has always been a traditional role within nursing practice, but seldom are nurses hired for their professional services outside of nursing. In an entrepreneurial position such as that of the forensic psychiatric APN role, the nurse may be hired as a consultant on a case, usually to perform a forensic assessment and provide a professional opinion. This may entail a verbal discussion, a written report, testimony in court, or any combination of the three.

Muller-Smith (2006) used the acronym PULSE to work effectively in an independent consulting role (see the definition of PULSE in Box 13.5).

Box 13.5 PULSE

P	People the nurse will work with directly. Power bases within the organization. Politics of how decisions are made.
U	Understanding the scope of the consultation, limitations, and time frame.
L	Listen. Learn about the problem. Let the client define the priorities.
S	Stay focused on the problem and watch for roadblocks.
E	Expertise and experience are applied to develop solutions.

CIVIL COMPETENCY

Principles of Civil Competency

Civil competency is a legal concept (rather than a clinical one) that becomes relevant when important legal decisions need to be made regarding an individual: specifically, should the decisions be made by the individual or another person, such as a guardian. A person is deemed competent if he or she is able to act or make decisions in a particular context and possesses the cognitive resources to understand the likely consequences of those decisions. The reference to the particular context is important because competence is not global, but rather pertains to specific acts or situations. A person may be competent for one level of employment but not another. A different person may be competent to live independently, but not to refuse medical treatment. Competency comprises several clearly defined areas (see Box 13.6).

Just as an individual's competence is related to context and is situation specific, it is also temporally specific. Competency will be reevaluated and reinstated depending on the nature of the condition responsible for compromised function. Reevaluation is likely when the stability of the impairment pertains to but is not limited to medical decisions, independent living, employment, and child custody matters.

A legal guardian may be appointed as a surrogate decision maker when the court determines that a person is incompetent with regard to a specific context in question. The appointed guardian is responsible for the best interests of the individual, or ward, he or she represents. The guardian has the legal authority to make decisions concerning the ward, and the guardian's responsibilities and decision-making authority is dependent upon the extent of the ward's impairment.

A general guardian is responsible for the personal, legal, and financial well-being of an individual, such as the parent of an underage child. A special guardian with limited decision-making authority may be assigned to an individual with circumscribed impairment. For example, a special guardian may be responsible for the financial interests of the ward, but have no authority over the ward's living arrangements. An ***ad litem* guardian** has power over a single action or a single interest of an individual, such as the person's last will and testament. The *ad litem* guardian is often appointed to represent the best interests of a child at the time of a divorce, in child custody hearings, abuse or neglect allegations, and juvenile delinquency cases.

The ward's interests are usually categorized as person and property. A guardian may be responsible for interests of the ward that involve the person, such as the ward's medical treatment or living arrangements. Hence, the "guardian of person" is responsible for the ward's physical well-being. Conversely, the guardian may be responsible only for the property assets of the person, such as the ward's inheritance or financial settlements. A guardian responsible for the financial and property resources of the ward is referred to as a **conservator** or "guardian of the property."

The court appoints a legal guardian when one was not appointed by a responsible family member or by the person himself or herself. Legal guardians are often volunteers, social workers, or attorneys, depending on the area of interest. Family members may request guardianship for the parents of an adult child with a developmental disability or the adult child of a parent whose cognitive function has declined and who failed to complete a **power of attorney** (a legal document authorizing another person to act on one's behalf).

Conditions of Impairment

The competency of an individual is determined by the court. Medical testimony is heard, and all pertinent information that may influence the court's decision is considered. The

---

Box 13.6   Defined Areas of Competency

1. Fiduciary competency, which is the ability to make financial decisions, such as the allocation of financial resources.
2. Testamentary competency, which is the ability to sign legal documents, such as a will, and to understand the implications and potential ramifications of providing the signature.
3. Criminal competency, which is competency at the time of the offense, appreciation of the illegality of the offense, and the ability to waive Miranda rights.
4. Competency to stand trial, ability to consult with/refuse legal counsel, and presence of mind to understand the proceedings and sentencing.
5. Competency to consent to medical treatment, which includes the acceptance or rejection of medical treatment.
6. Competency to live independently.
7. Competency to maintain employment and perform the tasks satisfactorily (Franzen, 2003; Slovenko, 2006).

(Data taken from Franzen, M.D. (2003). Neuropsychological evaluations in the context of competency decisions. In A.M. Horton, Jr. & L.C. Hartlage (Eds.), *Handbook of forensic neuropsychology.* New York: Springer Publishing; Slovenko, R. (2006). Civil competency. In I.B. Weiner & A.K. Hess (Eds.), *The handbook of forensic psychology,* (3rd ed.). Hoboken, NJ: John Wiley & Sons.)

Case Study

A Question of Competency

The adult children of 85-year-old Mr. P have petitioned the court to have their father declared incompetent to make financial, personal, and medical decisions. They have requested that the eldest son be named legal guardian for the remainder of Mr. P's life.

The adult children are concerned about their father's decision to marry a 65-year-old widow, whom he has known for only 2 months. They claim that the woman is a "gold-digger" who only wants access to Mr. P's modest estate. They also note that Mr. P has been having decisional difficulties of late. They state he has been acting unusually extravagant and that he had always been conservative throughout his life. As one example, they state that Mr. P would have remortgaged his home last year to go on an extensive cruise had they not intervened and convinced him that he could not make the monthly payments. The adult children feared their father could have lost his home, especially since his forgetfulness has caused him to be delinquent in his property taxes this past year. They also note that Mr. P had recently been diagnosed with colon cancer, but that he refused both surgical and medical interventions.

Mr. P states that he loves his children dearly, but they simply do not understand the needs of an old and dying man. He states he knows his memory is not what

it used to be and that he frequently misplaces things, but that he still knows what's going on. He states he is an old man who has already made his peace with God and that he lived a good life and was blessed with a good family. He missed his beloved wife who died 10 years ago, but he does love his intended, with whom he wants to spend his last days.

Mr. P's medical records note the following: moderately active 85-year-old male who lives in a two-bedroom, ranch home; hygiene and dress appropriate; ADLs met with some difficulty; history of hypertension, diabetes, and coronary artery disease with increasing noncompliance with medications; recently diagnosed with Stage III colon cancer and refuses treatment; no past history of mental illness or substance abuse.

Discussion Questions:

1. How would competency/incompetency be assessed?
2. Describe the roles of the nurse generalist and the advanced practice forensic nurse, generalist and advanced practice psychiatric nurse, primary care advanced practice nurse (for those in this role) for both the plaintiff (adult children) and the defense (Mr. P).

nature of the debilitating condition is of particular importance. The majority of defendants involved in criminal proceedings who are found incompetent have a combination of low IQ, psychotic symptoms, and/or affective disorder.

There are several classes of conditions that result in impairment and therefore are likely to result in the appointment of a guardian. One class includes conditions that have stable and significant impairment and little likelihood of improvement. This first classification would include developmental disabilities such as mental retardation, chronic and persistent mental illness (certain forms of schizophrenia), and irreversible brain damage. Second, competency would be assessed in persons with progressive, degenerative diseases such as Huntington's chorea, Alzheimer's disease, or HIV/AIDS. Third in the classification of conditions for which competency hearings are performed involves diseases or impairments with a sudden onset. Included in this group would be neurological disease or dysfunction, motor vehicle accidents involving brain injury or coma, and certain forms of mental illness.

In addition, treatable infections/diseases for which cognitive impairment is sustained may lead to the need for competency hearings. This class of impairment differs from the others in that the prognosis may include substantial recovery, at which time the determination of incompetence may be overturned.

Competency Evaluation Considerations

One primary factor to consider during the competency evaluation is the nature of the impairment and the likely course of the condition over time. There are also other factors that influence the cognitive resources and adaptive functioning of the individual. The clinician should make every effort to ensure that the information obtained in evaluations is accurate and thorough, particularly since there may be a restriction of rights following the evaluation. Recommendations and predictions based on the evaluation must be appropriate and serve the best interests of the individual. Information that is typically obtained includes current cognitive functioning of the individual. If the impairment is progressive in nature (such as in the case of AIDS or Alzheimer's), then recent cognitive functioning is also relevant. Cognitive functioning is often determined through neuropsychological assessment batteries that are administered and interpreted by a neuropsychologist or other professional trained in the administration of such assessments.

Assessment batteries may include the Brief Neuropsychological Cognitive Exam (BNCE) and the Dementia Rating Scale (DRS). Both scales assess current cognitive functioning across several domains. Both the BNCE and the DRS have demonstrated sound psychometric properties and are used in a variety of settings to quickly and accurately determine the cognitive functioning of an individual.

In addition to assessments of cognitive functioning, the adaptive functioning, or ability to perform day-to-day tasks, is also assessed. Adaptive functioning is determined through behavioral observations, corroborative materials obtained from individuals who have regular contact with the subject, and interviews with the subject. Again, the evaluation of competency must take into account the skills being questioned, such that deficits in other, irrelevant areas are not influential in the decision-making process.

To complete the assessment, there are additional factors that might be taken into account during the evaluation. Impairment-related factors that should be evaluated include the etiology of the impairment, whether it is stable, progressive, or treatable, as well as any subsequent and likely prognosis. Impairments that are severe, stable, and degenerative should be interpreted differently than those that are acute, unstable, and treatable. The history of the functioning of the individual should be incorporated into the evaluation, as well as the resources available to the subject (e.g., social supports, financial situation, treatment options). However, although historical information is often reviewed, the competency determination is actually based on current functioning.

An additional factor to consider in a competency evaluation is the validity of the information obtained from the subject and the corroborating sources. The subject may be motivated to perform poorly or inaccurately, depending on the possible outcomes of the evaluation. The subject's ability to stand trial may be in question, so he or she may be motivated to appear more impaired so as to avoid being tried as a competent defendant. On the other hand, an individual attempting to maintain an independent living situation would be motivated to perform to the best of his or her ability. Several tests of malingering (a purposeful behavior exhibited for a specific reason) exist to measure the validity of the subject's performance, but an awareness of the various motivational factors at work is also necessary. These tests are intended to detect the degree of motivation present and any efforts to manipulate test results. Typically, if the examinee's performance on such measures indicates that malingering is suspected, the evaluation is considered invalid.

Restoration of Competency

The restoration of competency as determined by the court may be possible for individuals with treatable conditions for which improved function is conceivable. If indicated, the court would order a hearing, and the reasons for the request to restore competency would be heard. If the court finds the evidence of improvement to be compelling, then the need for guardianship may be dismissed or modified. The decision to restore competency is based on the degree of improvement. If the ward has fully regained his or her capacity to make decisions, then he or she could have full restoration of rights. If the improvements were circumscribed to a few areas, but some deficiencies remained, then the order of incompetency would be modified, and the rights would be restored to the ward, to the extent possible. Given that the ward's decision-making abilities may improve, the assessment of his or her functioning is ongoing, with regular annual reviews being held before the court.

Competency to Proceed and Criminal Responsibility

Competency and criminal responsibility are two different issues. Competency refers to the "here and now" ability of an offender to function, such as competency to stand trial or to plead guilty (**competency to proceed**). Other types of criminal competency evaluations include: competency to waive Miranda warnings; competency to confess; competency to waive trial by jury; competency to waive counsel; competency to testify; competency to be sentenced; and competency to be executed. **Criminal responsibility**, as in the insanity defense, refers to the offender's **mental state at the time of the offense (MSO).** The MSO is determined through a series of three interviews. The first focuses upon historical information about the subject, the second examines the mental state at the time the offense occurred, and the third assesses the subject's current mental state. Factors such as planning the offense, awareness of the criminality of the act(s), and degree of self-control are rated to determine if a mental disorder caused cognitive impairment at the time of the offense.

Competency to Proceed

Competency denotes the person's capacity to function knowingly and meaningfully in a legal proceeding, understanding the legal proceedings, communicating with attorneys, appreciating one's role in the proceedings, and making legally relevant decisions. Competency to stand trial (CST) is also termed "fitness" in some jurisdictions and serves four legal purposes. First, being fit to stand trial safeguards the accuracy of the criminal adjudication; second, it guarantees a fair trial; and third, it preserves the dignity and integrity of the legal process. Finally, fitness ensures that the defendant knows why he or she will be punished if found guilty. Trying incompetent defendants violates their constitutional rights, including the 14th Amendment right to due process. A CST evaluation may be the most common forensic psychiatric evaluation, and 2% to 8% of all felony defendants are referred for competency evaluations.

All states now have competency statutes that are either exact or modified versions of the original Dusky standard, which was the standard for competency to stand trial set by the U.S. Supreme Court in *Dusky v. U.S.* in 1960. The standard is whether a defendant has adequate present ability to consult with his or her attorney with a reasonable degree of rational understanding of the proceedings. It is not sufficient that the defendant be oriented to time, place, and some events. Concerns about a defendant's competence may arise at different stages of the judicial process. Therefore, competency to proceed may be reevaluated at any time during the criminal proceedings if the defendant appears to be exhibiting signs of mental illness. For example, defendants may require brief competency assessments while awaiting trial if they exhibit bizarre behavior. Requests for evaluations may also come from the defendant's defense attorney or the court. Assessments may include a mental status exam (MSE), clinical interview, and psychological tests.

Specific tests used in competency to proceed to trial evaluations include the Competency Screening Test (CST) and the Competency Assessment Instrument (CAI). In a study by Nottingham and Mattson (2005), 50 male residents of a state forensic unit were administered the CST. The residents were later interviewed by the forensic team to determine whether they were competent to stand trial. Results showed that the CST correctly predicted the competency recommendations of the forensic team in 82% of the 50 cases. The data were consistent with previous research and suggest that the CST be further investigated as a preliminary screening instrument in the determination of competency to stand trial. Good internal consistency is reported for the CAI scales (Cronbach's $\alpha = 0.52$ to 0.93), test-retest reliability (scales ranged from 0.42 to 0.78), and validity and thus should be useful in efforts to accurately determine competency.

Competence to proceed determines the defendant's capacity in the present and must be determined each time he or she goes to court. A previous determination of incompetence does not preclude a subsequent finding of competency in a later, unrelated case. No person may be tried if found incompetent, and the court remands incompetent defendants to suitable facilities for treatment to regain competency.

Forensic psychiatric mental health nurses can function as competency therapists. The nurse must remain objective, however. Competency therapy to assist a person in regaining competency to stand trial is not a form of psychotherapy. The nurse performs the assessment at the request of a client who is a member of the court, not at the request of the defendant.

Criminal Responsibility

The law recognizes that the responsibility for committing a crime depends on two factors. First is *actus reus,* which is the physical action (or omission) that makes one liable for a crime. Second is **mens rea,** which means that the accused had the mental capacity to have intended to commit the act or have foreseen its consequences. Intent is a top priority in murder cases because it helps separate different degrees of homicide, from negligence for manslaughter to premeditation for first-degree murder.

Sanity is a legal, not clinical, term related to a plea of **not guilty by reason of insanity (NGRI).** Sanity evaluations may be entered into evidence at a criminal trial to help a judge or jury determine whether a defendant is criminally responsible for an alleged offense. The definition of legal sanity varies from one jurisdiction to another, but it usually denotes the defendant's ability to tell right from wrong with respect to the offense. Forensic psychiatric mental health nurses need to be aware of the standard that applies in their jurisdiction. Most jurisdictions also view insanity; automatism (somnambulism, hypnotic states, fugues, epilepsy, and metabolic disorders); and diminished capacity (impaired mental state short of insanity) as separate defenses. A defense of diminished capacity is typically used to aid in determining the degree of the offense or the punishment.

Although the insanity defense traces back to biblical times, it emerges in its modern form in the 1843 case of Daniel M'Naghten. M'Naghten was found insane for mistakenly killing the secretary of British Prime Minister Robert Peel in an assassination attempt on Peel. The House of Lords then set the parameters for the insanity defense that dominated Anglo-American jurisprudence for more than a century. To prevail, defendants must have a mental illness or defect so severe that they did not understand the "nature and quality of the act" or did not know it was wrong. This defense started to evolve in the United States in 1962, when some states adopted the approach of the Model Penal Code developed by the American Law Institute. The code expanded the M'Naghten rule beyond the defendant's understanding of the act to include the inability "to conform his conduct to the requirements of the law."

The Durham Rule (1954) went further and stated that there is a causal relationship between the mental disease and the act, yet this rule was rejected in 1972. In 1962, the American Law Institute issued the Model Penal Code, based on the M'Naughten rule and the irresistible impulse standard of 1929. The M'Naughten rule stated that a defendant is not responsible for his or her criminal conduct if, as a result of **mental disease or defect,** the defendant lacked substantial capacity to appreciate the criminality of the act or conform his or her conduct to the requirements of the law. The irresistible impulse standard recognizes the ability of the defendant to distinguish right from wrong at the time of the offense, but affirms that he or she could not control the impulse to commit the crime due to some mental disease or disorder. Further clarification came about with the 1962 McDonald modification, which stated that the mental diseases or defects must substantially impair mental or emotional processes and impact one's behavior.

Demands for abolition of the insanity defense surfaced in 1982 after John Hinckley was found not guilty by reason of insanity in his assassination attempt on President Ronald Reagan. The defense survived, but many jurisdictions reduced the M'Naghten rule to the defendant's understanding of right and wrong. The Hinkley case also resulted in a change in the burden of proof, which shifted from prosecutors to defendants in most states and supplemented the NGRI verdict with a **guilty but mentally ill (GBMI)** verdict. Some states also changed the standard of proof from a preponderance of evidence to clear and convincing evidence.

Currently, all insanity standards require that the defendant had a mental disease or defect at the time of the offense. However, the terms "mental disease" and "mental defect" do not equate with particular disorders listed in the *Diagnostic and Statistical Manual IV-Text Revised* (DSM-IV-TR) (2000), which is used by mental health professionals to describe psychiatric diagnoses by diagnostic criteria and gives information about the disorders. Courts typically rule that serious psychotic and mood disorders qualify as a mental disease and mental retardation qualifies as a mental defect. However, the courts do not usually qualify personality disorders, paraphilias (sexual deviations), and voluntary intoxication as a disease or defect.

The forensic psychiatric mental health nurse reviews all pertinent medical and legal records and performs a MSE, an interview, and psychological testing of the offender. An instrument that may be used for assessment is the Rogers Criminal Responsibility Assessment Scales (R-CRAS) (Rogers and Sewell, 1999). The five graded scales, reliability, organicity, psychopathology, cognitive control, and behavioral control, have 30 items each. Construct validity of the R-CRAS was examined in a reanalysis of 413 insanity cases with six separate discriminant analyses to address major components of insanity evaluations. The analyses yielded highly discriminating patterns (M hit rates of 94.3%) and accounted for a substantial proportion of the variance (M = 63.7%), supporting the predicted relationships between individual variables and the discriminant functions. The researchers also found the R-CRAS variables useful for the assessment of insanity and found that the variables contributed substantially to the determination of criminal responsibility.

The forensic psychiatric nurse uses various tools during the assessment interview to determine the presence of the following:

- Signs of irresistible impulse, such as inability to defer the act
- Signs of the defendant knowing the act was wrong by demonstrated efforts to avoid prosecution (wearing gloves during commission of the offense, falsifying information) or disposal of evidence (hiding the body, removing fingerprints)
- Efforts to avoid apprehension (fleeing)

FORENSIC ASSESSMENT OF SEX OFFENDERS

Standards are often refined and clarified following a major publicized crime, such as Hinkley's assassination attempt of President Reagan. Policy development and passage of new laws are subsequently generated due to public outcry and fear for individual and community safety.

Megan's Law and the Adam Walsh Law

Subsequent to the rape and murder of 7-year-old Megan Kanka, the state of New Jersey led the United States in sex offender legislation with the passage of Megan's Law in 1994. The law requires law enforcement officials to notify the public of convicted sexual offenders who live in the local community. The law was prompted, in part, by the public awareness of the fact that Megan's murderer had previously pled guilty to the attempted aggravated sexual assault of another young girl. Megan's death was considered by many to have been preventable, since the offender had a previous guilty plea for a similar act. Supporters of the law argued that parents have the right to know if a dangerous sexual predator lives in their neighborhood.

Two years later, the federal government required every state to enact similar laws. Upon release from prison, convicted sex offenders are required to notify local law enforcement of their address. The types of sex offenders that are required to adhere to this law, and the period of time for which it applies, vary by state, but it is approximately 10 years.

Proponents of Megan's Law argued that the purpose of the law was to enhance public safety, not to punish or harass the offenders. Critics of the law, however, argued that people convicted of consensual acts or public nudity (e.g., streaking, skinny dipping, and public urination) should not be lumped together with dangerous sexual predators. More importantly, others argued that the most dangerous offenders are unlikely to register or may provide false information. The registered offenders are more apt to be law-abiding and less threatening. Further criticisms have been generated by civil rights activists and law enforcement officials who purport that the registries provide vigilantes with the means to find the offenders and harass, injure, and even kill them. Several states have reported crimes that target sex offenders who are registered.

Despite the efforts made by each state to monitor and track convicted sex offenders, many offenders evade the registries, and their whereabouts remain unknown to legal authorities. As many as 100,000 convicted sex offenders were unaccounted for nationwide in 2006. The lack of funding necessary to develop a more comprehensive and effective tracking program for missing convicted sex offenders who have evaded registering resulted in President George W. Bush signing the Adam Walsh Child Protection and Safety Act into law in 2006. Under this law, a national sex offender registry was created that required each state to follow the same criteria for posting offender information on the Internet. This law also provided more clarity and categorized offenders into three tiers according to the severity of the crime. The most dangerous offenders are in Tier III, and they are required to register for life (or 25 years for juvenile offenders) and update their whereabouts in person every 3 months. Failure to do so is a felony offense. Tier II offenders must register in person every 6 months for 25 years, and Tier I offenders must do so annually for 15 years.

Pathways to Offending

What factors lead an individual to become a sexual offender is an empirical question that has attracted considerable scientific attention over the past several years. Several theoretical models focus primarily on a single or small cluster of causal factors (Box 13.7). One line of theorists implicate biological mechanisms such as genetic determinants, hormone imbalances, or both, as being responsible for the onset of sexually aggressive and sexually deviant behavior. Other researchers have found structural brain abnormalities to be associated with sexual aggression.

An alternative causative pathway posits that issues of attachment and early social development are responsible for sexual dysfunction later in life. Some researchers have found that insecurely attached boys with emotionally unsupportive parents are more likely to become sexual predators later in life. Consequences of the negative attachment style may also include problems with intimacy in adulthood. Attempts to establish loving relationships are thwarted by fears of rejection and may lead to abusive behavior. Similarly, other developmental variables have been associated with sexual violence. Children who were raised in an abusive or violent household, or who were exposed to social environments that promote criminality, aggression, defiance, and the inferiority of women, are linked with sexual violence. In accordance with social learning theory, children observe and learn from their social environments. If childhood social environments include violence, abuse, and the degradation of women, then the propensity to mimic those behaviors is strengthened. For these reasons, several theorists have argued that the graphic violence on television, in conjunction with the portrayal of women as submissive and sexualized, can serve to desensitize children to violence and promote sexual aggression.

Although each of these theories has established supportive evidence, none of them are able to account for all instances of sexual violence. The etiological pathways to

---

Box 13.7   Theoretical Components that Contribute to Sexual Aggression

- Biological components: hormonal imbalances and neurological abnormalities
- Developmental vulnerabilities: a history of abuse, neglect, violence, abandonment
- Interpersonal problems: social skills deficits, lack of empathy, history of rejection, social isolation
- Cognitive distortions: justification of sexual aggression and deviant behavior, negative beliefs about women
- Contextual or proximal factors: increased stress, negative emotion, emotional instability, poor impulse control, intoxication that contributes to the breakdown of inhibitions

sexual offending are multiple and complex. More recent models attempt to incorporate several, or all, of these individual factors. Examples of such integrated models will be described; however, a comprehensive review of each model is beyond the scope of this chapter. There is also a great deal of overlap among theories.

One of the earliest multifactor theories focused specifically on the etiological factors involved in child molestation. In the precondition theory, Finkelhor suggested that four underlying motivations precipitate the sexual offense, and each one is necessary for the offense to take place. According to the precondition theory, the offender finds sex with children to be emotionally satisfying (emotional congruence); the offender is aroused by the child (sexual arousal); the offender is unable to satisfy sexual needs in socially acceptable ways (blockage); and the offender must be able to overcome sexual inhibitions (disinhibition). Once the offender is motivated (e.g., targets a child, is aroused by the child), disinhibited (e.g., intoxicated, under stress, experiences poor impulse control), and able to overcome the child's resistance (e.g., become friends, give gifts, gradually escalate sexual behaviors, etc.), then the offense will occur.

Another multifactor theory of child molestation is the quadripartite theory. The quadripartite theory suggests that offenders exhibit an underlying personality disposition that acts as a precursor, or vulnerability, to offending. When this underlying precursor is combined with situational factors, then the offense will occur. The situational factors include sexual arousal, cognitive distortions or beliefs that justify sexual aggression, and emotional dysregulation.

Hall and Hirshman's quadripartite theory incorporates both underlying personality factors as well as current situational factors in their etiological explanation of sexual offending. A similar theory is the integrated theory of Marshall and Barabee. The integrated theory suggests that distal, developmental factors interact with more proximal, situational factors to set the stage for sexual offending. Negative events in childhood, such as punitive or negligent parenting, physical or sexual abuse, and emotional or physical conflict between parents, may result in the cognitive perception or attitude that interpersonal relationships are dysfunctional and painful. As a result, social and self-regulation skills are impaired. Marshall and Barabee claim that these developmental stressors predispose the individual to behave in antisocial ways. The negative attitudes about social relationships are well-established by the time an individual has reached adolescence. The neural structures responsible for sexual arousal are the amygdala and hypothalamus, the same neural structures associated with

aggression. For adolescent males who are predisposed toward aggression, the pubertal influx of sex hormones may act as an associated link between sexual arousal and aggression. If the young men experience rejection from women due to their social and self-control deficits, they may begin to view women with hostility and anger. Anger may result in sexual fantasies that incorporate violence and aggression, which are rehearsed through masturbation. Adult women come to be viewed as rejecting and threatening, so the individual targets children, who are seen as safe and nonthreatening. The offender is able to regain a sense of power and masculinity, while releasing sexual tension and experiencing personal intimacy when he targets children. The distal vulnerability factors, such as an abusive childhood or negative relationship experiences, then interact with proximal situational factors of stress, emotional instability, intoxication, an available victim, and the result is the sexual offense. The sexual offense is reinforced by the sexual gratification, intimacy, and sense of power that maintain the sexually deviant behavior.

Evaluation of Sex Offenders

The advanced practice forensic psychiatric nurse determines whether a sex offender meets the criteria for a mental disease/defect or personality disorder that places the person at risk for sexual offending and thereby determines whether the person is following a sexual deviant (paraphilic) pathway or antisocial **pathway to offending.** Offenders who follow a sexually deviant pathway to sexual offending have intense sexually arousing fantasies, sexual urges, or behaviors that generally involve nonhuman objects. Fantasies include the suffering or humiliation of themselves or their partners, children, or other nonconsenting persons. Such fantasies occur over a period of 6 months or more. For example, an adult offender sexually assaulted his 7-year-old niece for a period of 2 years. He has no history of any other criminal or juvenile delinquent behavior. He is most likely following a sexually deviant pathway, possibly pedophilia.

Offenders who follow a generally antisocial pathway to sexual offending have a pervasive pattern of disregard for, and violation of, the rights of others. Their behaviors fall into patterns that include failing to conform to social norms with respect to lawful behavior, impulsivity, frequent deceit and manipulation for personal gain, irritability, aggression, recklessness, irresponsibility, and risk-taking behaviors. If on this pathway, the offender may have raped an adult stranger, but the offender also has a history of juvenile delinquency, chronic lying, relationship and employment problems, and a history of other criminal activity besides the rape. For example, an adult male sexually assaults both his school-age daughter and his wife. He has a history of substance abuse and numerous nonsexual crimes committed both as a juvenile and an adult. He is most likely following an antisocial pathway.

Etiological theories of sexual offending are important because they help clinicians to better understand how and why an individual becomes a sexual offender. However, by establishing the causal pathways associated with deviant sexual behavior, it may also be possible to identify the risk factors for offending (and reoffending) to both prevent future offenses and provide effective treatment for sex offenders.

Risk assessment includes the identification of static and dynamic risk factors. Historical characteristics that cannot be altered, such as age of the offender, gender of the victims, relationship between the offender and the victims, and prior offense history, are referred to as **static risk factors.** Attitudes and characteristics that can change throughout a person's life are termed **dynamic risk factors.** Dynamic factors can be further categorized as stable or acute. Stable dynamic factors include deviant sexual preferences and practices and victim blaming, whereas acute dynamic factors include intoxication preceding the offense.

The two predominant methods of assessing risk of offending are actuarial risk assessment and clinical judgment. **Actuarial risk assessment** incorporates risk factors that have been identified through scientific research into an actuarial measure. Based on the individual's score on the measures, the probability of reoffending is calculated. These actuarial measures rely almost exclusively on static, or unchanging, factors, such as criminal history, the nature of the offense, age at time of offense, etc. Examples of actuarial risk assessments are the STATIC-99 and the Minnesota Sex Offender Screening Tool (MnSOST-R). STATIC-99 is an instrument designed to assist in the prediction of sexual and violent recidivism for sexual offenders. This risk assessment was developed by Hanson and Thornton (1999) based on follow-up studies from Canada and the United Kingdom, with a total sample size of 1301 sexual offenders. The STATIC-99 consists of 10 items and produces estimates of future risk based upon the number of risk factors present in any one individual. The risk factors included in the risk assessment instrument are the presence of prior sexual offenses, having committed a current nonsexual violent offense, having a history of nonsexual violence, the number of previous sentencing dates, being younger than 25 years old, having male victims, having never lived with a lover for 2 or more consecutive years, having a history of noncontact sex offenses, having unrelated victims, and having stranger victims.

The MnSOST-R consists of 16 items that measure dynamic, criminal, chronic, offender-related, and unstable lifestyle variables. Two reliability studies present evidence that attest to the reliability of raters using the MnSOST-R. The Minnesota study yielded a reliability coefficient of 0.76, whereas the Florida study yielded a reliability coefficient of 0.86. The validity indices for the MnSOST-R in a cross-validation study ($r = 0.35$; ROC AUC = 0.73) are comparable to those reported for similar sex offender actuarial risk assessment tools.

Other assessment tools include the Rapid Risk Assessment for Sex Offense Recidivism (RRASOR), which correlated at 0.27 with sexual recidivism; the Violence Risk Appraisal Guide (VRAG), which was developed to determine risk for violent recidivism for males who have committed a violent offense that was either sexual or nonsexual in nature; the Sex Offender Risk Appraisal Guide (SORAG), which has 14 items in total (10 identical to VRAG items) and was developed to predict offenders' probability for committing sexual and sexually violent offenses.

An alternative assessment method involves using clinical judgment. This method involves the collection of interview materials and offender criminal records. Once the relevant information has been collected and reviewed, the clinician arrives at a judgment about the offender's likelihood of reoffending. Factors that are often considered include criminal history, psychiatric diagnosis, social supports, and relationship stability. Considerable overlap exists among clinicians' impressions of the factors most predictive of future offending. The factors that were identified as valid clinician impressions included degree of insight (does the offender view himself as dangerous, violent, impulsive, have negative attitudes such as antisocial beliefs); the presence of mental illness; impulsivity; and failed treatment efforts.

Alternatively, research suggests that clinical judgments are subjective, lack reliability, and are often inferior to actuarial measures. The empirical and professional trend has been to integrate the clinical judgment and risk assessment tools to maximize predictive power and accuracy. One example of an integrated approach is the Clinically Adjusted Actuarial Approach. The actuarial measures, as well as clinical judgments, dispositional factors (e.g., an antisocial, angry, or impulsive personality), and contextual factors (e.g., intoxication, stress, availability of a victim), are incorporated. Other theorists have attempted to integrate static, unchanging factors (e.g., developmental adversity) with dynamic, contextual factors. For instance, Hanson and Harris incorporate "acute dynamic risk factors," which they define as factors that may signal that an individual is highly likely to commit an offense in the near future. Examples of these risk factors include fluctuating mood states, substance abuse, a humiliation or rejection experience, or the availability of a child/victim.

Overall, the integration of actuarial and clinical approaches, static and dynamic factors, and dispositional and contextual factors appears to be the current trend. The ultimate goal, both empirically and clinically, is to achieve a comprehensive approach to risk assessment that will result in more accurate predictions and appropriate treatment methods.

EVIDENCE-BASED FORENSIC MENTAL HEALTH NURSING

There are numerous roles that may lie ahead for forensic psychiatric mental health nurses, including working in mental health and drug courts, in violence and recidivism prevention, with victims of violent crimes, and in civil cases, such as child custody and elder law issues. However, it is critical that forensic psychiatric mental health nurses establish themselves as a distinct subspecialty of both forensic and psychiatric nursing. There is a need to differentiate the roles of the generalist and specialist nurse, with clear delineations in the scope and standards of practice for both levels. It would also be prudent to develop more stringent educational standards so that APNs are better prepared for the forensic psychiatric role, including forensic assessment for civil competency, competency to proceed, criminal responsibility, and the evaluation and treatment of sexual and other offenders. The recent development of the doctor of nursing practice (DNP) degree creates an ideal environment for this type of education.

Case Study

RISK OF RECIDIVISM

(Please note that specific charges and agency names have not been used due to their differences throughout jurisdictions nationwide.)

Mr. C is a 45-year-old male who is currently serving 5 to 10 years incarceration for sexually abusing his three biological daughters, ages 5, 8, and 9 years at the time of the abuse. He is presently up for parole and presents for evaluation of recidivism risk. Mr. C pled guilty to charges involving fondling of his 5-year-old daughter and oral sex with the older daughters. Child pornography possession charges were dropped as part of the plea bargain. The incidents took place over a 3-year period, following Mr. C's loss of his job as a long-distance truck driver, a job that he held for 15 years and lost because the company went out of business. He has no previous offenses as an adult or as a juvenile and has incurred no misconducts during his incarceration. There is one Child Abuse Agency Report from when Mr. C was 23 years old that claimed he fondled his then 7-year-old niece; the claim was not substantiated, and charges were not filed. Mr. C has no history of substance abuse or treatment for mental illness. Mr. C began sex offender treatment during his incarceration, but has not completed it.

Mr. C's history is remarkable for the following: he is the youngest of five siblings in an intact family. Both his parents are deceased, but he has kept in contact with his siblings, even through his incarceration. He denied ever being sexually, physically, or emotionally abused by his parents, but states his baseball coach fondled his genitals on several occasions when he was about 12 to 14 years old. He graduated high school and worked steadily at a factory before being employed as a trucker, a job he pursued because it was much better pay for his family, despite his frequent absences.

Mr. and Mrs. C married when he was 28. She was 25. His first experience with sexual intercourse was with Mrs. C on their wedding night because, according to Mr. C, he is a very religious person and wanted to wait until he was married. The marriage produced three daughters, the victims in the above-noted offense. Mrs. C filed for divorce immediately after Mr. C was incarcerated and has filed for sole custody of their children. Mr. C states that he plans to fight his ex-wife for custody because he has learned his lesson and would never touch them again.

Discussion Questions

1. Does Mr. C meet the criteria for a mental illness/defect or personality disorder that can cause him to sexually reoffend? (Use the following categories in the DSM-IV-TR: Paraphilias, Antisocial Personality Disorder, Personality Disorder Not Otherwise Specified [NOS]).
2. Use the brief history above and the STATIC-99 to assess Mr. C's risk of reoffending (realize that this is only a partial assessment and a learning exercise). (STATIC-99 coding rules and scoring sheet may be found at http://ww2.ps-sp.gc.ca/publications/corrections/pdf/Static-99-coding-Rules_e.pdf.)
3. Discuss possible nursing roles for this case: correctional health nurse, generalist forensic nurse, forensic nurse specialist, advance practice psychiatric nurse.

Evidence-Based Nursing Practice

Forensic psychiatric nursing research is still in its infancy, and nurses can incorporate evidence-based principles from other disciplines, such as psychiatry, psychology, and criminal justice, into practice. Doing so allows for more professional forensic assessments while fortifying the forensic psychiatric mental health nurse's role as an expert witness.

The wealth of opportunities for forensic psychiatric mental health research is endless, both for the role of the forensic psychiatric mental health nurse and for forensic psychiatric issues. For example, more research is needed regarding the treatment of sex offenders, particularly those with learning disabilities. A *Cochrane Review* summary of the treatment of sex offenders noted that, while there are currently a variety of treatment approaches (medication and talk therapy) for sex offenders, little is known about their success rate. Sex offenders with learning disabilities pose challenges, and talk therapies need to be modified to account for the offender's limited understanding. The reviewers noted that they could find no randomized controlled trial evidence to guide in the treatment of learning disabled sex offenders.

CONCLUSIONS

Forensic psychiatric mental health nursing is a challenging, though satisfying, career path for nurses. It provides an avenue for entrepreneurship for the individual nurse and a path for nursing to take in a field once dominated by other disciplines. Forensic psychiatric mental health nurses play an important role in the criminal justice system and may be involved in the assessment of an individual's competency to stand trial, evaluation of an offender's mental state during commission of a crime, and determination of a sex offender's likelihood of recidivism.

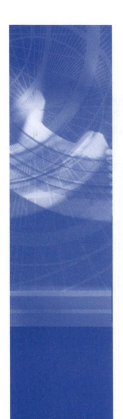

EVIDENCE-BASED PRACTICE BOX

Research Question: Does group therapy as opposed to individual therapy for mentally ill forensic patients increase competency to stand trial?

P = mentally ill forensic patients
I = group therapy
C = individual therapy
O = increased competency
T = within 1 year of treatment

Database(s) to Search: Lexis-Nexis

Search Strategy: Because of the small chance of finding research articles using the terms that are more popular—"mentally ill," "forensics," and "competency"—to find articles that talk about all three subjects, "AND" the terms and limit results to the desired publication date.

Selected References From Search:

1. *Drug Week* editors. (2009). Forensic science: Findings from S.B. Billick and co-researchers advance knowledge in forensic science. *NewsRx.com & NewsRx.net.* Retrieved August 14, 2009.
2. Erickson, S.K. (2008). The myth of mental disorder: Transsubstantive behavior and taxometric psychiatry. *Akron Law Review, 41*:67-112.
3. Cremin, K.M., Philips, J., Sickinger, C., & Zelhof, J. (2009). Ensuring a fair hearing for litigants with mental illnesses: The law and psychology of capacity, admissibility, and credibility assessments in civil proceedings. *Journal of Law and Policy, 17*(2):455.

Questions Used to Discern Evidence:

Choose two studies among the studies listed, read about them, and answer the following questions:

1. What are the differences between the two studies in the design, methods, and results?
2. What are the similarities between the two studies in the number of subjects, measures used, and interventions, if any?
3. What skills do you think you need to learn to practice psychiatric forensic nursing?

REVIEW QUESTIONS

1. A forensic psychiatric mental health nurse maintains the same type of therapeutic relationship between client and nurse as the traditional psychiatric nurse treatment approaches:
   A. True.
   B. False.

2. Collateral information obtained by a forensic psychiatric mental health nurse may *not* include interviewing the client due to which of the following:
   A. Principles of consultation
   B. Competency evaluation
   C. Fifth Amendment
   D. Criminal responsibility

3. Forensic psychiatric mental health nurses are involved in all of the following *except*:
   A. Evaluation of sex offenders
   B. Substance abuse counseling
   C. Risk assessment determination
   D. Collection of physical evidence from crime scenes

4. Factors that contribute to recidivism (reoffending) include:
   A. Homelessness
   B. Good social skills
   C. Job training
   D. Strong support systems

5. If a person is determined to be able to make his or her own decisions, that person is:
   A. Legally impaired
   B. Reliable
   C. An *ad litem* guardian
   D. Competent

6. Adaptive functioning is partially determined by observing and interviewing the subject:
   A. True
   B. False

7. The mental state at time of offense (MSO) is determined by the subject's:
   A. Use of a weapon during commission of a crime
   B. Awareness of the criminality of an act
   C. Blood alcohol level
   D. Criminal record

8. The law that requires public notification of convicted sex offenders living in a local community is:
   A. Megan's Law
   B. Sex Offender Registry Law
   C. Public Access Law
   D. Adam Walsh's Law

9. Offenders who follow a sexually deviant pathway to offending are *not* likely to fantasize about harming themselves or others.
   A. True
   B. False

10. Risk factors that contribute to a sex offender's likelihood of recidivism (reoffending) include all of the following *except*:
    A. Prior sexual offenses
    B. History of nonsexual violence
    C. Current age greater than 30 years
    D. Having male victims

References

Abrams, A.A. (2002). Assessing competency in criminal proceedings. In B.V. Dorsten (Ed.), *Forensic psychology: From classroom to courtroom*. New York: Kluwer Academic/Plenum Publishers.

American Academy of Psychiatry and the Law. (1995). *Ethics and guidelines for the practice of forensic psychiatry*. Bloomfield, CT: American Academy of Psychiatry and the Law.

American Psychiatric Association (2000). Diagnostic and Statistical Manual-IV-TR. Washington D.C.: American Psychiatric Association.

American Psychiatric Association. (2006). *Training in subspecialties: Forensic psychiatry*. Retrieved December 28, 2007, from http://www.psych.org/edu/subspecialties.cfm

Anonymous. (2006). The evolving insanity defense. *The American Bar Association Journal, 92*:37.

Ashman, L., & Duggan, L. (2002). Interventions for learning disabled sex offenders. *Cochrane Database of Systematic Reviews, 2*. Art. No.: CD003682. DOI: 10.1002/14651858.CD003682.pub2.

Blackburn, R. (2000). Foreword. In D. Mercer, T. Mason, M. McKeown, et al. (Eds.), *Forensic mental health care*. Edinburgh: Churchill Livingston, pp. xi-xii.

Boersma, R. (2002). Forensic psychiatric nursing: Role development in the United States. *National Forensic Nurses' Research & Development Group Newsletter, 6*:1-2.

Bonnie, R.J. (1992). The competence of criminal defendants: A theoretical reformulation. *Behavioral Sciences and the Law, 10*:291-316.

Burnard, P. (1992). The expanded role of the forensic psychiatric nurse. In P. Morrison & P. Burnard (Eds.), *Aspects of forensic psychiatric nursing*. Aldrershot, UK: Averbury, pp. 139-154.

Brooke, P. (2006). Legal and ethical guidelines for safe practice. In E. Varcarolis, V. Carson, & N. Shoemaker (Eds.), *Foundations of psychiatric mental health nursing: A clinical approach*, 5th ed. Philadelphia: Saunders Elsevier, p. 119.

Burrow, S. (1993). The role conflict of the forensic nurse. *Senior Nurse, 13*:20-25.

Cashen, A. (2006). Extreme nursing: Forensic adolescent mental health nursing in Australia. *Journal of Child and Adolescent Psychiatric Nursing, 19*(3):99–102.

Coram, J. (1993). *Role development within a new subspecialty: Forensic nursing*. Unpublished master's thesis. Washington State University, Spokane, WA.

Coram, J. (2006). Psychiatric forensic nursing. In E. Varcarolis, V. Carson, & N. Shoemaker (Eds.), *Foundations of psychiatric mental health nursing: A clinical approach*, 5th ed. Philadelphia: Saunders Elsevier, pp. 623-631.

Ennis, B.J., & Hansen, C. (1976). Memorandum of law: Competency to stand trial. *Journal of Psychiatry and Law, 4*:491–512.

Fethouse, A. (2003). Competency to stand trial. *Behavioral Sciences and the Law, 21*:281–283.

Follet, M. (1940). As cited in Mintzberg, H., Dougherty, D., Jorgensen, J., et al., (1996). Some surprising things about collaboration: Knowing how people connect makes it work better. *Organization Dynamics, 25*(1):30-71.

Franzen, M.D. (2003). Neuropsychological evaluations in the context of competency decisions. In A.M. Horton, Jr. & L.C. Hartlage (Eds.), *Handbook of forensic neuropsychology*. New York: Springer Publishing.

Gardner, D. (2005). Ten lessons in collaboration. *Online Journal of Issues in Nursing, 10*(1). Retrieved December 12, 2007, from http://www.nursingworld.org/MainMenuCategories/ANAMarketplace/ANAPeriodicals/OJIN/TableofContents/Volume102005/No1January31/tpc26_116008.aspx

Gray, B. (1989). *Collaborating*. San Francisco: Jossey-Bass.

Greenburg, S.A., & Shuman, D.W. (1997). Irreconcilable conflict between therapeutic and forensic roles. *Professional Psychology: Research & Practice, 28*(1):50-57.

Hanson, R.K., & Harris, A. (1998). *Dynamic predictors of sexual recidivism*. Ottawa: Solicitor General of Canada. Retrieved from http://ww2.ps-sp.gc.ca/publications/corrections/199801b_e.pdf

Hanson, R.K., & Thornton, D. (1999). Static-99: Improving actuarial risk assessments for sex offenders. *User Report 99-02*. Ottawa: Department of the Solicitor General of Canada.

International Association of Forensic Nurses & the American Nurses Association. (1997). *Scope and standards of forensic nursing practice*. Washington, DC: American Nurses Association.

International Association of Forensic Nurses. (2006). About forensic nursing. Retrieved December 12, 2007, from http://iafn.org/about/aboutWork.cfm

James, D., & Glaze, L. (2006). *Mental health problems of prison and jail inmates*. U.S. Department of Justice, Bureau of Justice Statistics, Special Report NCJ 213600, revised December 14, 2006.

Lindeke, L., & Seickert, A. (2005). Nurse-physician workplace collaboration. *Online Journal of Issues in Nursing, 10*(1). Retrieved January 2, 2008, from http://www.medscape.com/viewarticle/499268

Martin, T. Something special: Forensic psychiatric nursing. *Journal of Psychiatric and Mental Health Nursing, 8*:25-32.

Mason, T. (2002). Forensic psychiatric nursing: A literature review and thematic analysis of role tensions. *Journal of Psychiatric and Mental Health Nursing, 9*:511-520.

Mattis, S. (1988). *Dementia rating scale professional manual*. Odessa, FL: Psychological Assessment Resources.

McNeil, D., Binder, R., & Robinson, J. (2005). Incarceration associated with homelessness, mental disorder, and co-occurring substance abuse. *Psychiatric Services, 56*:840–846.

Muller-Smith, P. (2006). Independent nurse consultant. *The Oklahoma Nurse, 51*(3):26.

Nicholson, R.A., & Kugler, K.E. (1991). Competent and incompetent criminal defendants: A quantitative review of comparative research. *Psychological Bulletin, 109*:355-370.

Nolan, P. (1993). *A history of mental health nursing*. London: Chapman Hill.

Nottingham, E., & Mattson, R. (2005). A validation study of the Competency Screening Test. *Law and Human Behavior, 5*(4):329-335.

Perlin, M. (1995). *1995 cumulative supplement to mental disability law: Civil and criminal,* (vol. 1). Charlottesville, VA: Michie.

Peternelj, C., Hufft, A., Connolly, P., et al. (2003). The role of the forensic nurse in Canada: An evolving specialty. In D. Robinson & A. Kettles (Eds.), *Forensic nursing and multidisciplinary care of the mentally disordered offender*. Philadelphia: Lippincott, Williams & Wilkins, pp. 192-212.

Richardson, J. (2006). *Sex offender risk assessment*. Institute of Public Policy. University of Missouri–Columbia. Retrieved from http://www.mosac.mo.gov/Documents/SOrisk-assessment.pdf

Rogers, R., & Sewell, K. (1999). The R-CRAS and insanity evaluations: A re-examination of construct validity. Rogers Criminal Responsibility Assessment Scales. *Behavioral Science and the Law, 17*(2):181-194.

Shelton, D. (2003). The clinical practice of juvenile forensic psychiatric nurses. *Journal of Psychosocial and Mental Health Services, 41*(9):42-53.

Slovenko, R. (2006). Civil competency. In I.B. Weiner & A.K. Hess (Eds.), *The handbook of forensic psychology*, 3rd ed. Hoboken, NJ: John Wiley & Sons.

Tonkonogy, J. (1997). *The brief neuropsychological cognitive exam*. Los Angeles: Western Psychological Services.

Varcarolis, E. (2006). Developing therapeutic relationships. In E. Varcarolis, V. Carson, & N. Shoemaker (Eds.), *Foundations of psychiatric mental health nursing: A clinical approach*, 5th ed. Philadelphia: Saunders Elsevier, pp. 155-170.

West, S., & Noffsinger, S. (2006). How to assess a defendant's mental state at the time of the offense. *Journal of Family Practice, 5*(8). Retrieved January 1, 2008, from http://www.jfponline.com/Pages.asp?AID=4312

Wrightsman, L., Greene, E., Nietzel, M., et al. (2002). *Psychology and the legal system*, 5th ed. Belmont, CA: Wadsworth.

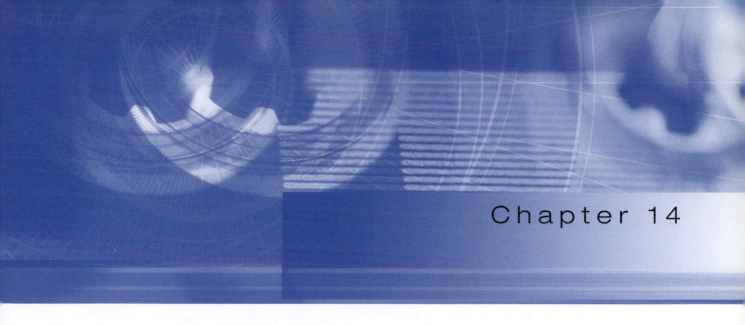

Chapter 14

CORRECTIONAL NURSING

Anita Hufft

"All life is an experiment. The more experiments you make the better."
Ralph Walso Emerson

Competencies

1. Relating standards of practice to the constitutional and ethical mandates to provide health care to individuals detained in secure settings within the criminal justice system.
2. Prioritizing nursing roles and interventions based on characteristics and needs of offenders.
3. Identifying multiple levels of vulnerability, culture, and risk associated with offender populations in jails and prisons.
4. Selecting nursing interventions that maximize security and safety within secure settings.
5. Promoting empowering and effective nursing strategies within collaborations with other staff and professionals in secure health-care settings within the criminal justice system

Key Terms

Access to care
Evidence-based correctional nursing
Factitious disorders
Incarceration
Malingering
Offender management
Ordered care
Professional judgment
Secure settings
Stress management

INTRODUCTION

One of the most significant demographic trends affecting public policy and health-care costs in the United States during the past 30 years has been the exponential growth of the number of people who are incarcerated. A study by the Pew Charitable Trust Public Safety Performance Project projected an increase in the inmate population at a rate three times faster than the growth of the overall population in the United States, which is expected to cost states more than $27 billion. More than 1.7 million inmates are expected to populate the prisons and jails of the United States by the end of 2012, and there are over 2.2 million Americans incarcerated on any given day. The nation's population, by comparison, is projected to grow by 4.5% in that time.

Over $3.3 billion was spent on inmate medical care in 2001. States are projected to spend up to $27.5 billion on the new inmates, including $12.5 billion in construction costs, according to the study. Currently, men outnumber women in prison nearly 14 to 1. In the next 5 years, the number of women inmates is projected to increase by 16% compared with a 12% increase for men. These individuals have health-care needs that will be met through an extensive and complex system of correctional health care, and that care will be provided by correctional nurses.

Correctional nursing practice is determined by the unique nature of the correctional practice environment and characteristics as well as the needs of the inmate client. A significant factor influencing the practice of correctional nursing is the impact of inmates' constitutional rights and court principles on nursing practice in the correctional setting. Upon entry to a correctional setting, inmates lose their rights to basic freedoms and live under supervision and control of a governing agency. Inmates must rely on correctional authorities to meet their medical needs, and courts have interpreted the Eighth Amendment to the U.S. Constitution to mean that failure to provide convicted and pretrial inmates with necessary medical care and treatment is cruel and unusual punishment. Established principles of constitutional law require correctional facilities to provide inmates with necessary dental, medical, psychiatric, and psychological treatment.

Competent nursing practice in correctional settings requires collaboration in the decision of *what is medically necessary care* for each detained individual. Nurses are responsible for ensuring that those individuals in their care are not subjected to deliberate indifference to a serious medical need. To reliably determine appropriate care in the context of correctional settings, an evidence base for that care is essential.

EVIDENCE-BASED CORRECTIONAL NURSING PRACTICE

Evidence-based correctional nursing practice integrates individual clinical expertise with the best available external clinical evidence from systematic research and institutional data sources relevant to correctional health care. Evidence-based correctional nursing is characterized by the use of empirically validated processes that facilitate conscientious, explicit, and judicious application of clinical expertise, patient hopes and values, and the best available clinical evidence from systematic research.

Clinical expertise for correctional nursing requires the requisite knowledge and experience to make correct decisions in a specific clinical situation at the right time. When there is insufficient research guiding decision making related to specific clinical problems, clinicians must rely on only clinical expertise to support their decisions. The first step in developing clinical expertise as a correctional nurse involves understanding what is known and not known and identifying strengths and weaknesses in relation to correctional health care.

"Understanding the rules" is the foundation for successful correctional nursing, and evidence for practice must relate to and complement the regulations inherent in any correctional setting. Rules for correctional nursing practice are established through the body of policies, procedures, and regulations governing specific jurisdictions of correctional health care. Just knowing the "rules" is not enough. The nurse must understand who developed the rules and if the rules are valid and up to date. Upon what body of evidence, ethical principle, or legal statute were the rules based? Placing the procedural guidelines, policies, and procedures in an evidence-based context is a critical component of the role socialization for correctional nursing. A correctional nurse expert questions knowledge, learns new information, and questions the validity and reliability of the data that contribute to making decisions.

Whether acknowledged or not, personal values dramatically affect correctional nursing practice as individual nurses bring personal biases and stereotypes to the care of inmates. The clinical decision-making process is guided by both the objective and subjective interpretation of assessment data, and it will rely heavily on the presentation of symptoms and communications of the inmate. How these data are interpreted depends on the experiences of the nurse and the ability of the nurse to frame interpretation of inmate health status and need in terms of evidence and fact, rather than a belief system built on television programming, experience as a victim, or other nonscientific sources. Clinical expertise in correctional nursing is not necessarily a function of seniority or experience. Expert knowledge, along with experience in successful problem solving, is the basis for correctional nursing expertise. Evidence-based correctional nursing depends on a comprehensive orientation to the principles and "rules" of correctional nursing practice and access to scientific data sources supporting practice. A critical aspect of successful correctional nursing practice is the availability of senior nursing mentors who value evidence-based practice and who have been successful in achieving desired clinical outcomes with inmate patients.

Evidence-based correctional nursing practice is based on the principle that there are levels of evidence and some forms of evidence that are more informative for clinical decision making than others. Correctional nurses must consider research conducted in correctional settings with correctional populations and related research, along with the best available data that allow for a consideration of potential costs, benefits, and harms that could result from nursing decisions and interventions. Evidence-based correctional nursing involves a thoughtful consideration of diagnosis, causation, treatment, prevention, harm, guidelines, cost-effectiveness, and more. The correctional nurse expert develops skills in adapting general scientific knowledge to solving problems in the correctional health setting.

Populations Served by Correctional Nurses

Populations served in correctional settings present unique challenges for nurses, including knowledge of inmate characteristics so that the nurse may appropriately assess inmate health needs and care priorities. Jails differ from prisons in that jails incarcerate people awaiting trials, people serving less than 1-year sentences, and people serving parole or probation violations. Jail populations tend to have high rates of substance abuse, mental illnesses, and infections and chronic diseases. Few people serving jail terms receive health interventions addressing the physical and psychosocial problems that contributed to their incarcerations in the first place.

The ability of the correctional nurses to intervene successfully with patients in a sensitive, creative, and responsible manner is contingent upon the ability to base care on scientific and other evidence-based knowledge and extend their roles to include personal advocacy for culturally competent care for inmates. Current population statistics indicate that the diversity of inmate populations will increase, emphasizing the subpopulations within correctional health-care systems and the unique health needs and challenges they represent.

Elderly

As mandated sentences for drug-related offenses continue to grow, along with an increase in mandatory length of sentences across all offenses, there has been a "graying" of the inmate population. Recent literature defines older offenders as those over the age of 50, based on the fact that the aging process is observed to be accelerated in the inmate population secondary to lifestyle, long-term substance abuse, poor nutrition, poor dental hygiene and lack of access to health-care services, lack of exercise, and the stress of **incarceration.** This premature aging is reflected in the estimation that inmates are, on average, 10 to 15 years older, physiologically, than their chronological age. Gerontological care and end-of-life care are essential components of correctional nursing. In addition to gerontological health problems related to aging, such as cardiovascular and musculoskeletal changes, compared to younger offenders, older offenders experience increased social isolation, depression, and risk of suicide. The British Geriatric Society identified characteristics of high-quality service for older inmates in a report based on the assessment of patient outcomes in geriatric medicine. Indicators of quality correctional health care include (1) adequate access to acute teams specializing in gerontological care; (2) policies for the referral and transfer specific for older inmates; (3) access to rehabilitation services for stroke and common orthogeriatric problems; (4) care protocols specific to falls, cerebrovascular disease, incontinence, osteoporosis, delirium, fractured neck of femur, and Parkinson's disease. Also included as elder-specific care requirements were professional in-service training for clinicians and support staff not trained in gerontology, programs of health promotion and preventive health care specific to elderly, and quality assurance indicators.

The need for long-term care nursing services among aging inmates requires an expansion of models of comprehensive health care in correctional settings. The World Health Organization conceptual model of functioning and disability provides a useful framework for gerontological rehabilitation, integrating complex body functions and structures, health conditions, individual activities and participation in life situations, and environmental and personal factors. Research confirms that favorable outcomes among persons with stroke and hip fracture are more likely when inpatient rehabilitation services are implemented, rather than rehabilitation in a nursing home setting. This document serves as an essential reference for the development of gerontological protocols for the systematic approach to assessment, prevention, and management of comorbid conditions frequently found in elderly, including skin breakdown and development of decubiti, incontinence and bladder problems, and pneumonia.

Correctional nurses promote health and provide elder-specific care by establishing and overseeing nursing specialty clinics for such problems as hypertension and wound and foot care. Training in advanced cardiac life support, mental health screening, and suicide risk assessment is an essential component of correctional nursing staff development programs in settings in which elderly inmates are detained. Psycho-education priorities for elder inmates include healthy aging, recreational adjustment programming, and wellness adaptation to institutionalization. Correctional nurses provide leadership in the area of developing staff, updating correctional and health-care staff on healthy aging and the aging process, and advocating for administrative responses to specialized care and staffing, along with institutional physical facilities adapted for elder mobility and function.

Women

Women constitute about 6% of the prison population in the United States, and the rate of growth is accelerating. Between 1980 and 1993, the rate of incarceration for women prisoners increased by 313%. However, due to the low numbers of incarcerated women compared with men, little research has been done on the health status and health needs of incarcerated women.

Women entering the criminal justice system come from conditions of poverty and prejudice, and many have histories of sexual abuse, battery, and substance abuse. Women in prison often present with serious health problems, including HIV, tuberculosis, and hepatitis. Most are imprisoned for nonviolent drug-related crimes. Women inmates tuberculosis, of color present with histories of discrimination, and all women inmates are at risk for a lack of basic medical care. More than half are unemployed at the time of their arrest, and 30% receive welfare. Incarcerated women have a high rate of HIV infection, 35 times the rate of the general population. However, few incarcerated women receive treatment or antiretroviral medications while in jail, and many institutions do not have sufficient HIV risk reduction or treatment programs to sufficiently address the health needs of this population.

Many incarcerated women have experienced physical or sexual abuse, and the majority have a history of mental illness. As many incarcerated women are mothers, they face additional emotional stress and worry concerning the care and well-being of their children. The prison health-care system is often inadequate, punitive, and dehumanizing, and women rarely receive adequate treatment for drug problems or other health issues. Research is needed to address these concerns and to serve the unique health needs of women while in prison in hopes of allowing them to leave prison in better health than they entered and decrease the risk of reincarceration.

Parasuicidal behavior—nonfatal, intentional, self-injurious actions—most frequently occur in female correctional populations with characteristics of borderline personality disorder. Actually viewed as maladaptive life-preserving measures, parasuicidal behavior is considered to be as stressful for the staff as for the inmates. Parasuicidal behavior differs from suicide attempts in that the intent is not death, but rather alleviation of intense anxiety and the desire to "feel." Efforts to control and prevent this behavior have usually focused on the removal of opportunities through the control of activity; promotion of physical activity; and limitation of access to means of self-harm such as utensils, pencils, hairpins, and fingernails. Roth and Presse describe an "intensive healing program" in which dialectical behavior therapy is used to develop a therapeutic healing environment characterized by "cheerleading" the patients to reinforce learned adaptive behaviors and appropriate coping strategies.

Most incarcerated women have substance abuse problems and/or have committed drug-related crimes. There are unique characteristics of addiction among women and across ethnic groups of women that affect their patterns of addiction and needs related to recovery. Women tend to become addicted faster than men, and they require gender-specific substance abuse treatment to successfully abstain and heal. In addition to addictions problems, women in prison have high rates of interpersonal violence as victims of sexual, physical, and emotional abuse. The likelihood of a dual diagnosis in which the addiction serves as a source of "self-care" is common in incarcerated women. Gender-specific health programs have been developed based on the evidence from numerous studies of substance abuse treatment and dual-diagnosis treatment modalities. Among the strategies considered important for women's care are same-gender therapists; involvement of family and focus on parenting role; comprehensive services, including literacy and community skills training; and focus on the development of relationships. Women's health care in prison focuses on outcomes of primary health care, psychiatric care, substance abuse treatment, reproductive health, integration of family roles, and the development of life skills.

Youth

The most severe sanction that a juvenile court can impose entails the restriction of a juvenile's freedom through placement in a residential facility. Usually, such placement occurs after a youth has been convicted of an offense; however, a youth may also be held in detention after arrest or during court proceedings. In a few cases, jurisdiction over the youth might be transferred to criminal court, which then carries out processing and sentencing.

Between 1999 and 2004, the adult jail population increased 19%, whereas population of those under the age of 18 dropped 25%. The decline was driven by the reduction in the number of under-18 inmates held as juveniles, with increased numbers of adolescents being sent to adult facilities. At the present time, all U.S. states allow certain juveniles to be tried in criminal court as adults, and nearly 9 in 10 are held as adults. When incarcerated with adults, juveniles are at an increased risk for rape, assault, and suicide. Mirroring the adult correctional population, juveniles in custody are overrepresented by blacks, Asians, Hispanics, and American Indians.

Juveniles in custody generally serve much shorter sentences and are often moved between several residential facilities, making the establishment of a health-care provider relationship difficult. The prison or detention system serves "in loco parentis," taking custody of the minor offender and responsibility for health, welfare, education, and general well-being of children who are in varying stages of growth and development. The assessment and care protocols used by correctional nurses working with juvenile offenders reflect this diversity and reflect age and developmentally appropriate standards of care and health milestones. Many juveniles in custody have significant educational, mental health, medical, and social needs, which has led to the observation that the juvenile justice system is a default placement for youth who can't read or write.

Juveniles are required to attend school while in custody, and other than medical emergency care, health interventions must be scheduled around educational priorities. Major health-care needs for juveniles focus on health promotion (immunizations, health screening, and health education), prevention and treatment of physical injuries, acute illnesses such as upper respiratory infection and gastroenteritis, and headaches. Communicable diseases, especially sexually transmitted diseases, hepatitis, and positive tuberculosis testing are prevalent in this population. Although rates of HIV infection are relatively low in adolescents, participation in high-risk behaviors exposing them to HIV is high. Juveniles who present with chronic conditions such as obesity, asthma, allergy, and diabetes need specialized care and often are referred to outsourced clinics or visiting specialists.

Up to two thirds of youth in corrections are detained due to mental health problems; they are referred to juvenile detention centers without criminal offenses charged against them because there are insufficient mental health services available in the community. While most juvenile offenders are held in facilities that screen for mental health needs and suicide risk, there is a shortage of mental health services to treat them.

Predominant mental health problems in juvenile corrections include attention-deficit/hyperactivity disorder, conduct disorder, oppositional-defiant disorder, and depression. Trauma is considered a factor in the development of conduct disorders and other mental health issues experienced by adolescents in corrections, accounting for symptoms of lack of empathy, impulsivity, anger, acting out, and resistance to treatment. Juveniles in corrections experience higher rates of psychiatric hospitalizations, and recent research documents increasing rates of post-traumatic stress disorder (PTSD) among youths. Particularly prevalent among girls, PTSD has been linked to violent behavior. Prudent practice would include careful screening for PTSD among all adolescents demonstrating mental health symptomatology. Among youth in correctional facilities, 65% to 70% meet criteria for a mental health disorder.

The female juvenile offender is likely to have been sexually or physically abused, to come from a single-parent home, and to lack appropriate social and work-related skills. She is likely to be under age 15 and more likely a woman of color. Most female juvenile offenders are retained on status offenses, noncriminal behavior such as running away from home, incorrigibility, truancy, and curfew violation. Young women involved in delinquent behaviors tend to be arrested for gender-sensitive offenses of prostitution, embezzlement, forgery, and counterfeiting. While young women are still less likely than young men to be delinquent, in recent years involvement in violent delinquency has significantly increased. Many state service delivery systems, which often underestimate the numbers of female juveniles that will be admitted to their facilities, are not prepared to deal effectively with female offenders in custody.

Homosexual Inmates

Homosexuals are probably represented in the correctional population in numbers approximating the general population, although no conclusive data are available due to the difficulty sampling and measuring homosexuality related to possible fear of sexual predation and variation in the definition of homosexuality. While homosexual activity in prisons is condemned and prohibited by formal prison policy, it is encouraged and promoted by the environmental and social structures supporting prison subculture. There are different types of homosexual activities in prison. One type of homosexual activity involves predatory behavior of heterosexuals reacting to the constraints of prison life that prohibit heterosexual liaison: sexual expressions with members of the same sex are means of satisfying sexual urges. In many instances of same-gender sexual activity, sex is considered a commodity to be used for the "purchase" of goods and favors. At other times, sex is used as a means of establishing and maintaining power. Another type of homosexuality involves those gays and lesbians who had homosexual relationships outside of prison.

Homosexual activity among female offenders is generally less aggressive than for males and involves needs for attention and affection; relatively low numbers of women report initiation of sexual coercion by other women inmates. Newly admitted offenders, who are new to the correctional system, may be sought out by older offenders looking for a sexual union. Older offenders will ingratiate themselves by offering cigarettes, money, drugs, and other favors and then demand sexual favors in return. The inmate code calls for the payment of debt, and the new inmate is therefore obliged to perform sexual favors or be subject to inmate "justice."

While most sexual aggressors do not consider themselves homosexuals, and sexual release is not the primary motivation for sexual attack, many aggressors continue to participate in gang rape activity to avoid becoming a victim of rape. It is estimated that 12% of all hate crimes are perpetrated against males believed by their attackers to be homosexuals. This aggression often continues into the correctional setting against the homosexual offender.

Research has confirmed that not only gender, but also race, homosexual behavior during incarceration, and remaining sentence time had statistically significant effects on inmates' attitudes toward homosexuality. Incarcerated men were more likely than incarcerated women to have homophobic attitudes; black inmates were more tolerant of homosexuality compared with white inmates; and inmates who had engaged in homosexual behavior during incarceration were less likely to have homophobic attitudes than those who had not. Finally, those who had longer remaining sentence times were more likely to have negative attitudes toward homosexuality compared with those with shorter remaining sentence times. Other research has confirmed that, although heterosexuality is viewed as the "right sexual orientation," homosexual relationships occur in prisons among individuals who consider themselves "straight" to define roles in an institutional setting that organizes behavior and roles according to absolute power, deprivation, and coercion. Situational homosexuality is commonly defined as sexual activity with partners of the same sex that occurs not as part of a gay identification, but because the participants happen to find themselves in a

single-sex environment for a prolonged period. Formal in-depth interviews were conducted with 20 self-identified homosexuals, and interviews and extensive case studies were conducted with four homosexual couples involved in ongoing sexual relationships. Statistical data were based on two questionnaires (surveys of sexual behavior) and on observations of the prison scene. Although subtle changes within the prison were noted, sexual assaults and the pattern of forcing sexual favors from newcomers resulted in the common pattern of homosexuals pairing for protection. Except for church services, no organized social groups for gays are provided in the prison. The apparent lack of positive gay identities in prison maintains a social milieu that works to feminize and stereotype homosexuals. For many gays confined to prison, the lack of alternative role models, the apparent apathy of the prison staff, and the neglect until recently of the external gay and straight community to the plight of prison homosexuals appear to maintain a prison environment that exploits homosexuals. From a gay liberationist point of view, prison remains restricted and bleak. The prison environment tolerates homosexuality but does not yet support the formation of a gay subculture or support group. This discussion challenges the present dichotomizing of prison homosexuality into true and situational categories, a division that dominates the prison literature. The only crucial dichotomy is between those who come to see themselves as homosexual and those who do not.

Mentally Disordered

The prevalence of mental health problems among offender populations is overwhelming; 10% to 15% of persons in jails or prisons have a serious mental illness, and approximately two million people in the United States are in jails and prisons. Men who have been incarcerated have higher rates of mental illness and suicide, and all inmates have poorer access to mental health care than the general population. Factors affecting inmate use of mental health care while in prison include previous history with the mental health care system and trust of the health-care providers.

Many individuals make their way into the criminal justice system because there is inadequate mental health care in the community. When their mental health deteriorates and behavioral problems emerge, often the jail or prison becomes the substitute mental health care institution. Juveniles with mental health problems reflect a growing population in corrections, and, as with adults, present along the continuum of mental disorders, including depression, bipolar disorder, attention-deficit/hyperactivity disorder (ADHD), substance abuse disorders, suicidal behavior, self-injurious behavior, PTSD, and psychosis. The correctional health setting needs to emphasize structured needs assessment within custody and community settings in conjunction with a care program approach to provide continuity of care.

There is a growing body of research documenting the mental health needs of women offenders. Bloom, Owen, and Covington identified a relationship between substance abuse, trauma, and mental health, common characteristics among women offenders. The links between these factors represent an important development in correctional mental health care, acknowledging that significant numbers of women offenders have experienced trauma and that these traumatic experiences are critical factors in the development of physical and mental health problems. Correctional nurses must compensate for the gaps that exist in mental health care, physical health care, prevention, follow-up, and transitional services for women across the criminal justice spectrum.

While different in nature, male prisoners have high rates of interpersonal trauma and high levels of psychological distress. Offenders are reluctant to engage in mental health care because most are men, and men are less likely to seek help than are women. In addition, family and social networks are often not available to serve as a support system. Low rates of disclosure to health professionals and reluctance to seek help have also been noted in male and female victims of sexual assault and victims of domestic violence, with men being significantly less likely to disclose traumatic and distressing early experiences than are women. Offenders seeking care have complex social and psychological problems, high rates of drug and alcohol misuse, low compliance with treatment, and ambivalence toward figures of authority.

CORE ELEMENTS OF CORRECTIONAL HEALTH CARE

Core elements of correctional health care are useful categories to use when organizing knowledge from which to practice correctional nursing. First, correctional nurses are not only bound by the professional standards of nursing, but also by the legal obligation to provide care and avoid "deliberate indifference" in the administration of care to inmates. Whatever the limitations of the resources or legal status of the inmate, consideration of efficiency and cost-effectiveness must be balanced against the standard of human action. Second, theory, knowledge, and valid clinical protocols form the basis of medical and health-care practice in correctional settings. Sources such as the Centers

for Disease Control and Prevention (CDC), health-care accrediting agencies, and professional bodies must be accessible so that the correctional nurse can transfer guidelines and standards to daily practice. Third, the most vital of all core elements of correctional health care, health-care staffing, is frequently the responsibility of nursing and involves collaboration with other health-care professionals and correctional administration in the assignment of appropriate individuals for triage, diagnosis, and treatment of inmates. In correctional facilities, the health-care authority is the physician. All health professionals must be licensed, and inmates should not provide health care unless they are in a certified vocational training program. While staff-to-inmate ratios are not specified, it is incumbent upon nurses to be knowledgeable about prevailing patient assignment ratios and staff mix to ensure safe patient care.

Fourth, correctional health-care settings must provide for direct care/emergency care, and fifth, provide nonemergency care. Components of nonemergency care in correctional settings include the following: intake procedures and medical screening; daily sick call and daily visits to segregated inmates (those confined and separated from the general inmate population); communicable disease and infection control; mental health care; dental care; and other special population needs, such as chronic and terminal care. Sixth, support services included in the core elements of correctional health care involve laboratory and diagnostic services, ongoing professional development programs for nurses and other health-care providers, prevention training for inmates, and pharmacy services. Seventh, quality assurance data include statistical reporting that becomes part of the evidence base upon which health-care protocols and practices are developed. Correctional nurses provide leadership for the implementation of these seven core elements; the degree to which correctional nurses are knowledgeable regarding the theoretical, research, and legal bases that serve as the foundation for the implementation of the elements determines the degree of accountability for practice and predictability of quality patient outcomes.

PROFESSIONAL SOCIALIZATION OF CORRECTIONAL NURSES

Professional socialization is the process by which individuals acquire the specialized knowledge, skills, attitudes, values, and norms needed to perform their professional role. In addition to the specific skills employed in correctional health care, professional socialization also requires the development of ethical values as well as an understanding of the complex needs of human beings encountered as patients within the correctional system. There are segments of our society that view inmates in prisons and jails as outcasts, those persons for whom punishment, degradation, and deprivation are not only acceptable, but appropriate. These beliefs are part of the culture in which correctional nurses exist.

While there is a scientific basis for the practice of nursing, correctional nurses often practice in a manner reflecting their previous experiences in nursing education or other practice sites. When this skill set does not overlap the requirements specific to the care of inmates, the provision of quality care and the feelings of control over practice can suffer. Control over practice is fostered when correctional nurses accept responsibility for inmates' care, if they have access to ideas, if there is a mentor in place to reflect clinical expertise, and if they see research utilization as congruent with their role. Research utilization includes both the development of the science of nursing as well as the application of that knowledge to the nursing care provided in practice.

Research has confirmed the need for expanded postbaccalaureate professional development for correctional nurses. Increasing the knowledge base supporting correctional nursing practice has the potential to positively affect levels of clinical competency, which in turn leads to better patient outcomes. Current basic nursing education programs do not usually include correctional nursing components and do not encourage entry into correctional settings.

Qualifications of correctional nurses vary greatly from setting to setting. The gap between service and education continues to grow as nursing education is more established in baccalaureate and higher degree programs within the United States. Clinical placements or didactic instruction in correctional nursing is rare within formal nursing programs, so most nurses practicing in correctional settings have been socialized through on-the-job training and continuing professional development programs offered either by the institution or by their professional organizations.

The primary source of correctional nursing role development occurs through the American Correctional Association (ACA) and the National Commission for Correctional Health Care (NCCHC). Nurses working in correctional settings should join their professional organizations so that they will have access to professional networking, updates in correctional health care, and certification education and credentialing. With the move to greater integration of health and prison health care, opportunities, greater use of interdisciplinary and interagency

teaching and learning opportunities should take place within clinical settings. Membership in professional organizations not only provides correctional nurses with access to professional guidelines and standards, but also protects them from undue coercion to perform inappropriate duties and provides access to confidential advice, counsel, and support.

STANDARDS OF PRACTICE

The American Nurses Association's second revision of *Scope and Standards of Nursing Practice in Correctional facilities*, first released in 1995, was updated in 2007 and is the professional reference for the role of the correctional nurse in the United States. The *Scope and Standards* describes the context of correctional nursing practice as patient care within the distinctive environments of the criminal justice system, including juvenile detention centers and substance abuse treatment facilities. Registered nurses in this field must demonstrate the essence of nursing in practice settings and work environments for which health care is not a primary mission, delivering adequate and humane levels of health care in an unbiased and nonjudgmental manner.

An registered nurse (RN) in any corrections setting must be prepared to practice across a wide range of clinical applications. The corrections nurse must address patient needs presented in the correctional setting, including women's health problems and health promotion needs and the spectrum of health-care needs dictated by stage of growth and development (from pediatric through geriatric) and end-of-life care. Correctional nurses apply concepts of primary health care, including ambulatory care, community health, emergency health care, occupational health, public health, and school nursing. The *Scope and Standards of Practice* articulates the essentials of the correctional nursing specialty, its activities and accountabilities at all practice levels and settings, and serves as the foundation for professional socialization of correctional nurses and the identification of core knowledge for which correctional nurses need an evidence base.

The "culture shock" experienced by nurses working in correctional settings is reflective of the stress encountered in the unique environment of the criminal justice system in which nurses care primarily for a disadvantaged community of offenders. Prisons and jails are inherently coercive institutions that, for security reasons, exercise nearly total control over their residents' lives and the activities of all persons within the institution. The lack of resources for correctional health care is accompanied by staffing patterns that require nurses to specialize in everything and in nothing. Nurses working in correctional environments are presented with patient needs requiring knowledge in varying specialties. The challenge of providing expert care in medical, surgical, psychiatric, and community health nursing to a very high-risk, high-need, and high-security population results in correctional nursing stress and role inadequacy, which in turn can increase job dissatisfaction and turnover rates. This pattern of work in correctional nursing can be the source of negative professional self-concept and a stigmatization of the role of correctional nurse.

Standards for correctional nursing practice are sources of role expectations for the developing correctional nurse and include those from the ANA Scope and Standards of Practice in Correctional Facilities, the Principles of the American Correctional Health Service Association, and the National Commission for Correctional Health Care. Aims of practice standards are to provide benchmarks against which the correctional nurse can preserve professional autonomy in the structured environment of corrections.

Nursing education traditionally has not included content or competencies directly related to correctional nursing practice. The unique experiences and demands of correctional nursing dictate formal professional socialization in order to appropriately prepare practitioners for successful nursing. Nurses who work in correctional environments face particular challenges and issues that are part of the broader field of correctional health care. Prior experience and sources of primary socialization have been found to play a role in the shaping of perceptions that guide correctional nursing practice. The overarching issue of security provides the context in which all correctional nursing occurs, dictating the need for acceptance and comfort working within specific policies and procedures that may restrict movement, communications, and even the type of equipment that can be used.

ETHICAL AND LEGAL FOUNDATIONS OF CORRECTIONAL NURSING PRACTICE

Ethical foundations for nursing practice provide the basis for answering the question "what should I do?" Ethics is about making decisions to act well, to act morally, and to act humanely. Defining parameters of "acting well" within the context of correctional nursing involves consideration of the legal, as well as the moral, justifications for interpretation of professional standards intended to guide nurses in the prevention of illness, the alleviation of suffering, and the protection, promotion, and restoration of health in the

care of inmates. Ethical obligations and duties, along with the interpretation of nursing's commitment to society, is provided in the ANA Code of Ethics, which expands on concepts of medical ethics and bioethics and focuses on problems coming from the conflicting rights and obligations of correctional nurses, inmates, other correctional staff, the correctional system, and the public. Correctional facilities, such as prisons, jails, and juvenile detention, are some of the most complex settings in which to provide health services. The difficulty of the environment, poor health status, and compromised access to health services add to the complexity of this practice and pose confounding legal and ethical issues for all concerned.

A code of ethics is a set of principles that guides the conduct of a group of professionals and establishes moral duties and obligations in relation to clients, institutions, and society. One of the characteristics of the American Correctional Health Services Association (ACHSA) is the development and adoption of a code of ethics with the purpose of identifying fundamental values of correctional health professionals and ethical conflicts in the correctional health-care setting (Box 14.1).

Distinguished from codes for individual professional disciplines, the correctional health-care ethical code addresses the practice of many health-care disciplines, including, physicians, nurses, physician assistants, psychologists, pharmacists, social workers, nutritionists, health information specialists, and administrators. The fundamental values reflected in the ethics code are derived from the culture and experience of health professionals; the duties and obligations toward the correctional institution; the codes of ethics of the professional disciplines; and international principles of law and ethics, such as the World Medical Association Declaration of Tokyo, the United Nations Principles of Medical Ethics, the United Nations Standard Minimum Rules for the Treatment of Prisoners, and the International Council of Nurses Statement of the Role of the Nurse in Care of Detainees and Prisoners. Correctional health professionals are obligated to respect human dignity and act in ways that merit trust and prevent harm. They must ensure autonomy in decisions about their inmate patients and promote a safe environment.

BOUNDARY VIOLATIONS

As in any health-care setting in which professional nurses work, appropriate communication and the avoidance of social relationships in deference to professional relationships is essential. Safety and security depend upon nurses and inmate patients knowing as little about each other as possible.

Box 14.1   ACHSA Obligations of the Correctional Health Professional (1990)

1. Evaluate the inmate as a patient or client in each and every health-care encounter.
2. Render medical treatment only when it is justified by an accepted medical diagnosis. Treatment and invasive procedures shall be rendered after informed consent.
3. Afford inmates the right to refuse care and treatment. Involuntary treatment shall be reserved for emergency situations in which there is grave disability and immediate threat of danger to the inmate or others.
4. Provide sound privacy during health services in all cases and sight privacy whenever possible.
5. Provide health-care to all inmates regardless of custody status.
6. Identify yourself to patients and do not represent yourself as other than your professional license or certification permits.
7. Collect and analyze specimens only for diagnostic testing based on sound medical principles.
8. Perform body cavity searches only after training in proper techniques and when not in a patient-provider relationship with the inmate.
9. Avoid any involvement in any aspect of execution of the death penalty.
10. Ensure that all medical information is confidential and health-care records are maintained and transported in a confidential manner.
11. Honor custody functions but not participate in such activities as escorting inmates, forced transfers, security supervision, strip searches, or witnessing use of force.
12. Undertake biomedical research on prisoners only when the research methods meet all requirements for experimentation on human subjects and individual prisoners or prison populations are expected to derive benefits from the results of the research.

It is therefore incumbent upon the nurse to recognize the "need to know" versus "the desire or interest to know" facts about patients. In most cases, nurses do not need to know the offending behavior that led to incarceration. Boundary violations are often the product of unnecessary and destructive social relationships between caregiver and patient. Boundary violations are inappropriate and destructive behaviors between a caregiver and a patient, characterized by close social interaction for the purpose of personal benefit and reward, rather than therapeutic outcome.

The most extreme example of boundary violation in correctional settings is participation of a nurse in contraband and illegal activity on behalf of an inmate. Long before inappropriate intimacy or sexual contact occur in a helping relationship, a variety of boundary crossings or violations often occur. Inappropriate touch is only one form of boundary violation. Boundary violations include intimate communications such as secret keeping and gossiping, disclosure of personal information, gift giving, and granting favors or special treatment. These actions represent breakdowns in the professionalism of the relationship and, as such, often undermine the health outcomes of the patient. Intense friendships and enmeshed relationships between nurse and patient divert goals from health care to personal gain. Boundary violations may be present if any of the following occur: (1) nurse retains relationship with patient, without referral or discharge when patient is clearly ready for discharge; (2) nurse creates nontherapeutic dependency of the patient on the nurse; (3) a distrustful patient behavior emerges that did not previously exist (as when a previously cooperative patient demands to be seen only by one nurse); (4) there is a sudden disruption of family visits and an increase in visits to the nurse; and (5) the inmate patient displays anger, loss of self-esteem, depression, and other psychological distress not previously observed or previously resolved.

Correctional nurses seldom begin a correctional nursing career with the theoretical knowledge or experience to address boundary violations in clinical practice. Role socialization processes, perceptions of professionalism, and gender issues, along with the atmosphere of the correctional environment, are factors that predispose correctional nurses to boundary violations.

Ethical practice involves the identification of individuals at risk for misconduct, along with intervention with those individuals. Ethical practice is more than a function of personality. There are significant sociological forces that affect conduct in **secure settings**; character, alone, is not a good predictor of who will engage in correctional forms of misconduct. The correctional environment creates a captor-captive situation that presents the opportunities and triggers for ethical misconduct. Specific policies prohibiting fraternization among staff and inmates help to limit misconduct, but violations of professional standards are constant antagonists to the implementation of evidence-based practice.

Violations of organizational rules and regulations for personal gain are common forms of corruption in corrections. Administrators can be complicit in the denial of ethics problems due to the overwhelmingly negative impact such problems have on the maintenance of respect, order, and the control needed in correctional settings.

Corruption through friendship occurs when the policies and practices in the work environment fail to adequately distinguish roles of the correctional nurse and staff from those of the inmates. The correctional nurse experiences a conflict of loyalties, and the working conditions predispose the nurse to feelings of vulnerability or powerlessness.

Corruption through reciprocity occurs when the correctional nurse ignores minor infractions of inmates in return for compliance or cooperative behavior related to health care. Inmates may advise correctional nurses that inmates will "look out for them" and keep them safe. This can be a powerful incentive in settings where hostage situations or riots occur.

Corruption through default occurs because of indifference, laziness, or naiveté on the part of the correctional nurse. When inmates are used as care providers for other inmates or have other duties in the infirmary or prison health-care setting, they may encroach on the duties of the nurse, expanding their presence and freedom of movement within the health-care setting, increasing access to contraband, and possibly increasing unobserved behavior. Inmates can take advantage of such positions by stealing health supplies and drugs, exerting control over other inmate patients, and running illegal operations such as prostitution and loan sharking out of the health-care unit.

Risk of professional misconduct in a total institution exists where values and mores of the external community may be perceived as remote and irrelevant (Box 14.2). Theft, trafficking in contraband, or sexual favors are common dangers for nurses who do not prepare sufficiently for the inappropriate behaviors on the part of inmates. Fraternization, which can be defined as illegal or inappropriate familiarity in an inmate-staff relationship, may very well be the central issue behind most ethical problems in corrections. Many correctional systems have made fraternization an important part of their anti-corruption policies, and at the extreme end, serious felonies exist, making some forms of fraternization, such

as sexual contact, a crime, punishable by 20 years of imprisonment or more. Less extreme forms of fraternization (such as meeting with an inmate when they get out) usually result in dismissals or resignations, frequently accompanied by requiring the ex-employee to sign a form stating that he or she will never work in a department of corrections facility again.

Familiarity, as opposed to fraternization, refers to knowing the inmates' habits, demeanor, and behavior. It is a valued skill among correctional nurses and increases ability to supervise inmate behavior. Favoritism is not professional, but exists in all correctional health settings. Most correctional nurses have their "favorite" inmates: ones they talk to the most, to whom they give special attention, or whom they try to protect from harm or manipulation by other inmates or staff. The "snitch" system that exists in correctional environments reinforces favoritism and exists to promote a sense of respect, trust, and cooperation among some inmates and a means to manipulation among others.

Undue familiarity is illegal or inappropriate familiarity between an inmate and a staff member; it occurs when inmates know the employee's personal business. It is the prisoner's familiarity with an employee's personal habits, demeanor, behavior, or problems, and it represents a breakdown in the professional and ethical boundaries between prisoners and nurse. Correctional nurses are vulnerable to certain "divide and conquer" games by inmates in this regard due to the relative power struggle that occurs when inmates perceive weakness or ambiguity in the assumption of role identity and role mastery in the nurse. When inmates use personal differences among staff as a way to elicit the discussion of personal issues, their goal is to manipulate for personal gain. Inmates will use age, race, gender, religion, marital status, health, or background as issues that trigger emotional attachments with nurses. They will exploit any personal or professional weakness among staff and will make up lies about any employee who doesn't seem to have any inadequacies. They will also exploit any job dissatisfaction among employees. They will do anything to detract from the professional environment, including slang, stereotypes, flattering, or seductive comments (Box 14.3).

A staff pattern that results primarily from close proximity to inmates has been called the "poor devil syndrome." With this syndrome, nurses view the inmate as a "victim" and begin feeling sorry for him. A related variation is the rescuer syndrome, which describes the attraction of nurses to the correctional role. Wanting to help poor, unfortunate people who just happen to have gotten into trouble with the law, nurses gravitate to a position in

---

Box 14.2 Examples of Professional Misconduct Common in Correctional Settings

- Abuse of inmates
- Inappropriate relationship with inmates
- Smuggling contraband
- Fiscal improprieties
- On-duty misconduct
- Off-duty misconduct
- Investigative violations or fixing a ticket for an inmate

(Data taken from del Carmen, 2004.)

Box 14.3 Exploitation of Relationships: Inmate Types

■ *Predators*. These are inmates who are not truly seeking relationships, but rather prey. It is a game to them, and it is their method of survival while in prison. Any staff person they have "gotten over" on is a "trophy" to them, used to obtain status among other inmates or used to turn into the administration as a way to improve their chances for early release. This is perhaps the largest group of exploitative inmates.

■ *Lookers*. These are good-looking inmates who are groomed and dress well, are well-spoken, and are intelligent. They will try to exploit their appearance, portray themselves as victims, and lie by half-truth or omission. Their game involves getting you to join them in pointing out the inadequacies of other staff and/or inmates and eventually joining them on a journey to learn about each other or learning in general (education). These inmates make you believe that no others have ever understood each other the way you two do. They elicit your assistance in escape plans or for a place to live when they get out.

■ *Leaders*. These are usually inmate gang leaders with a narcissistic self-image who see themselves as different (superior) from other inmates, and they have either helped staff significantly in some way or simply have developed the admiration of staff as role models. Power and pleasure are their aims. Staff are an object to be used in their power games. They have no remorse and are most likely to use staff to smuggle contraband.

■ *Snitches*. These sociopsychologically sophisticated types have fooled even the most experienced employee and will turn someone over in a heartbeat. They manage to stay out of trouble all the time, operate very independently, and have their "game" down so well that it can be described as a "network" of employees being manipulated, some in short-term cons and others in long-term con games that take years to develop.

which they can save the inmate. Compassion and understanding on the part of the caregiver are necessary components to the management of inmate health needs; however, they can become the means by which inmates engage staff to develop trust, to share inappropriate information, or to provide favors. All caregiver occupational groups are vulnerable to this syndrome.

Emphasizing risks of inmate predatory behavior provides a substantial challenge to the correctional nurse. Protection against exploitation from inmates must be balanced with the responsibility to protect and care for inmates. Nurses are often the first staff to detect improper or

inadequate treatment of inmates, and it is their responsibility to take appropriate action to safeguard inmate rights. Often cited as the conflict between custody and the caring role, conflict experienced by correctional nurses can occur when the nurse assumes prison security obligations such as body cavity searches and punitive segregation supervision, which directly violate the mandates of prescribed ethical conduct for health-care staff in general and nursing in particular.

A significant influence on the practice of correctional nursing in the United States has been the establishment of the constitutional right to care in the *Estelle vs. Gamble* decision. The Eighth amendment to the U.S. Constitution in 1791 prohibited "cruel and unusual punishment," and from this basic right have emerged three rights that are applied to correctional health care: access to care, ordered care, and professional judgment.

Access to care requires that nurses know which patients need immediate attention and which can wait. All correctional institutions must maintain the ability to address emergencies and provide for sick call. Access to medical specialists and inpatient hospital treatment is guaranteed by the Eighth Amendment.

Ordered care must be carried out. Once an order for care is written by an authorized health-care professional for a serious condition characterized by pain, discomfort, or threat to good health, expedient care must be provided.

Professional judgment concerning the nature and timing of medical care is made by medical personnel, not by correctional personnel.

CHARACTERISTICS OF THE CORRECTIONAL SETTING AND HEALTH-CARE IMPLICATIONS

In closed or total institutions such as prisons and jails, perception of power and expected role can result in exploitation and abuse of the underclass. This phenomenon was first explained in the classical work of Erving Goffman, *Presentation of Self in Everyday Life*. In this book he explains the nature of total institutions, such as jails and prisons, in terms of the breakdown of the barriers ordinarily separating three spheres of life (sleeping, playing, and working).

Total institutions distort the usual roles that individuals assume and do not allow the transitions or relief from personal expressions of identity, which can result in aberration of roles and distortion of emotions and values. St. Pierre suggests conclusion power, surveillance, and disciplinary techniques are used at all levels of health-care management to control and contain both human resources and costs. This can result in the use of power as an agent of an individual's sense of moral authority, and the methods by which the authority is executed can become more harmful than the behavior over which the nurse or other health-care provider or correctional officer power is being exerted. All aspects of life are conducted in the same place and under the same central authority. Each phase of the member's daily activity is carried out in the immediate company of a large group of others, all of whom are treated alike and required to do the same thing together. All phases of the day's activities are tightly scheduled, with one activity leading at prearranged time into the next, the whole sequence of activities being imposed from above by a system of explicit formal rulings and a body of officials. The enforced activities of the total institution are brought together into a single rational plan purportedly designed to fulfill the official aims of the institution.

Expectations of the correctional nursing role include skills and competencies and the predisposition to address common characteristics and needs of inmates presented in high-risk health problems, as well as frequent maladaptive behaviors of manipulation, malingering, and factitious disorders. Manipulation among inmates involves the conscious and unaltruistic use of destructive or self-oriented relationships or behavior to establish power, achieve goals, or create chaos. Manipulation is a way of life and a primary means of goal-oriented behavior and satisfaction for many inmates, among whom personality disorders are overrepresented compared to the general population. The primary aims of manipulation are usually directed at securing privileges to which inmates are not eligible, escaping the boredom of daily routine in correctional settings, establishing or maintaining a sense of power, or creating and sustaining social boundaries that increase perceptions of self-esteem and self-image. The inmate-nurse encounter is viewed as an ideal setting in which to achieve these goals.

Major socialization goals for the correctional nurse include learning responses to manipulative behavior. Evidence from research in correctional and psychiatric settings suggests techniques for recognizing manipulation and dealing positively with this behavior. It is essential that the correctional nurse not take such behavior on the part of inmates personally. Studies of correctional clinical settings indicate that nurses who have histories of past trauma or maladaptive interpersonal relationships are particularly vulnerable to manipulation and seduction by inmates, thus it is important for the correctional nurse to

frequently use introspection and self-reflection, along with clinical supervision (the oversight and evaluation of one's clinical practice by an expert mentor), to identify personal areas of vulnerability. Maintaining a matter-of-fact, nonjudgmental approach decreases the perception on the part of the inmate that the nurse is an "easy target." Skills in systematic physical and mental assessment based on fact and direct observation and the consistent application of policies and procedures strengthen the diagnoses and foundations upon which nursing judgments are based, reducing the likelihood of manipulation.

Malingering and **factitious disorders** are diagnoses applied more frequently in correctional populations than in general populations. Malingering is the "intentional faking of physical or psychological illness or symptoms for intentional personal gain." Malingering can take the form of one of the categories of self-directed violence and is a consideration when assessing potential for suicide among inmates. Because of the high priority for prevention of self-harm and suicide in prison and jails, correctional nurses spend significant time and energy assessing presentation of symptoms and complaints in the consideration of malingering. Malingering cannot be "treated" as it is not officially a psychiatric disorder; however, it is a behavior that must be assessed by correctional nurses, and its occurrence may be decreased with appropriate response by the health-care staff. The ability to identify malingering as a distinct clinical syndrome is critical to successful response.

Little research has been done on the characteristics, process, and prevalence of malingering and self-mutilation in corrections that lead to clear implications for prevention and intervention. As the boundaries between malingering, factitious disorder, other forms of self-harm, and suicidal intent are not always clear, correctional nurses must accept the inevitable error in assessment and response. Situations commonly scrutinized for malingering include presentation of superficial slashing or cutting and claims of suicidal ideation by inmates who perceive they are in a dangerous situation with other inmates. Other suspicious presentations in which malingering should be considered include intractable back pain with no accompanying trauma or other explanation; refusal to undergo extensive, painful diagnostic testing when claims of injury or trauma are presented; significant discrepancies between presentation of claims of symptoms and assessment data; or a lack of cooperation during a nursing evaluation and nonadherence to treatment.

The correctional setting is characterized by violence, trauma, and victimization. Violence is the intentional and malevolent physical injury of another mitigated by anger-motivation or goal-orientation, without adequate social justification. Anger is considered an antecedent to criminal behavior, and an understanding of the role of violence, trauma, and victimization, as they occur and characterize the correctional health-care setting, is essential to developing an evidence base for correctional nursing practice. While anger control or anger management is viewed as the most common treatment of violent offenders, there is relatively little literature to support the efficacy of such treatment.

Several factors converge in the prison environment to magnify the prevalence and importance of violence and victimization as critical themes of everyday life. Hostility is considered negative or distrustful beliefs about others and may also be antecedent to violent behavior, but it is not the same as violence. Controlling violence and anger are constant themes in correctional services.

Violence has been identified as a public health hazard in the United States by the American Medical Association and represents a major concern for correctional settings. Violence is a learned behavior and can be exaggerated in the total institutional setting of the prison or jail. Evidence suggests that this environment provides the opportunity for the adoption of victim and abuser roles among inmates and among staff. There is a connection between abuse and criminality. Women and young adults with a history of childhood physical and sexual abuse have elevated rates of arrest for crimes against persons. In addition, inmates who have previous experience of abuse have higher rates of substance abuse, emotional problems, and interpersonal problems.

The deviant behavior exhibited by inmates can occur as a result of the labeling they received early in life. Deviant self-identity serves as a foundation for criminal activity that is reinforced in the absence of alternative role models among most inmates. Deviant behavior has the goal of not only the disruption of social order and defiance of authority, but also the expression of self-identity and deviant group norms. Deviant behavior may be criminalized (as in the case of theft of a car by an individual with an antisocial personality disorder) or medicalized (as in the case of theft of alcohol by an alcoholic or drug addict trying to self-medicate). In either case, the individual comes to prison with learned behaviors to either attempt to control or to treat, and the distinctions must be clear to correctional nurses so that they may appropriately intervene and effectively collaborate with correctional staff.

Assessment and management of violence and victimization in correctional settings are critical skills for the correctional nurse and are based on evidence that includes identification of dynamic environmental factors contributing to violence, personal characteristics of the inmate and nurse that may contribute to violence and aggression, and interventions likely to decrease the incidence of violence and aggression in correctional health-care settings. Anger, antisocial personality style, and impulsivity are predictors of institutional aggression. Targeting behavior through interdisciplinary approaches to anger management are frequently used strategies to reduce institutional violence and reoffending.

Most anger management programs incorporate components of identification and modification of anger arousal levels, the rehearsal of alternative thinking, and **stress management.** Contemporary approaches to anger management incorporate stages of change. Preparing for change incorporates helping patients to increase their motivation and awareness of their anger. The changing stage includes assertiveness training, the avoidance and escape from anger-arousing situations, and a "barb exposure technique" that triggers patients' anger and then teaches them to relax. Accepting and adjusting to change requires inmates to reconceptualize their anger triggers, forgive others, and avoid carrying a grudge against those who might anger them. Maintaining the change through anger management treatment requires a long-term plan. Relapse prevention training focuses on identifying and managing new triggers that might reignite anger, particularly differentiating those that are part of the correctional setting and those that are not.

Emerging evidence suggests that anger management is not an effective intervention for all inmates and may actually exacerbate anger in some individuals. Anger management classes have been found to reduce feelings and expressions of anger only in those who are motivated to change; inmates with lack of impulse control and strong aggressive tendencies are not good candidates for such programs. Inmates with severe anger issues often have mental health and substance abuse problems that complicate their care. Use of anger therapy groups for this type of individual is not only a waste of time and resources, it may also be harmful.

For those for whom anger management is helpful, the use of group therapy, although economical, may not be an effective strategy. Open expressions of hostility and anger do not relieve stress and pressure of anxiety related to anger, and they may actually increase the likelihood that anger will be expressed since the group setting provides opportunities for the reinforcing of anger and hostility among its members. For correctional settings using anger management programs, the following have been empirically supported: relaxation coping skills, cognitive interventions for behavioral coping, social skills training, and problem-solving skills training.

Short-term psychopharmacology is used in situations in which the offender is acting in a seriously threatening manner to self or others. This primary goal is control, and the choice of medication must be one of rapid onset of action. Intramuscular injection is almost always the preferred method of administration, and correctional nurses must master containment and medication administration methodologies in collaboration with other members of the health-care team. Correctional nurses will provide leadership in times of medical and behavioral crisis in correctional health settings, mandating safe treatment for the inmate patient and the staff as well as objective and caring analysis of the situation. The ability to relate an individual's behavior to possible etiology without prejudging the value of that person is essential to maintaining a caring milieu. Because violent episodes are so often volatile and stressful, correctional nurses need to mentally "rehearse" responses to crises and think through expected responses on a regular basis to increase the likelihood of successful intervention. Among recent drugs reviewed for efficacy in controlling violence, quetiapine has been demonstrated to decrease hostility, impulsivity, and aggression (and subsequent violence) in individuals with severe personality disorder.

Sexual victimization in prisons is a complex problem affecting inmates, staff, and the public and occurs as nonconsensual sexual acts, abusive sexual contacts, staff sexual misconduct, or staff sexual harassment. Nonviolent offenders are more likely to become the victims of sexual assault in prison than are those who have been convicted of more serious crime. Young first-time offenders and inmates with mental illnesses are at greatest risk of sexual victimization in jails and prisons. The prevalent victim profile for which vigilance is needed is young, small, white, with feminine physical features and body movements and a person with no prison experience, friends or companions, or social support. Girls who were victimized before age 12 are at a much higher risk for sexual abuse, including prison rape, as an adult.

It is estimated that the total number of inmates who have been sexually assaulted in the past 20 years exceeds 1,000,000. Most prison staff are not adequately prepared to prevent, report, or treat inmate sexual assaults, and prison rape often goes unreported, leaving victims untreated or undertreated for the physical and psychological effects of rape.

The consequences to the public carry over to the release of the victim and perpetrator of prison rape, both of whom are at risk for continuing the cycle of violence, increasing likelihood of repeat offenses, spread of communicable diseases, and return to prison. Brutalized inmates are more likely to commit crimes when they are released.

Consequences of rape are gender based, with female inmates experiencing the highest rates of communicable disease and psychological trauma. Current studies confirm prison rapes have racial implications, indicating a prevalence of predominantly black perpetrators on white victims nationwide for the last 40 years. It is recommended that the inmate classification system be reviewed in order to separate sexual aggressors from the general nonviolent prison population and possible segregation by race to reduce racial tensions that are magnified in total institutional settings.

The effects of prison rape extend beyond imprisonment and include severe physical and psychological responses that decrease an inmate's ability to maintain employment and integrate into society. Victims of prison rape are more likely to become homeless or require government assistance. Prison rape exceeds the level of homicides and other violence against inmates and staff and the risk of insurrections and riots. Faced with overwhelming frustrations related to the detection and treatment of prison rape, the correctional nurse may feel inadequate and unable to respond. However, deliberate indifference to the risk of sexual assault constitutes a violation of the United States Constitution and prisoners' rights to protection from cruel and unusual punishment.

After more than four decades of research, it is still unclear how much rape and sexually violent activity occurs in prisons, jails, and other corrections facilities in the United States. What is clear from research is that, as with rape outside correctional settings, prison rape goes largely unreported. Of the hundreds of studies in institutional corrections, less than 25 research studies have been conducted on prison rape. Of those studies, some asked inmates to describe their victimizations, including nonconsensual activities other than rape, while others examined official reports filed by inmates. Because none of these studies were national in scope, it remains difficult to estimate the extent of the problem. A meta-analysis of this research estimates 1.91% lifetime prevalence for all inmates in the United States. In 2004, the Bureau of Justice Statistics (BJS) examined administrative records from adult and juvenile facilities at state and local levels. According to these official records, slightly more than 8000 male, female, and juvenile inmates—or 0.005% of the total incarcerated population—reported that they had been victims of sexual violence while incarcerated. An even smaller percentage of inmates' claims were substantiated.

The Prison Rape Elimination Act (PREA) of 2003 states that 13% of all inmates have been raped in U.S. prisons and jails. The most recent research estimates less prevalence of rape, whether inmate-on-inmate or staff-on-inmate sexual misconduct. Whether the number of prison rapes is large or small, the Prison Rape Elimination Act of 2003 requires that federal, state, and local correctional facilities maintain and enforce a zero-tolerance policy on sexual assault, including inmate-on-inmate and staff-on-inmate misconduct. The National Institute of Justice (NIJ) was given the task under PREA to conduct research on rape in prisons, jails, and lock-up facilities.

Although rates of inmate-on-inmate violence are reported to be very high and 1 in 22 incarcerated men and women report they were sexually assaulted while incarcerated in U.S. prisons, inmate education and prevention programs are sometimes stifled by inmate culture. Inmates report having difficulty differentiating consensual, coercive, and predatory sex in prison, and they state they cannot relate to the terms that correctional officers and health staff use. Risk assessment is a priority for correctional nurses as it is estimated that a relatively small percentage of inmates are responsible for about 75% of the prison rapes.

Prevention of prison rape requires an extensive orientation of all new correctional nursing staff and on-going training that includes a rigorous examination of a code of ethics. Nurses need to be involved in the development of protocols for assessment of risk, classification, and cell assignments of inmates. There should be provisions for protective custody for inmates at risk for victimization, along with single bed cell space. Procedures should be in place for inmates to request a change in housing, and detection devices, such as cameras, recorders, key issuance logs, and sign-in logs should be in place. Forensically trained nurses without conflict of interest should be available to provide a sexual assault examination, and specified mental health teams should be available to investigate allegations of rape. Protocols must be in place for infectious disease testing, prevention of pregnancy for female inmates, and post-trauma counseling. There should be clear protocols for who authorizes the collection of evidence, and the policies should specifically prescribe the duty to report.

Treatment response to prison rape is a collaborative effort, and correctional nurses must be clear on their roles and the manner in which they can support the roles of others. Confidentiality is the foundation of anti-sexual violence initiatives, and client-counselor privilege can create a challenge in prison settings. Communications between sexual assault advocates/counselors and inmate clients are generally held confidential; however, if correctional officers perceive a threat to the facility, they may request privileged information. Openness and sharing information is an expectation in most prisons to maintain safety for staff and inmates. Correctional nurses are in a position to support the work of sexual assault advocates, providing them information on prison culture and protocols.

Inmate support groups are effective strategies for rape trauma aftercare. However, in prison settings, confidentiality is almost nonexistent when organizing group activities, and this fact needs to be acknowledged. Correctional nurses can create environments within the healthcare settings or within other settings in the prison to ensure privacy during the sessions, even if the entry and exit from the meetings cannot be anonymous. Purposive selection of survivors of sexual assault can be used to develop health promotion groups that are not labeled with terms such as "victims" or "sexual assault."

In some settings, female inmates are particularly vulnerable to sexual harassment and abuse by corrections and health-care staff. The number of female prisoners is increasing, and many of these women report a history of sexual assault. Youth in detention facilities are vulnerable to abuse, including sexual abuse from other adolescents and staff. Many survivors of prisoner rape blame themselves: males feeling they have been "stripped of their manhood" and gay men blaming their sexual orientation for the rape, women having their mistrust of men and authority figures reinforced, and youth affirmed in their belief that no one can care for them. Correctional nurses are situated within the correctional system in a position to identify those at risk, provide education to maintain vigilance, and institute effective and timely responses to injury and outcomes of sexual assault.

Nursing goals focus on the reduction of violent events and prevention of harm. Correctional nurses must be knowledgeable regarding stages of escalating violence, use of body language and voice tone to adjust behavior, and methods for organizing the environment and inmate housing to reduce opportunities and stressors linked to violence. Violence prevention programs aimed at high-risk inmates are based on social learning and social information-processing theories that assume the inmate's past violent behavior is learned through modeling, reinforcement, and cognitive mediation. The violence prevention methods aim to achieve changes in attitudes and behaviors through modifications of self-responsibility and control.

MENTAL HEALTH CARE IN PRISONS AND JAILS

More than half of U.S. prison and jail inmates have symptoms of a mental health problem, but fewer than one third of those with problems are getting treatment behind bars.

Based on a survey of nationally representative samples, the Bureau of Justice Statistics estimated that 56% of the nation's 1.25 million state prisoners, 64% of its 747,000 jail inmates, and 45% of its 156,000 federal prisoners reported treatment for or symptoms of major depression, mania, or psychotic disorders such as hallucinations or delusions in the last year.

Treatment behind bars is available to most state prisoners: 34% of those reporting symptoms, compared with 24% of the troubled federal prisoners and 17% of jail inmates with problems. The most common treatment was a prescribed medication: 27% of state, 19% of federal, and 15% of jail inmates problems. Mental health problems predominating in the correctional setting and for which inmates may present for care include inability to control behavior, physical health concerns, negative affect, interpersonal relationships, and institutional relations. Potential barriers to accessing prison mental health services are common in correctional settings and relate to the stigmatization of mental illness and the concern for self-preservation.

While jails are legally required to provide mental health treatment, the availability of treatment and the ability to access these services vary across facilities. Furthermore, little is known about the impact of mental health treatment on an inmate's mental health during incarceration. Prisoners with substance abuse and mental health problems have the most problematic health profiles and more extensive health services utilization. Correctional nurses using the case management approach will organize care with the knowledge that most prisoners will return to the community at some point in time. Effective correctional health may lead to better community health; therefore, effective coordination of care/services from institution to community could reduce health-care costs to both correctional and community health-care systems.

The prison environment can have a negative effect on mental health due overcrowding; presence of violence; and frustrations from restrictions on movement, decision making, and freedom to associate. Social isolation and lack of personal space and privacy can be part of an inmate's prison experience. The increased risk of suicide in prisons (often related to depression) can be an outcome of the cumulative effects of the prison environment.

As mentioned previously, when the community does not provide adequate mental health care, prisons can become the mental health-care system. In some instances, people with severe mental disorders are inappropriately locked up in prisons simply because of the lack of mental health services. Persons with substance abuse disorders and mental disorders are frequently involved in minor offenses and sent to prison rather than treated for their disorder.

Long periods of isolation with little mental stimulus contributes to poor mental health and leads to intense feelings of anger, frustration, and anxiety among inmates with mental health problems. Prisoners abuse drugs to relieve boredom. Correctional nurses will monitor the environment for factors that can be changed to minimize the negative effects of the setting.

SUICIDE IN PRISONS AND JAILS

Among prison inmates, the rate of suicide is approximately 1.5 times that of the general population. Among jail inmates, the rate increases to 5 times that of the general population. The highest rate of suicide among those in custody occurs in individuals who, immediately after being taken into custody and placed in a lockup facility, are left alone. Often these individuals may be experiencing mental health problems or may be withdrawing from alcohol or drug intoxication. Rates of suicide among juvenile males, closely related to drug use and depression, steadily rises from age 11 to 21. Juveniles in custody who are housed in adult jails are 19 times more likely to commit suicide while behind bars than are young people in the general population, and they are 36 times more likely to kill themselves in an adult jail than young people held in juvenile facilities. Suicides in jails are heavily concentrated in the first week spent in custody (48%), with almost a quarter of suicides taking place on the day of admission to jail (14%) or on the following day (9%).

While deaths of juveniles in custody are rare, it is a devastating event for staff and juvenile offenders alike. Accidents and suicides account for most deaths of juveniles in custody, with an average of 28 deaths per year. Suicide is the most commonly reported cause of death among juveniles in custody, usually 2 to 4 weeks after incarceration, usually preceded by previous deliberate self-harm.

A major challenge in correctional health care is prevention of suicide. Environmental and situational factors in correctional settings affect the incidence of suicide and self-harm, and the correctional nurse is part of the health-care team charged with the assessment, treatment, and prevention of suicide and self-harm. Differentiating the suicide attempt and self-harm is an essential skill of the correctional nurse who uses such tools as the assessment of lethal behavior and wound patterning.

Although jails and suicides are closed, secure, and controlled environments, social and logistical characteristics complicate efforts at suicide prevention. Attitudes among many correctional and health-care staff perpetuate messages that suicide prevention is futile, that if inmates want to die, they will eventually succeed. In addition, many staff do not perceive that suicide prevention is "their job." Suicide attempts are often viewed as "attention getting" behaviors. Interventions to prevent suicide in correctional settings include surveillance of fatal and nonfatal injuries, mental health screening, professional development and staff training, symptom and stress management, and critical incident management.

Suicide in Jails

Jails are the point of highest risk for suicide in the correctional system; risk of suicide is comparable to community risk by offender classification category in prisons. The two primary causes of jail suicides are considered to be (1) environmental and (2) situational. The jail environment is conducive to suicidal behavior. The jail inmate generally has a distrust of authority figures, including health-care providers, and has a fear of the unknown. Experiencing a complete lack of control of their present and future, jail inmates are isolated from social support systems and may be experiencing shame of incarceration and the dehumanizing nature of the jail policies and procedures.

Jail inmates enter the correctional setting in the middle of a personal crisis that may be exacerbated by recent use and abuse of alcohol and other drugs that can remove inhibitions to destructive impulses. They are more likely than the general public to be experiencing crises related to loss of stabilizing resources and relationships, victimization, difficult legal situations, and difficulty coping with the environment.

Small jails have the highest risk of suicide; the larger the correctional facility, the less likely the suicide incidence. This is further complicated by the fact that smaller facilities are less likely to have the personnel to provide the types of surveillance and intervention necessary to affect suicide and self-harm.

Risk factors associated with jail suicide include the following characteristics: male gender, white, violent offender (but detained on nonviolent offense), and younger than 18 or older than 55 years. Most jail suicides occur in the first week of incarceration, with over 50% of jail suicides occurring in the first day. Inmates undergoing initial adaptation to the correctional setting are vulnerable to the multiple demands required of them; if they are placed in isolation, jail inmates respond even more negatively to the incarceration experience. Most suicide completers have histories of previous suicide attempts. A significant risk factor for suicide is intoxication; over 60% of jail suicide victims in one study were intoxicated at the time of confinement. Other common risk factors are history of mental illness, history of prior suicide attempts, being housed

in isolation or a single cell, and loss of support systems and resources. Suicide rates increase as time in jail increases, secondary to failure to cope with stressors of confinement. Feelings of victimization and hopelessness are common among those who attempt or commit jail suicides. Staff may disregard suicide attempts among inmates with antisocial personality disorder, assuming the behavior to be attention-getting or manipulation. For this reason, all self-injury should be screened as suicide attempt until demonstrated otherwise, and a history of self-harm should be considered evidence of risk for suicide.

Suicide prevention should begin at the top, with administrators and staff in positions of authority asserting that suicide is not tolerated, that suicide can be prevented, and that suicide is not good for the inmates, for the staff, or for society. Key components of successful suicide risk reduction are integrated in a team effort and include available resources delineating policies and protocols, regular training, screening, housing, and supervision. Correctional nurses should take leadership in establishing a culture and milieu that discourage and prevent suicide by focusing on staff training. Intake screening tools should include specific data related to history and current thoughts of suicide. Initial screening should be done by mental health staff or psychiatric nurses, but all health-care staff and correctional staff have roles in the continuing assessment of suicide risk.

Upon admission, a thorough physical and mental status assessment confirms the presence of risk factors for suicide, such as intoxication or depression. Nurses should always verify whether the inmate was on suicide watch prior to confinement in the receiving institution. It is important to not only ask the questions regarding suicidal ideation and suicidal behaviors, but also to observe for signs and symptoms of mood changes related to depression, despair, anxiety, and hopelessness: these are the clues to risk of suicide. It is important not to discontinue surveillance of inmates whose depression appears to be improving. Sudden mood improvement may be a signal that antidepressant therapy is working, elevating not only mood but energy levels to the point that the inmate has the ability to carry out a suicide plan. Another explanation for the sudden mood change may be the relief an individual experiences after the decision to die has been made. These situations warrant very careful observation.

Contrary to common practice, research confirms decisions about restraints, isolation, and removal of personal objects should depend on the individual situation and not be a routine measure. Inmates in isolation are at increased risk for suicide. It is preferable to house suicidal detainees in the general population or in a protective housing such as a medical unit or infirmary. A suicide-resistant environment is free of obvious protrusions that could be used as suspension points for hanging, provides for full visibility for staff observation, has tamper-proof light fixtures and electrical outlets, and has no areas or surfaces that provide a mechanism for hanging or self-infliction of cuts.

Supervision of inmates whose condition has been determined to be at risk for suicide occurs at two levels. Close observation is used for inmates who are not actively suicidal but express suicidal thoughts and/or have had recent history of self-destructive behavior. Actively suicidal inmates are provided continuous surveillance. Continuous observation can be supplemented with closed circuit TV, but this does not replace direct personal contact. Jails require closer supervision than prisons and other secure environments, particularly during the first 1 to 2 days of confinement.

Effective multidisciplinary communication is essential to the prevention of suicide in prison. Issues of power, personality, mutual respect, and control can become barriers to effective information sharing between the disciplines, preventing the necessary assessment data from being used to determine appropriate observation level and intervention. It is important to listen carefully to the observations of any staff that have direct communications or contact with the inmate. Inmates will not share critical information if they perceive staff will respond in humiliating or punitive ways when they disclose suicidal or self-harm thoughts or activities. Responses to suicide risk should be uniform across the setting so that there is reasonable expectation for consistent treatment.

Upon detection of a suicide attempt, intervention must be immediate, as death or permanent disability can occur in a matter of minutes. Fatality can be as high as 79%; those who are alive when they reach an acute care setting capable of providing ventilator-dependent services have increased survival rates of up to 80% and higher.

While **"no-suicide contracts"** have not been demonstrated to affect suicide rates, most practitioners use them, particularly in nontreatment settings, citing benefits related to establishment of trust and interpersonal alliances between patient and caregiver and as a means to interact therapeutically with the patient. Used as a means to explore patient feelings and motivation, the "no-suicide" decision procedure can serve as a means to qualitatively monitor the degree to which an inmate is at risk and therefore be referred for suicide watch. It can also be used as a patient management approach, setting boundaries for self-destructive behavior that are understood by inmate and nurse.

Only about 10% of suicide attempts in correctional settings are by hanging, but hangings account for over 80% of the suicide deaths. Prevention of hanging should focus on the removal of the means by taking away access to ropes, belts, flex, and ligature points such as beams, banisters, hooks, knobs, and trees. Hanging events can be survived, even when the victim has been suspended for up to 5 minutes or more. Protocols for staff responsibilities should be known by everyone because any one of the staff could be the first responder to a suicide attempt. In a hanging, the first response is to stabilize the neck, cutting off the ligature but not the knot (this is for forensic evidence). In addition to the initiation of cardiopulmonary resuscitation and establishment of an IV, baseline blood should be drawn and a history of the patient position, knot placement, drop, and type of ligature should be documented.

When an inmate dies of suicide, staff are usually traumatized, and it is essential that nurses be involved in the development and use of critical incident stress management teams. Involvement in trauma such as suicide increases personal risk in a setting already at higher risk for stress, injury, and violence. An administrative review will be conducted to provide an objective analysis of the circumstances surrounding the incident, whether jail or prison procedures were followed, and if sufficient training has been offered to involved staff. A complete analysis of the medical and mental health care received by the victim will include nursing actions. Correctional nurses will be responsible for the assessment of suicide risk, actions taken to reduce risk, reporting and documentation, and intervention to treat the victim.

Successful suicide prevention programs include the availability of 24-hour access to a mental health professional for feedback on assessment data and recommendations for mental health services for those inmates considered to be at risk by health-care staff and correctional officers. Additionally, community-based services are increasing their communications and collaborations with prisons and jails to provide a continuous documentation of assessments, services, and plans of care for individuals inside and outside the correctional system. All jail and prison staff should be required to receive annual training related to mental health assessment and screening for risk for suicide, along with emergency response protocols. Some institutions are developing laminated cards for staff to carry that alert them to the identifying characteristics of inmates at risk for suicide. Many states are partnering with universities and colleges to augment mental health care, providing psychologists, physicians, nurses, and social workers to perform assessments, screenings, and care planning for at-risk inmates.

While we do not have sufficient scientifically confirmed evidence regarding self-inflicted death in custody to develop truly effective preventive strategies, nursing can access available evidence from which to develop best current practices in suicide prevention in jails. There are five steps to developing evidence-based correctional nursing interventions in the prevention of jail suicide: (1) defining the question, (2) collecting evidence, (3) performing a critical appraisal, (4) integrating the evidence and patient factors to make and carry out the decision, and (5) evaluating the whole process. An analysis of national data on prisons identified the effects of institutional conditions such as deprivation and overcrowding in jails and prisons and their interaction on the likelihood of prison suicide. Jails differ from prisons in that jails incarcerate people awaiting trials, people serving less than 1-year sentences, and people serving parole or probation violations. Jail populations tend to have high rates of substance abuse, mental illnesses,

infections, and chronic diseases. Few people serving jail terms receive health interventions addressing the physical and psychosocial problems that contributed to their incarcerations in the first place.

Enhanced mental health and social services for inmates with life sentences and long-term offenders, along with elderly offenders, is aimed at reducing risk for suicide among these populations. Some programs use other inmates to assist in suicide observations, especially when inmates are placed in the general population. Inmates are chosen who receive "gatekeeper" training and act as volunteers to talk with suicidal inmates. Through this approach, the inmates gain better communication skills, greater self-esteem, and purpose. They are prepared to intervene in situations of grief, depression, and self-harm.

Case Study

SUICIDE PREVENTION TRAINING

You are a new staff member assigned to a county jail in a rural area of the state and have been given responsibility for managing the suicide prevention training of the nursing staff. Two recent suicide completions have left the unit in chaos and confusion. An initial assessment indicates the nursing staff is uncomfortable doing mental status evaluations and is reluctant to call in social workers, psychologists, and physicians on weekends. The correctional staff voice interest in helping you take action (Table 14.1).

TABLE 14.1 **Research-Based Actions**

Research and Evidence	Action
Suicides occur 24 hours a day; there is no one time at which the risk is highest.	Correctional officers and staff will make rounds every 30 minutes throughout the night and observe all prisoners in cells every 30 minutes 24 hours a day.
Most jail suicides occur in the first 24 hours and decrease as time from entry into system increases.	Review intake procedures to ensure intensive, comprehensive screening for suicide risk; provide close surveillance for all new prisoners (present for less than 48 hours). Remind staff to listen to arresting officers or transport officers carefully for any information about the prisoner's behavior prior to admission.
The major psychiatric diagnosis of prisoners who commit suicide is drug and alcohol dependence and psychiatric disorders of affective disorder and schizophrenia.	Contact community and other resources to provide detoxification treatment and services to prisoners with a history of alcohol or drug abuse. Explore possibility of opiate-addicted prisoners having access to methadone treatment and not losing their priority if on a waiting list for treatment in community facilities. Organize detoxification training for nursing staff. Meet with psychologist, social worker, and/or psychiatrist to determine who will be points of contact for suicide assessment and placement of prisoners on suicide watch, covering 24 hours a day, 7 days a week. Provide training for nursing staff. Explore links with community-based mental health treatment providers and increased use of fax, computer, and telephone communications to facilitate rapid, effective communications for continuity of care for prisoners who have received a mental health assessment or treatment prior to incarceration.

Research and Evidence	Action
	Collaborate with mental health care providers to integrate screening, assessment, and treatment planning into routine nursing activities.
Recognition and treatment of depression are related to reduced suicide rates in jails and prisons.	Provide a schedule of training, along with posted information regarding signs and symptoms of depression.
Most suicides in jails are by hanging; other methods include jumping from an exposed platform. The most common methods of hanging include ligatures (ropes, belts, flex) and ligature points (beams, banisters, hooks, doorknobs, and trees). Fifty percent of hanging suicides are not fully suspended; ligature points below the head level are commonly used, and relatively minimal neck pressure is required to cause death by hanging. Survival is possible even after 5 minutes of suspension.	Set up schedule for risk assessment for means for suicide. Limit access of prisoners to ligature points or other means for hanging. Install Plexiglass barriers in areas where suicidal prisoners are housed. Rounds during sleep periods should ensure that the prisoners' heads and necks are visible. All staff should be trained in emergency recovery and CPR with neck protection methods. Emphasize immediate transport to hospital. Secure "cut-down tools," specialized knives built to hook on to cloth to cut through fibers quickly, so that they cannot be used by inmates as a weapon.
Isolation is related to increased suicide attempts and successful suicides.	House inmates in multiple-occupancy cells; restrict use of single-cell occupancy to those areas of high surveillance only. Consider housing suicidal inmates together for social housing and surveillance.
Traumatic life events (divorce, abuse, new criminal charges) are associated with suicide risk.	Review intake screening and assessment tools to ensure sufficient psychosocial and mental health history is provided to identify high-risk prisoners.
Critical incident management has been associated with decreased vicarious traumatization and reductions in suicide completions in some settings.	Collaborate with mental health staff to create effective strategies for critical incident management and integration of nursing staff in organization and management of process.
The great majority of all suicides in prison are preceded by previous suicide attempts and/or self-injury.	Record and take seriously all self-harm. Do not assume that self-mutilation or other self-harm is just for "attention"; educate staff to be observant and conservative in assessing suicide risk.
Bullying is associated with suicide.	Train staff to observe inmate-on-inmate interpersonal behavior and take claims of bullying seriously; share with correctional staff to gauge their readiness to provide surveillance.

CORRECTIONAL WORKING CONDITIONS AND HEALTH PATTERNS IN CORRECTIONS

Environments for correctional health care are characterized by isolation, scarce resources and the need to carefully allocate those resources, and staff that are generally underprepared for their responsibilities. Correctional nurses must have access to resources such as rape kits, postassault services, and therapy for substance abuse and mental health problems, in addition to the general medical services that are customary in primary health-care settings and emergent care settings in jails and prisons.

Organizational issues affecting quality of care in correctional health-care settings, extrapolated from studies of forensic psychiatric settings, include mandatory overtime, staff injuries, and violence that can affect not only staff morale and performance, but also outcomes of care. Staffing patterns and nurses' working conditions are risk factors for health-care–associated infections as well as occupational injuries and infections. As inmate populations increase beyond capacity, correctional health-care services are characterized by chronic conditions of understaffing, complicating planning and efforts to respond to health-care emergencies or emerging infectious diseases or other health issues. Evaluations of soon-to-be-released inmates concluded that improving the health care of inmates can benefit public health in two important ways: (1) reducing the transmission of communicable disease to others in the community from inmates who are released with untreated conditions and without having participated in disease prevention programs and (2) reducing the financial burden on the public associated with treating released inmates who return to the community with undiagnosed or untreated communicable disease, chronic disease, and mental illness, thereby freeing up resources for other worthy public health initiatives.

It is incumbent upon correctional nurses to provide leadership in the application of effective strategies to reduce the transmission of communicable diseases through aggressive and effective identification of at-risk inmates and effective treatment management during incarceration. Voluntary HIV counseling and testing can be effective if accompanied by sufficient intensity of counseling. Counseling and testing are not effective methods for managing HIV risk behavior or transference unless significant time for explaining and describing consequences of response options, along with implications of inaction, is provided.

Strong testing and counseling models for communicable disease, for HIV prevention, and substance abuse treatment care have been demonstrated to be effective in correctional settings. Substance abuse treatment in prison decreases drug dependency and use, reduces recidivism rates, and is cost effective. Discharge planning is a critical component in the containment of infectious disease and continuation of treatment adherence after release. Standards and guidelines for the treatment and follow-up of infectious diseases presenting in correctional settings is updated regularly by the Centers for Disease Control and Prevention and the National Commission for Correctional Health Care (2002a, 2002b).

Offender management involves the use of inmate classification, which is the assignment of a label indicating assessment of inmate behavior and risk. There are two levels of classification: internal classification determines placement within the correctional institution, whereas external classification determines custody level and institutional placement. The anticipation of problem behavior and special needs is an essential component of classification, and nursing assessment may be a critical input to the assessment of inmate status. Such factors as needs for mental health and medical care are areas in which nurses can provide data. Placement on medical units should not be used for administrative segregation, disciplinary segregation, or protective custody. Studies of classification indicate there is no one effective model for inmate classification; each facility needs to develop the best model for its population. While there is some speculation that the prison environment itself serves as a mediator of criminal behavior, research by Camp and Gaes confirmed that inmate behavior is not dependent upon the classification

level of institution to which they are assigned. However, the prison environment has been shown to have deleterious effects on mental health.

Vicarious Traumatization

The cumulative impact of dealing with inmates whose life experiences are characterized by abuse, trauma, and violence, and whose daily lives reflect that history, can be a burden to those nurses who care for them. Vicarious traumatization, also referred to as secondary trauma, is an occupational hazard that is largely unrecognized and unaddressed in correctional nursing. It can be experienced by any clinician who works with traumatized individuals, whether victims of child maltreatment, domestic violence, victims of torture, or victims of large-scale disasters. Those who work with trauma victims, and who have a personal trauma history, show more negative effects from their work than do those without a personal trauma. Vicarious traumatization among professionals working with victims results from the inability of the health-care provider to process the traumatic clinical material they hear. Vicarious traumatization has symptoms that are similar to post-traumatic stress disorder.

Implementation of a public health model for correctional health care provides for early detection, diagnosis, treatment, education, and post-release follow-up for inmates. Collaborations with community health centers provide inmates with medical and case management services, integrating a continuum of care from corrections to community and containment of communicable and chronic conditions such as HIV/AIDS and other serious illnesses. Such programming has been demonstrated to be effective in providing sustained care and risk-reduction education, as well as in reducing recidivism rates.

Upon release from prison, few inmates identify health care as a priority need. While no single problem emerges as a high priority among all former inmates, housing, unemployment, and education are common issues for adults and adolescent males. The high rates of hypertension, HIV, homelessness, and substance abuse, particularly among ethnic minorities, highlight the need to focus on strong case management and referral systems for these individuals upon release from prison.

Basic offender management programs include substance abuse treatment, mental health services, educational and vocational programs, cognitive-behavioral programs, family interventions, special needs services, and balanced supervision strategies. This array of programming is best implemented by applying principles of effective correctional intervention. Interventions and strategies that have evidence to support positive outcomes among inmates include increasing their skills, competencies, adjustments, and stability—all critical components of health promotion. Correctional nurses most effectively affect inmate health and long-term well-being by carefully prioritizing health promotion programming based on an assessment of relative risk of specific outcome in the population served, the perceived need for services, and the ability of the inmate population to respond positively to intervention.

A qualitative analysis of the impact of prison programs in which inmates train dogs suggests these programs have the potential to break down barriers of fear and mistrust between staff and inmates. There is additional evidence supporting the relationship between inmate participation in dog-training programs and a reduction in recidivism and behavioral infractions. Correctional nurses may consider the institution of such programs, if feasible, in the treatment plan for inmates in mental health promotion programs whose goals might include impulse control, behavior management, and relationship building.

EVIDENCE-BASED RECOMMENDATIONS FOR CORRECTIONAL HEALTH-CARE MANAGEMENT

Institutional practices in correctional settings directly affect nursing roles and quality of care. Sick call triage is an event in most correctional settings characterized as inadequate and inefficient. Often cited as a barometer of quality of prison health-care services, sick call has been identified as being sensitive to the overall population density of the correctional institution. Effective organization, efficiency, and effectiveness in delivery of timely and proper care are essential components of sick call in prison. In 2004 the Florida Correctional Medical Authority survey of medical and mental health care provided in its prisons reviewed efforts to ensure provision of a constitutionally adequate level of basic medical care consistent with minimum standards accepted in the community at large. Specific issues were identified as critical to the preservation of expected health-care outcomes. To ensure continuity of care, a coordinated process for transferring inmates among institutions is necessary. Documentation of transfer requirements and patient status upon referral, exit, and entry should be overseen by professional nursing staff.

Role Conflict: Custody and Caring

Successful collaboration and clinical competency within the correctional health system depends on recognition of the role expectations of the correctional nurse, necessary and required performance standards, and clear distinctions between the role of the nurse and the other staff, particularly corrections staff. Correctional officers are primarily concerned with the security of the facility. They focus on maintaining order, keeping everyone safe through vigilance, and keeping rules enforced. **Role strain** is experienced by an individual when incompatible behavior, expectations, or obligations are associated with a single social role. Role strain occurs when the demands of the correctional nurse role require responses that are beyond the capabilities of the nurse or that exhaust the coping and problem-solving resources of the nurse. Role stress is the result of role strain, and it is a state in which the correctional nurse experiences personal loss and reduced performance in response to the demands of the correctional nursing role. Individual responses to professional role strain include specific factors of role overload, role expectation conflict, inter-role distance, resource inadequacy, role stagnation, and role isolation as predictors of role stress leading to job dissatisfaction, decreased productivity, poor organizational morale, and eventual departure.

Stress is the physical or psychological tension derived from demands that exceed available resources. Often misinterpreted as an all-around nuisance, stress can bring about both positive and negative results. When experienced in the right proportions, it can inspire a worker to perform better. Because of these physical and psychological detriments, negative shifts in behavior can occur. Burned-out workers have been known to escape from their troubles through drug and alcohol use.

While all nurses are at risk for stress, correctional nurses are particularly vulnerable to role stress and role strain. Correctional nurses' stressors and the sources of conflict for correctional nursing staff can include too many tasks and too heavy of an everyday workload, conflicting demands from colleagues and superiors, incompatible demands from their different personal and organizational roles, inadequate resources for appropriate performance, insufficient competency to meet the demands of their role, inadequate autonomy to make decisions on different tasks, and a feeling of underutilization.

To decrease incidents of burnout among correctional nurses, roles must be clearly delineated, differentiating the "caring" from the "custody" roles. Implementation of evidence-based practice interventions that increase the probability of treatment success among inmates provides support for the valuing of the nursing role in the correctional setting.

Few university courses offered specifically target how to deal with offenders in a confined setting. With this in mind, nursing staff should receive continuing training that covers inmate manipulation and coping techniques for negotiating resistant and confrontational behavior. Stress management workshops could be implemented that focus specifically on overcoming the difficulties of interacting with problem offenders. To enhance job stimulation and meaning, staff should be updated frequently on scholarly and scientific publications that discuss advancements and current issues in offender care. A similar motivation tool resides in permitting and encouraging nurses to conduct research experiments that relate to their job functions. For example, compiling information and statistics on what is and is not working in a program can reveal how to be more productive. The creation of empirical evidence for practice provides an alternative to the boredom of routine work, presenting challenges and adding variety, which, in turn, promotes more interest in and involvement with correctional nursing.

Research Spotlight on Correctional Nursing Education

The competency framework used by Storey and Dale outlined 45 competencies that were thematically grouped into 11 sections: communication and relationships; assessment; care planning, implementation, and evaluation; health and primary health care; discharge and community support; providing and developing therapeutic environments; safety; helping manage change and loss; staff support; professional development; and management. These groupings reflect the fundamentals of nursing practice, and given that introducing a competency framework into practice would require demonstration of successful role performance within these dimensions, it would provide some assurance that nurses held the capacity to carry out the tasks in a competent manner to a given standard. It is suggested, therefore, that implementing the framework would have the effect of driving up standards and consequentially improving patient care by providing a more certain skill base within the clinical setting.

CONCLUSIONS

The exponential growth rate of the incarcerated in the United States has created the need for a health-care system to address inmates' constitutional rights to necessary medical care and treatment. Correctional nurses are pivotal in the delivery of safe and cost-effective health care to individuals detained in secure settings within the jails and prisons of the United States. Clinical expertise for correctional nursing requires the requisite knowledge and experience to make correct decisions in specific clinical situations, mitigated by the characteristics and needs of inmates. Balancing personal values, societal mandates, and professional codes for correctional nursing is extremely stressful to correctional nurses. Understanding the special populations served in correctional settings includes understanding patterns of health and disease prominent in correctional settings, such as high rates of substance abuse, mental illnesses, infections, and chronic diseases, as well as the physical and psychological trauma associated with incarceration. Emerging populations presenting health-care challenges include elderly, women, and juveniles. Confined settings are challenged to provide care to significant numbers of inmates with HIV, tuberculosis, and hepatitis. To deal with recurring issues of inmate patient management problems, malingering, and manipulative behavior, correctional nurses must develop excellent assessment and critical thinking skills to differentiate actual and created symptoms.

Long-term planning and coordination of care with community health-care providers is essential for public health, as most inmates are released into communities either on parole or at completion of sentences. Education and career socialization and planning are priorities for correctional nurses. Nursing and health research findings, along with professional standards of care, are part of the evidence base from which they deliver safe and cost-effective health care in correctional settings.

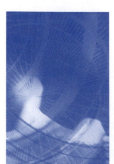

EVIDENCE-BASED PRACTICE

Reference Question: Are there legal defenses for women who kill their abusers?

Database(s) to Search: PubMed, LexusNexis

Search Strategy: Use the MeSH term '"jurisprudence" to cover issues of law for this question. Use "OR" with the MeSH terms "battered women" and "spouse abuse" to create one large set of articles talking about women. Use "AND" with the women and jurisprudence set, then limit according to your preferences.

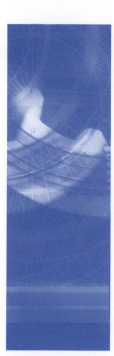

EVIDENCE-BASED PRACTICE *(continued)*

Selected References From Search:

1. Phillips, N.D. (2009). The prosecution of hate crimes: The limitations of the hate crime typology. *Journal of Interpersonal Violence, 24*(5):883-905.
2. Plumm, K.M., & Terrance, C.A. (2009). Battered women who kill: The impact of expert testimony and empathy induction in the courtroom. *Violence Against Women, 15*(2):186-205.
3. van Wormer, K. (2009). Restorative justice as social justice for victims of gendered violence: A standpoint feminist perspective. *Social Work, 54*(2):107-116.

Questions Used to Discern Evidence:

Choose two studies among the studies listed, read about them, and answer the following questions:

1. What are the differences between the two studies in the design, methods, and results?
2. What are the similarities between the two studies in the number of subjects, measures used, and interventions, if any?
3. What competencies do you need to acquire in working with abused women who kill their abusers?

REVIEW QUESTIONS

1. Demographic and public policy shifts in the United States have led to:
   A. Reduction of incarcerated persons in federal facilities but growth in state facilities.
   B. Growth of incarcerated persons in federal facilities but reduction in state facilities.
   C. Stable but concerning numbers over the past 30 years.
   D. Projected growth at three times that of the general population.

2. Correctional nursing practice is influenced by:
   A. Lack of constitutional rights of inmates that limit health care provided to them.
   B. Health care that is a dire medical necessity.
   C. Principles of constitutional law that require provision of dental, medical, psychiatric, and psychological care.
   D. Eighth Amendment requirements to modify care to inmates when cost is in question.

3. Which of the following statements is true?
   A. Personal values of the nurse have no effect on correctional nursing practice.
   B. Clinical expertise in correctional nursing comes with seniority.
   C. Expert knowledge and successful problem solving is the basis for correctional nursing.
   D. Correctional nursing care is guided by law and access to care, not by evidence.

4. Which of the following is true regarding women's health in correctional facilities?
   A. Women make up 6% of the prison population, and the numbers are rapidly increasing.
   B. Women's health in prison is the most frequently researched.
   C. Women who are incarcerated rarely have the life-threatening health problems that men do.
   D. Incarcerated women are generally more violent and dangerous than male prisoners.

(review questions continued on page 278)

5. The majority of adolescents in correctional facilities:
   A. Just need discipline and guidelines for behavior disorders.
   B. Are not in need of serious medical or mental health care.
   C. Have access to abundant services that exist but are seldom used for their health care.
   D. Should be prudently screened for post-traumatic stress disorder that could lead to violent behavior.

6. Core elements of correctional health care are categories for organizing knowledge for practice and include all of the following *except:*
   A. There is a legal obligation to provide care and avoid deliberate indifference.
   B. Theory, knowledge, and protocol have little place in standards of correctional nursing care.
   C. Laboratory, diagnostic, and emergency care are mandatory components of correctional health care.
   D. Awareness of patient-to-staff ratios are mandatory for safety.

7. Special issues that are experienced by correctional nurses do *not* include:
   A. Culture shock that reflects the stress of caring for the disadvantaged.
   B. Supportive and collaborative nature of prison and jail administration, staff, and patients.
   C. Limitation of resources for health-care provision, including staff.
   D. Role socialization for nurses working in secure environments.

8. Boundary violations are a breakdown in professionalism and may result when which of the following occurs?
   A. An inmate demands to be seen by one nurse only.
   B. Sexual intimacy occurs between inmate and staff member.
   C. The nurse refers and discharges a patient when patient is clearly ready.
   D. A cooperative inmate requests to be seen by one nurse only.

9. Fraternization is:
   A. Not a crime but an ethical issue.
   B. An inmate-staff relationship such as a sexual relationship.
   C. The same thing as favoritism or familiarity.
   D. Seldom addressed in correctional policies.

10. The U.S. Constitution prohibits cruel and unusual punishment for inmates, which has led to the emergence of which of the following inmates' rights?
   A. Access to care, ordered care, and surgical care equal to the public at large.
   B. Access to care, ordered care, and professional judgment.
   C. Ordered care, professional judgment, and reasonable emergency care.
   D. Access to cost-effective care, reasonable preventive care, and care mandated by correctional personnel.

References

Adams, K., & Ferrandino, J. (2008). Managing mentally ill inmates in prison. *Criminal Justice and Behavior, 35*(8):913-927.

American Academy of Pediatrics Committee on Adolescence. (2001). Health care for children and adolescents in the juvenile correctional care system: A policy statement. *Pediatrics, 107*(4):799-803.

American Nurses Association (ANA). (2007). *Scope and standards of practice for nurses.* Washington, DC: ANA.

Anno, B.J. (2001). *Correctional health care: Guidelines for the management of an adequate delivery system.* Chicago, IL: National Commission on Correctional Health Care.

Arehart-Treichel, J. (2004). Risk of prison suicide highest in first week. *Psychiatric News, 39*(9):16.

Austin, J. (2003). Findings in prison classification and risk assessment. *Prisons Division-Issues in Brief.* Washington, DC: National Institute of Corrections.

Beck, A.G., & Hughes, T.A. (2005). *Sexual violence reported by correctional authorities, 2004* (NCJ 210333). Washington, DC: US Department of Justice, Bureau of Statistics.

Beckett, J., Peternelj-Taylor, C., & Johnson, R.L. (2003). Growing old in the correctional system. *Journal of Psychosocial Nursing, 41*(9):12-18.

Bender, E. (2004). Averting prison suicides requires special strategies. *Psychiatric News, 39*(24):15.

Berk, R., Ladd, H., & Graziano, H. (2002). A randomized experiment testing inmate classification systems. Retrieved February 2, 2008, from http://repositories.cdlib.org/cgi/viewcontent.cgi?article=1126&context=uclastat

Berk, R.A., Kriegler, B., & Baek, J.H. (2006). *Forecasting dangerous inmate misconduct.* Los Angeles, CA: University of California Policy Research Center.

Beyea, S.C., & Nicoll, L.H. (2000). Clinical expertise and research findings: Understanding the fit. *AORN Journal, 71*(2): 41, 413.

Blaauw, E., Aresman, E., Kraaij, V., et al. (2005). Traumatic life events and suicide risk among jail inmates: The influence of types of events, time period and significant others. *Journal of Traumatic Stress, 15*(1):9-16.

Bloom, B., Owen, B., & Covington, S. (2003). *Gender-responsive strategies: Research, practice and guiding principles for women offenders* (HIC Accession Number 018017). Washington, DC: U.S. Department of Justice, National Institute of Corrections.

Bonner, R.L. (2006). Stressful segregation housing and psychosocial vulnerability in prison suicide ideators. *Suicide and Life Threatening Behavior, 36*(2):250-254.

Britton, D.M., & Button, A. (2005). Prison pups: Assessing the effects of dog training programs in correctional facilities. *Journal of Family Social Work, 9*(4):79-95.

Bureau of Health Information and Policy. (2005). *Evidence-based practices for healthiest Wisconsin, 2010.* University of Wisconsin Population Health Institute. Retrieved from http://dhfs.wisconsin.gov/statehealthplan/practices/

Bureau of Justice Statistics. (2004). *Data collections for the prison rape elimination act of 2003* (NCJ 206109). Washington, DC: U.S. Department of Justice, Bureau of Statistics.

Bureau of Justice Statistics. (2008). *Prison statistics summary findings.* Retrieved from www.ojp.usdoj.gov/bjs/prisons.htm

Camp, S.D., & Gaes, G.G. (2004). *Criminogenic effects of the prison environment on inmate behavior: Some experimental evidence.* Retrieved March 1, 2008, from www.bop.gov/news/research_projects/published_reports/cond_envir/camp_gaes_c&d.pdf

Clawson, E. (2006). *Increasing public safety and reducing recidivism by enhancing offender success—Evidence based practices in offender management.* Presented June 29, 2006, Center for Effective Public Policy. Retrieved July 7, 2007, from www.tennessee.gov/correction/criminaljustice/Evidence-Based%20Practice-RFINAL_2.pdf

Colwell, B. (2007). Deference or respect? Status management practices among prison inmates. *Social Psychology Quarterly, 70*(4):442-460.

Conner, K.R., & Goldston, D.B. (2007). Rates of suicide among males increase steadily from age 11 to 21: Developmental framework and outline for prevention. *Aggression and Violent Behavior, 12*(2):193-207.

Conroy, M.A., & Kwartner, P.P. (2006). Malingering. *Applied Psychology in Criminal Justice, 3*(3):29-51.

Cornell Law School. (2005). *Prison rape elimination: Findings of Congress.* Retrieved on March 8, 2008, from www.law.cornell.edu/uscode/uscode42/usc_sec_42_00015601——000-.html

Crawford, N. (2003). Helping inmates cope with prison life. *Monitor on Psychology, 34*(7):1-3. Retrieved from www.apa.org/monitor/julaug03/helping.html

Daniel, A.E. (2006). Preventing suicide in prison: A collaborative responsibility of administrative, custodial, and clinical staff. *Journal of the American Academy of Psychiatry and the Law, 34*:165-175.

Deffenbacher, J.L., Oetting, E.R., & DiGiuseppe, R.A. (2002). Principles of empirically supported interventions applied to anger management. *The Counseling Psychologist, 30*(2): 262-280.

DeLisi, M., Berg, M.T., & Hochstetler, A. (2004). Gang members, career criminals and prison violence: Further specification of the importation model of inmate behavior. *Criminal Justice Studies, 17*(4):369-383.

Dial, K.C., & Worley, R. (2008). Crossing the line: A quantitative analysis of inmate boundary violators in a southern prison system. *American Journal of Criminal Justice, 33*:69-84.

Dixon, A., Howie, P., & Starling, J. (2005). Trauma exposure, posttraumatic stress, and psychiatric co-morbidity in female juvenile offenders. *Journal of the American Academy of Child and Adolescent Psychiatry, 44*(8):798-806.

Drye, R.C. (2005). No suicide decision. *Psychiatric News, 40*(22):36.

Edens, J.F., Poythress, N.G., & Watkins-Clay, M.M. (2007). Detection of malingering in psychiatric unit and general population prison inmates: A comparison of the PAI, SIMS and SIRS. *Journal of Personality Assessment, 88*(1):33-42.

Edwards, P. (2002). *Active ageing: A policy framework.* Geneva, Switzerland: World Health Organization, Noncommunicable Disease and Health Promotion Department.

Eliason, M.J. (2006). Are therapeutic communities therapeutic for women? *Substance Abuse Treatment, Prevention, and Policy.* Retrieved August 1, 2007, from www.substanceabusepolicy.com/content/pdf/1747-597X-1-3.pdf

Flores, J.R. (2008). *Girls study group: Understanding and responding to girl's delinquency* (NCJ 218905). Washington, DC: U.S. Department of Justice, Office of Justice Programs, Office of Juvenile Justice and Delinquency Prevention.

Forsyth, C.J., Evans, R.D., & Foster, D.B. (2002). An analysis of inmate explanations for lesbian relationships in prison. *International Journal of Sociology of the Family, 30*(1):66-77.

French, M.T., Zavala, S.K., McCollister, K.E., et al. (2006). Cost-effectiveness analysis of four interventions for adolescents with a substance use disorder. *Journal of Substance Abuse Treatment.*

Gaes, G.G., & Goldberg, A.L. (2004). *Prison rape: A critical review of the literature* (NCJ 213365). Washington, DC: U.S. Department of Justice, National Institute of Justice.

Gear, S. (2005). Rules of engagement: Structuring sex and damage in men's prisons and beyond. *Culture, Health and Sexuality, 7*(3):195-208.

Gilmartin, K., & Davis, R.M. (2004). *The correctional officer Stockholm syndrome: Management implications.* National Institute of Corrections, First Annual Symposium on Now Generation Jails. Retrieved from www.emotionalsurvival.com/stockholm_syndrome.htm

Goffman, E. (1959). *The presentation of self in everyday life.* Garden City, NY: Doubleday Anchor Books.

Greve, W., Enzmann, D., & Hosser, D. (2001). The stabilization of self-esteem among incarcerated adolescents: Accommodative and immunizing processes. *International Journal of Offender Therapy and Comparative Criminology, 45*(6): 749-768.

Grimes, J.C. (2008). Prisoner HIV program leads to continuum of medical care after release. Retrieved May 10, 2008, from www.eurekalert.org/pub_releases/2008-05/l-php050708.php

Gunnell, D., Bennewith, O., Hawton, K., et al. (2005). The epidemiology and prevention of suicide by hanging: A systematic review. *International Journal of Epidemiology, 34*:433-442.

Hammond, S. (2007). *Mental health needs of juvenile offenders.* National Conference of State Legislatures Criminal Justice Program Briefing Paper. Retrieved from www.ncsl.org/programs/cj/juvenilejustice.htm

Hayes, L.M. (2007). Reducing inmate suicides through the mortality review process. In R.B. Greiginger (d.), *Public health behind bars: From prisons to communities.* New York: Springer.

Hensley, C., Castle, T., & Tewksbury, R. (2003). Inmate-to-inmate sexual coercion in a prison for women. *Journal of Offender Rehabilitation, 37*(2):77-87.

Hensley, C., & Tewksbury, R. (2002). Inmate-to-inmate prison sexuality: A review of empirical studies. *Trauma, Violence & Abuse, 3*(3):226-243.

Holloway, J.D. (2003). Advances in anger management. *Monitor on Psychology, APA Online, 34*(3). Retrieved February 2, 2007, from www.apa.org/monitor/mar03/advances.html

Howells, K., & Day, A. (2003). Readiness for anger management: Clinical and theoretical issues. *Clinical Psychology Review, 23*:319-337.

Howells, K., Day, A., Williamson, P., et al. (2005). Brief anger management programs with offenders: Outcomes and predictors of change. *Journal of Forensic Psychiatry & Psychology, 16*(2):296-311.

Hufft, A. (2000). Multidisciplinary care of the mentally disordered offender in the USA. In D. Robinson & A. Kettles (Eds.), *Multidisciplinary care of the mentally disordered offender.* London: Kingsley Publishers.

Hufft, A. (2004). *Characteristics and performance expectations of forensic psychiatric nurses: A comparison of disciplines of nursing and forensic psychology.* Presented at the Applied Psychology Symposium. Valdosta State University, Valdosta, GA.

Hufft, A., & Kite, J.J. (2003). Vulnerable and cultural perspectives for nursing care in correctional systems. *Journal of Multicultural Nursing & Health, 9*(1):18-25.

Institute of Medicine. (2000). *To err is human: Building a safer health system.* Washington, DC: National Academy Press.

James, D.J., & Glaze, L.E. (2006). Mental health problems of prison and jail inmates. *Bureau of Justice Statistics Special Report* (NCJ 213600). Washington, DC: U.S. Department of Justice.

Jesperson, A. (2006). Treatment efficacy for female offenders. *Lethbridge Undergraduate Research Journal, 1*(1):1-11.

Kaminski, M.M. (2003). Games prisoners play: Allocation of roles in a total institution. *Rationality and Society, 15*(2):188-217.

Kantor, E. (2006). HIV transmission and prevention in prisons. HIV INSite. Retrieved July 30, 2007, from http://hivinsite.ucsf.edu/InSite?page=kb-07-04-13

Kay, S. (1991). *The constitutional dimensions of an inmate's right to health care.* Chicago: National Commission on Correctional Health Care.

Kroll, J. (2007). No-suicide contracts as a suicide prevention strategy. *Psychiatric Times, 24*(6):11.

Kruttschnitt, C., & Hussemann, J. (2008). Micropolitics of race and ethnicity in women's prison in two political contexts. *British Journal of Sociology, 59*(4):709-728.

Laffan, S. (2005). The inside look on correctional nursing: A unique nursing specialty. *New Jersey Nurse.* Retrieved from http://findarticles.com/p/articles/mi_qa4080/is_200501/ai_n11826429

Lee, J.B., & Bartlett, M.L. (2005). Suicide prevention: Critical elements for managing suicidal clients and counselor liability without the use of a no-suicide contract. *Death Studies, 29*(9):847-865.

Lindquist, C.H., & Lindquist, C.A. (2007). Gender differences in distress: Mental health consequences of environmental stress among jail inmates. *Behavioral Sciences and the Law, 15*(4):503-523.

Lopez-Williams, A., Stoep, A.V., Kuo, E., et al. (2006). Predictors of mental health service enrollment among juvenile offenders. *Youth Violence and Juvenile Justice, 4*(3):266-280.

McKinney, E.B. (2008). Hard time and health care: The squeeze on medicine behind bars. *Virtual Mentor, 10*(2):116-120. Retrieved from http://virtualmentor.ama-assn.org/2008/02/msoc2-0802.html

Moloney, K.P., Vanden Bergh, B.J., & Moller, L.F. (2009). Women in prison: The central issues of gender characteristics and trauma history. *Public Health, 123*(6):426-430.

Morgan, J., & Hawton, K. (2004). Self-reported suicidal behavior in juvenile offenders in custody: Prevalence and associated factors. *Crisis: The Journal of Crisis Intervention and Suicide Prevention, 25*(1):8-11.

Morgan, R.D., Steffan, J., Shaw, L.B., et al. (2007). Needs for and barriers to correctional mental health services: Inmate perceptions. *Psychiatric Services, 58*:1181-1186.

Morris, J., & Forsyth, D. (2005). Specialist medical input to residential and nursing home residents position statement. *British Geriatrics Society Newsletter Online.* Retrieved from www.bgsnet.org.uk/Jan05NL/12_specialist_input.htm

Morrison, E., Morman, G., Bonner, G., et al. (2002). Reducing staff injuries and violence in a forensic psychiatric setting. *Archives of Psychiatric Nursing, 16*(3):108-117.

Mueser, K.T., & Taub, J. (2008). Trauma and PTSD among adolescents with severe emotional disorders involved in multiple service systems. *Psychiatric Services, 59*:627-634.

National Commission on Correctional Health Care (NCCHC). (2008). *Standards for health services in prisons.* Chicago: NCCHC.

Nurse, J., Woodcock, P., & Ormsby, J. (2003). Influence of environmental factors on mental health within prisons: Focus group study. *British Medical Journal, 327*:480-487.

O'Connell, K.L. (2006). *Suicide prevention in correctional settings: Best practices.* Presented at the Indiana Department of Corrections Suicide Prevention Summit March 1, 2006, Indianapolis, IN.

O'Connor, T. (2006). Advanced topics in correctional ethics. *MegaLinks in criminal justice.* Retrieved June 6, 2007, from www.apsu.edu/oconnort/3300/3300lect06a.htm

Odgers, C.L., Burnette, M.L., Chauhan, P., Moretti, M.M., & Reppucci, N.D. (2005). Misdiagnosing the problem: Mental health profiles of incarcerated juveniles. *The Canadian Child and Adolescent Psychiatry Review, 12*(1):26-29.

Page, S.A., & King, M.C. (2008). No-suicide agreements: Current practices and opinions in a Canadian urban health region. *The Canadian Journal of Psychiatry, 53*(3):169-175.

Plugge, E., & Fitzpatrick, D.N. (2009). The impact of imprisonment on health—What do women prisoners say? *Journal of Epidemiology and Community Health, 63*(9):749-754.

Potter, R.H. (2003). Discharge planning and community case management of HIV-infected inmates: Collaboration enhances public health and safety. *Corrections Today, 65*(6): 80-85.

Pratt, D., Piper, M., Appleby, L., et al. (2006). Suicide in recently released prisoners: A population-based cohort study. *The Lancet, 368*(953):119-123.

Proctor, J. (2004). *The impact of imprisonment on women's health and health care*. Unpublished conference paper. Retrieved July 6, 2008, from www.allacademic.com/meta/p_mla_apa_research_citation/1/0/9/3/6/p109368_index.html

Quinn, M.M., Rutherford, R.B., Leone, P.E., et al. (2005). Youth with disabilities in juvenile corrections: A national survey. *Exceptional Children, 71*(3):339-345.

Reimer, G. (2008). The graying of the U.S. prisoner population. *Journal of Correctional Health Care, 14*(3):202-208.

Rold, W.J. (2008). Thirty years after *Estelle v. Gamble*: A legal retrospective. *Journal of Correctional Health Care, 14*(1):11-20.

Ross, T., & Pfafflin, F. (2007). Attachment and interpersonal problems in a prison environment. *Journal of Forensic Psychiatry & Psychology, 18*(1):90-98.

Roth, B., & Presse, L. (2003). Nursing interventions for parasuicidal behaviors in female offenders. *Journal of Psychosocial Nursing, 41*(9):20-29.

Rowe, C.L., Wang, W., Greenbaum, P., et al. (2008). Predicting HIV/STD risk level and substance use disorders among incarcerated adolescents. *Journal of Psychoactive Drugs, 40*(4):503-512.

Sabol, W.J., Couture, H., & Harrison, P. (2007). Prisoners in 2006. *Bureau of Justice Statistics Bulletin* (NJC 219416):1-26.

Sachdeva, R.K., & Wanchu, A. (2006). Women's issues in HIV infection. *JK Science, 8*(3):129-132.

Schafer, P. (2003). When a client develops an attraction: Successful resolution vs. boundary violation. *Journal of Psychiatric and Mental Health Nursing, 4*(3):203-211.

Shelton, D. (2003). The clinical practice of juvenile forensic psychiatric nurses. *Journal of Psychosocial Nursing and Mental Health Services, 41*(9):42-53.

Sickmund, M. (2005). *Deaths in custody, 2004*. Retrieved July 3, 2008, from www.aca.org/research/pdf/Research_Notes03_07.pdf

Sijuwade, P.O. (2007). General systems theory and structural analysis of correctional institution social systems. *Journal of Social Science, 14*(2):163-167.

Snyder, H.N., & Sickmund, M. (2006). *Juvenile offenders and victims: 2006 national report*. Washington, DC: US Department of Justice, Office of Justice Programs, Office of Juvenile Justice and Delinquency Prevention.

Souryal, S. (2006). *Ethics in criminal justice: In search of the truth* (3rd ed.). Cincinnati, OH: Anderson Publishing.

St. Pierre, I. (2008). Managing nurses through disciplinary power: A Foucauldian analysis of workplace violence. *Journal of Nursing Management, 16*(3):352-359.

Stone, P.W., Clarke, S., Cimiotti, J., et al. (2004). Nurses' working conditions: Implications for infectious disease. *Emerging Infectious Diseases*. Retrieved from www.cdc.gov/ncidod/EID/vol10no11/04-0253.htm

Thomas, J., & Allen, R.S. (2002). *Quetiapine use in patients with severe antisocial personality disorder*. Paper presented at the 26th National Conference on Correctional Health Care, October 19-23, Nashville, TN.

Tripodi, S.J., & Bender, K. (2007). Inmate suicide: Prevalence, assessment and protocols. *Brief Treatment and Crisis Intervention, 71*(1):40-54.

U.S. Department of Justice, Office of Juvenile Justice and Delinquency Prevention. (2009). *Statistical briefing book: Juvenile justice system structure and process*. Retrieved from http://ojjdp.ncjrs.org/ojstatbb/structure_process/index.html

Wagoner, L. (2004). Predicting violent behavior among inmates: Washington Correctional Institute's development of a risk protection tool. *Corrections Today*. Retrieved March 1, 2008, from http://goliath.ecnext.com/coms2/gi_0199-2612986/Predicting-violent-behavior-among-inmates.html

Warren, J. (2008). *One in 100: Behind bars in America 2008*. Washington, DC: The Pew Charitable Trust Public Safety Performance Project. Retrieved from www.pewcenteronthestates.org/uploadedFiles/8015PCTS_Prison08_FINAL_2-1-1_FORWEB.pdf

Wener, R.E., & Keys, C. (2006). The effects of changes in jail population densities on crowding, sick call, and spatial behavior. *Journal of Applied Social Psychology, 18*(10):852-866.

Williams, N.H. (2007). Prison health care and the health of the public: Ties that bind. Atlanta, GA: The National Center for Primary Care, Morehouse School of Medicine. Retrieved from www.communityvoices.org/Uploads/TiesThatBind_00108_00150.pdf

Wolf, N., Blitz, C.L., Shi, J., et al. (2006). Sexual violence inside prisons: Rates of victimization. *Journal of Urban Health: Bulletin of the New York Academy of Medicine*. Retrieved from www.google.com/search?q=Blitz%2C+Shi%2C+Bachman+%26+Siegel&rls=com.microsoft:en-us&ie=UTF-8&oe=UTF-8&startIndex=&startPage=1

World Health Organization, Department of Mental Health and Substance Abuse. (2007). *Preventing suicide in jails and prisons*. Geneva, Switzerland: World Health Organization.

Zimbardo, P. (2007). *The Lucifer effect: Understanding how good people turn evil*. New York: Random House.

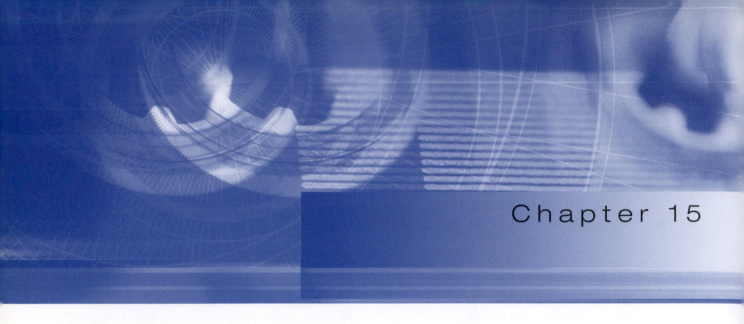

Chapter 15

The Forensic Nurse as a Legal Nurse Consultant

Nursine S. Jackson

"Small opportunities are often the beginning of great enterprises."
Demosthenes

Competencies

1. Describing professional roles and responsibilities of the legal nurse consultant (LNC).
2. Analyzing the elements of negligence (duty, breach of duty, proximate cause, and damages) in a professional malpractice case.
3. Evaluating the issues in selecting computer hardware and software to enhance performance.
4. Synthesizing the need and critical use of scientific literature as the evidence base in LNC practice.

Key Terms

Bates stamping
Breach of duty
Damages
Demonstrative evidence
Duty
Discovery
Focus groups
Legal nurse consultant
Medical chronology
Negligence
Proximate cause

INTRODUCTION

A **legal nurse consultant (LNC)** is a nurse who is knowledgeable in many aspects of law, nursing, and medicine, as well as the social influences controlling and affecting patient care, legal claims, and litigation. In the 1970s, LNCs slowly started finding their niches and defining their roles by trial and error in law offices handling *personal injury* cases. Personal injury is an area in civil law that includes medical negligence cases, injuries resulting from automobile accidents, and various other acts of negligence. Over time, the legal nurse consulting skills have been found to be applicable in many other practice settings.

Evaluating for medical errors has historically been the most common area of law for LNC involvement. The LNC is challenged to assist in determining what went wrong, to "discover" the dynamics that led to the clinical incident or misadventure: the shortcuts born of short staffing, the inadequately prepared nurse reassigned from another unit, the inaccessible physician, the misunderstood behaviors of patients that interfere with care. The LNC must then determine what injuries and damages flowed from the event. It is the role of the LNC to explore in detail the medical records and tease the facts from the printed pages, bring the details and facts to light, and then to make those facts accessible.

ROLES OF THE LNC

In addition to a law office setting, a nurse with the LNC skill set might be employed in an acute health-care setting, as a risk manager, in quality assurance, in health-care administration, or as a patient representative. The LNC may have a role in insurance companies and in worker's compensation, as a case manager and in claims analysis, monitoring for appropriateness of diagnostics and treatments rendered and appropriateness of billing. The LNC may be involved in the development of health-care policy in the government and private sector. LNCs are frequently employed by government agencies and state or federally funded health programs to screen for evidence of abuse and fraud in Medicare cases and other health and legal issues.

The LNC has a key role in education settings where children with disabilities (physical, psychological, and cognitive) and their families seek appropriate educational support. The knowledge base for educators, administrators, and attorneys is commonly insufficient to translate a student's complex needs into practical plans that permit the individual with special challenges to learn. The nurse's role in this setting is to help others understand the implications of each individual's disability and the legal responsibilities of all parties in providing appropriate services based on the client's need.

The LNC role evolved and became more widely recognized and used in the 1990s, leading to many nurses in more traditional roles seeing the LNC as an appealing alternate role. As this new professional career path arose, private educational facilities and university-based nursing programs responded to the increased demand to educate and certify LNCs, thus creating opportunities for LNC educators as the curriculum continues to evolve. Likewise, educational preparation and certifying qualifications of an LNC educator remain in development.

The role of the LNC as a researcher is the least established of the roles within this specialty. The LNC commonly uses skills and ability to identify, read, and interpret peer-reviewed research publications and literature to establish the elements (or lack thereof) in a legal case. There are countless issues that could greatly benefit from investigation by the LNC professional, including data collection for research purposes. Researchers need to explore ways of testing the feasibility and effectiveness of interventions related to LNC practice. Utilization of the scientific literature as evidence when researching forensic health care or medical legal issues is the critical base of the LNC practice.

The settings in which LNCs practice are varied. LNCs might work in traditional roles within a health-care institution, or may work ad lib from a home office, or in an office that is remote from their employer's facility. The LNC work may be full or part-time and is often done while maintaining an active clinical practice. Attorneys or other employers may hire LNCs to perform tasks that are beyond the scope of their in-office salaried staff and then craft a working relationship to complement the needs of both the employer and the LNC. The LNC with an entrepreneurial spirit finds flexibility in this role that is not found in the more traditional nursing positions.

PROFESSIONAL TASKS AND RESPONSIBILITIES

There is a common thread throughout LNCs' professional responsibilities. Regardless of the practice setting, the common thread is the careful and thorough organization and review of the client's health records. A thorough overview of common role responsibilities of the LNC professional is provided next.

Medical Records Organization

LNC tasks and responsibilities may come from many sources. A common example starts with a client walking into a plaintiff's attorney's office and telling a story of a catastrophic injury or death of a loved one, which was an unexpected outcome, often under suspicious circumstances. In turn, the attorney may call upon the LNC to interview the client and/or review medical records to try to identify whether medical errors caused this questionable outcome. A risk manager may be called in to investigate an untoward event that unfolded on the hospital unit resulting in an injury that may result in problems for the hospital. An insurance agency may assign a "claim" to an LNC and ask for an investigation to determine whether the negligent event and the injuries claimed should be covered under the terms of the insurance policy.

Attorneys, hospital risk managers, insurance claims agents, and others may hire an LNC for a project, but they do not know what to ask for. Commonly they will say, "Tell me what is in there and organize it, so I can find it." On occasion, employers will ask for a specific task, for example, to identify all of the injuries suffered as a result of an automobile accident or to determine whether the labor nurse's failure to appreciate an abnormal fetal heart tracing contributed to a delay in delivering the baby.

The physical project is presented to the LNC as hard copies of the medical records in a disorganized pile without any dividers. The stacks of records related to a medical case in question must be organized into recognizable formats of hospital or medical office medical charts to facilitate review. As the LNC initially reviews the documents provided, he or she maintains checklists to keep track of which records have been provided and which records need to be requested or retrieved from another provider. The records are organized, and medical record tabs and dividers are inserted. The medical records are then paginated, using a method known as Bates stamping. **Bates stamping** (also known as Bates numbering, Bates branding, or Bates coding) is the task of placing identifying numbers and/or date and time marks on images and documents as they are scanned or processed.

Organizing the charts and papers may be viewed as a pathway toward a legal outcome. The LNC may have to map out a pathway through all case materials to the outcome so that the legal team has access to the "facts" and may develop the knowledge needed to navigate effectively. The LNC creates a table of contents (Table 15.1) with lists of the health-care providers, dates of hospitalizations, procedures, office visits, and what happened at each visit. The tables of contents serve as a guide as the LNC reviews medical records and related documents.

TABLE 15.1

TABLE OF CONTENTS

Client: Jane Doe	SS# 123-32-4567
DOB/Age: 11/23/41 - 66 yo	Date of Incident: 12/25/95 - 12/29/95
Created 1/4/2008	

TABS	DOCUMENT	PAGES
I.	MEDICAL CHRONOLOGY	30
II.	CAST OF CHARACTERS	5
III.	LITERATURE REVIEW	
IV.	HOSPITAL POLICIES AND PROCEDURES	

V.	DEPOSITIONS
	A. Defendant Doctor
	  1. Deposition Preparation
	  2. Deposition Transcript
	  3. Summary of Transcript	

VI.	MEDICAL RECORDS
	A. St. Somewhere Hospital, Anywhere, USA
	  Hospitalization
	  Diagnosis: Intractable Back Pain
	  12/25/2006 through 12/29/2006
	  [add1 records requested - incl. nursing notes and graphics]
		69

	B. Autopsy
	  Anywhere County Pathologist, Joe Bow, MD
	  12/29/06
		12

Confidential Work Products - Law Offices of John Lawyer, PC

The final format of the organized records might be old-fashioned hard copies in three-ring binders. The records may also come as electronic PDF files (portable document files) that are bookmarked and have key issues highlighted and explanations inserted in text boxes or "sticky notes" on each key page of the medical record on the file.

Medical Chronologies and Timelines

Creating timelines or medical chronologies of events leading to an outcome is the most common responsibility assigned to and performed by an LNC. The LNC extracts the key facts from the medical records, depositions, itemized statements, and many other sources to form medical chronologies so that a reader can glean the highlights or facts of the case and then readily locate the primary source from which the information was extracted. The chronologies also can be presented in graphic forms, such as timelines, that outline and illustrate the sequence and relationships of the critical events.

The LNC will configure an individual format and style for the chronology with one of the many software options available. Software programs commonly used to develop medical chronologies include (but are not limited to) Microsoft Word, Corel WordPerfect, and Microsoft Excel. Sometimes the chronologies are in the form of Macintosh documents, as Macs become more common in law offices. Specialty software developed for the production of medical chronologies and timelines may further facilitate this aspect of the LNC's role. Table 15.1 is one example of a format for a **medical chronology,** in which the LNC entered data into CaseMap (a Lexis-Nexis product), then converted it into a four-column Word table with the following content:

1. Date and time
2. An excerpt of the health-care record with an identifying header using the name of document from which the excerpt was taken, as well as the facility name and the author of the health-care record
3. Page number cited
4. LNC comments and analysis.

There is no "correct" format for medical chronologies. Different formats may be used for different cases, and different formats may be used within one individual case. The detailed verbatim extraction of text from a medical record, as in Table 15.1, may be appropriate to illustrate the details of the target incident that resulted in the litigation. More general summaries of previous hospitalizations may be appropriate to more concisely illustrate the patient's baseline status prior to the incident that led to litigation (Table 15.2).

Furthermore, when the nursing or medical documentation of anatomy and physiology or pharmacology in the medical records needs further explanation for clarity, images and explanations can be embedded directly into the chronology (Table 15.3).

As the LNC performs case development, mechanisms that would most clearly illustrate medical issues should be considered throughout the process. If the case were to go to trial, the LNC would be instrumental in developing the trial exhibits. (See more about exhibits and demonstrative evidence later in this chapter.) For trial, the medical chronology can be converted into a timeline to illustrate a specific element of time. The CaseMap program by Lexis-Nexis CaseSoft is one example of many medical chronology software programs available that has a companion product. For instance, TimeMap, a companion to CaseMap, converts data into a timeline. The data entered can then be modified as needed to make the facts clear to readers.

There is no right or wrong way to develop a timeline for demonstrative evidence and to communicate to the legal team. In court, many juries and attorneys have expressed that color and a technically glitzy presentation

Case Study

Timeline or Lifeline?

In the following case exhibit, a 56-year-old man suffered multiple perforations of his coronary artery, as well as his common iliac artery, during an angioplasty. The following timeline illustrates events, signs, and symptoms intended to demonstrate the interventionist's delayed response to decedent's hypotension. Part of the timeline (not included here due to space constraints) went on to show that the interventionist persisted in performing two additional angioplasties, in spite of the persistent hypotension caused by exsanguination. The goal of the timeline was to depict the delayed appreciation of the bleeding in a setting of dramatic signs and symptoms of shock. The arterial perforations resulted in delayed diagnostics, followed by insufficient resuscitation efforts, causing this patient's death. The LNC's assignment was to communicate this complicated course as succinctly as possible in a timeline.

(case study continued on page 286)

Case Study

TIMELINE OR LIFELINE? (continued)

In the course of preparing for this same jury trial, several timelines (each undergoing countless revisions) were developed in an attempt to communicate the facts of this case. Another timeline, using a Microsoft Excel spreadsheet, showed the decedent's blood pressure and heart rates throughout the angioplasty. Excel software converts the numeric entry into a graphic depiction illustrating the deteriorating vital signs over time, as seen in Figure 15.1.

WAYNE HEAD
Blood Pressure during Cath Surgery
10/31/2002
Source: Conscious Sedation Printout (Exhibit #10)
Arterial BP's: Procedure Log

Date	Time	Systolic	Diastolic	Arterial (systolic)	Arterial (dyalstolic)	Heart rate	Comments
10/31.02	1:04:40 PM	172	107			59	
	1:09:00 PM	173	114			70	
	1:14:01 PM	175	105			74	
	1:17:00 PM	157	110			77	
	1:28:01 PM	133	88			65	
	1:33:01 PM	143	94			66	
	1:38:00 PM	153	105			44	
	1:43:01 PM	179	106			70	
	1:48:01 PM	148	102			95	
	1:53:01 PM	178	120			79	
	1:57:04 PM	160	112			118	
	1:59:43 PM	156	107			85	
	2:09:01 PM	114	70			77	
	2:14:01 PM	108	76			80	
	2:19:01 PM	112	81			109	
	2:22:52 PM	75	43			74	
	2:25:13 PM	74	45			76	
	2:27:42 PM	84	53			77	
	2:31:45 PM	92	46			72	
	2:36:00 PM	93	52			75	
	2:40:15 PM	77	43			76	
	2:41:25 PM	75	44			76	
	2:43:57 PM	79	51			86	
	2:44:41 PM	84	56			87	
	2:45:29 PM	85	59			87	
	2:46:01 PM	87	61			65	
	2:46:38 PM	91	65			86	
	2:47:23 PM	82	57			141	
	2:48:23 PM	84	40			69	
	2:49:30 PM	62	39			87	
	2:51:45 PM	82	47			111	
	2:52:31 PM	79	50			52	
	2:53:17 PM	74	50			87	
	2:53:59 PM	81	44			86	
	2:55:00 PM	67	41			84	
	2:56:05 PM	65	34			83	
	2:57:08 PM	70	42			84	
	2:58:45 PM	81	53			83	
	3:04:42 PM			62	39		
	3:05:22 PM			68	45		
	3:05:27 PM			70	44		
	3:06:26 PM			71	45		
	3:07:18 PM			92	49		
	3:07:49 PM			93	51		
	3:09:58 PM			74	45		
	3:12:02 PM			86	48		
	3:13:42 PM			77	43		
	3:16:38 PM			68	38		
	3:19:02 PM			78	45		
	3:19:27 PM			76	42		
	3:20:49 PM			78	43		

■ **FIGURE 15.1** Excel timeline.

TABLE 15.2   **Detailed Medical Chronology With Verbatim Excerpts From Medical Records**

Date/Time	Document	Cite	LNC Comments/Analysis
3/20/07 02:10	**City Hospital Emergency Department, Nurses Notes, Nancy Nurse, RN** "Knife-like pain over sternum today—intermittent in nature/steady since 10:30 p.m. Emesis × 2. Patient states pain radiates from chest down to stomach. Color pale—skin warm and dry." Implement chest pain protocol.	A3	Though this pain is not "classic" cardiac pain, it was very good nursing judgment to implement the chest pain protocol because of decedent's age and risk factors. Unfortunately, only the first set of laboratory results and baseline EKG were obtained, and serial studies were not drawn. This omission probably resulted in missing the diagnosis of his serious myocardial infarction.

TABLE 15.3   **Medical Chronology With Narrative Summary Providing Overview of a Medical Record**

Date/Time	Document	Cite	LNC Comments/Analysis
3/17/80 through 4/24/07	**JB, MD, Family Physician, 123 Hospital Way, Pittsburgh, PA** The medical records provided by this family physician demonstrate that he served as Mr. B's primary care physician for 27 years. These office records document regular exercise, healthful living, and good health maintenance, until weight gain following a back injury lead to his development of diabetes. His diabetes was documented as being well-controlled with oral medications. He had no other noteworthy past medical history, operations, or hospitalizations. He was married with three healthy adult children and employed as a fireman until his retirement 2 years prior to the events leading to litigation. These records reflect that he remained active in his retirement, doing physical labor, helping his son build a garage, and doing bookkeeping for his son's business.	B	Even though this decedent was retired, significant damages flowed from his death from negligent care. There is no evidence in this record of culpable conduct, that is, he had good health practices and did not smoke or engage in practices that a jury would perceive as self-abuse that may have contributed to his bad outcome. Even after his retirement, he continued to make valuable contributions to his community and his offspring, and he left a dependent wife behind; therefore damages flowing from his death are significant.

TABLE 15.4   **Medical Chronology With Medical Illustrations and LNC Commentary**

Wed 01/25/2006 3:30 p.m. ET	**ED Nurse Progress Note, KM, RN**	**Hospital #2, Pg 31**
	X-ray shows right tibial plateau fracture. C/O pain 9 out of 10. Pain meds given. Pt states meds work for short x. **R. pedal pulse now not palpable.** Able to Doppler the AT [anterior tibial pulse] and PT [posterior tibial], but neither is palpable. Continues to feel light touch, wiggle his toes and dorsiflex his foot. **Toes purple and cool to touch. Vascular surgeon paged.**	

LNC Comments

What this nurse is describing is the loss of circulation to the foot as a result of his developing compartment syndrome. Compartment syndrome may be seen in patients that sustain the type of trauma that results in tibial plateau fractures. Muscle fascia creates a closed space, a compartment, that contains the muscles, blood vessels and nerves. When trauma causes the muscles to swell within the enclosed space, the pressure in the compartment builds and compresses the nerves and blood vessels. If the pressure is not relieved within 4 to 6 hours, permanent injury can occur.

The symptoms described at 3:30 p.m. suggest that the swelling within the compartment had become so serious that the arterial flow to the foot was compromised. At this point, the nerves were still viable, as reflected by the nurse's observation that he can still move his foot, wiggle his toes, and has sensation, but time was critical to relieve the compartment syndrome and to restore blood flow to the lower leg.

of the facts using trial software kept their attention and enhanced their comprehension of the issues. Others have responded that simplicity is best.

The "best" presentation of facts will be determined by the skills of the presenter and the needs of the audience. Familiarity with the attorney, mediator, and judge and/or jurors in the venue of a case is the best guide for the LNC to develop exhibits that are appreciated. **Focus groups,** such as mock trials or e-trials, allow the attorney to pre-try a case and get feedback from a jury composed of people from the venue in which the case is to be tried. This method is an invaluable means to get feedback to help craft the best demonstrative aids. The LNC can participate in mock trials, just as in the pretrial support and in the actual trial.

CASE ANALYSIS

Law offices may seek the services of an LNC to provide a medical-legal summary or case analysis to help determine whether the facts of each case support the legal elements required for a viable case. The LNC performs a case analysis to flesh out the elements of a case based on the following elements or principles.

- Duty
- Breach of duty
- Causal connection (proximate cause)
- Damages

To proceed with a meritorious negligence lawsuit, all of the legal elements must be present. Only a very small percentage of potential clients bringing complaints to a plaintiff's attorney will actually have the facts that fulfill the requisite legal elements that would allow a negligence case to go forward. It is often the role of the LNC in a plaintiff's law practice to first interview the client and determine whether additional investigation is warranted and then to obtain and review the key medical records

to help determine whether the case investigation should proceed. The LNC does not determine case "merit." Only an expert witnesses can establish whether the elements of the case are present, that is, whether a case is meritorious. In contrast, the LNC will initially determine whether the case is likely to have the elements required for a legal case to proceed. The LNC identifies other issues that impact on the quality of the case. Commonly, the case analysis determines the likelihood of subsequent case development.

The following definitions are the elements of a negligence case. There is also a brief explanation of associated LNC activities to evaluate the presence or absence of each element.

Duty is a requirement that a person act toward others and the public with such watchfulness, attention, caution, and prudence as a reasonable person in the same circumstances would act. The LNC may participate in finding evidence to establish the level of accountability to which defendants could and should be held. LNC responsibilities may include finding information about physician's membership in professional associations, insurance companies, institutional or individual medical professional's Web sites, or advertisements that may help define the defendant's duty to the patient. The LNC's research may include searching for resources that provide the training and certifications each putative defendant has or should have. This information is important because physicians with different levels of training and certifications are held to differing levels of accountability; for example, a specialist is held to a higher level of accountability than someone with general training.

The LNC may also search for information about defendant institutions, associations, and other providers. A hospital advertising itself as specializing in treating strokes will be held accountable, both legally and by a jury, to properly treat a patient presenting with a stroke. The HMO advertising that it provides comprehensive care with top specialists on staff would be expected to perform appropriate diagnostics and provide timely consultations

Case Study

WRONGLY PLACED THERMOTHERAPY

Mr. M, suffering from benign prostatic hypertrophy, went to a urologist seeking an intervention to relieve his bothersome symptoms. This surgeon was performing post-market research of a new technology called water-induced thermotherapy and recommended this intervention to Mr. M. Something went terribly wrong, and the catheter heater that was supposed to shrink his prostate instead burned his bulbar urethra distal to the prostatic

urethra where it was supposed to be placed on the prostatic tissue. The case went to trial, and the jury was clearly captivated when the plaintiff's current treating urologic surgeon did a freehand drawing as he explained Mr. M's injuries from the negligent placement of this device. He drew images of the stricture that recurred every 6 to 12 months, and he provided cystoscopic images of the same segment of the urethra that had been burned.

with the specialists, so when HMO members' health problems demonstrate a need for diagnostics and specialists, their care should not be limited to that provided by the primary care provider.

Breach of duty is failure to exercise the care toward others that a reasonable or prudent person would exercise in the same circumstances or take an action that such a reasonable person would not take.

Negligence is the term commonly used to describe that a breach in duty occurred and that there was a failure to live up to the "standard of care."

A physician, nurse, or other health professional is expected to exercise the degree of skill, learning, and care possessed by physicians, nurses, and other professionals in circumstances similar to the professional whose conduct is in question, giving due regard to the advanced state of the profession at the time of the treatment. In some states a professional expert can only serve as an expert against a like-trained professional and must be actively working in or have recent experience in a similar clinical setting.

The LNC's responsibility in case analysis is to use available resources to determine the standard of care for all providers and assist in determining whether negligent care was rendered by any of the health-care providers. If the LNC is working for the plaintiff, his or her case analysis may determine whether the case is developed further. If the LNC is working for the defense, his or her analysis may determine how the case is developed, which experts should be engaged to address each issue or claim of negligence, and whether the case should be aggressively defended or settled.

Resources that the LNC may use to describe the standard of care in a given community for a specific medical issue might include the following:

- Guidelines, publications, and Web sites of medical and nursing professional associations
- Chapters in well-respected texts
- Scientific research published in peer-reviewed journals
- Lecture material and/or consultations with experts in the community
- Requirements defined by third-party payers, departments of health, the Joint Commission, and other credentialing bodies.

Learning to identify high-quality research and articles is within the scope of practice for the LNC. The LNC should pursue course work such as statistics and other classes designed specifically to assist the LNC in dissection and analysis of research.

An LNC should not overlook the value of networking with other LNCs and physicians in person, at meetings and lectures, or on legal nurse consultant and legal

medicine Web sites. Other professionals involved in legal consulting provide a rich source of information to enhance case development.

The scientific medical evidence is the base for best practices of care and influences the minimum standards for practice. The LNC incorporates all levels of evidence as resources; no single resource establishes standards. For example, the American Cancer Society publishes guidelines for breast cancer surveillance (Box 15.1), but the actual plan of care that is appropriate for each individual is based on the individual's risk factors, clinical presentation, and to a large degree, what is available in the community in which the patient is being treated.

The LNC should be familiar with the standard of care used at the time of the incident being litigated. As an example, guidelines for breast screening with MRI as an adjunct to mammography are evolving. Several studies have demonstrated the ability of MRI screening to detect cancer with early-stage tumors that are associated with

---

Box 15.1   Guideline Example: American Cancer Society Guidelines for the Early Detection of Cancer

The American Cancer Society recommends these screening guidelines for most adults.

Breast Cancer

- Yearly mammograms are recommended starting at age 40 and continuing for as long as a woman is in good health.
- Clinical breast exam (CBE) is recommended about every 3 years for women in their 20s and 30s and every year for women 40 and over.
- Women should know how their breasts normally look and feel and report any breast change promptly to their health-care provider. Breast self-exam (BSE) is an option for women starting in their 20s.

The American Cancer Society recommends that some women, because of their family history, a genetic tendency, or certain other factors—be screened with MRIs in addition to mammograms. (The number of women who fall into this category is small: less than 2% of all the women in the United States.) Talk with your doctor about your history and whether you should have additional tests at an earlier age. For more information, see *Breast Cancer: Early Detection*, available from the American Cancer Society at http://www.cancer.org/Cancer/BreastCancer/MoreInformation/BreastCancerEarlyDetection/index

(From: The American Cancer Society.)

better outcomes, but this evidence has not yet resulted in changes in the standard of care for breast screening. Until the evidence becomes accepted and results in assimilating the intervention into practice, one might see guidelines being implemented differently in different settings. An MRI of the breast might be readily implemented to evaluate a suspicious mass in a medical center, whereas a rural community facility's standard practice may be to provide compression views and ultrasound and rarely offer the option of MRI. While most states' statutes apply national standards to all similarly trained medical professionals, consideration must be given to the practices and facilities available in a community when evaluating its standard of care. Several states still have "locality rules," so that the physicians and nurses in these states are held to the standards practiced in those communities and not to national standards.

The legal definition of *injury* is any harm done to a person by the acts or omissions of another. Injury may include physical hurt as well as damage to reputation or dignity, loss of a legal right, or breach of contract. If the party causing the injury was either willful (intentionally causing harm) or negligent, then he or she is responsible (liable) for payment of damages for the harm caused.

Sometimes injuries may be easily documented through radiology images, photos, or videos. Injuries might be also demonstrated through some of the following methods:

- Diagnostic studies
- Medical records
- Photos or videos
- Client testimony
- Employer's, friend's, family's testimony
- Medical bills

- Medical illustrations or demonstrative evidence
- Scientific research that supports the LNC's findings and addresses best practice guidelines for diagnosis and treatment

Other times, however, such injuries as psychological scarring, pain, and mild brain injuries are more challenging to illustrate. The LNC may have the responsibility for identifying the best manner in which to illustrate injuries that are not apparent.

The next case study is an example of incorporating images in a medical summary to orient the reader to the anatomy that has been injured.

Proximate cause is an act that results in an event, particularly an injury due to negligence or an intentional wrongful act. To prevail (win) in a lawsuit for damages due to negligence or some other wrong, it is essential to claim (plead) proximate cause in the complaint and to prove in trial that the negligent act of the defendant was the proximate cause (and not the approximate cause) of the injury to the plaintiff (person filing the lawsuit). Some states recognize that an event may have more than one proximate cause; thus, the plaintiff need not prove it was "the" proximate cause. Rather, the plaintiff must prove that it was "a" proximate, direct, or legal cause, that is, a "substantial" injury-producing cause, not the "sole" producing cause.

Proximate causation is frequently difficult to establish because often there is a comorbidity or intervening cause that comes between the original negligence of the defendant and the injured plaintiff, which may confound causation. If the intervening cause either reduces the amount of responsibility, or if this intervening cause is the substantial reason for the injury, then the defendant will not be liable at all.

Case Study

INCORPORATING MULTIPLE TRAUMA

M.K., 42 years old, was critically injured in the rollover crash of a SUV in the early morning of January 24, 2007. She was an unrestrained rear-seat passenger, who was reportedly ejected 20 feet from the vehicle that rolled over multiple times.

By the time the medics transported her to **Medical Center** at 7:45 a.m., her mental status changed and she had become combative and was screaming. A quick survey revealed that she had suffered **multiple trauma** to her **head, face, back, abdomen, chest, right hand, and left lower leg.** She had bloody drainage from her right ear, and she was diaphoretic,

a sign of shock. She did not follow commands, even when a French interpreter came to assist in communicating and giving commands in her native tongue.

On the initial evaluation her pupils were equal, although her gaze was off to the right; within 30 minutes, her pupils became unequal (L: 2 mm reacting briskly; R: 4 mm reacting very sluggishly).

Following his initial survey examination, the emergency physician sent her for a battery of radiological studies, which revealed multiple fractures, including burst fractures of her thoracic spine.

Case Study

SEVERE HYPOXIC ENCEPHALOPATHY

The decedent, Mrs. J., was an 80-pound elderly women with liver disease, who became confused following a hip replacement. Caregivers did not assess for hypoxia or other possible causes for her mental status changes, but based on a remote history of alcohol abuse, they treated Ms. J. for delirium tremens at the same time they treated her postoperative pain. Her physicians and nurses administered multiple agents with respiratory depressant effects over a short period of time, after which Mrs. J. suffered a respiratory arrest.

There was no other etiology for her respiratory arrest identified, nonetheless the plaintiff had the burden of proving that the negligent administration of multiple sedating medications in a very small patient with poor liver function caused her respiratory arrest, which in turn caused a severe hypoxic encephalopathy and her subsequent death.

Damages are monetary compensations awarded by a court in a civil action to an individual who has been injured through the wrongful conduct of another party. Damages attempt to measure in financial terms the extent of harm a plaintiff has suffered because of the defendant's actions. Both the defense team and plaintiff's team perform analyses to determine objective evidence of the case's worth. They may compile spreadsheets specifying medical costs and all other damages that flowed from the injuries from the time of the event and into the future to which monetary values can be assigned. An LNC familiar with the case is in the best position to analyze itemized statements from institutions that treated the victim to determine which charges were related to care for injuries flowing from negligent acts. The LNC reviews itemized statements from provider institutions and/or from third-party payers such as Medicare and then separates the related costs from costs for care provided for comorbidities unrelated to the litigation.

All LNC work products should be designed to allow a direct cut-and-paste into future documents. Accordingly, spreadsheets summarizing medical costs incurred as a consequence of the purportedly negligent act should include information that will be needed later in the litigation process. For example, interrogatories provided to the plaintiff by each defendant will request the names and contact information of all of the providers of services (physicians, hospitals, ambulance companies, medical equipment suppliers, home health nurses, and others); dates of service; descriptions of services provided; and charges for services. Anticipating this discovery demand, the spreadsheet listing past medical costs should include this information.

Once the plaintiff is awarded a settlement or wins a jury verdict, a third party, such as Medicare or Medicaid, may demand repayment for related medical care for which they have paid. In other words, they will exert a lien against any recovery, which must be repaid. Anticipating lien issues, the spreadsheet may also include a breakdown of payments made by third-party payers (health insurance companies, Medicare, Medicaid).

Ultimately, this cost analysis is used to value the case, that is, to help determine a dollar value for settlement negotiations, and to anticipate liens that reimburse recovery costs. For example, if there is a $1,000,000 lien as a result of payments for medical care from Medicare, settling a case for $1,000,000 will not assist the injured person to recover or restore quality of life.

Tools commonly used by LNCs to develop spreadsheets representing costs include tables on word-processing programs or financial software that allows the development of spreadsheets. Figure 15.2 used Microsoft Excel.

Future Damages

A life care planner is an expert who may be brought in as a "damages expert," that is, the expert witness who will outline the costs that the injured person may face in the future as a result of the injury caused by negligence. A life care planner may be an LNC or may have other training and experience, such as in vocational rehabilitation. This expert will compile a list of projected costs for future diagnostics, medical and nursing care, appliances, home modifications, special services required, and all costs that flow from injuries resulting from negligence for the remainder of the injured person's life.

Damages may be objective figures. For example, a 42-year-old husband and father who is disabled, preventing him from engaging in his professional career, may have damages that include 23 years of work loss. In contrast, a retired person who has been rendered quadriplegic may only have damages related to pain and suffering. A child or retired person without dependents, who died as a

Dates of service	Provider Name & Address/ Description treatments rendered	Charges for service	#1 Rental car insurance	#1 Payor: Amount paid	#2: Medicaid	#2: Payor: Amount paid	#3 Outstanding balance owed
11/24–12/3/02	Private Diagnostic Clinic Extensive X-rays of body; Treat ankle, lip wound; ankle cast	4,840.00	Alamo, Any Town, USA 12345	848.92			3,991.08
11/24/02	GHP. MD Diagnostic X-ray	371.00	Alamo, Any Town, USA 12345	355.32	Medicaid NY	132.48	15.68
11/24/02	County EMS: P.O. Box 1181 Any Town, USA 12345 Amb Srv., ER Trans	330.00	Alamo, Any Town, USA 12345	164.70			165.30

■ **FIGURE 15.2** Past medical costs spreadsheet.

result of medical error, may have only burial costs and, as defined by many state's statutes, have no other objective value.

Many individuals who have been disabled or killed as a result of negligence may have no work loss, no out-of-pocket payments for medical care, and no other easily measurable costs. The LNC has the challenge of identifying and illustrating the less tangible damages, the pain and suffering of the injured, and losses of the negligence victim's dependent survivors. One means of demonstrating the difficulties and suffering caused by the injuries can be day-in-the-life videos. For example, videos of débridement of a victim injured as a result of a flawed product exploding, a demonstration of emptying a colostomy for a patient who suffered a delayed appreciation of a bowel obstruction, and a film of the modifications made to an existing home and the activities of daily living for a person who was rendered quadriplegic may convey the seriousness of the pain and suffering resulting from negligence.

Another example of the varied and creative means used by the LNC to illustrate damages includes presentation of a person's preinjury activity and behavior through use of school and gym records or by using previous employers to testify to preinjury activities and abilities. Various means of illustrating a victim's preinjury status can be used and then contrasted against post-event limitations. A plaintiff who sustained a "mild" brain injury may look normal to a jury, even though he has lost his executive functions, his ability to multitask, his frontal inhibitions, his social controls, etc. An employer who had to dismiss the plaintiff from his job after the event, when the plaintiff had previously been a productive and valued employee, could be an excellent witness. The employer can describe the effects of the frontal brain injury that precluded the plaintiff from returning to his preinjury employment role. Family members may attest to the injured party's inability to maintain relationships, his quick anger, his bad judgments, his inability to follow through to complete tasks as

he had in the past, even though he "looks just fine." The LNC, more than anyone on the legal team, is likely to have the insight to assist with the development of these aspects of the case.

The LNC can present the scientific evidence from the literature following a demonstration of the damages to support the plaintiff's position. An appraisal of the literature on intervention studies that compares treatments with study populations that have similar diagnoses may support the position that such limitations exist, last a lifetime, and are costly to the injured and to their families. Furthermore, presenting a summary of publications that list verdicts and settlements in similar cases and/or in the same venue provides additional means of supporting the damages. Recommendations for determining the value cannot be taken out of context, but rather are viewed with literature on other cases with similar circumstances to improve outcomes.

LNC Work Product

After the LNC extracts the facts of the case, the next challenge is to develop a working theory of what actually happened that may have led to the negative outcome. The LNC must identify and interpret gold standard literature, guidelines, policies and procedures, and other relevant resources to illustrate the standard of care that applied to the medical issues in each instance. Presenting the expected minimal standard of care in a given situation with a specific diagnosis is the foundation for explaining negligent care or deviations from standard of care.

Evidence-based practice is based on the specific question, such as "What treatment is typically provided to individuals with the diagnosis X?" The literature on diagnosis X is retrieved and critically appraised and summarized. When the injured person with diagnosis X appears to have received very divergent treatment, then the care may not have met the standard. The LNC must access the current scientific research *at the time of the event* to determine if the science at that time supports the claim being made.

Viewed from another perspective, an insurance company may argue that further damages do not need to be paid to the injured person and that the financial cost is not consistent with their guidelines. The LNC may be called upon to illustrate the case on behalf of the injured or on behalf of the insurance agency. Scientific literature may be used to support or refute (depending on the side making the argument) whether similar persons in a variety of studies with diagnosis X have gained full recovery in the given time frame, whether additional therapeutic interventions are warranted, and/or whether family financial support is appropriate to fulfill the contractual commitment of the insurer.

The LNC may work with an expert witness to assist in the analysis of the facts of the case. In yet another role, the LNC may testify in court as a fact witness to explain health-care issues in support of the theory of the developed case. The LNC may need to assist the expert in accessing and illustrating the scientific evidence to establish what the standard of care was and explain the deviations from the standard of care that caused the injuries and resultant damages caused by the injury.

The analysis provided by a skilled LNC extends far beyond the assessment of the elements of the case. The analysis includes identifying the case's strengths and weaknesses, which may depend on the human elements and social and political circumstances at the time, in addition to how the facts affect the legal elements of the case. The LNC considers the credibility of the plaintiff and how a jury in the venue in which the case will be tried might perceive him or her or specific issues of the case. Also, the LNC should be attuned to related issues from the news media that could sway public opinion and affect the objectivity of potential jurors. For example, a jury may not believe that the brain damage suffered by a baby born to an uneducated, unemployed, single mother with a history of drug abuse was caused by a mismanaged labor and delivery, no matter how compelling the facts.

The trial team may bring in a professional jury and trial adviser (which is another role for an LNC, although many other professionals also perform this role) to help prepare for trial and jury selection. Trial preparation may include holding a mock trial or focus group to get feedback from mock jurors on the best way to present the case to a jury of their peers. An LNC may orchestrate the mock trial or serve as a support person, as in a real trial.

The LNC has the burden, duty, and challenge to visualize all pathways and viewpoints of the entire map of the case. More importantly, the LNC must strategize a plan to deal with the human elements that more often make or break a case.

In practice, a case typically presents in the form of an uninspiring 12-inch stack of $8 \times 11\frac{1}{2}$ inch paper, black print on white pages. The story buried within must be uncovered and revealed by the LNC. Questions arise: Why did that nurse chart that at 2 a.m. a 52-year-old male patient was complaining of "10 out of 10 tearing chest pain, radiating to his back," yet did not report this noteworthy event to the physician or her supervisor? What was the reason that the nurse removed the call bell from the wall of a new immigrant woman from Africa, who was screaming with pain during labor—pain that was later discovered to be due to a uterine rupture?

Case Study

ABSENCE OF DAMAGES IN A NEGLIGENCE CASE

A registered nurse presented to a law office due to her concerns that a serious medical error occurred in the care of her mother when she was hospitalized following a motor vehicle accident. During the hospitalization for multiple physical injuries, her mother, Mrs. S., had a central intravenous (IV) line, drainage tubes, and a gastric feeding tube. During Mrs. S.'s bath, when she was turned by one of the nonprofessional nursing staff, several of the tubes and IV lines became disconnected. This staff person hurriedly reconnected several leaking lines just as Mrs. S.'s daughter entered the room to visit her mother. Mrs. S.'s daughter immediately saw that the gastric feeding solution had been misconnected to the central IV line, and promptly turned off the infusion tube feeding before it entered Mrs. S.'s body.

Because the misconnected lines were contaminated, Mrs. S.'s physician removed the lines and ordered the reinsertion of a new central IV line, which is a surgical procedure. Mrs. S. was elderly and frail and had to endure several attempts before a successful replacement of the central IV line was accomplished.

The Analysis of the Legal Elements

1. Was there negligence?

Yes. The nonprofessional nursing staff person was not trained to connect IV lines and should never have

(case study continued on page 294)

Case Study

ABSENCE OF DAMAGES IN A NEGLIGENCE CASE (continued)

reconnected them. Perhaps she should not even have been moving the critically ill patient with so many lines without having the assistance of a registered nurse. Additionally, the products used provided a foreseeable problem. The use of connection devices for the central IV line and gastric feeding tubes that have the same size and type of connectors created a dangerous situation that set the patient and nursing staff person up for a potentially disastrous occurrence.

2. Was there an injury?

Yes. Mrs. S. experienced suffering with the multiple attempts to successfully replace the central IV line, and there were financial consequences to having to have a new central line placed. However, the entry of tube feeding into Mrs. S. was interrupted by Mrs. S.'s daughter before the infusion entered her veins, and no infection or embolus resulted from misconnection of the lines. The potentially life-threatening consequences were averted. Although Mrs. S., an elderly, frail woman with poor venous access, was placed at risk for infection, dehydration, vascular injury, air emboli, pneumothorax, etc., none of the potential risks came to fruition.

3. Did the negligence cause the injury; that is, was there a proximate cause?

Yes. The negligent misconnection of the lines resulted in the removal of the central IV line and reinsertion, at the risk and suffering of Mrs. S.

4. Were there damages?

Yes. The cost of replacing the central IV line included the cost of the supplies and the cost of skilled medical staff to place the line in a surgical procedure. Mrs. S. experienced pain, fear, and apprehension during the replacement of the central IV line. Mrs. S. was placed at risk for many potential problems, but none were realized.

5. Is this a case?

This case is not economically feasible to develop. While there was clear negligence, that is, plugging a gastric feeding into a central IV line, no significant damages flowed from this negligence. If the tube feeding had entered Mrs. S.'s vein, it likely would have caused a catastrophic outcome, but it did not. The injuries that resulted were suffering, relatively minor costs, and the inconvenience of having a new line placed.

Despite the negligent act, there are insufficient damages to justify the expense, the tens of thousands of dollars, that will be required for the case development.

Conclusion

This case clearly shows negligence but has insufficient damages to justify the cost of developing a medical negligence suit.

DEVELOPING THE CASE

Assisting in Developing Legal Documents

Legal writing should be concise and clear, using short words, short sentences, short paragraphs, and be devoid of statements of personal belief. Nurses need to write objectively in short declarative sentences. This practice may be the greatest challenge the LNC encounters when transitioning from the bedside to the legal nursing role. Good medical documentation may incorporate the use of a shorthand that does not translate well into the legal arena. The LNC must develop work products in a format that allows relevant data to be transferred directly into legal documents. The LNC should be responsible for putting the finishing touches on all legal documents created. Additionally, the LNC may perform the final editing of the

legal documents developed by the attorneys and paralegals. This is done to ensure that language excerpts from the medical records and work products and images contained in final drafts of legal documents accurately reflect the medical facts, expert testimony, and legal theories of each case. The legal writing skills of the LNC are a critical and vital asset to the legal team.

Legal documents such as affidavits of merit, complaints, interrogatories, bills of particulars, requests for production of documents, motion papers or briefs, expert witness reports, and pretrial statements may have different names in different venues, but all will benefit from a skilled LNC's involvement.

The LNC may translate the medical and technical language into legal language, comprehensible to the attorneys, adjusters, judge, and jury. The LNC tends to be most familiar with the case, so he or she is often the best person team member to define the "elements" of the case after the facts are sorted out and analyzed.

Each state has a unique format for presenting the medical history of events, issues of negligence, injuries, and damages. The LNC involved in generating even the most basic case analysis should be familiar with the legal documents required so that the work products produced can be easily assimilated into legal documents.

Collaborating With Expert Witnesses in the Case

The LNC may often participate in locating and working with experts who are engaged to help analyze and support the legal cases through expert reports and testimony. LNCs may have a lucrative expert business in which their sole services are to identify the appropriate expert to develop and support a case, to put the attorney in touch with individuals with the necessary expert qualifications, and to serve as an interface to make certain that the experts make themselves available to the attorneys or facilities in need of support.

Once an expert is brought into the case, as part of the legal team the LNC serves as the interface between the law office or facility and the expert who has been hired. The LNC may also be responsible for performing background checks on experts engaged by the LNC's office and those engaged by their adversaries. The work involves reviewing experts' publications, the sources illustrating their opinions, and even their lectures or lecture materials. The LNC may collect and review deposition and court transcripts generated by each expert.

Communicating

Maintaining a clear and consistent line of communication is vital, whether the LNC acts as the coordinator of the case development or has a peripheral role. The LNC needs to consider communication options that will most effectively and efficiently keep work on track and remain in line with the needs and expectations for the legal team. Communications in legal work are frequently discoverable or able to be obtained by the opposing side, thus care should be taken when creating written documents, including e-mails.

The LNC must be sensitive to documentation of communications and have knowledge of communications that are not allowed. A member of the plaintiff's team cannot call a defendant asking for more medical records once the case is in suit. The LNC must be sensitive to specific issues associated with the communication form chosen. Quickly composed e-mails that can be sent with the touch of a button can be seen as insulting. Poorly edited communications may reflect unprofessionalism rather than the sharp professional image an LNC would prefer to convey.

Forming a "Cast of Characters"

During the process of reviewing the medical records and related documents, the LNC may identify and compile a list of key people and witnesses in the case. This information can come from intake interviews, medical records, depositions, itemized statements, and the stacks of notes and papers provided by the plaintiffs or defendants. The list might include the lay people and professionals (e.g., family members, employers, and friends, family physician) who were part of their client's pre-event life and could attest to his or her baseline activity status. Other people who should be listed are defendants, laypersons, and professionals who witnessed the target events. To illustrate damages flowing from the injury, home health nurses, therapists, and others who are most knowledgeable about the effects of the inflicted injuries and damages should be noted.

Identifying persons who witnessed events and obtaining their contact information in a timely fashion is important because over the years that case development takes, it inevitably becomes more difficult to identify and find target witnesses. As the case development progresses, expert witnesses for both the plaintiff and defense and additional professionals and lay damages witnesses will be added to the list.

The information provided in the cast of characters can be as simple as providing only their names and roles in the case. This work product can become increasingly complex as needed and can be expanded to list all kinds of useful information, for example, credentials and certifications of key professional witnesses and defendants, the page numbers of the medical records and documents that relate to each witness, contact information for witnesses, and more, as case needs dictate. Figure 15.3 is an actual work product showing (as requested by the attorney) who the plaintiff's attorney should consider naming as defendants and who might be good witnesses to depose.

Performing Literature Reviews

The LNC often reviews the literature that supports and/or refutes the medical and legal theories of a case. The legal team depends on medical records, testimony of witnesses, and other documents to better understand the events that led to the litigation, and they can only theorize as to what actually happened. The LNC may need to find literature to help accurately describe a medical pathway from the causal event to the negative outcome. The literature may

CAST OF CHARACTERS

Decedent: R.C.	DOB - Age: 11/3/57 - 49yo
Dates of Events: 5/21/07 & 6/11/07 to 6/12/07	SS# 123-45-2862

Created: December 7, 2007

Name	Role in Case	Defendant	Depose?
Regional Medical Centers	Facility that employed negligent radiologist and nurses, where the diagnosis of decedent's aorta-enteric fistula was negligently delayed *(Health Grades list them as providing substandard care as per Medicare and Medicaid services in 2003-2005 in their ability to diagnose and treat in time.)*	Y	
J.T., RN	Nurse on Med Surg floor on the morning shift, caring for him through to his arrest		Y
W.C., MD	Radiologist who interpreted CT of abdomen and pelvis ~ 11 pm on 6/11/07 *(not certified and not listed on hospital website - probably not an employee)*	Y	
E.T.G., MD/City Surgical Group	General Surgeon from whom he sought first opinion on treatment of his aneurysms		
F.T.Y., MD	Attending MD/surgeon for his terminal admission	Y	
H.S., RN	ED Nurse on admission in 6/11/07		?
M.M., MD	Radiologist consulted for second opinion/over-read of CT abdomen in the morning of 6/12/07 (time of consult is in dispute)	Y	
M.M., RN	Nurse who did ED assessment in the early morning of 6/12 - documenting pain as 0, unlikely		
M.C.P., MD/Vascular and Vein Specialist	Vascular surgeon who performed the aorta-bi-iliac bypass graft	?	
P.P.T., MD	Vascular surgeon who was consulted too late to intervene on 6/12/07 Bio provided on hospital website: 　Medical School: University of _ College of Medicine 　Residency: _ Medical School - General Surgery 　Fellowship: University of _ Medical Branch Hospitals 　- Thoracic Surgery 　Board Certifications: General Surgery & Thoracic 　Surgery 　Specialty: Cardiac Surgery 　Heart and Vascular Center 　137 _ Drive, 　Anytown, USA 12345		Y
R.J.P., MD	Emergency Physician on admission in 6/11/07	?	
J.S.R., MD	Performed Autopsy, County Office of the Coroner		

Confidential Work Product - Law Offices of John Lawyer, PC

■ **FIGURE 15.3** Cast of characters.

corroborate or refute the truth of a witness's testimony and credibility as to the accounting of events. An LNC needs to become skilled at Internet and library searches for supporting informational resources and scientific literature. After compiling the relevant literature, the LNC is also responsible for developing a mechanism to educate the attorney and the legal team and to help them translate complex medical information into a form that a jury, judge, or insurance adjuster can understand.

If LNCs do not have electronic access to a medical library through their employers, alumni or professional associations, or other resources, then access through a subscription service is needed. Fast access is available to the most current medical guidelines, full-text articles, textbooks, and searches of the gold standard literature through such services as MDConsult.com and UpToDate.com. In addition to becoming familiar with a nearby medical library, the LNC should also use an article retrieval service to find scientific articles and book chapters that are not otherwise accessible. Such resources do not eliminate the need for access to a quality medical library, but they significantly reduce the frequency of time-consuming trips to the library.

Much information is readily available to the LNC without subscribing to services and without engaging a skilled librarian to locate the needed resources and scientific research. The first step in performing research begins with deciding which Internet search engines to use. Using multiple search engines such as Google, Google Scholar, Yahoo, Ask, and AltaVista increases the likelihood of gaining access to the information. Accurate and current medical science may be searched most efficiently with PubMed, the search engine for the U.S. National Library of Medicine and the National Institutes of Health. Customizing a search technique or style is critical to maximizing the results.

The best practice is to regularly use different sites to learn which is best for specific types of searches. The function of medical search sites is actually quite diverse, although on the surface it may appear similar. Different rules and procedures (explained within the help menus) exist to analyze queries and the resulting output. With practice, the LNC will learn to select the site best designed for each query and how to search most effectively on each site. An LNC's skill in accessing medical research, then in comprehending and applying it to the case, is critical. The LNC must know how to apply scientific research as evidence of best practice to effectively assist in the resolution of medical legal cases.

Explaining Findings to the Attorney and the Legal Team

The goals for implementing the research should be clearly defined at the initiation of work on a case because the types of information and the format of the information provided must be tailored to the needs of the person using it. For example, in some situations, perhaps early in case development when the team is trying to gain an overview of the relevant medical literature, the LNC might be asked to provide a compendium of excerpts from gold standard literature demonstrating evidence, pro and con, regarding the key medical issues in the case.

The LNC may later need to provide full texts of articles for the attorney examining witnesses in depositions and trial. To show how the literature affects the case, the LNC may create tutorials, using medical record excerpts interspersed with medical illustrations and citations from respected periodicals and texts to educate and orient the legal team.

In preparing to examine witnesses, in addition to the information compiled in the cast of characters, the LNC may compile a list of each expert's publications and may provide full texts of publications directly relevant to the case. Additionally, compiling other works by or reflecting the work of each expert, such as lists of lectures given and research performed, and even obtaining lecture handouts, deposition transcripts, letters to the editor, etc., will help the legal team anticipate the opinions the experts may hold. Compiling the requisite information is insufficient if the attorney cannot readily access the document needed. As always, providing a table of contents as a road map to expedite locating a document that meets a particular need makes an LNC indispensable

Incorporating Findings and Illustrations into Work Products

The LNC's work product should effectively illustrate a review of scientific literature and show whether violations in the standard of care that are claimed in the lawsuit are consistent with the literature. Likewise, the LNC should compile literature that supports or refutes injuries and damages claimed. The effectiveness of the LNC's presentation of the literature findings may determine whether or not damages should be paid to the injured person. A variety of sources can be used.

For example, a 52-year-old man faced worsened prognosis as a result of a 3-year delay in diagnosing his colon cancer. The worsened prognosis resulted in a more difficult treatment regimen that was needed for the late stage of the cancer when it was diagnosed. To show the causative relationship of delay in diagnosis, worsened prognosis, and more difficult treatment, the LNC used two resources, the American Cancer Society and AdjuvantOnline.com to illustrate damages. These resources were also used by the treating oncologist in documenting his patient's worsened prognosis due to a delay in diagnosing cancer of the colon.

Before relying on these resources for projecting prognoses, the LNC would need to verify that the expert witnesses, and the medical community in general, would concur that the literature was considered reliable for the medical issue of the case; however, for purposes of the initial case investigation, these resources were satisfactory.

LNCs could illustrate standards of care by compiling good-quality scientific research studies. In selecting the appropriate studies to represent practice guidelines and protocols relevant for each case, the quality of the study design (for example, systematic reviews, meta-analyses, and randomized controlled trials) and the appropriateness of the interpretation of the data must be considered, along with the similarity of the samples and variables to the plaintiff and facts of the case. When relevant literature of the highest quality is accessed and the LNC has a full understanding of the development of evidence-based care, a presentation can be very influential when presented and explained to the legal team and the courts.

Creating Exhibits

Educating the attorney and the entire legal team regarding the medical procedures and terms related to the case generally requires creating or finding exhibits and tutorials. The LNC considers how to distill complex medical concepts down to a point where they can be communicated succinctly to a lay audience. Effective exhibits will help this process. The initial goal is to educate the legal team about requisite pathophysiology, procedures, medical equipment, guidelines and standards, medical warnings about a product or procedure, and the associated significant medical information that is relevant to the case. With such materials conveniently accessible, the team members can refresh their understanding of the medical issues of the case and proceed fully informed about the preparation of the case. They may also use the information in exhibits to communicate with the experts, with opposing counsel, and then ultimately with the judge, jury, insurance adjustor, or mediator.

Exhibits that prove to be effective in communicating relevant medical issues can be turned into demonstrative evidence for trial. **Demonstrative evidence** may comprise actual objects, pictures, models, and other devices that are intended to clarify the facts for the judge and jury and explain how an accident occurred, the actual damages, medical problems, and methods used to commit an alleged crime or negligent act. Many of exhibits are not supposed to be actual evidence, but rather aids to understanding.

A variety of resources support the development of good-quality informative displays. Vendors' booths at national meetings and advertisements in professional journals often have useful information. Demonstrative evidence can be x-rays that are color coded to enhance findings, re-creations of fires or mechanisms of accidents, and plastic models of relevant anatomy.

Exhibits can be as simple as enlarged copies of key medical records on foam board, overhead projections, or PowerPoint presentations. The LNC may use complex trial software, such as Trial Director or Sanction, loaded with all of the scanned medical records, legal documents, exhibits, deposition transcripts, and other evidence, so that all documents, work products, and exhibits are readily accessible during the trial.

The LNC should be familiar with resources and collect ideas for exhibits while pursuing continuing education,

so that when needs arise for exhibits, the LNC can draw from multiple resources at hand to find the best means to communicate an image. The LNC should gather contacts such as medical illustrators and exhibitors and create a database of resources for developing exhibits. Developing exhibits commonly falls to the LNC, who is aware of the key issues of the case that need to be demonstrated and who has insights into how to educate non–health-care professionals about science and medical issues.

Providing Support at Depositions, Mediations, and Trial

Once the case is moving forward toward a resolution, which may take 2 to 5 (in some situations, even 8 or more) years, the legal team needs to have a working file with key documents readily accessible, along with organized work products to educate, to refresh memories, and to bring new team members up to speed quickly. There will be planning conferences, depositions and ongoing phone exchanges, and court appearances in the years leading up to settlements, mediations, or trials. The LNC can facilitate these exchanges by arming the attorneys or legal representatives with knowledge so that they have a better command of the medical vocabulary and pronunciations, comprehend the relevant medical concepts, and have ready access to the documents and information needed. All the knowledge and insight that an LNC acquires during case development is worthless if it is not accessible to the attorney or member of the legal team who needs to apply it. Possibly the biggest challenge to the LNC is to figure out how to convey the requisite information.

During depositions, mediations, or trial, the LNC needs to make sure the key documents and work products are current, accessible, and in a form that can be used. When trial is anticipated, since most litigation takes years to complete, all health records need to be updated and all the experts and other witnesses need to be brought up to date with changes in status and additional information obtained in **discovery**. Poor or late communications may leave the LNC in trial with his or her expert on vacation in another country.

The best-laid plans can be undermined by technical glitches, such an overloaded and sprung three-ring binder that spews its contents, leaving the attorney with a disorganized mess of papers, or critical electronic documents loaded onto a laptop for an attorney who doesn't have access to an electric outlet. An LNC is often the coordinator who verifies everything is in place for trial and that everything has a back-up plan. A checklist of trial preparation can help keep this demanding and busy process on track (Box 15.2).

Box 15.2   How to Prepare for Trial

I. Developing a timeline for trial preparation
   A. Make list of what needs to be done
   B. Update calendar to trigger alerts for due dates
   C. Coordinate trial preparation responsibilities with trial team
   D. Meet with trial team to define strategy to accomplish what has to be done for trial
   E. Develop contact list of everyone involved in the trial, including attorneys involved, witnesses, etc.

II. Trial preparation activities in which the LNC may have a vital role
   A. Medical record preparation
      a. Verify completeness
      b. Organize material
      c. Complete copy of medical records to attorney and experts
      d. Verify that appropriate discovery has been completed
   B. Witness handling
      a. Compile witness list and contact information
      b. Verify their availability for trial
      c. Review their role in trial and verify they have related documents
      d. Provide expert work
      e. Review opinions/testimony in this case
      f. Obtain prior related opinions/testimony
      g. Perform review of the literature regarding each professional witness
   C. Demonstrating damages
      a. Finalize spreadsheets of medical costs
      b. Verify that life care plan regarding future costs is complete and appropriate
      c. Obtain lien information
   D. Attorney preparation
      a. Develop trial binder with critical documents
      b. Review literature on the issues in the case and summarize
      c. Review issues of case
      d. Teach the attorney the pathophysiology and language of the case
   E. Exhibit preparation
      a. Develop or organize development of trial exhibits and demonstrative evidence
      b. Develop PowerPoint exhibits for opening and closing statements
      c. Coordinate with experts to have medical illustrations and tools available to help them illustrate the case
   F. Legal document preparation
      a. Verify that the requisite legal documents filed are current and appropriate
      b. Finalize expert reports and verify they are served in a timely manner
      c. Prepare pretrial statements
      d. Participate in planning/writing pretrial motions
   G. Jury selection
      a. Perform research regarding type of jury needed in the specific case
      b. Participate in jury consultant preparation
      c. Compose questions for voir dire
   H. Organize for trial
      a. Plan for transporting trial exhibits/supplies
      b. Plan for trial support professionals
      c. Plan for order of trial
      d. Contact all witnesses and have them on standby
      e. Plan transportation/accommodations

Each case has unique needs, but typically the attorney will need easy access to the following documents: (1) a hard copy of key medical records for each witness; (2) a complete set of medical records in hard copy; (3) an outline of evidence needed from each witness; (4) relevant literature, guidelines, and resources; (5) expert reports and curriculum vita; (6) abstracted depositions or full depositions with key phrases tabbed or bookmarked; (7) photos, medical illustrations, and/or tutorials; and (8) medical chronologies and other key work products, as defined by the case needs.

The LNC may sit beside the attorney at trial or in deposition to provide key documents and reminder notes for questions to ask. The LNC often assists in developing and managing the exhibits and presentations used in the opening and closing statements and may assist in handling the witnesses and communicating with everyone involved

in trial support. Orchestrating a trial requires extraordinary organizational, communication, and management skills, as well as a full command of the facts, the medicine, and related technical knowledge.

SUMMARY OF LNC ROLES AND RESPONSIBILITIES

LNCs have been established as a professional role since the 1970s, yet their value goes unrecognized by many attorneys who do not know how to use them. The LNC may be used as a glorified secretary relegated to organizing and retrieving medical records or performing random paralegal tasks rather than performing the unique responsibilities of legal nurse consulting. As with many advanced nursing roles, the LNC may need to teach the attorney or legal representative what is needed and how to use the LNC's work products to facilitate the legal preparation of a case work.

Case examples that may benefit from the work of an LNC include the medical malpractice or personal injury cases, toxic torts (e.g., black mold, asbestosis), drug liability, products liability, cases with medical issues (driving under the influence, psychologically or mentally impaired defendant), and education cases. A variety of types of cases in which a medical issue is intertwined with a legal issue can be found in the files of the LNC.

Clear goals for development of the end products useful to the attorney on a specific case should be an initial step. Systematically, goals for case development will be revised as the case proceeds. The LNC needs to work within the budget and time constraints that are allotted. The LNC often serves as the case coordinator to keep case development organized and efficient. Producing a work product of the highest quality facilitates the work process, spurring on the entire legal team to do its best.

TECHNICAL INFRASTRUCTURE RESOURCE

The paperless office is a reasonable goal, and the LNC with no computer skills would be greatly challenged. The LNC skill levels span the spectrum. The computer-illiterate LNC may work around the lack of skill and still meet the employers' needs. Essentially, all law offices are computerized, so LNCs must adapt or be constrained in their functional ability. There are some basic requirements for the LNC's office.

Powerful computer that is dedicated to LNC practice. Many nurses ease into the LNC work gradually, starting their LNC practice using whatever computer the family has available. This could end the career of an LNC abruptly. If the LNC sends a virus to a law office within an e-mail or work product, or if confidentiality is breached by family members and friends accessing the home computer, it is unprofessional. A computer without the requisite organizational and safety features of a professional computer or by the use of free word-processing software could make the electronic LNC work product unusable.

Word-processing software. In the early days of law office computing, Corel WordPerfect cornered the law office market. In the last decade, many law offices have transitioned to Microsoft Word and others have changed to Macs. An independent LNC working with multiple law offices may find a need to use both common word-processing programs. LNCs may need to be functional, if not fluent, in both Word and WordPerfect so that they may provide work products that are compatible with the programs used in the various law offices with whom they work.

Free software programs that are preinstalled on computers and programs that are downloaded from the Internet may be incompatible with the standard law office word-processing programs. Electronic documents created using free software may be cumbersome for the law office to use. The goal in producing work products is to facilitate the legal processes. A law office may have to scan and convert hard copy to an electronic form with optic character recognition (OCR) to create an electronic form and have access to the LNC work product; this could lead to a document losing its formatting when it is opened on the law office computers. The law office may seek an LNC who creates a more accessible product rather than one who uses a program that creates more work.

Antivirus software that automatically updates and creates firewalls. Antivirus software is mandatory for every professional creating and sharing electronic work products. It is critical to purchase the most current version of an antivirus software with recognized efficacy (e.g., AVG, Norton by Symantec, McAfee) and set it to automatically retrieve updates from the Internet to maintain the most current antivirus prescriptions available and to run regularly. A computer virus or worm can corrupt data or cause devastating changes to the hard drive. They can also cause more subtle problems, making a computer run slowly and send e-mails containing the virus or worm to every address in your contact file. While the various anti-virus software programs are not infallible, they reduce the likelihood of contracting a virus or worm.

Quality printer/scanner/fax machines. Multifunction machines are problem solvers and space savers for the office. They can reproduce copies in addition to printing, collating, scanning, and faxing. Decisions can be reached regarding ink-jet versus laser, flatbed versus paper feeder, cost comparison of the printer and refill cartridges by reading consumer guides, joining office technology chat groups, and talking to sales people in local office supply stores. In contrast to the professional computer that truly needs to be dedicated to the LNC user, the printer can be networked to other computers. Alternatively, electronic copies of files may be carried to the local copy center and printed.

Quality Internet service provider and e-mail applications. LNCs need high-speed access to research, e-mail, and the wide array of Internet services. The LNC role consists of researching medical issues, standards of care, expert information, and scientific literature for which high-speed

Internet access at the office is imperative. Many electronic files are conveyed as e-mail attachments both to and from the LNC, and the Internet service provider (ISP) used should have the capability to manage larger files. Another thing to consider is that an e-mail address conveys an important message, and the LNC's contact information should reflect professionalism (DrCraneLNC@gmail.com) and not frivolity (Flowerchild@hotmail.com).

A backup system. The use of a dedicated computer reduces the risk of losing or corrupting data, but data still need to be backed up regularly to another source. A routine backup of data to an external hard drive is a safeguard that protects against such losses if the main computer is destroyed. An on-site backup system is insufficient for a professional with irreplaceable electronic files, and an off-site storage site is necessary to protect data from fires, thefts, or other catastrophic occurrences.

Other tools for the LNC. The following tools that may comprise the LNC's arsenal include a laptop computer with protective carrying case, PalmPilot, tape recorder, litigation bags/luggage and cases/briefcases/exhibit carrying cases, and a quality digital camera and videocam. The LNC may need these tools if required to attend medical examinations with clients, provide attorney support during depositions at the office and for trials, and perform initial interviews with plaintiff and other tasks.

Software and Formatting Methods

e-Organization
Before opening the first work product file, a plan should be in place for naming conventions for files. Identify the product file most likely to be needed. Produce and establish file names to use consistently, for example, "Chrono" for medical chronology, "T of C" for tables of contents, "Initial Analysis," and "Lit Review" for literature review. Create an organization chart or tree of directories for electronic file storage so that files can be readily retrieved.

Managing Medical Records and Documents

Space limitations for storing paper files, the logistics of keeping track of documents, and environmental concerns all factor into how an LNC chooses to manage documents. The practical reality is that some law offices have evolved to deal solely with electronic files. Many businesses choose the ease and cost-savings of providing records and documents as electronic documents appended to e-mails or by mailing CDs via U.S. Postal Service. However, it is easier and faster to flip through hard copies to try to find a specific fact. Consequently, many law offices provide hard copies of records and documents. It is realistic to anticipate that the documents in an LNC's office will be a composite of medical records in three-ring binders and loose pages within accordion binders that require both shelf and drawer space, as well as electronic files. Similarly, most law offices may want work products provided in both hard-copy and electronic format. Hence, the LNC needs to develop a system for safe storage and easy retrieval of all the different formats of documents. Likewise, a mechanism for archiving and secure disposal of hard copies and CDs is mandatory at the completion of cases.

A portable document file (PDF) is smaller and more stable, so it is unlikely to become corrupted when e-mailed. It doesn't lose its formatting when opened on another computer or printed from another printer, and it is more difficult to alter. A paperless office, where all medical records and other documents are ultimately scanned and stored as PDF files, can be set as the ultimate goal. With this in mind, the LNC needs to be equipped with software to manage PDF files, which is the standard for managing and archiving documents and forms. Adobe Reader is free as a download from Adobe.com, but additional software is needed to paginate PDF files; to shuffle, add, or delete pages; to make notes on the records; and to bookmark key pages. Adobe Acrobat and PaperPort are the industry standards for creating and working with PDF files, though an Internet search for "create pdf" will yield many other options.

Keeping Work Products Safe and Accessible

Creating the work product is only the first step in the LNC being an asset to a case. Storing the products so they are readily retrievable is another goal. Many new products can be expansions of old products. To be able to retrieve old work products, files need to be archived properly after cases are closed. Additionally, carefully stored and filed documents also need backup systems to keep them safe. Fires, thefts, and computer viruses have devastated businesses. On-site backup to an external hard drive or laptop and off-site storage for current work and archived work must be part of the office system of a competent LNC.

THE LNC IN PRACTICE

The LNC in the Law Firm

The process for practice is essentially the same whether the LNC is employed by firms representing the plaintiff or defense. To be profitable, nurses in defense firms are more likely to have to account for, and bill for, every 6-minute segment of their work day. Differences in roles and job descriptions come from the personalities and skills of the people who make up each legal team. Some legal teams include one attorney, a secretary, and the LNC. In others, paralegals and associate attorneys, or partners, may be part of the team. LNCs may find the role limited to ordering and organizing medical records if they have less-developed skills, and they will miss out on the rich case analysis and development.

Attorneys need to be taught how to best use an LNC to enhance the legal practice. The LNC needs to learn his or her capabilities and skills and enhance those skills more specific to the LNC role to assimilate into the team most productively. Job descriptions should not be static. The learning curve may be steep for a nurse beginning legal analysis after doing bedside care for years. Gaining confidence to reach out to experts takes time and hard work. Skill acquisition should include computer skills, legal writing, and research skills. The LNC acquires the requisite skills in a way that may be foreign to a hospital nurse, who may be fed continuing education. The LNC clinical knowledge must be kept current by reading research, texts, and attending conferences.

The LNC in the Health-Care Setting and the Insurance Industry

LNCs who work in risk management, quality assurance, and as case managers, claims adjustors, etc., are more likely to step into an established role with a job description than the LNC who is hired into a health-care system or a law firm. Health-care system roles tend to be more rule bound by the institutional credentialing agencies, by policies and procedures, and by the round-the-clock shift work mentality. LNCs in health-care systems may also find it challenging to develop writing and research skills. They have an ongoing challenge to maintain current clinical knowledge and skills despite the fact that they may not be clinically active in the LNC role. The LNC is more likely to have a pay scale comparable to hospital nurses and have health-care benefits, but not have weekend and shift work.

The LNC as an Independent Contractor

One of the biggest challenges in establishing an independent practice is the bookkeeping portion of a business. Use of business software, such as Quicken or Quickbooks, often gets neglected when the LNC is focusing on other skills. The significant financial expenditures needed to take LNC courses, purchase basic equipment, and set up an office may not be offset by income for years. Challenges for the entrepreneur include whether to use contracts and request retainers, insurance for LNC practice, separation of family and business in the home office, and liabilities of the self-employed. The independence and freedom gained by having an independent practice may be a double-edged sword for many embarking on the LNC professional course.

The LNC as Educator

The term "LNC educator" may be thought of as one LNC educating another. In practice, the LNC has many non-LNC students, including the attorney and legal team with whom he or she collaborates on each case, the injured person, the judge, the jury, and even the general public, who needs to know how this legal process serves them as health-care consumers. Because the learning needs of the "students" are so diverse, teaching tools and goals and outcomes have to be developed and revised constantly. It is likely that the LNCs who think of themselves first and foremost as educators and role models develop the most effective practice patterns and have the most successful and fulfilling practices.

The LNC as Researcher

The role of the LNC researcher is virtually uncharted territory. Limitations imposed on the researcher within the privacy mandates of the medical-legal world pose even more challenges than in the medical world. Not only is the researcher constrained by the Health Insurance Portability and Accounting Act (HIPAA) and the need to protect private medical information, but also there is an added level of secrecy within legal proceedings. Legal actions may take many years to resolve, so key information needed for the research process may be tied up for a long time and delay publications of research findings. The LNC as a researcher may chart a research pathway that is less traveled by other nurses in the area of root cause analysis of malpractice cases that involve a nurse.

The first published study of LNCs was a survey conducted by a practicing LNC of 14 years. The author collected data through a survey of nurses who worked in the legal arena as expert witnesses, consultants, or both. A random selection of 400 of the 600 members in "a specialty organization" were mailed survey questionnaires with forced-choice questions about their biographical information, professional practice in medical records review, analysis and research, medically related correspondence, liaison activities, and specialized assistance. There were 239 usable responses, and this provided the initial insight into the type of nurses who worked in LNC practice, their education, clinical backgrounds, and the scope of their LNC practices.

Several years later, the American Association of Legal Nurse Consultant (AALNC) Certification Board performed a "practice analysis" to define the role of the LNC to develop a certification examination that would measure competent performance within the occupation. The survey measured the frequency and rated the importance of activities performed by LNCs, as well as the knowledge they deemed necessary that the LNC possess to perform successfully. The methodology employed was a combination of logical analysis and activity inventory. The sample was self-selected AALNC members who returned mailed surveys from 36 states, the District of Columbia, and Canada. They found the highest ranked activities and knowledge of LNCs as follows, and then weighted the questions on the certification examination accordingly.

The LNC activity statements were ranked with the 10 highest ranked activities as follows:

1. Maintain confidentiality in your practice
2. Develop and maintain professional client relations in written and verbal communications
3. Extrapolate key information from health-care documents
4. Summarize medical records and other case documents as work products
5. Prepare detailed chronologies/timelines of the medical record information as work product
6. Evaluate cases to determine causation
7. Organize the health-care records of the plaintiff as part of the case analysis (tied)
8. Educate the client about health-care aspects of the case (tied)
9. Generate written reports on areas of liability as work product
10. Evaluate cases to determine areas of liability

The highest ranked areas of knowledge and ability were reported as follows:

1. Medical terminology
2. Written communications
3. Analytical thinking skills, rules of confidentiality, ethical principles (tied)
4. Verbal communication skills
5. Rules of professional conduct
6. Anatomy and physiology
7. Organizational skills

In a literature search, no published research on LNC practice was found until 2007 when Constantino (2007) with a transdisciplinary team (a physician, a nurse, and a lawyer) performed an analysis of 20 moot malpractice cases decided in 2005, entitled *Acting On Evidence: A Root Cause Analysis of Malpractice Cases*. A brief abstract of the research is presented in Box 15.3.

Box 15.3   Research Exemplar

Background

The global focus on the business of caring and patient safety place an enormous burden on health-care staff with patients 24/7. The fundamental reason for the breakdown of a system in any practice setting has a "root cause." Root cause analysis is one way of learning the reason(s) for the failure or breakdown of a process (error) in a health-care system. The work was done as a transdisciplinary project in the department of health and community systems in a university school of nursing (Datillo & Constantino, 2006).

The Problem

The problem of errors was underscored by tragic high-profile malpractice cases nationally and internationally: 80,000 to 98,000 people die in U.S. hospitals due to errors, with an estimated cost of $17 to $29 billion. Performing a retrospective

root cause assessment and analysis of malpractice cases was needed. Our specific aims are to: (1) review moot malpractice cases decided by the Allegheny County Common Pleas Court, (2) classify the sentinel event that led to the malpractice outcome, (3) develop a framework for categorizing contributing and mitigating factors, (4) perform mixed methods analysis, and (5) disseminate findings (Datillo & Constantino, 2006; Kohn, Corrigan, & Donaldson, 2000; Harris, Westfall, Fernald, et al, 2006).

Method

Twenty malpractice cases decided in the Common Pleas Court of Allegheny County in 2005 wherein a nurse was named among the defendants were reviewed using a grounded theory method of data collection and analysis (Waltz, Strickland, & Lenz, 2005). Specifically, focus was on the court's opinion in the concepts and phrases used in its findings.

(box continued on page 304)

Box 15.3 Research Exemplar (continued)

Assessment of Problem and Analysis of Its Causes

Mixed methods analysis was used to integrate qualitative and quantitative techniques for data collection and analysis. Five attributes in designing mixed methods studies were considered: (1) rationale for mixing methods, (2) techniques used, (3) priority given to quantitative versus qualitative research, (4) sequential or concurrent implementation, and (5) phase at which the integration occurred. Twenty malpractice cases were reviewed where physicians and nurses were defendants (Cresswell, Fetters, & Ivankova, 2006).

Strategy for Change

The outcomes and prevention and intervention strategies derived from the cascade of events leading to the malpractice suit were traced through documents filed in court related to the case. Data elements, significant attributes of qualitatively or quantitatively derived errors, and categorization of contributing or mitigating factors are described.

Measurement of Improvement

In Constantino (2007) evidence of meaningful collaborative transdisciplinary team (two nurses, one physician, two lawyers) was shown. The team designed a project analyzing moot malpractice cases where a nurse is mentioned as a defendant or one of the defendants in the case. Analyzing malpractice cases needs to be based on careful and thoughtful planning, design, and evidence. Results of mixed methods data collection and data analyses may be translated globally to hasten the application of evidence-based research into practice.

Results

Communication problem or lack of communication (40%, $n = 8$) ranked the highest root cause of the 20 cases,

followed by medication errors (25%, $n = 5$), procedural non-compliance (20%, $n = 4$), lack of competence (15%, $n = 2$), and lack of leadership/improper delegation (10%, $n = 1$).

Changes

As a result of this study, the transdiciplinary team (TT) was expanded to include a patient advocate. The TT needs to be transparent in their activities to maintain trust and confidence among other disciplines and consumers.

Lessons Learned

Quality and safety in health-care settings is not a single profession's responsibility. A transdisciplinary team is needed for health-care systems to act based on evidence in response to consumer demands for quality and safety. Using a transdiciplinary team to examine malpractice cases provides a greater perspective on policy development and staff training. A more diverse team will enhance the breadth and depth of the analysis, including the five levels of harm.

Message to Others

Other service settings, for example, first responders and community agencies, should heed the fundamental root cause for the breakdown in any system. Life-saving patient safety solutions by the World Health Organization will be presented.

LNCs are in unique positions to lead a transdisciplinary research team that examines the root cause of an event within health-care systems that leads to the catastrophic cascade of events leading to litigation. Furthermore, the research team may analyze the systems breakdown that allowed the medical misadventure to occur. The transdisciplinary team research could take the final steps to design evidence-based policies and procedures correcting the systems that failed.

Researchable questions might address the effectiveness of LNCs in optimizing their work and work products. The years of experience in nursing practice and education, along with self-esteem and confidence, are invaluable tools for the LNC. Attorney satisfaction with various aspects of LNC work product is paramount in this competitive, collaborative LNC role. Effectiveness of equipment, tools, and instruments used in practice needs to be evaluated and vetted. Exploring issues of plaintiff or defendant satisfaction in legal outcomes when an LNC is involved in a lawsuit would be a valuable research question. Evidence-based LNC practice will sharpen tools when randomized clinical trials in LNC quality outcomes are performed.

Conclusions

The LNC role is entrepreneurial and has vast potential. The LNC can create a role that is an indispensable part of the legal team. The LNC can use and share health and scientific knowledge with other professionals, the courts, and the public.

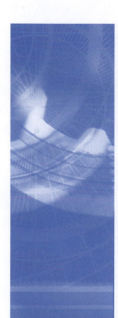

EVIDENCE-BASED PRACTICE

Example Search Terms: Searching articles or research studies on legal nurse consulting or articles or research by legal nurse consultants could begin with choosing search terms. The search terms used were: "legal nurse", "consultant", or "legal nurse research".

Database(s) to Search: LexisNexis, PubMed

Search Strategy: Using LexisNexis Academic, select "Power Search" and then the radio button for "Natural Language." Insert the terms "legal nurse" in the search box and then "consultant" in the "Required Terms" box. The results are well over 500. In PubMed you can simply enter "legal nurse consultant" as a phrase and limit to the year of your interest.

Direct Resources: http://aalnc.org/edupro/journal.cfm, *The Journal of Legal Nurse Consulting*, http://lncezine.com leads to http://www.legalnurse.com

Selected References From Search:

1. Bemis, P.A. (2008). Nurses in the legal field. *RN, 71*(6):20-21.
2. Masoorli, S. (2005). Legal issues related to vascular access devices and infusion therapy. *Journal Infusion Nursing, 28*(3 Suppl):S18-21; quiz S33-16.
3. Meiner, S.E. (2005). The legal nurse consultant. *Geriatric Nursing, 26*(1):34-36.
4. Milazzo, V.L. (2007). Legal nurse consultants keep the healthcare system healthy. *Imprint, 54*(1):46-49.

Questions Used to Discern Evidence:

Choose two studies among the studies listed, read about them, and answer the following questions:

1. What are the differences between the two studies in the design, methods, and results?
2. What are the similarities between the two studies in the number of subjects, measures used, and interventions, if any?
3. What skills do you need to learn to practice forensic nursing as a legal nurse consultant?

REVIEW QUESTIONS

1. A legal nurse consultant can demonstrate "damages" by:
   A. Producing supportive services and supplies used by the plaintiff.
   B. Developing a spreadsheet to demonstrate medical costs incurred as a result of injuries from a negligent act.
   C. Developing a video of the victim's family.
   D. Performing a review of the expert's publications and prior court testimony.

2. An important role of the legal nurse consultant is to:
   A. Determine where to file the complaint.
   B. Conduct depositions during the discovery process.
   C. Provide gold standard literature to assist in illustrating the standard of care.
   D. Serve as a paralegal/secretary for the attorney in the law office setting.

(review questions continued on page 306)

3. Certification for the LNC:
  A. Is mandatory to work in a law firm as a legal nurse consultant.
  B. Is available only through the American Nurses Credentialing Center of the ANA.
  C. Reflects that an LNC has extensive experience in the role of LNC.
  D. Can come from many sources and may have little correlation with the LNC skill level.

4. Word-processing software that should be used to develop all work products for law offices is:
  A. Corel WordPerfect.
  B. Microsoft Word.
  C. Freeware that came on the computer.
  D. Whatever yields a product that the law office can access without corruptions.

5. Challenges commonly encountered by LNCs in practice include:
  A. Developing good paralegal practice skills.
  B. Deposing expert witnesses.
  C. Finding the causal connection between the negligent care and the injury.
  D. Teaching the attorney defensive nursing practice.

6. Work products that LNCs are commonly asked to produce include:
  A. Medical chronologies.
  B. Professional licenses of all defendants.
  C. Disorganized medical records.
  D. List of jurors in the case.

7. Tasks LNCs perform at trial time may include all of the following *except*:
  A. Writing complaints.
  B. Finding or developing medical exhibits.
  C. Recording key damages.
  D. Drafting closing arguments.

8. An LNC is:
  A. A registered nurse who is knowledgeable in many aspects of law, nursing, and medicine, as well as the social influences controlling and affecting patient care, legal claims, and litigation.
  B. A nurse who serves as a secretary in a large law corporation.
  C. A clinical nurse who served as a witness in a landmark case.
  D. A nurse who reviews evidence of child abuse.

9. The most important goal for the LNC is to:
  A. Organize and verify that key medical records have been obtained.
  B. Interview defendants.
  C. Interview plaintiffs.
  D. Communicate with opposing counsel, judge, jury, and insurance adjustor or mediator.

10. Exhibits that prove to be effective in communicating relevant medical issues can be turned into:
  A. Pictorial evidence.
  B. Demonstrative evidence.
  C. Formal evidence.
  D. Informal evidence.

11. Maintaining a clear and consistent line of communication is vital, whether the LNC acts as the coordinator of the case development or has a peripheral role. Communications in legal work are frequently:
  A. Undiscoverable.
  B. Unobtainable by the opposing side.
  C. Discoverable or obtainable by the opposing side.
  D. Converted as the property of the court.

References

Adobe Systems, Inc. (2003). PDF as a standard in managing and archiving documents and forms. Electronic version. Retrieved January 30, 2008, from http://www.adobe.com/enterprise/pdfs/managing_archiving.pdf

Cohen, S. Freehand drawing of bulbar stenosis. Unpublished law office work product for the Law Offices of Mark R. Bower, New York, NY.

Constantino, R.E. (2007). A transdisciplinary team acting on evidence through analysis of moot malpractice cases. *Dimensions of Critical Care Nursing 26*(4):150-155.

Constantino, R.E., & Bricker, P.L. (1997) Social support, stress, and depression among battered women in the judicial setting. *Journal of the American Psychiatric Nurses Association, 3*(3):81-88.

Datillo, E. & Constantino R.E. (2006). Root cause analysis and nursing management responsibilities in wrong site surgery. *Dimensions of Critical Care Nursing,* 25:1-5.

Faherty, B. (1995). LNCs: Who are they? *Journal of Nursing Law*, 2(1):37-49.

Fandray, S. (2007). A day in the life of an in-house defense LNC. *LiNC*, pp 9-11. Electronic version. Retrieved November 23, 2007, from http://www.pittsburghchapteraalnc.org/the%20LiNC%20%20%20final%20%20%20spring%202007.pdf

Farlex, Inc. (2008). *The Free Dictionary*. Retrieved April 10, 2010, from http://legal-dictionary.thefreedictionary.com/But+for+causation

Forrest, B. (2006). Excel time line. Unpublished law office work product. Schlender Law Office, Mountain Home, ID.

Jackson, N.S., & Bower, M.R. *Roser v. Benedictine Hospital and Leftowitz, MD*. Affirmation in Opposition to Defendant Dr. Leftowitz's cross motion. November 24, 2004.

Jackson, N.S., Boyd, J., & Gardner, S. *Considering a career as a LNC*. About LNCing: Website of the Pittsburgh chapter of AALNC. Retrieved November 23, 2007, from http://www.pittsburghchapteraalnc.org/about%20LNCing.htm

Law.com Dictionary. (2010). Retrieved April 10, 2010, from http://dictionary.law.com/default2.asp?selected=486&bold=%7C%7C%7C%7C

Magnusson, J.K., & Garbin, M. (1999). LNC practice analysis summary report. *Journal of Legal Nurse Consulting,* 10(1):10-18.

Parisi, V. (2005). Life care plan for therapy for child with brachial plexus injury. Unpublished law office work product by Valpar Consultants, Inc. for the Law Offices of Mark R. Bower, PC, New York, NY.

Peterson, A.M. & Kopishke, L. (Eds.) (2010). Legal Nurse Consulting Principles. 3rd Ed. New York: CRC Press.

Peterson, A.M. & Kopishke, L. (Eds.) (2010). Legal Nurse Consulting Practices. 3rd Ed. New York: CRC Press.

Saslow, D., Boetes, C., Burke, W., et al. (2007). American Cancer Society guidelines for breast screening with MRI as adjunct to mammography. *California Cancer Journal for Clinicians*, 57(2): 75-89. Retrieved April 10, 2010, from http://caonline.amcancersoc.org/cgi/content/full/57/2/75

Smith, R.A., Cokkinides, V., & Brawley, O.W. (2008). Cancer screening in the United States, 2008: A review of current American Cancer Society guidelines and cancer screening issues. *California Cancer Journal for Clinicians*, 58:161-179. Retrieved April 10, 2010, from http://www.cancer.org/docroot/ped/content/ped_2_3x_acs_cancer_detection_guidelines_36.asp

Taylor, J.F. (2010). *Utilizing the power of the web: Medical resources for attorneys*. Retrieved April 10, 2010, from http://www.attorneysmedicalservices.com/medinf.html

Wikipedia: The free encyclopedia. (2010). Bates numbering. Retrieved April 10, 2010, from http://en.wikipedia.org/wiki/Bates_numbering

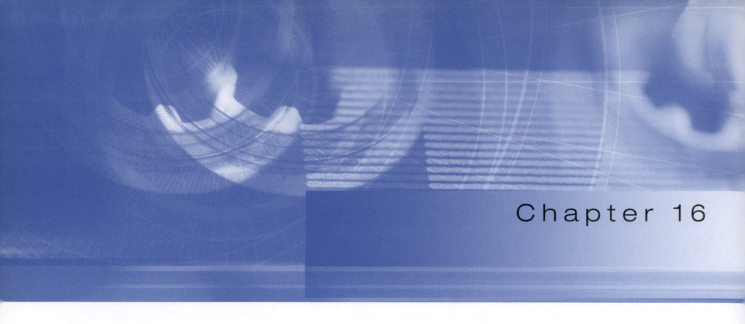

Chapter 16

EVIDENCE: FORENSIC NURSING IN THE EMERGENCY AND ACUTE CARE DEPARTMENTS

Angie Primeau and Daniel J. Sheridan

"Everything is determined, the beginning as well as the end, by forces over which we have no control. It is determined for insects as well as for the stars. Human beings, vegetables or cosmic dust, we all dance to a mysterious tune, intoned in the distance."

Albert Einstein

Competencies

1. Understanding the evolution of emergency-based forensic programs.
2. Listing specific patient populations served by emergency department (ED) nurses with forensic training.
3. Understanding the importance of written and photographic documentation in the medical records.
4. Assessing for intimate partner violence using reliable and valid tools.
5. Identifying barriers to conducting intimate partner violence assessments.
6. Describing the types of injuries associated with intimate partner violence.

Key Terms

Documentation
Evidence collection
Forensic nurse examiner
Forensic photography
Intimate partner violence
Secondary victimization
Sexual assault forensic examiner
Sexual assault nurse examiner

INTRODUCTION

Thousands of times every day across North America, persons injured in the commission of a crime are evaluated and treated in emergency departments (EDs) and acute care settings. These patients include victims of child abuse and neglect, family violence, intimate partner violence, abuse and neglect of the elderly and the disabled, and sexual assault. In addition, victims of random stranger-to-stranger and gang violence seek emergent care. Every time patients victimized by violence in the community arrive in the emergent care setting, they bring parts of the crime with them and sometimes literally in them.

While highly skilled in providing emergent medical and nursing care, many ED and acute care nursing staff are not trained to preserve valuable evidence to document the histories of assault in a forensically useful manner. However, with the steady growth of ED-based forensic nursing programs and ongoing forensic nursing continuing education events, the ED and acute care nurse is now beginning to recognize **evidence collection** and preservation as part of the nursing role.

In fact, the Emergency Nurses Association (ENA) has developed a position statement on forensic evidence collection recognizing the ED nurses' role in evidence collection, written and photographic documentation, court testimony, and collaboration with law enforcement and social service agencies. Although faculty in schools of nursing seldom possess forensic nursing expertise, there is a growing interest in offering courses that include principles of evidence collection and other forensic nursing skills and competencies, and textbooks are beginning to include chapters that focus on forensic nursing. Additionally, some state boards of nursing have mandated continuing education in evidence collection for nurses who work in the ED.

The purpose of this chapter is to present a brief history of the development of forensically focused nursing programs in emergent care settings and to explore, from an evidenced-based perspective, the efficacy of these programs. The current trend to expand **Sexual Assault Nurse Examiner** (SANE) programs to serve other victimized patient groups, as well as barriers to implementing hospital-based forensic practices, will be discussed.

DEVELOPMENT OF HEALTH-CARE–BASED VIOLENCE INTERVENTION PROGRAMS

The Evolution of Intimate Partner and Family Violence Programs

Forensic nursing was being practiced in ED and acute care settings long before it was identified as a nursing specialty. In 1975, an ED nurse at the Hennepin County Medical Center in Minneapolis, Minnesota, created the first hospital-based program focused on providing specialized care and advocacy services to patients experiencing **intimate partner violence** (IPV). The program had one paid staff nurse and multiple volunteer advocates. By the mid-1990s, this one program had served over 2500 abused women and had expanded its services by providing a battered elder women's support group.

Approximately 10 years later, in January 1986, in a nearby hospital in Minneapolis, Susan Hadley created WomenKind at Fairview Southdale Hospital. This program's goals were to provide advocacy and safety planning for abused women presenting to the ED for care as well as to educate ED staff on assessing for domestic violence. Domestic violence is used by one person in a relationship to control another and can include physical assault, sexual abuse, as well as emotional, psychological, and financial abuse. WomenKind is still providing advocacy-based victim services today.

In July 1986, in Chicago, Illinois, Daniel Sheridan created the Family Violence Program (FVP) at Rush-Presbyterian-St. Luke's Medical Center in a funded partnership between the ED Nursing Division and the Department of Social Work. This nurse-coordinated program provided specialized nursing care and advocacy services to patients presenting with injuries from any form of family violence and sexual assault. The services included obtaining and documenting extensive histories around the reported abuse, photographic documentation of injuries, and referrals to community-based programs and resources. Other services included maintaining a cadre of advocates to respond to sexual assault cases as well as to provide educational outreach training throughout the medical center and community. In 1993, the FVP stopped providing services during a hospital-wide restructuring.

In 1994, Susan Dersch, a registered nurse with a women's health background, created the Assisting Women with Advocacy, Resources and Education (AWARE) Program at Barnes and Jewish Hospital in St. Louis, Missouri. The AWARE Program provides patient advocacy and education to health providers to view domestic violence as a major health issue that extends far beyond just an ED focus. Dersch still coordinates the AWARE Program, which has established institutional longevity.

STATE OF THE SCIENCE

Olive (2007) performed a meta-analysis review of evidence-based literature on care of ED patients who experienced domestic violence in the United Kingdom and United States and found the data indicated that at least 6% of ED patients had experienced IPV in the past year. IPV is abuse that occurs between two people who are in a close relationship; the term *intimate partner violence* is often used interchangeably with that of *domestic violence*. She reported that the actual number of IVP cases is probably higher as a result of ED personnel primarily screening patients for whom there were higher degrees of suspicion of IPV occurrence rather than doing routine assessments on all patients, which could uncover additional cases. The data indicated that abused women who felt that they were not taken seriously or were not identified as abused by the ED staff had negative perceptions of their care.

Anglin and Sachs (2003) systematically reviewed the ED literature from 1980 through 2002 looking for evidence linking ED screening for IPV with decreased morbidity and mortality. Over 330 articles were found on the topic, of which only 20 met the inclusion criteria, which was having an intervention using an outcome that determined decreased prevalence or improved burden of suffering. They designed their study to build on a controversial 1996 report produced by the U.S. Preventative Services Task Force (USPSTF) on domestic violence screening in general medical settings. The task force concluded there was not enough evidence to recommend for or against routine screening for IPV. Anglin and Sachs also found insufficient evidence for or against routine IPV screening, but still recommended health-care providers routinely ask questions about IPV because of the high burden of suffering victims experience.

Houry et al. (2008) identified that the USPSTF report was deficient because it did not include an assessment of the safety of IPV screening itself. To fill that gap, the researchers performed research with patients ($n = 6328$) who were triaged in a large, urban ED during study hours. Seventy percent ($n = 3083$) agreed to participate in the study, of which 2134 answered questions on the computerized survey related to IPV. Of the 2134 patients who answered questions about IPV, 548 (26%) screened positive for IPV during the past year.

Follow-up interviews were conducted with 281 patients identified as having experienced IPV (216 in person and 65 via telephone). None of the participants ($n = 3083$) expressed any safety issues or emotional distress after participating in the computer screening. However, two participants who were interviewed in person reported that they had recurring negative emotional thoughts, and one participant interviewed via the telephone reported a verbal argument with her partner about chores after she returned home from the ED. Houry and colleagues also found no increase in 911 emergency calls for IPV in the local police district in the 6 months following the ED visits. The 131 patients who reported IPV had contacted community

resources during the 3-month follow-up period. The researchers concluded there were no significant adverse events to participating in the screening for any of the patients who screened positive for IPV.

The Michigan Department of Community Health created the Michigan Intimate Partner Violence Surveillance System linking IPV cases from the prosecutor database to ED visits. Kothari and Rhodes (2006) conducted a retrospective observational case series reviewing one county's ED visits from 1999 through 2001 looking for female IPV victims. Of 964 female IPV victims in the prosecutor IPV database, 64% ($n = 616$) had been seen in at least one ED within the past year for a medical reason, but not necessarily for injuries from abuse. The study demonstrated that physicians almost never documented a negative screen for IPV, but performed relatively well regarding following up on positive screens conducted by the nurses.

Screening Issues

Screening is defined as the "systematic application of a test of inquiry to identify individuals at sufficient risk of a specific disorder to benefit from further investigation or direct preventative action." It is a procedure used in health-care settings to identify a problem and provide an intervention designed to reduce prevalence and risk of that problem. Screening for IPV has many barriers to implementation in health-care practices. As stated earlier, the most recent USPSTF report still has no recommendations regarding routine screening for IPV due to insufficient evidence that it reduces morbidity and mortality. Therefore, some health-care providers and institutions struggle with the dilemma of whether to screen or not to screen. IPV is a major public health problem and not a disease. Therefore, it is not best practice to evaluate the efficacy of IPV intervention studies based on a medical disease model such as that used by the USPSTF.

Barriers to Conducting IPV Assessments

Emergency departments are the third most common source of help for patients suffering from IPV, following law enforcement and family and friends. In the United Kingdom, forensic patients experience an average of 35 incidents of abuse prior to seeking medical help.

When forensic patients enter an ED, they are often overlooked, and abuse is frequently misdiagnosed as a wide array of health conditions that are associated with abuse and neglect. Injuries suffered by those affected by IPV reach far beyond the abusive act itself and impact physical, psychological, and mental health. Brain injury, hypertension, obesity, hearing loss, thyroid dysfunctions, gastrointestinal disorders, sleep disturbances, and gynecological illnesses are physical health conditions linked to IPV. IPV has also been related to increased rates of HIV and STI infection, substance abuse, alcoholism, risky sexual behaviors, spontaneous abortion, fetal death, and preterm birth.

Accompanying these physical conditions, there are many psychological illnesses that are correlated to IPV, including depression, anxiety, post-traumatic stress disorder, and suicidal ideation. Although identification of IPV may be difficult, the associated health conditions necessitate the accurate identification and diagnosis of IPV and the need for interventions.

Furthermore, health-care providers, including nurses, may impose barriers that influence patient disclosure of IPV and subsequent nursing care. Providers may face factors such as having a personal history of abuse that may interfere with their ability and willingness to provide screening and care to patients suffering from IPV. Provider education can also influence patient care. Medical and nursing schools provide little education on domestic violence or sexual abuse; therefore, providers may feel as though they do not possess sufficient knowledge and skills to address this issue.

Many providers also fear involvement with the justice system. When caring for patients who experience IPV or sexual assault, the likelihood of court subpoenas and required testimony increases. Providers may fear loss of professional certification or licensure following civil torts, which creates hesitance to care for IPV patients. Along with fear of the justice system, providers have fears of offending their patients and creating a hostile patient-provider relationship. Some providers believe questions regarding IPV are too personal and patients can easily take offense.

Additionally, there is frustration among providers when patients do not comply with prescribed treatments or interventions. Those suffering from IPV often are dependent on their partner and may return to the abusive relationship multiple times. Patients experiencing IPV may not seek counseling services or legal assistance due to isolation and restrictions enforced by the partner. They may have multiple hospitalizations related to abusive episodes. Providers may have a hostile bias when caring for these patients due to their not leaving the relationship and seeking help as the provider suggests. These barriers and biases produce resistance to the successful implementation of routine screening for IPV.

Sheridan (2007) has identified barriers to women leaving abusive relationships:

1. Fear of further harm or being killed by the abuser.
2. Limited finances making leaving difficult.
3. Wanting the children to have a father in the home.
4. A faith-based belief that marriage is for life, even when being abused.

5. Family pressures to maintain the relationship.
6. Lack of family support.
7. Having limited friends or social support secondary to being isolated.
8. Forgiving the abuser when he says he is sorry for beating her.

Despite these barriers, most current literature supports the implementation of routine IPV assessments as well as the need for further research to develop evidence-based interventions and more standardized assessment tools. Screening has been shown to produce positive patient outcomes through providing validation, acknowledging abuse, and increasing self-esteem. In addition, assessing for IPV enhances patient trust in the patient-provider relationship and confidence in health-care institutions.

The literature supports mandatory routine IPV assessments in every health-care institution for every person, regardless of age, gender, or ethnicity. The literature recognizes there is a current gap of research in evidenced-based interventions within clinical practice that reduces the patient's risk for IPV recurrence, but no studies have shown negative patient outcomes from IPV screening. Patients may feel uncomfortable disclosing information to providers, yet disclosure itself has not been shown to increase IPV prevalence.

While more research on effective IPV assessment tools is needed, there are reliable and valid IPV tools in common clinical use. Versions of the Abuse Assessment Screen (AAS) have been used in clinical research for over 10 years. Sheridan et al. advocate for the use of the six-item AAS (Fig. 16.1). No matter what IPV screening tool is used, with any "yes" answer, the ED or acute care nurse needs to have additional reliable and valid IPV tools available to identify women at risk for homicide, such as the Danger Assessment (DA; Fig. 16.2) and the HARASS (Harassment in Abusive Relationships: A Self-report Scale; Fig. 16.3) tools.

THE DEVELOPMENT OF SEXUAL ASSAULT FORENSIC EXAMINER AND FORENSIC NURSE EXAMINER PROGRAMS

Prior to the development and proliferation of Sexual Assault Nurse Examiner (SANE) programs in the late 1990s, patients victimized by sexual assault would suffer long ED wait times, substandard medical care, and hostility from medical and legal personnel responsible for conducting a forensic examination or investigation. Most

Abuse Assessment Screen
NRCVA. (1988)

Violence is very common in today's world and it can overlap into our homes. Because violence affects so many people, I now routinely ask all my patients (clients) a few questions about violence in their lives.

All couples argue now and again, even the best of couples.

1. When you and your partner argue are you ever afraid of him (her)?

2. When you and your partner verbally argue, do you think he (she) tries to emotionally hurt/abuse you?

3. Does your partner try to control you? Where you go? Who you see? How much money you can have?

4. Has your partner (or anyone) ever hit, slapped, kicked, choked, pushed, shoved, or otherwise physically hurt you?

5. Since you have been pregnant (when you were pregnant), has your partner ever hit, slapped, kicked, choked, pushed, shoved, or otherwise physically hurt you?

6. Has your partner ever forced you into sex when you did not want to participate?

With any yes, say thank you for sharing. Can you tell me more about the last time?

The Nursing Research Consortium on Violence and Abuse (1988) encourages the reproduction, modification, and/or use of the Abuse Assessment Screen in routine screening for domestic violence.

■ FIGURE 16.1 Abuse Assessment Screen (NRCVA, 1988).

examinations and treatment were completed by non-forensically trained physicians who would provide incomplete and inconsistent care. Patients would leave the ED feeling depressed, helpless, violated, and reluctant to seek further assistance.

In the late 1970s, innovative nurses created the first Sexual Assault Nurse Examiner/Forensic Nurse Examiner (SANE/FNE) programs to train and certify nursing professionals to become skilled in performing quality forensic medical-legal examinations to meet the complex needs of patients suffering from violence and to collect evidence usable in court cases: in 1976 in Memphis, Tennessee; 1977 in Minneapolis, Minnesota; and 1979 in Amarillo, Texas. The development of the first SANE programs in the 1970s coincided with the development of Rape Victim Advocate programs, an outgrowth of the then-burgeoning women's movement. In addition, the 1970s gave rise to the development of the first standardized sexual assault evidence collection kits and the recognition of the importance of collecting deoxyribonucleic acid (DNA) as evidence.

When the sexual assault evidence kits were first introduced into EDs, physicians were the health-care providers designated to obtain the victimized patient's history of assault and collect the evidence. The forensic medical examination in many hospitals was delegated to the inexperienced medical intern or resident on call at the time or rotating through the ED on a temporary basis. Also present during each examination would be a regularly assigned, usually very experienced ED nurse who would coach the physician through every step of the examination. Out of necessity, ED nurses would have to constantly train every group of physicians rotating through the ED on how to complete a sexual assault evidence kit.

The first SANE programs around the country used standing orders in their EDs or community-based settings and had experienced nurses perform the forensic examination. The purpose of these programs was to minimize substandard care by providing consistent, objective, and comprehensive medical assessments, including physical and emotional treatment of reported victims, to meet the needs of these forensic patients. Goals included minimizing trauma experienced by patients during the examination and facilitating connections to community resources.

DANGER ASSESSMENT

Jacquelyn C. Campbell, Ph.D., R.N.
Copyright, 2003

Several risk factors have been associated with increased risk of homicides (murders) of women and men in violent relationships. We cannot predict what will happen in your case, but we would like you to be aware of the danger of homicide in situations of abuse and for you to see how many of the risk factors apply to your situation.

Using the calender, please mark the approximate dates during the past year when you were abused by your partner or ex-partner. Write on that date how bad the incident was according to the following scale:

1. Slapping, pushing; no injuries and/or lasting pain
2. Punching, kicking; bruises, cuts and/or continuing pain
3. "Beating up"; severe contusions, burns, broken bones
4. Threat to use weapon; head injury, internal injury, permanent injury
5. Use of weapon; wounds from weapon

(If **any** of the descriptions for the higher number apply, use the higher number.)

Mark **Yes** or **No** for each of the following. ("He" refers to your husband, partner, ex-husband, ex-partner, or whoever is currently physically hurting you.)

_____ 1. Has the physical violence increased in severity or frequency over the past year?
_____ 2. Does he own a gun?
_____ 3. Have you left him after living together during the past year?
        3a. (If have never lived with him, check here ____)
_____ 4. Is he unemployed?
_____ 5. Has he ever used a weapon against you or threatened you with a lethal weapon?
        (If yes, was the weapon a gun? ____)
_____ 6. Does he threaten to kill you?
_____ 7. Has he avoided being arrested for domestic violence?
_____ 8. Do you have a child that is not his?
_____ 9. Has he ever forced you to have sex when you did not wish to do so?
_____ 10. Does he ever try to choke you?
_____ 11. Does he use illegal drugs? By drugs, I mean 'uppers' or amphetamines, speed, angel dust, cocaine, 'crack', street drugs or mixtures.
_____ 12. Is he an alcoholic or problem drinker?
_____ 13. Does he control most or all of your daily activities? For instance: does he tell you who you can be friends with, when you can see your family, how much money you can use, or when you can take the car? (If he tries, but you do not let him, check here: ____)
_____ 14. Is he violently and constantly jealous of you? (For instance, does he say "If I can't have you, no one can.")
_____ 15. Have you ever been beaten by him while you were pregnant?
        (If you have never been pregnant by him, check here: ____)
_____ 16. Has he ever threatened or tried to commit suicide?
_____ 17. Does he threaten to harm your children?
_____ 18. Do you believe he is capable of killing you?
_____ 19. Does he follow or spy on you, leave threatening notes or messages, destroy your property, or call you when you don't want him to?
_____ 20. Have you ever threatened or tried to commit suicide?

_____ Total "Yes" Answers

Thank you. Please talk to your nurse, advocate or counselor about what the
Danger Assessment means in terms of your situation.

■ **FIGURE 16.2** Danger Assessment (Courtesy of Jacquelyn C. Campbell, Ph.D., R.N., Copyright, 2003).

The very first SANEs worked in isolation until the late 1980s when Gail Lenehan, then editor of the *Journal of Emergency Nursing (JEN)*, published the first list of 20 SANE programs around the country. In 1992, 72 nurses from SANE and other violence programs around the country met in Minneapolis and created the International Association of Forensic Nurses. The term *forensic nursing* was coined and defined by Virginia Lynch in the late 1980s to describe the application of the nursing process to public or legal proceedings and the application of forensic health care to the scientific investigation of abuse and violence-related trauma and/or death.

With the creation of IAFN and publications in various journals, especially in the *Journal of Emergency*

Nursing (JEN), the importance of SANE/FNE programs was recognized by other communities. Similar programs began to develop across the United States and Canada. By 1996, 86 SANE/FNE programs had been developed, and by 1999, there were 116 functioning SANE/FNE programs. In 2005, there were 419 active SANE/FNE programs in the United States and 42 in Canada. As of 2009, the IAFN estimates that there are more than 500 functioning SANE/FNE programs in the United States and Canada.

Harassment in

Abusive

Relationship:

A

Self-report

Scale

Many women are harassed in relationships with their abusive partners, especially if the women are trying to end the relationship. You may be experiencing harassment. This instrument is designed to measure harassment of women who are in abusive relationships or who are in the process of leaving abusive relationships. By completing this questionnaire, you may better understand harassment in your life. If you have any questions, please talk with the service provider who gave you this tool.

Harassment is defined as: a persistent pattern of behavior by an intimate partner that is intended to bother, annoy, trap, emotionally wear down, threaten, frighten, terrify and/or coerce a women with the overall intent to control her choices and behavior about leaving an abusive relationship.

There are no right or wrong answers. Do not put your name on the from. The instrument takes about 10 minutes to complete.

For each item, circle the number that best describes how often the behavior occurred. Next, rate how distressing the behavior is to you. If the behavior has never occurred, circle 0 (NEVER) and go to the next questions. If the question does not apply to you, circle NA (NOT APPLICABLE). If you are still in the relationship please circle below MY PARTNER. If you have left the relationship, please circle below MY FORMER PARTNER.

THE BEHAVIOR MY PARTNER MY FORMER PARTNER (circle one)	0 = Never 1 = Rarely 2 = Occasionally 3 = Frequently 4 = Very Frequently NA = Not applicable **How often does it occur?**	0 = Not at all distressing 1 = Slightly distressing 2 = Moderately distressing 3 = Very distressing 4 = Extremely distressing NA = Not applicable **How distressing is this behavior to you?**
1. Frightens people close to me	0 1 2 3 4 NA	0 1 2 3 4 NA
2. Pretends to be someone else in order to get to me	0 1 2 3 4 NA	0 1 2 3 4 NA
3. Comes to my home when I don't want him there	0 1 2 3 4 NA	0 1 2 3 4 NA
4. Threatens to kill me if I leave or stay away from him	0 1 2 3 4 NA	0 1 2 3 4 NA
5. Threatens to harm the kids if I leave or stay away from him	0 1 2 3 4 NA	0 1 2 3 4 NA
6. Takes things that belong to me so I have to see him to get them back	0 1 2 3 4 NA	0 1 2 3 4 NA
7. Tries getting me fired from my job	0 1 2 3 4 NA	0 1 2 3 4 NA
8. Ignores court orders to stay away from me	0 1 2 3 4 NA	0 1 2 3 4 NA
9. Keeps showing up wherever I am	0 1 2 3 4 NA	0 1 2 3 4 NA
10. Bothers me at work when I don't want to talk to him	0 1 2 3 4 NA	0 1 2 3 4 NA
11. Uses the kids as pawns to get me physically close to him	0 1 2 3 4 NA	0 1 2 3 4 NA
12. Shows up without warning	0 1 2 3 4 NA	0 1 2 3 4 NA

■ **Figure 16.3** HARASS (Copyright 1998, Daniel J. Sheridan, Ph.D., R.N. The HARASS instrument can be used without copyright permission in any clinical setting. Anyone interested in using the HARASS instrument in a research project is requested to contact the author at dsheridan@son.jhmi.edu.).

THE BEHAVIOR MY PARTNER MY FORMER PARTNER (circle one)	0 = Never 1 = Rarely 2 = Occasionally 3 = Frequently 4 = Very Frequently NA = Not applicable **How often does it occur?**	0 = Not at all distressing 1 = Slightly distressing 2 = Moderately distressing 3 = Very distressing 4 = Extremely distressing NA = Not applicable **How distressing is this behavior to you?**
13. Messes with my property (For example: sells my stuff, breaks my furniture, damages my car, steals my things)	0 1 2 3 4 NA	0 1 2 3 4 NA
14. Scares me with a weapon	0 1 2 3 4 NA	0 1 2 3 4 NA
15. Breaks into my home	0 1 2 3 4 NA	0 1 2 3 4 NA
16. Threatens to kill himself if I leave or stay away from him	0 1 2 3 4 NA	0 1 2 3 4 NA
17. Makes me feel like he can again force me into sex	0 1 2 3 4 NA	0 1 2 3 4 NA
18. Threatens to snatch of have the kids taken away from me	0 1 2 3 4 NA	0 1 2 3 4 NA
19. Sits in his car outside my home	0 1 2 3 4 NA	0 1 2 3 4 NA
20. Leaves me threatening messages (for example: puts scary notes in the car, sends me threatening text messages or letters, sends me threats through family and friends, leaves threatening messages on my cell phone or telephone answering machine)	0 1 2 3 4 NA	0 1 2 3 4 NA
21. Threatens to harm our pet	0 1 2 3 4 NA	0 1 2 3 4 NA
22. Calls me on the telephone and hangs up	0 1 2 3 4 NA	0 1 2 3 4 NA
23. Reports me to the authorities for taking drugs when I don't.	0 1 2 3 4 NA	0 1 2 3 4 NA
Additional harassing behaviors not listed above: 24. _____	0 1 2 3 4 NA	0 1 2 3 4 NA
25. _____	0 1 2 3 4 NA	0 1 2 3 4 NA

Please answer a few additional questions:

_____Your age in years

Check the statement that best describes you:

☐ Married, living with an abusive partner

☐ Single, living with an abusive partner

☐ Married, living apart from an abusive partner

☐ Single, living apart from an abusive partner

How long were in the above relationship? _____

Are you still in the relationship?   ☐ Yes   ☐ No

If you have left the relationship, how long have you been out? _____

What is your approximate annual income? _____

How many years of school have you completed? _____

Check the statement that best describes you:

☐ Asian/Pacific Islander

☐ Black/African American

☐ Caucasian/White

☐ Hispanic

☐ Native American/American Indian

☐ Other _____

■ **FIGURE 16.3**—cont'd

While most SANE/FNE programs have unique aspects and services that vary depending on institutional affiliations, most programs are consistent in offering the following services:

- Obtaining a thorough history
- Conducting a head-to-toe physical examination
- Treating assessed injury or injuries
- Collecting and preserving evidence
- Creating thorough, unbiased written documentation
- Providing detailed forensic photography
- Providing prophylactic treatment for possible sexually transmitted infections (STIs)
- Obtaining STI cultures
- Administering emergency contraception medications for pregnancy prevention
- Providing crisis intervention as indicated
- Performing safety planning
- Providing postexamination assistance, such as new clothing, accessibility to showers, and hygienic supplies
- Providing referrals to community resources for counseling, medical follow-up, and housing
- Testifying in court as fact or expert witnesses.

In addition, some SANE/FNE Programs provide:

- Free HIV testing
- HIV prophylaxis

Individual and/or community education on safe sex practices, pregnancy options, and STIs, as well as prevention of future victimization.

SANE versus SAFE versus FNE

SANE is the acronym most often used to describe programs providing specialized care to patients reporting sexual assault. However, some programs are called SAFE (**Sexual Assault Forensic Examiner**) programs to allow for forensically trained physicians and physician assistants to conduct program-based examinations. Registered nurses in Maryland and New Jersey are licensed to perform sexual assault examinations and are called **forensic nurse examiners** (FNEs), with board of nursing certification as either a FNE-A, licensed to conduct forensic examinations on adolescent/adults (age 13 and older), or FNE-P, licensed to conduct forensic examinations on children (age 12 and younger).

ED-based, forensically trained nurses are increasingly being used to provide in-depth, forensic nursing care to a growing number of patients presenting for care from other types of abuse and neglect besides sexual assault. For example, Mercy Medical Center in Baltimore,

Maryland; Winchester Medical Center in Winchester, Virginia; and Christiana Hospital in Wilmington, Delaware, routinely provide specialized forensic nursing assessments and care to a variety of victimized patients, such as those experiencing IPV, elder abuse, and child abuse.

When studies compared traditional ED forensic sexual assault services to SANE/FNE program services, it was shown the SANE/FNE programs delivered more consistent evidentiary collection and documentation of injuries, as well as minimized secondary victimization to patients. **Secondary victimization** is described as negative behaviors and/or comments that make sexual assault survivors feel they are to blame or have caused the assault. Also, SANE/FNE programs more consistently provided patients with testing and prophylaxis for STIs and pregnancy in addition to educating on safe sex practices and safety planning. Patient care is provided in a compassionate, nonjudgmental fashion that is patient-centered, and patients report feeling more informed, in control, respected, safe, and cared for when treated by SANE/FNE nurses.

ANONYMOUS ("JANE DOE") REPORTING

In the United States, approximately one third of women experience physical or sexual abuse at some point during their lives, and up to 84% of cases remain unreported to police. To receive federal STOP Violence Against Women Formula Grant Program funding, the Violence Against Women and Department of Justice Reauthorization Act of 2005 mandated that by January 2009 all states were required to offer free forensic physical examination and evidence collection to sexual assault victims regardless of whether women chose to involve law enforcement or not.

The Violence Against Women Act recognizes that victims of sexual assault may feel fearful, overwhelmed, and resistant to informing law enforcement of the assault right away. This act enables them to have medical treatment and evidence collection in a timely manner, as well as additional time to decide whether or not to pursue legal action. The implementation of the act was intended to improve health care for persons suffering from sexual assault as well as to gain greater understanding of its actual prevalence.

To date, no research has been published addressing the significant change in how patients are evaluated by sexual assault programs since the enactment of this requirement. Research at the programmatic, local, regional, state, and federal level is needed to determine how many more patients victimized by sexual assault are receiving a forensic examination. In addition, research will be needed to explore how many cases of "anonymous" examinations convert to being investigated by the police and prosecuted in the courts.

INTERNATIONAL STUDIES OF FORENSIC NURSES IN ED SETTINGS

In South Africa, "violence and trauma victims are flooding the health-care system." ED nurses in the Durbin, South Africa, area who had at least six months experience completed a 40-item survey about the role of forensic nurses in ED settings. The results were disappointing. The study demonstrated that forensically trained nurses in Durban, South Africa, "are almost nonexistent." The respondents recognized the need for forensic training and were very excited about eventually having a forensic nurse specialist assigned to the ED who could educate other nurses to improve forensic nursing care. While the nurse respondents acknowledged their lack of training in forensic evidence collection, they responded in the survey that the ED physicians had even less forensic knowledge. In one case, a nurse wrote "some doctors are clueless."

A study conducted in the Netherlands had experienced ED physicians, ED nurses, forensically trained physicians, and students look at a series of color photographs of a variety of patients throughout the lifecycle with abuse-related injuries. Understandably, the providers with forensic training were the most accurate in assessing, correctly identifying, and documenting the injuries and the students the most inaccurate. However, there was no significant difference in the assessments conducted by experienced ED nurses and experienced ED physicians. The study concluded that there was an imminent need for more training around forensic health care and abuse identification by health professionals, including ED nurses and physicians.

ISSUES AFFECTING ALL FORENSIC NURSING PROGRAMS

Throughout the United States, mandatory reporting laws pertaining to IPV lack standardization and can differ between states. It can be difficult for health-care providers to understand when and what types of abuse need to be reported. For example, all U.S. states have statutes indicating specific persons (such as social workers, teachers, medical personnel, and law enforcement) who are required to report child maltreatment, and 18 states have laws requiring any person who suspects child abuse or neglect to report it. Yet, not all states have mandatory reporting for elder abuse and neglect, and there is much confusion in the reporting laws concerning abuse reports and neglect of younger disabled and vulnerable adults. A key role for a forensically trained nurse in the ED or acute care setting is to stay abreast of laws that address mandatory reporting to authorities.

There is also a lack of standardization among institutions for IPV screening questions or whether the questions are being asked at all. Nurses provide interventions in hopes of decreasing the prevalence or stopping the problem entirely. When patients screen positively for IPV, health-care providers express frustration due to the lack of available effective, evidence-based interventions. Health-care institutions also lack protocols regarding what interventions to incorporate into patient care. Lack of protocols creates greater uncertainty among health-care providers who may consider whether to screen at all and which interventions, treatments, and referrals to complete. One explanation for the lack of available evidence-based interventions when treating forensic patients is the lack of violence education offered to health-care providers. Medical and nursing schools provide little education on IPV, and continued education in violence is optional after a degree is obtained. Providers may not feel as though they have sufficient knowledge and skills to address this issue due to their lack of education.

TYPES OF INJURIES

Whether a health-care institution has an ED-based or acute care–based formal forensic nursing program or it only provides registered nurses with additional forensic training, it is critical for the nurses to use correct forensic terminology. The following is a brief review of the most commonly used medical forensic terms.

Abrasion

An abrasion, often called a scratch or scrape, is a superficial injury to the epidermis layer of the skin caused by friction or rubbing from a rough object. Abrasions can appear in all sizes and shapes, depending upon the object applying force.

By examining the injury closely, the provider will note that one edge of the wound contains connected abraded epithelium that can be used to determine the direction of the applied force. If this injury has not been thoroughly cleaned, trace evidence of the object causing injury or the surrounding environment can be found within the wound bed. The presence or absence of trace evidence in a wound can add to or subtract from the consistency or credibility of the history being given by the patient and/or the person(s) accompanying the patient.

Avulsion

An avulsion is the complete tearing away of a structure or part, often caused by shearing, tearing, or blunt force energies. While there are orthopedic-related avulsion injuries, forensically trained nurses are more likely to see avulsed or partially avulsed skin from assault-related traumas. Partial avulsions have been described as skin tears. Skin tears usually occur over hands, forearms, and bony prominences, but they can be seen anywhere blunt force is applied.

Bruise/Contusion

Blunt force or compression-related trauma can result in destruction of blood vessels in any tissue of the body. This damage causes a leakage of red blood cells into surrounding tissues, resulting in a discoloration of the area called a bruise or contusion. Bruises are often accompanied by other symptoms such as pain, swelling, and induration of the area.

Many research studies have been conducted attempting to determine the exact age of a bruise, yet results found that trying to accurately date a bruise either by direct examination or via photographs was not possible. Bruises to the skin have a relatively predictable color change pattern of turning from red, to black and blue, to bluish-green, to greenish-brown, to brownish-yellow, to yellow, to light yellow, then into fading. However, every person will transition through these stages at different rates because of gender, normal physiological changes of aging, quantity of adipose tissue, administered medications, and the body's immune response. Without a reliable history, it is not scientifically possible to accurately date when a bruise occurred purely by its appearance. However, a clinically experienced nurse can document if the age of the bruise is consistent with the history being provided. If the nurse cannot assess if the bruise is consistent or not consistent with the presenting history, it would be prudent to only describe the bruise in detail.

Laceration

A laceration is the splitting of tissue resulting from blunt or shearing force trauma. Many medical personnel inaccurately document any open wound to the skin as a laceration. Unlike cuts or incisions, lacerations have jagged edges, varying wound depths, and are often found over bony prominences. They are frequently accompanied by bruising of surrounding tissues. Upon close examination of the wound depth and edges, the direction of the applied force can sometimes be determined.

Cut/Incision

A cut or incision is an injury created by a sharp object resulting in a wound with smooth edges and depths correlating with the object used. They can be caused by various objects such as knives, glass, razors, or even paper. Like abrasions, some objects can cause a clustering of epithelium cells at one end of the wound, revealing the direction of force applied. A cut or incision that is deeper than it is wide is often called a stab wound. A stab wound is also classified as a penetrating wound—a wound that enters, but does not exit, a body part. A wound passing completely through a body part is called a through-and-through wound or a perforating injury and could include, for example, a sharp object (sword), a pointed object (spear), or a bullet. Body piercing is an example of a perforating injury.

Ecchymosis

Often misinterpreted and mislabeled as bruising, ecchymosis is the subcutaneous leakage of released red blood cells from damaged blood vessels. Unlike bruises, areas of ecchymosis are usually nonpainful and nonindurated, lack distinct outer margins, and spread in the direction of gravity. Discoloration under the skin from a venipuncture or arterial puncture is best described as an "ecchymotic lesion," since the blood leaked from the blood vessel into surrounding tissue. Blood vessel leaks from needle punctures can be rapid, contain significant volume, and be painful to the touch. The blood under the skin from a contusion (blunt or squeezing force trauma) can be pulled downward by gravity, causing a much larger area of discoloration. The point of impact is the bruise; however, the discolored, gravity-dependent dispersion of blood should be documented by the ED nurse as ecchymotic spread.

Patterned Injury

Patterned injuries (or geometrically patterned injuries) have identifiable markings of the specific object that caused the injury, or they are so unique that a specific cause is known. Patterned injuries often involve bruising or burns, but they can include abrasions, incisions, or lacerations. If the ED nurse, based on training and experience, is professionally comfortable with identifying a specific patterned injury, the nurse can document descriptions of these injuries in connection with the known or most likely cause by using the word *like*. For example, the nurse could document "three purplish, circular fingertip-*like* bruises to the upper inner arm" or "two cord-*like* circular, red abrasions in a circumferential pattern around the neck" to help describe what object was most likely to have caused the injury or if the patterned injury is consistent with the history being provided. If the nurse is not comfortable in attributing an injury to a specific mechanism of injury, the nurse should only thoroughly document the injury in writing and via photographs as to its location, color, size, shape, and whether it is painful or not.

Petechia

A petechia is a small, pinpoint, nonelevated, purplish spot caused by hemorrhagic ruptures of capillaries due to significant increases in vascular pressure. Accidental or intentional strangulation and suffocation can cause facial petechiae, as can other more common activities, such as vaginal birthing, strenuous bowel movements, severe vomiting, aggressive screaming, coughing, or sneezing. It is important that the nurse differentiate between petechiae to sclera (which are more pinpoint or rashlike in nature) and conjunctival hemorrhages, which can cause all or parts of the eye to be solid red in color.

Slap Injury

When slapped, especially administered to a flat body surface, the resulting injury is uniquely patterned. These injuries will initially present as a raised, generalized reddened area on the skin that is very painful to the touch, often in an outline of a hand and often documented as a welt. As the injury heals, the resulting bruises centrally fade to show the pattern of finger outlines. When a slap injury occurs over the ear, the eardrum will show signs of trauma, such as being reddened or ruptured.

Firearm Injury

Firearm injuries are frequently seen in ED or trauma-related health-care settings. They are caused by high-velocity blunt force trauma from projectiles of a gun or rifle. The type of injury is directly related to the distance between the person injured and the gun fired. If a person is shot with the gun pressed against the skin, examination of the injury will reveal a brand of the gun's muzzle. If a handgun is shot from close range (up to 4 feet), it will cause a circular burn of gunpowder residue on the skin, also called *stippling*. If the shot is taken from greater distances, a small circular wound will be present.

Due to the high velocity behind the object causing this type of injury, wounds often come in pairs: entrance and exit wounds. Data demonstrate that health-care providers cannot accurately distinguish between entrance and exit wounds and therefore should not label these injuries as such: providers should only document the location and characteristics of the wounds.

Bite Mark

Human bite marks present as an oval or circular bruise surrounded by two opposing arch-like abrasions. Occasionally, a bite from one person to another could leave incisor punctures, partial avulsions, complete avulsions, and finger amputations. The area between the bite arches can be a good location to collect DNA evidence, usually from the saliva of the biter. The abrasions are also good evidence to photograph because they are a direct imprint of the biter's tooth pattern or dental signature. A forensic odontologist may be able to use photographic images of bite wounds to link the bite pattern to the individual who caused it. Using a right-angle ruler and taking photographs from a 90-degree angle to the skin can greatly assist the forensic dentist.

Strangulation

Strangulation, choking, and suffocation are unique and should not be used interchangeably, even though all result in loss of or decreased oxygen to the brain. Suffocation involves obstruction of the mouth and nose (or covering a tracheostomy, if present), preventing air from entering the lungs. Choking involves the blockage of the airway by an object lodged in the retropharyngeal area or upper airway. Strangulation involves constricting the vessels of the neck and/or the airway by external forces.

Strangulation injuries are often associated with IPV and are a risk factor for intimate partner homicide of women. There are three general types of strangulation: (1) manual, (2) ligature, and (3) mechanical. Manual and ligature strangulation are often associated with IPV. Brain trauma can occur from one or more of these causes:

1. The jugular veins become occluded, causing blood to back up into the cranium and triggering depressed respirations, unconsciousness, and then death.
2. The carotid arteries become occluded, causing rapid loss of consciousness and death of brain cells from lack of oxygenated blood to the brain.
3. The airway becomes occluded, preventing adequate respirations and leading to hypoxia and then death.

Manual strangulation involves compressing a person's neck with any part of the body and could include using hands, "head-lock" arm holds, "head-lock" leg or "scissor" holds; leaning on the neck; or stepping on the neck. Manual strangulation injuries can present as finger-like linear or fingertip-like circular bruising, with or without fingernail-like abrasions to the neck. When fingernail-like abrasions are present, it is usually from the victim trying to pry the assailant's hands or ligature away from the neck.

In a study of about 300 manual strangulation cases, about 50% of victims had no visible bruising after the assault, and 67% developed no symptoms. The absence of physical findings does not mean the patient was not strangled, however. Bruising visible enough to be photographed was found in only 15% of the cases. Patients reporting strangulation did have other symptoms, including pain (point tenderness), raspy voice, sore throat, difficulty swallowing, changes in perceived voice quality, coughing, nausea and vomiting, headaches, ear pain, lightheadedness, and reported loss of consciousness. As a victim becomes unconscious from strangulation, the person may lose control of his or her bowel and bladder. It is critical the ED nurse ask, in a sensitive manner, about all of the above possible sequelae from being strangled, including possible incontinence.

Ligature strangulation involves wrapping and compressing a cord-like object around the neck. This mechanism exerts compressive forces to the blood vessels of the neck as well as the airway. Ligature strangulation can often leave patterned circumferential bruises and/or abrasions around the patient's neck.

Recent advances in use of alternate light sources (ALSs) during forensic examinations have been shown clinically to highlight strangulation-related bruises to the body not visible to the naked eye. However, to date, there are no evidence-based studies documenting the accuracy of ALS usage on known injury areas.

DOCUMENTATION

Importance of Documentation

Complete and accurate written and photographic **documentation** is of vital importance for health-care providers. It provides an explanation of the patient's physical, psychological, and emotional condition, and the patient's progress throughout the patient's hospitalization or visit. If there is a misuse of medical terminology or absence in documentation, it can negatively affect the outcome for forensic patients that choose to pursue legal action for their assault.

Written Documentation

Forensic patients will present for medical care with a wide array of symptoms. It is essential to patient care that health-care providers document the physical and emotional condition thoroughly, as well as use appropriate medical diagnoses. Failure to document this information correctly can produce discrepancies that can be viewed as violations by the Joint Commission.

Written documentation in the ED or acute care record also needs to be viewed as valuable evidence and must be free of bias and subjectivity. Words such as "alleged," "claims," "refused," and "uncooperative" should be avoided. For example, a nurse would never consider writing "alleged chest pain" as the chief complaint. Similarly, the ED nurse should never document "alleged sexual assault," "alleged child abuse," or "alleged domestic violence" in the medical record.

If a nurse documents that a patient is "claiming" something happened, the bias embedded in that word implies that the patient is not believable. The word "refused" should never be used in medical documentation either. The bias in charting suggests good patients do what health providers ask while bad patients "refuse" providers' advice. Instead of charting that a patient "refused" to make a police report, the nurse should write, "Patient states he/she does not want to make a police report." Starting a note with "Patient said . . ." or "Patient states . . ." or "Patient reports . . ." is free from any bias. Whenever possible, document verbatim the history of the actual assault and do not sanitize or "medicalize" the patient's words.

Every injury needs to be described in detail, including its size, shape, color(s), and location. Document if the injury is painful to touch, firm on palpation (indurated), and if the injury has a distinct margin. Document if the injury is patterned resembling a particular object and if there are multiple visible injuries in various degrees of healing.

Written documentation also includes the use of body maps to identify the extent and location of each injury. Cuts, bites, bruises, burns, fractures, dislocations, punctures, areas of bleeding, and other types of injuries need to be counted, described, and illustrated on readily available body maps.

Photographic Documentation

Taking photographs of all injuries should be a routine practice in ED and acute care settings. Photographic documentation can enhance injury description and medical documentation of a patient's physical condition. It provides a record of the direct observation of the patient at the time of examination. **Forensic photography** is a process in which photographs are taken and can be used in future legal proceedings. In many institutions, taking a patient's photograph requires informed consent by the person being photographed.

There are multiple forensic photography techniques to establish a "true and accurate" photographic record of an injury. The "rule of thirds" is a technique in which the nurse photographer takes a sequence of photographs—first from about 6 feet away, then 4 feet away, and finally about 2 feet away. The first image should be a full body photo to establish identity and placement of injuries. This sequence allows correct anatomic placement of the injury or injuries on the body.

Serial photography, taking a series of photographs over time, is used to document wound-healing progression. For many years, forensic photographers used 35-mm SLR or Polaroid cameras. Polaroid cameras and film are no longer widely used, nor are 35-mm cameras; both have been replaced by digital cameras. While 35-mm film cameras produce excellent quality images of injuries, it is not known until the film is developed if the camera actually captured the injury. As a result, digital cameras have become widely accepted as the forensic photography norm. Practitioners are able to view images within an instant and take additional photographs if the images are unclear.

A national trend is being seen to meet contemporary demands for using digital evidence: JPEG digital images are attached to unalterable raw file images as digital evidence. In addition, the state of information technology and medical health information has led to many forensic medical records being stored along with the photographic images in secure portals. Forensic medical images and records can be stored indefinitely and accessed as needed by police and other forensic professionals prior to court proceedings.

CONCLUSIONS

Forensic nursing in emergency and acute care departments has dramatically improved patient care for persons affected by violence through the development of SANE/FNE programs and also through much-needed additional training and education for providers, institutions, and communities. With the implementation of the forensic nursing programs, patients no longer suffer from delayed wait times, substandard evidence collection and treatment, or hostility from medical professionals. Instead, patients receive a thorough head-to-toe physical examination, complete documentation of abuse and injuries, and evidence collection and preservation.

As of January 5, 2009, the Anonymous "Jane Doe" Reporting Act enables all patients to be treated free of charge, regardless of police approval or investigation. Patients who are fearful and resistant to seeking police intervention immediately after an assault can still receive timely and needed medical treatment and evidence collection. Victims can take additional time to decide whether or not to involve police. However, to date, there is no research published pertaining to changes in patient care since the implementation of this act or the number of patients who choose to involve police at a later time.

Even with these improvements in practice, there remains a gap in evidence-based literature pertaining to effective interventions to decrease the prevalence, morbidity, and mortality of IPV and sexual assault. Currently, the majority of the published literature is of the highest evidence level. Research on IPV and sexual assault can be difficult due to the potential for increased IPV assaults, patient emotional trauma, and low follow-up rates. However, it is possible to initiate research at any level with appropriate clinical questions. Conducting research at the higher levels requires more time and effort to locate and interview participants and obtain required institutional approval for working with vulnerable populations. Yet, research by multidisciplinary professionals to enhance patient and health-care outcomes is a necessity in order to develop best practices from evidence-based patient care practices and interventions.

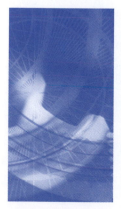

EVIDENCE-BASED PRACTICE

Reference Question: For female rape victims is Web-based social support more likely to prevent post-traumatic stress disorder (PTSD) from occurring than normal standard treatment when subjects participate within a year of the last incident?

P = female rape victims
I = Internet (web-based) social support
C = standard treatment
O = no PTSD
T = within year of last incident

Database(s) to Search: PubMed, PsychInfo, Cochrane Library

(evidence-based practice box continued on page 322)

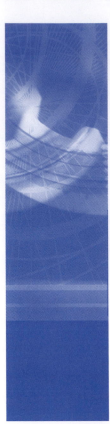

EVIDENCE-BASED PRACTICE *(continued)*

Search Terms: Use the MeSH terms "rape," "social support," "Internet," and "stress, disorders, post-traumatic" individually. Combine "Internet" AND "social support" AND "stress disorders, post-traumatic" with the "Internet" and "social support" set. Add "rape" to the search only if needed to decrease the number of results.

Selected References From Search:

1. Phillips, N.D. (2009). The prosecution of hate crimes: The limitations of the hate crime typology. *Journal of Interpersonal Violence, 24*(5):883-905.
2. Plumm, K.M., & Terrance, C.A. (2009). Battered women who kill: The impact of expert testimony and empathy induction in the courtroom. *Violence Against Women, 15*(2):186-205.
3. van Wormer, K. (2009). Restorative justice as social justice for victims of gendered violence: A standpoint feminist perspective. *Social Work, 54*(2):107-116.
4. van Straten, C.P., & Smits, N. (2008). Effectiveness of a web-based self-help intervention for symptoms of depression, anxiety, and stress: Randomized controlled trial. *Journal of Medical Internet Research, 10*(1):e7.

Questions Used to Discern Evidence:

Choose two studies among the studies listed, read about them, and answer the following questions:

1. What are the differences between the two studies in the design, methods, and results?
2. What are the similarities between the two studies in the number of subjects, measures used, and interventions, if any?
3. What competencies do you need to acquire in working with survivors with PTSD?

REVIEW QUESTIONS

1. The systematic application of a test of inquiry to identify individuals at sufficient risk of a specific disorder to benefit from further investigation or direct preventative action is:
   A. Screening.
   B. Assessment.
   C. Planning.
   D. Evaluation.

2. Sheridan (2007) clinically identified eight barriers to women leaving an abusive relationship, including fear of further harm, limited finances, wanting the children to have a father in the home, a belief that marriage is for life, family pressures to maintain the relationship, lack of family support, having limited friends or social support, and:
   A. Health-care providers' admonishment that abuse will stop if she gives in to abuser's demands.
   B. Forgiving the abuser when he says he is sorry for beating her.
   C. Family pressures to leave the relationship.
   D. Victim's knowledge regarding legal procedures.

3. The first Sexual Assault Nurse Examiner (SANE) programs around the country required that experienced nurses perform the forensic examination to maximize the quality of care by providing consistent, objective, and comprehensive medical assessments, including:
   A. Information on legal issues.
   B. Information on parenting.
   C. Information on finances.
   D. Physical and emotional treatment.

4. Patterned injuries or geometrically patterned injuries have identifiable markings of the specific object that caused the injury or are so unique that a specific:
   A. Perpetrator is known.
   B. Intent is known.
   C. Motive is known.
   D. Cause is known.

REVIEW QUESTIONS—cont'd

5. One explanation for the lack of evidence-based interventions available when treating forensic patients is the:
   A. Lack of funds and resources to assist survivors.
   B. Lack of violence education offered to health-care providers.
   C. Comprehensive care given to forensic patients.
   D. Lack of uniformity of rules and regulations in all jurisdictions.

6. If a provider documents a patient is "claiming" something happened, the bias embedded in that word implies that:
   A. The patient is gravely injured.
   B. The caregiver is not believable.
   C. The patient is not believable.
   D. Both patient and caregiver are believable.

7. Often misinterpreted and mislabeled as bruising, ecchymosis is the subcutaneous leakage of released red blood cells from damaged blood vessels. Unlike bruises, areas of ecchymosis are usually nonpainful and nonindurated, lack distinct outer margins, and:
   A. Spread in the direction of gravity.
   B. Spread in the direction opposite to gravity.
   C. Spread in all directions.
   D. Spread in no identifiable direction.

8. Strangulation injuries are often associated with intimate partner violence (IPV) and are a risk factor for intimate partner homicide of women. There are three general types of strangulation: manual, ligature, and:
   A. Chemical.
   B. Artificial.
   C. Staged.
   D. Mechanical.

9. A laceration is a/an:
   A. Superficial injury to the epidermis layer of the skin caused by friction or rubbing.
   B. Splitting of tissue resulting from blunt or shearing force trauma, resulting in injury with jagged edges and varying wound depth.
   C. Injury created by a sharp object, resulting in a wound with smooth edges and depths.
   D. Oval or circular bruise surrounded by two opposing arch-like abrasions.

10. The Violence Against Women and Department of Justice Reauthorization Act of 2005 mandated that by January 2009 all states are required to offer free forensic physical examinations and evidence collection to sexual assault victims regardless of whether women chose to involve law enforcement if states want to receive:
    A. Federal STOP Violence Against Women Formula Grant Program funds.
    B. United Nation's Trust Fund to End Violence Against Women funds.
    C. National Institute of Mental Health funds.
    D. National Institutes of Health funds.

References

Abdool, N.N.T., Curationis, M., & Brysiewicz, P. (2009). A description of the forensic nursing role in the emergency departments in Durban, South Africa. *Journal of Emergency Nursing, 35*(1):16-21.

Anglin, D. & Sachs, C.J. (2003). Preventive care in the emergency department: Screening for domestic violence in the emergency department. *Academic Emergency Medicine, 10*(10):1118-1127.

Antognoli-Toland, P. (1985). Comprehensive program for examination of sexual assault victims by nurses: A hospital-based project in Texas. *Journal of Emergency Nursing, 11*(3):132-135.

Bariciak, E.D., Plint, A.C., Gaboury, I., et al. (2003). Dating of bruises in children: An assessment of physician accuracy. *Pediatrics, 112*(4):804-807.

Berg, A.O. (2004). Screening for family and intimate partner violence: Recommendation statement. *Annals of Family Medicine, 2*(2):156-160.

Besant-Matthews, P. (2006). Blunt and sharp injuries. In V.A. Lynch & J.B. Duval (Eds.), *Forensic nursing*. St. Louis, MO: Elsevier Mosby, pp. 189-200.

Boyle, A., Robinson, S., & Atkinson, P. (2004). Domestic violence in emergency medicine patients. *Emergency Medicine Journal, 21*:9-13.

Campbell, J.C. (1995). Homicide of and by battered women. In J.C. Campbell (ed.), *Assessing dangerousness: Violence by sexual offenders, batterers, and child abusers.* Thousand Oaks, CA: Sage Publications, pp. 96-113.

Campbell, R., Patterson, D., & Lichty, L.F. (2005). The effectiveness of sexual assault nurse examiner (SANE) program: A review of psychological, medical, legal, and community outcomes. *Trauma, Violence, & Abuse, 6*(4):313-329.

Campbell, R., Townsend, S.M., Long, S.M., et al. (2006). Responding to sexual assault victims' medical and emotional needs: A national study of the services provided by SANE programs. *Research in Nursing and Health, 29*:384-398.

Centers for Disease Control and Prevention. (2006) Understanding intimate partner violence: Fact sheet. Retrieved July 22, 2009, from http://www.cdc.gov/ViolencePrevention/pdf/IPV-FactSheet.pdf

Cole, J., & Logan, T.K. (2008). Negotiating the challenges of multidisciplinary responses to sexual assault victims: Sexual assault nurse examiner and victim advocacy programs. *Research in Nursing & Health, 31*(1):76-84.

Davila, Y. (1991). Sexual assault nurse examiner resource list. *Journal of Emergency Nursing, 17*(4):31-35.

Emergency Nurse Association. (2003). Forensic evidence collection—Position statement. Retrieved August 29, 2009, from http://www.ena.org/about/position/position/Pages/Default.aspx

Glass, N., Laughon, K., Campbell, J.C., et al. (2008). Non-fatal strangulation is an important risk factor for homicide of women. *Journal of Emergency Medicine, 35*:329-335.

Golden, G.S. (2006). Bite mark injuries. In V.A. Lynch & J.B. Duval (Eds.), *Forensic nursing.* St. Louis, MO: Elsevier Mosby, pp. 147-156.

Hadley, S.M. (1992). Working with battered women in the emergency department: A model program. *Journal of Emergency Nursing, 18*(1):18-23.

Hadley, S., Short, L., Lesin, N., et al. (1995). WomenKind: An innovative model of health care response to domestic abuse. *Women's Health Issues, 5*:189-198.

Houry, D., Kaslow, N.J., Kemball, R.S., et al. (2008). Does screening in the emergency department hurt or help victims of intimate partner violence? *Annals of Emergency Medicine, 51*(4):433-442.

Jaffee, K.D., Epling, J.W., Grant, W., et al. (2005). Physician-identified barriers to intimate partner violence screening. *Journal of Women's Health, 14*(8):713-720.

Kothari, C., & Rhodes, K. (2006). Missed opportunities: Emergency department visits by police-identified victims of intimate partner violence. *Annals of Emergency Medicine, 47*:190-199.

Langlois, N.E., & Gresham, G.A. (1991). The ageing of bruises: A review and study of the colour changes with time. *Forensic Science International, 50*(2):227-238.

Ledray, L.E. (1993). Sexual assault nurse clinician: An emerging area of nursing expertise. In L.C. Andrist (Ed.), *Clinical issues in perinatal and women's health nursing.* Philadelphia, PA: Lippincott, p. 2.

Ledray, L.E. (1996). The sexual assault resource service: A new model of care. *Minnesota Medicine: A Journal of Clinical and Health Affairs, 79*(3):43-45.

Ledray, L.E. (1999). Sexual assault: Clinical issues: Date rape drug alert. *Journal of Emergency Nursing, 17*(1):1-2.

Ledray, L. (2005). Data on SANE programs crucial to refining the specialty, improving care. *Journal of Forensic Nursing, 3*(1):187-188.

Liebschutz, J., Battaglia, T., Finley, E., et al. (2008). Disclosing intimate partner violence to health care clinicians-what a difference the setting makes: A qualitative study. *BMC Public Health, 8*:229. Retrieved from http://www.biomedcentral.com/1471-2458/8/229

Logan, T.K., Cole, J., & Capillo, A. (2006). Program and sexual assault survivor characteristics for one SANE program. *Journal of Forensic Nursing, 2*(2):66-74.

Logan, T.K., Cole, J., & Capillo, A. (2007). Sexual assault nurse examiner program characteristics, barriers, and lessons learned. *Journal of Forensic Nursing, 3*(1):24-34.

Lynch, V.A. (1990). *Clinical forensic nursing: A descriptive study in role development.* Unpublished master's thesis. University of Texas Health Science Center at Arlington.

McDonough, E.T. (2006). Death investigation. In R.M. Hammer, B. Moynihan, & E.M. Pagliaro (Eds.), *Forensic nursing: A handbook for practice.* Boston, MA: Jones & Bartlett, pp. 401-485.

Minsky-Kelly, D., Hamberger, L.K., Pape, D.A., et al. (2005). We've had training, now what? Qualitative analysis of barriers to domestic violence screening and referral in a health care setting. *Journal of Interpersonal Violence, 20*(10):1288-1309.

Mosqueda, L., Burnight, K., & Liao, S. (2005). The life cycle of bruises in older adults. *Journal of the American Geriatrics Society, 53*(8):1339-1343.

Nash, K.R. & Sheridan, D.J. (2009). Can one accurately date a bruise? State of the science. *Journal of Forensic Nursing, 5*(1):31-37.

Olive, P. (2007). Care for emergency department patients who have experienced domestic violence: A review of the evidence base. *Journal of Clinical Nursing, 16*:1736-1748.

Pakieser, R.A., Lenaghan, P.A., & Muelleman, R.L. (1998). Battered women: Where they go for help. *Journal of Emergency Nursing, 24*(1):16-19.

Parker, B., & McFarlane, J. (1991). Nursing assessment of the battered pregnant woman. *Maternity Child Nursing Journal, 16*:161-164.

Patterson, D., Campbell, R., & Townsend, S.M. (2006). Sexual assault nurse examiner (SANE) program goals and patient care practices. *Journal of Nursing Scholarship, 38*(2):180-186.

Phelan, M.B. (2007). Screening for intimate partner violence in medical settings. *Trauma, Violence, & Abuse, 8*(2):199-213.

Plichta, S.B., Clements, P.T., & Houseman, C. (2007). Why SANEs matter: Models of care for sexual violence victims in the emergency department. *Journal of Forensic Nursing, 3*(1):15-23.

Reijnders, U.J.L., Giannakopoulos, G.F., & de Bruin, K.H. (2006). Assessment of abuse-related injuries: A comparative study of forensic physicians, emergency room physicians, emergency room nurses and medical students. *Journal of Forensic and Legal Medicine, 15*:15-19.

Sheridan, D.J. (1998). Health care-based programs for domestic violence survivors. In J.C. Campbell (Ed.), *Empowering survivors of abuse: Health care for battered women and their children.* Thousand Oaks, CA: Sage, pp. 23-31.

Sheridan, D.J. (2001). Treating survivors of intimate partner abuse: Forensic identification and documentation. In J.S.

Olshaker, M.C. Jackson, & W.S. Smock (Eds.), *Forensic emergency medicine*. Philadelphia: Lippincott, Williams, & Wilkins, pp. 203-228.

Sheridan, D.J. (2007). Treating survivors of intimate partner abuse. In J.S. Olshaker, M.C. Jackson, & W.S. Smock (Eds.), *Forensic emergency medicine* (2nd ed.). Philadelphia: Lippincott, Williams, & Wilkins, pp 203-228.

Sheridan, D.J., Nash, K.R., & Bresee, H. (2010). Forensic nursing in the emergency department. In P.K. Howard & R.A. Steinmann (Eds.), *Sheehy's emergency nursing: Principles and practice* (6th ed.). St. Louis, MO: Mosby-Elsevier, pp. 174-186.

Sheridan, D.J., Nash, K.R., Hawkins, S.L., et al. (2006). Forensic implications of intimate partner violence. In R.M. Hammer, B. Moynihan, & E.M. Pagliaro (Eds.), *Forensic nursing: A handbook for practice.* Boston, MA: Jones & Bartlett, pp. 255-274.

Sheridan, D.J., Nash, K.R., Poulos, C.A., et al. (2009). Soft tissue and cutaneous injury patterns. In C. Mitchell & D. Anglin (Eds.), *Intimate partner violence: A health based perspective.* New York: Oxford University Press, pp. 237-252.

Sheridan, D.J. & Taylor, W.K. (1993). Developing hospital-based domestic violence programs, protocols, policies, and procedures. *AWHONS Clinical Issues Perinatal Womens Health Nursing. 4*(3):471.

Shoffner, D.H. (2008). We don't like to think about it. Intimate partner violence during pregnancy and postpartum. *Journal of Perinatal & Neonatal Nursing, (22)*1:39-48.

Sievers, V. (2003). Sexual assault evidence collection more accurate when completed by sexual assault nurse examiners: Colorado's experience. *Journal of Emergency Nursing, 29*(6):511-514.

Soeken, K.L., McFarlane, J., Parker, B., et al. (1998). The Abuse Assessment Screen: A clinical instrument to measure frequency, severity, and perpetrator of abuse against women. In J.C. Campbell (ed.), *Empowering survivors of abuse: Health care for battered women and their children.* Thousand Oaks: CA: Sage, pp. 195-203.

Spangaro, J., Zwi, A.B., & Poulos, R. (2009). The elusive search for definitive evidence on routine screening for intimate partner violence. *Trauma, Violence, & Abuse, (10)*1:55-68.

Speck, P., & Aiken, M. (1995). 20 years of community nursing service. *Tennessee Nurse, 58*(2):5.

Strack, G.B., McClane, G.E., & Hawley, D. (2001). A review of 300 attempted strangulation cases. *Journal of Emergency Nursing, 21*(3):303.

Sternac, L., Dunlap, H., & Bainbridge, D. (2005). Sexual assault services delivered by SANEs. *Journal of Forensic Nursing, 1*(3):124-128.

Taliaferro, E., Hawley, D., McClane, G., et al. (2009). Strangulation in intimate partner violence. In C. Mitchell and D. Anglin (Eds.), *Intimate partner violence: A health-based perspective.* New York: Oxford University Press.

Thurston, W.E., & Eisener, A.C. (2006). Successful integration and maintenance of screening for domestic violence in the health sector. *Trauma, Violence, & Abuse, 7*(2):83-92.

Trautman, D.E., McCarthy, M.L., Miller, N., et al. (2007). Intimate partner violence and emergency department screening: Computerized screening versus usual care. *Annals of Emergency Medicine, 49*(4):526-534.

Violence Against Women Act. (2005). Title II—Improving services for victims of domestic violence, sexual assault, and stalking. H.R. 3402-34 – H.R. 3402-70. Retrieved August 29, 2009, from http://www.google.com/search? hl=en&source=hp&q=vawa+2005&aq=3&oq=VAWA& aqi=g4g-s1g1g-s1g3

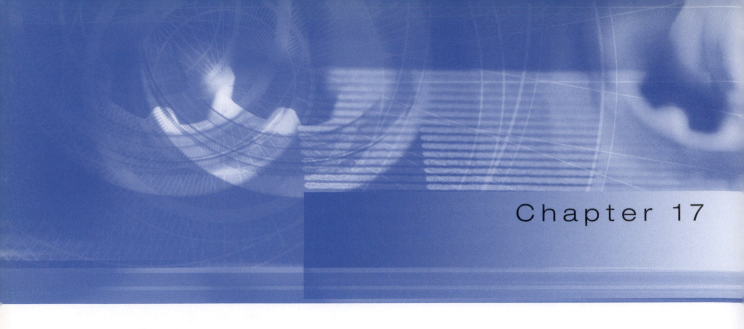

Chapter 17

ELDER ABUSE

Joyce P. Williams, Kathleen Thimsen, Angela Primeau,
Jocelyn Anderson, and David Williams

*"Everything that can be counted does not necessarily count; everything
that counts cannot necessarily be counted."*

Albert Einstein

Competencies

1. Describing the types of elder maltreatment, the category of abusers, and how abuse is perpetrated.
2. Recognizing risks and identifying injuries consistent with elder abuse.
3. Describing characteristics of adult vulnerable populations.
4. Identifying physiological changes associated with aging.
5. Differentiating between the Air Force patient screening model and civilian examples of screening.
6. Citing current research and best practices pertaining to intervention strategies.
7. Predicting risk factors for elder neglect.
8. Contrasting the differences between elder neglect and self-neglect.
9. Naming the most likely perpetrators of elder neglect.
10. Comparing reporting mechanisms among agencies.
11. Distinguishing the best practice to determine cause of death in the elderly.

Key Terms

Abandonment
Abuse
Ageism
Aging
Caregiver
Delirium
Elder maltreatment
Emotional abuse
Financial exploitation
Injury
Medical-legal autopsy
Neglect
Physical abuse
Polypharmacy
Respite care
Self-neglect
Sexual abuse
Social interaction
Social isolation

INTRODUCTION

The recognition of elder abuse and abuse of those nearing the end of life while providing routine health care is a means of primary prevention that can decrease the prevalence of abuse-related morbidity and mortality. Elder abuse identification did not become recognized as an issue until the 1970s. Researchers in England first made note of inadequate care provided to elders in the literature in 1975, with attention given to the topic in the United States following the 1978 Congressional hearings on domestic abuse.

Elder maltreatment, also referred to as **abuse** or neglect, may involve a single or repeated act of harm or distress against an elder by someone who is in a position of trust or responsibility. It is an issue thought to be a social dysfunction related to the population of the aging and their caregivers. There is limited literature on elder maltreatment, which has now become a public health problem across all communities and nations. Additionally, statistics on the health of the senior population are limited and thus not accurate enough to provide assistance in identifying potential vulnerabilities in an aging society. Erlingsson's (2007) review of the literature and study of evidence-based practices reported since the 1960s yielded a meta-analysis of 49 studies of elder maltreatment, identifying categories of abusers and how the abuse was perpetrated. However, only seven of the studies (14%) incorporated consistent use of reliable and valid data points and measurement tools. Limitations noted in the analysis were attributed to underreporting and a lack of standardized, objective reporting mechanisms. Yet, global reports showed a significant prevalence and incidence of maltreatment across numerous nations and diverse populations.

The National Center on Elder Abuse (NCEA) commissioned a National Elder Abuse Incidence Study (NEAIS) to estimate the incidence of abuse against elders and found approximately 450,000 older people were being abused in the United States in 1996. This number will likely grow as the predicted increase in the number of persons over the age of 65 is estimated to double over the next 30 years. In fact, the number of persons over the age of 65 is projected to be 25% of the U.S. population by 2050. As the senior population increases, so does the potential for elder maltreatment.

The identification of elder abuse has lagged in comparison with that of child abuse. For example, the first peer-reviewed article addressing child abuse by Kempe was published in 1962. Yet, it was not until 1975 that Baker and Burston first referred to the occurrence of elder abuse as "granny battering." The seminal work done by Baker and Burston created awareness of the problem and exposed the fact that older, vulnerable persons are prime targets for maltreatment.

Aging, or the process of growing old, has long been associated with a perception that advancing age is accompanied by chronic illnesses, altered mental status, frailty, and dependence on others for care. While these thoughts are stereotypical, the potential for vulnerability does exist and is quite high. Vulnerability makes those no longer able to advocate for or protect themselves prime targets for elder maltreatment.

A GLOBAL PROBLEM

The average age of the general population is increasing, with a projected global population of 1.2 billion people over the age of 60 by 2025, 80% of them living in the developing world. Increased education and awareness is required for all professionals to decrease the worldwide incidence and prevalence of elder homicides and abuse. Identification of warning signs or dangers associated with injury in elders is needed to aid in the prosecution of crimes against the elderly and to prevent injury and death. Throughout the world, abuse and neglect of older persons is largely under-recognized or simply disregarded. Unfortunately, no community or country in the world is immune from this costly public health and human rights crisis.

There is scant evidence-based practice literature addressing elder abuse. Statistical information on elder abuse has increased as awareness becomes more widespread, and educational programs and institutional guidelines mandate assessment and screening. However, research efforts and laws for the prevention of abuse toward the elderly continue to develop slowly. While some countries include abuse of the elderly under their legal statutes and have fully developed systems for reporting and treating cases of abuse, others have a much more limited response. Elders are vulnerable to a myriad of threats and negative events that begs for sensitization of the public to thwart the unnecessary exploitation of the elderly in all regions. Elder abuse and neglect is a hidden, unrecognized, and undiscussed matter. Raising awareness is promoted globally through Annual World Elder Abuse Awareness Day (WEAAD), first held in 2006, by the International Network for the Prevention of Elder Abuse (INPEA). Yet, in developing countries, there is no systematic collection of statistics or prevalence studies, crime or social welfare records, journalistic reports, or studies that provide scientific evidence that abuse, neglect, and financial exploitation of older people appear to be widely prevalent.

Normal Aging and Related Changes

There are several theories on aging that form the basis of defining and understanding the process. Zarit referred to biological aging as the structural and functional changes of the body occurring across the continuum. The basis of biological aging involves cell biology, replication, and mutation, which ultimately creates changes in bodily performance. The effect of free radicals from the environment alters metabolism of nutrients and production and absorption of vitamins, minerals, and other chemicals required for physical sustainability. Orgel proposed the error theory: this theory advances the idea that an error in protein synthesis is the first step in aging, illness, and death.

Another theory, on functional aging, by Birren and Renner involves the capacity of an individual to interact with others of the same age. They also described the roles and social habits of individuals in society as the sociological aging theory. Individual behavior, self-perception, and reaction to bodily changes are described by Gress and Bahr as psychological aging, whereas Stallwood and Stoll examined spirituality related to aging, focusing on relationships, the interaction of self with others, place of self in the world, and the self's worldview.

Nursing professionals should be knowledgeable about the theories of aging to critically evaluate findings of assessments. Assessing aging individuals may not include a focused or specific examination or evaluation of abuse; however, clinicians must bear in mind the potential for abuse in the presence of observed findings that are outside the usual and expected presenting signs, symptoms, complaints, and conditions. **Injury** (physical harm to the body or a body part) or alterations may be written off as age-related changes, when in fact the cause of the injury may actually be from abuse or neglect. The nurse, being an advocate, should fully assess and document the physical findings while also questioning the patient and caregivers about the injuries. It is necessary to compare location of injuries, responses, gestures, and consistency in the explanations with communicated explanations. However, one drawback to using this approach involves the lack of a reliable tool to use in patient examinations and interviews. Other factors include availability of adequate time to perform a comprehensive evaluation, as well as the skill level and competency of the nurse.

The physiological changes of aging and associated findings may also place individuals in a vulnerable state. Decline in health, mental, and mobility status decreases independence and accordingly increases dependency upon others. Being dependent creates not only the need for assistance and attention, but also increases the individual's response to the changes in life circumstances. Many individuals in dependent situations simply succumb to the lifestyle changes and become complacent, withdrawn, and tolerant of their plight, thereby becoming targets for abuse. Persons living in this type of environment often believe that living in a home-type environment, regardless of the tone and circumstances, is preferred over being "sent" to a nursing home. Yet, today's assisted living and supported living environments offer assistance in maintaining some degree of independence for as long as possible. Conditions that lead to facility placement are often due to the severe loss of self-care abilities. In fact, mobility, activity, and cognitive impairment are the leading causes of placement in a long-term care facility.

As seniors become immobile or inactive, there is decreased production of important growth factors and chemical nutrients that are necessary to sustain a healthy body. The physical, social, and mental functions also decline and result in diminished activity and mobility. Furthermore, mood dictates the level of **social interaction** (a dynamic, changing sequence of social actions between individuals or groups), which has been shown to decline after placement. Prolonged, unidentified, and untreated depression further exacerbates the vicious cycle of deterioration and may heighten dependence on others. Additionally, Rubin described the physiological changes related to bedrest, listing the many system-by-system alterations observed in healthy individuals after being restricted to bed.

Sensory alterations in the elderly also play a critical role in the health decline of the individual. Visual impairments such as cataracts, macular degeneration, and glaucoma change the behavior of a senior, contributing to mental and physical deterioration. For example, as visual acuity declines, appetite suffers as the individual eats less because of the inability to see the plate, utensils, and food. Decreased taste and smell sensory function contribute to anorexia that results in weight loss. Weight loss then brings about changes in the mouth, leading to dentures not fitting properly. Resulting nutritional deficiencies and hydration deficits place additional burdens on the gastrointestinal and renal systems, resulting in an accelerated cycle of decline. Additionally, the loss of auditory sensitivity results in withdrawal from social contact related to being unable to hear or only partially hear conversations; therefore, social interactions decrease. Often a senior with altered hearing may be thought to be demented based on inappropriate responses to questions or contributions to a conversation.

Medications used in the treatment of medical conditions in the elderly play an important role in restoring or maintaining health. Side effects of individual medications or the compounded interactions of multiple drugs, also referred to as **polypharmacy,** can result in deteriorating disorders and conditions. Toon presented his work on delirium and the anticholinergic effects of some medications, which can cause physical and mental impairment. Commonly prescribed medications (Box 17.1) create a disruption in the transfer of information through the synaptic channel. Drug molecules then accumulate and block the information being sent. This can present as symptoms of delirium and dementia-related behaviors, when in fact, they are simply side effects of a medication.

Delirium is an acute onset of confusion, disorientation, withdrawal, and lethargy. Instances of untreated and unresolved delirium can lead to what is interpreted as dementia.

Withdrawal of medications with anticholinergic effects may cause physical symptoms to worsen and additional symptoms to be present. The symptoms commonly associated with withdrawal are nausea, vomiting, diarrhea, tachycardia, bradycardia, as well as changes in respiratory rate and effort. Altered gait, communication disturbances, and hallucinations may also occur. These symptoms are temporary and will resolve once the accumulated molecular particles of the medication clear the synaptic junctions.

Comorbid conditions and treatments may create dysfunction in behaviors and systemic interactions that often render the elderly to a compromised state. It is critical for the forensic nurse to be knowledgeable about normal human physiology and the physiology of aging to detect and evaluate abuse and neglect in presenting signs and symptoms that may incorrectly be attributed simply to being elderly.

Box 17.1   Commonly Prescribed Medications for the Elderly

- Cimetadine
- Prednisolone
- Theophylline
- Ranitidine
- Nifedipine
- Furosemide
- Dipyridamole
- Codeine
- Captopril
- Warfarin
- Isosorbide

PREVALENCE AND TRENDS IN ELDER MALTREATMENT

It has been estimated that one to two million Americans over the age of 65 have been injured, exploited, or mistreated by someone on whom they depended for care or protection. Lachs and Pillmer found that 2% to 10% of elders are victims of some form of abuse. They include a disclaimer that the actual frequency is unable to be determined due to the lack of standardized methods of data collection and reporting. National reporting organizations and bureaus use various forms, data points, and reporting methods, which make it difficult to obtain a full understanding of the issue. The National Research Council (NRC) reported that no survey of the U.S. population has been done that can provide an estimate for the actual incidence of elder maltreatment.

DESCRIPTION OF THE ADULT VULNERABLE POPULATION

The NCEA report in 2003 indicated that the mean age of persons described as having been maltreated was 77.9 years. Self-neglect case reports indicate an average age of 77.4 years. In the United States, 66.4% of adult domestic abuse victims were white, 18.7% black, and 10.4% Hispanic. According to the U.S. Department of Justice (2006), the most frequent form of maltreatment is the violation of the right of decision making, by limiting free choice and the individual's right to self-determination.

DEFINITION OF ELDER MALTREATMENT

The NCEA defines seven different types of elder maltreatment (see Box 17.2). Categories of elder maltreatment are based on an analysis of the U. S. federal and state definitions that are now adopted by the NCEA.

Box 17.2   Types of Elder Maltreatment

- Physical abuse
- Emotional abuse
- Sexual abuse
- Financial exploitation
- Neglect
- Abandonment
- Self-neglect

Physical abuse is defined as the use of physical force that may result in bodily injury, physical pain, or impairment. Physical abuse may include, but is not limited to, such acts of violence as striking (with or without an object), hitting, beating, pushing, shoving, shaking, slapping, kicking, pinching, and burning. In addition, inappropriate use of drugs and physical restraints, force-feeding, and physical punishment of any kind also are also examples of physical abuse (Box 17.3).

Box 17.3 Signs of Maltreatment

- Bruises, black eyes, welts, lacerations, and rope marks
- Bone fractures, broken bones, and skull fractures
- Open wounds, cuts, punctures, untreated injuries in various stages of healing
- Sprains, dislocations, and internal injuries and bleeding
- Broken eyeglasses and frames, physical signs of being subjected to punishment, and signs of being restrained
- Laboratory findings of medication overdose or underutilization of prescribed drugs
- An elder's report of being hit, slapped, kicked, or mistreated
- An elder's sudden change in behavior
- Suicide attempt
- Evidence of alcohol or drug abuse
- The caregiver's refusal to allow visitors to see an elder alone

Sexual abuse is defined as nonconsensual sexual contact of any kind with an elderly person. Sexual contact with any person incapable of giving consent is also considered sexual abuse. It includes, but is not limited to, unwanted touching and all types of sexual assault or battery such as rape, sodomy, coerced nudity, and sexually explicit photography (see Box 17.4).

Emotional or psychological abuse is defined as the infliction of anguish, pain, or distress through verbal or nonverbal acts. Emotional/psychological abuse includes, but is not limited to, verbal assaults, insults, threats, intimidation, humiliation, and harassment. In addition, treating an older person like an infant; isolating an elderly person from his/her family, friends, or regular activities; giving an older person the "silent treatment"; and enforced **social isolation** (lack of contact with other human beings) are examples of emotional/psychological abuse. Confinement is also considered to be in the category of emotional abuse.

Box 17.4 Specific Signs and Symptoms of Elder Maltreatment

- Bruises around the breasts or genital area
- Unexplained venereal disease or genital infections
- Unexplained vaginal or anal bleeding
- Torn, stained, or bloody underclothing
- An elder's report of being sexually assaulted

Case Study

PARENTAL ABUSE BY FAMILY MEMBER WITH MENTAL ILLNESS

Harold is an 87-year-old widower living alone until his son Leo moves in to care for him. After 3 months, Harold is withdrawn, will not engage in eye contact, and has lost his eyeglasses. The ladies at his church bring him lunch on Sundays after the service. Over the last 4 weeks, Leo has told the church ladies that his father does not have an appetite and that they should stop bringing food. One of the ladies asks to see and talk to Harold. The son states that his father is napping; however, the ladies hear Harold calling for help. Leo still denies them entrance and slams the door in their faces. The ladies then call 911 and ask the police to check on Harold. The son denies the police access at first, but then allows them in after much discussion. The police find Harold in a chair in his bedroom. He is barely clothed, is covered with feces and urine, and is calling

out for help. Closer inspection finds him tied to the chair with belts and his arms and hands restrained with shoelaces. Harold is removed from the home and taken to the ED. Radiographs reveal that he has multiple healed fractures to both arms. Leo is taken into custody. Leo was homeless prior to his moving in with Harold. He has substance abuse problems and has untreated mental illness. He needed housing, shelter, and food to stay alive. He did not feel that living off of his father was at all abusive. Harold was returned to his home with the assistance of community care workers. Leo was court-ordered to a rehabilitation halfway house and ordered to have no further contact with his father. Harold returned home after a short stay in the hospital to resume his previous social life and was no longer suffering from the abuse and depression.

The abuser exerts power and control over the free will and social interactions of the older person.

Neglect is defined as the refusal or failure to fulfill obligations or duties to an elder for whom one is responsible. This may include neglect to provide financially for an elder or to ensure that safe housing, adequate food and water, clothing, and health-care needs are met.

Self-neglect is defined as behavior of an elderly person that threatens his or her own health or safety. A senior may refuse or fail to provide appropriate food, water, shelter, clothing, hygiene, medication, or safe living conditions for himself or herself. This involves a person's right to self-determination and creates a dilemma when an individual has impaired cognition, mental illness, or diminished decision-making capabilities. Each person has the right to self-determination, but when conditions and maladies diminish decision-making capacity, caregivers must determine the safest, most appropriate way to legally protect an individual from himself or herself. Self-neglect signs and symptoms should be evaluated during the assessment, as self-neglect is considered a reportable case of adult maltreatment. Interventions should begin with a comprehensive psychosocial evaluation in the presence of any of the findings seen in Box 17.5.

Box 17.5 Indicators of Need for Psychosocial Intervention

- Dehydration, malnutrition, untreated or improperly attended medical conditions, and poor personal hygiene
- Hazardous or unsafe living conditions/arrangements (e.g., improper wiring, no indoor plumbing, no heat, no running water)
- Unsanitary or unclean living quarters (e.g., animal/insect infestation, no functioning toilet, fecal/urine smell)
- Inappropriate and/or inadequate clothing, lack of the necessary medical aids (e.g., eyeglasses, hearing aids, dentures)
- Grossly inadequate housing or homelessness

Financial and material exploitation involves inappropriate use of an elder's funds, properties, or assets (Box 17.6). Families that have a vested interest in the financial arrangements of the elder person may take advantage of and exploit him or her in several ways: borrowing money using the excuse of buying food for the senior or helping to pay bills or using the senior's home and income to sustain a lifestyle otherwise not obtainable under the guise

Case Study

SELF-NEGLECT

Eileen is an 84-year-old widow, living alone in a mobile home, who has degenerative disc disease, COPD, and loss of mobility that requires her to use a wheelchair or walker. Eileen has a community caseworker who checks on her every 3 months (minimum state requirement). She is found repeatedly to be sitting in her wheelchair for days at a time, on a continuous basis. Eileen also has a history of not using her heating or air conditioning due to "not wanting to waste money," even in times of severe changes in temperature. A neighbor, who checks on Eileen once a week, provides food. On the last two encounters, the caseworker has found her on the floor, under her wheelchair. Eileen refuses emergent care or medical examination, as she fears nursing home placement. The last encounter required that a homecare nurse be called to assess Eileen as the temperature of the home was 107 degrees and the air conditioning was not being used. The nurse's evaluation revealed that Eileen had a body temperature of 103 degrees with a pulse of 130 and blood pressure of 70/30. It was also apparent to the

nurse that Eileen had fallen from her wheelchair several days before and had not been able to call for help. She had been incontinent of bowel and bladder. Her skin turgor was poor, with tenting for greater than 3 seconds. She had not had food or hydration for several days. She was in a right side-lying position. The wheelchair was on top of her, pinning her down and making it impossible to move. When the wheelchair was removed, findings revealed a pressure ulcer to the right side of the body that was evident to be the frame impression of her wheelchair. The left side of her body also showed signs of pressure ulcers to the shoulder, arm, hip, knee, and foot. Some areas of skin breakdown also showed necrosis of the tissue. Eileen refused to go to the ED: she cried, yelled, and pleaded to not have to go. EMS arrived, but she adamantly refused to go for evaluation and fluid rescue. The caseworker was advocating for Eileen by arranging for an increase in home services. The nurse knew that the patient needed emergency medical care or she would likely die. The nurse decided that Eileen had the right to refuse care but only if she was fully

(case study continued on page 332)

Case Study

aware of the consequences. The nurse decided to explain the options available to her so that she could indeed make an informed decision. The options set forth were to do nothing, stay in the home, but use air conditioning, hydrate, and eat three meals and snacks a day. The consequences of this decision would allow her to stay in her home, but due to the wounds and hydration status that were evident she would likely die. Another option was to go to the ED, be treated, and then transition to a rehabilitation facility for short-term therapy with a possible return to home. A third scenario involved a referral to hospice so that she could stay home and would not have to eat or drink unless she wanted to, but she would likely die within days. The final discussion with Eileen reiterated that she had options and the final decision was up to her. She then said, "I don't want to die; I will go to the hospital. I really didn't know that I was that sick."

of being there to "help" the parent or grandparent. A common method used to exploit seniors is to tell them that they owe money for repairs or bills, when in reality there are no bills or payments that need to be made. Another instance of exploitation of the vulnerable occurs when the "caregiver" family member or a stranger moves into the home; uses the income of the person; and denies the rightful senior food, water, hygiene, or health care. It is in this type of circumstance that, if the senior is hospitalized with a poor prognosis or grim outcome, often the abuser will request that extreme measures and life-prolonging activities be used. The rationale is that if the senior dies, access to the income

and living environment being exploited by the abuser will also be gone. This is one of the most unfortunate scenarios related to exploitation. There are a variety of common occurrences that are strong indicators of maltreatment.

Abandonment is the desertion of an elder (by whomever is responsible for the elder) in an environment that is not known or familiar to the person. Abandonment may be intentional or self-induced. Reports in the media have highlighted the plight of cognitively impaired elders who unintentionally leave home and cannot determine where they are or where their home is. Intentional abandonment occurs when a **caregiver,** someone who has primary responsibility for care of another, deliberately leaves the elder. This intentional and deliberate act of abandonment may be for personal gain or control over the elder. Interviewing the patient and/or responsible party, if found, is the only means to determine intent. Abandonment includes:

- Leaving the senior alone at a hospital, a nursing facility, or other similar institution without explanation or identifying information;
- Deserting an elder at a shopping center or other public location
- Reporting by an elder that he or she has been abandoned

Elder maltreatment cases can be multifaceted. Typical cases involve various types of maltreatment and events that make it difficult to identify the abuse in limited clinical or investigative encounters. Current investigation procedures and documentation will be discussed later in this chapter to exhibit the need for advancing research on scientific and clinically relevant parameters for reliable documentation of the maltreatment.

AGEISM

Ageism involves discrimination or prejudice against a particular age group. It is a contributing factor to elder

---

Box 17.6 Indicators of Elder Financial Exploitation

- Sudden changes in bank account or banking practice, including an unexplained withdrawal of large sums of money by a person accompanying the elder
- The inclusion of additional names on an elder's bank signature card
- Unauthorized withdrawal of the elder's funds using the elder's ATM card
- Abrupt changes in a will or other financial documents
- Unexplained disappearance of funds or valuable possessions
- Substandard care being provided or bills unpaid despite the availability of adequate financial resources
- Discovery of an elder's signature being forged for financial transactions or for the titles of his/her possessions
- Sudden appearance of previously uninvolved relatives claiming their rights to an elder's affairs and possessions
- Unexplained sudden transfer of assets to a family member or someone outside the family
- The provision of services that are not necessary
- An elder's report of financial exploitation

Case Study

ELDER MALTREATMENT BY A FAMILY MEMBER

Velma is an 88-year-old widow who resides in a federally funded housing project. Velma had become frail and had limited mobility, which prevented her from being able to ambulate outside of her home. A concerned neighbor had contacted Velma's doctor to request a homecare nurse. The nurse made the initial visit and found that Velma was bedfast in a second floor bedroom. The remainder of the house's first and second floor was inhabited by Velma's grandson and his friends. Velma's bed had a broken bed frame, which created a permanent Trendelenburg position. She had cans that she used for her toileting needs. The bedroom was infested with roaches and mice. It was evident that her right ankle wound was the result of a rat bite and that the rat had continued to gnaw at the necrotic tissue. Adult Protective Services was notified. The grandson had been collecting Velma's Social Security checks and was using them for his own benefit. The grandson also was living in Velma's home uninvited and unwelcome. Velma's rationale for not calling the authorities was that "at least I am in my own home."

This case demonstrates multiple forms of maltreatment that many elders are subjected to because they are not in a protective environment.

maltreatment and may help to explain underreporting and underidentification of victims of abuse and neglect. Early work done by Butler (1980) discussed the impressions and beliefs about aging. His coining of the word *ageist* refers to "the evaluative judgments toward a person or persons simply due to advanced age," which presumes that a vulnerable adult may be undertreated/overtreated and receive biased care and treatment, based solely on their advanced age. Attitudes toward old age were also discussed by Tuckman and Lorge in earlier works on the attitudes toward aging persons. A comprehensive and valid tool was devised to measure misconceptions and stereotypes about aged persons. The tool had 137 statements that were related to personality traits, physical characteristics, mental deterioration, and life questions. Results revealed that nearly all subjects believed that most elderly people are set in their ways and are conservative. Additionally, lack of attention to personal hygiene was a behavior unanimously agreed upon as being associated with being old. Although Tuckman and Lorge's work is not commonly used, their report of biased attitudes against the elderly is noteworthy. Furthermore, development of additional tools over five decades has resulted in such findings as having others complete one's sentences is more common for the older population than for any other stage of life. Additionally, Palmore's "Facts on Aging Quiz 1 and 2" are still in use today and are highly influential in aging sensitivity training. Palmore's work (1977) should be considered in the context of elder maltreatment because it brings forth the unconscious values and beliefs that people have toward the elderly by persons who regard themselves as "pro-ageists."

There is scant research on how seniors live, function, and maintain their independence. Many are health-oriented adults who are active socially, partake in mentally engaging lifestyles, and live independently or in retirement communities. Yet, common beliefs are that the majority of older adults reside in a long-term care facility, are completely dependent on others, and are socially withdrawn, and are either limited to a chair or are bedfast. This stereotypical belief is a stark contrast to reality in that less than 20% of seniors actually reside in a long-term care facility with round-the-clock care.

CLINICAL INTERVENTIONS

There are several key interventions that clinicians may use regarding elder maltreatment. Knowledge about conditions that increase the risk of abuse, indicators, context of abuse, and perpetrators are imperative to the clinicians' interpretation of clinical findings and physiological changes that may constitute maltreatment. The NCEA noted serious limitations on clinician knowledge regarding the risks, indicators, context of abuse, and perpetrator characteristics due to the lack of standardized protocols and assessment parameters on elder maltreatment. Limitations also include the lack of training and education for health-care providers in the recognition of characteristics that are hallmarks of maltreatment. Trained health-care providers are needed to ensure that abuse is properly identified and addressed.

Physiological, psychosocial, and emotional changes often associated with advancing age complicate identification of abuse or neglect. Many health conditions include signs and symptoms that may be presenting phenomena of abuse or neglect. Bruising, falls, fractures, or skin lesions identified with physical assessment are written off as minor complaints, side effects of medication, or complications of dementia or fragility. Also, findings associated with incontinence, falls, memory loss, and depression may be attributed to older age and dismissed. The same symptoms, when found in a younger population, would likely warrant a higher level of concern and be more likely to receive a work-up and discussion of treatment options. Rost and Frankel analyzed medical encounters of elderly patients ($n = 100$, ages 60 or older) and found that most were not successful in raising important medical and psychosocial problems in the context of health-care encounters. Health-care providers did not prompt patients to talk about new symptoms. If the patient did bring an issue to the health-care provider's attention, the issue was not explored thoroughly nor was there discussion or collaborative decision making. An example is an elderly woman who presents to her caregiver, who then reports that the patient had a fall. She has black eyes, multiple contusions, and bruised areas on her forearms. She weighs 78 pounds—10% less than she did at the previous medical encounter 6 months ago. Health-care providers often see such findings as age-related conditions and may not consider further investigation from a perspective of potential abuse.

A high-risk indicator of abuse for clinicians to be aware of includes social isolation of persons with or without short-term or permanent cognitive impairment. Also, recent change in circumstances or lifelong situations may also increase the chances of maltreatment. Additionally, elders with a personal or family history of domestic violence are at an increased risk for abuse and neglect. Examination of the aging person's experiences and interactions with family or caregivers with a history of personal or domestic violence may indicate dysfunction in the caring process that results in maltreatment. A qualitative phenomenological research study on abuse in residential and home care settings, where care was being provided by professional, licensed caregivers, showed that much abuse in residential centers is actually perpetrated by nurses, aides, and administrators in ways that they did not consider abusive. The maltreatment was justified as appropriate caregiver response, for example in response to a resident's behavioral outbursts, not following directions, or not being a "good" resident—one who is obedient. Responses were listed as threats to withhold care, food, water, social contact, or housing. Other responses included blatant disregard for providing personal hygiene, privacy, dignity, forcing activities, and by not addressing or relieving pain. None of the caregivers considered their responses to be intentional abuse.

Interpersonal relationships with family or caregivers that revolve around money and assets should also be evaluated. Financial well-being coupled with frailty creates a ripe medium for financial exploitation, which often accompanies other forms of maltreatment.

Longevity, quality, and value of an older person's life are concerns that will continue to be high priority as the fastest-growing sector of the population turns 60. Technological advances, medical innovations, improved treatments, and health promotion activities will all extend the life span. Eradication of diseases and maladies that once led to morbidity and mortality now add to longevity and create an extended timeline in which elders may become more and more vulnerable to maltreatment.

HEALTH-CARE PROVIDER TRAINING

In the United States, elder maltreatment investigators currently receive initial training, with updates on an annual basis. One training manual is a publication by Pritchard that incorporates role-playing, case examples and studies, handouts, exercises, and simulations. This training manual is a primer on identification and intervention in elder maltreatment. The manual is used for all investigators and case workers who perform evaluations after a complaint or those who do follow-up and surveillance on a continuing basis after a report has been filed. Elder abuse investigators typically perform their responsibilities under the state's department of public health, public aid, or Adult Protective Services. Laws and regulations that guide care, staffing, handling of complaints, and investigations are governed by state and federal regulations. Having regulatory and legal foundations affords thorough investigations and appropriate intervention activities, including civil and criminal penalties for harm, injury, or death of an elder.

SCREENING AND ASSESSMENT PROTOCOLS

Many states do not have standard data collection protocols, examination and observation tools, or procedures that objectively assign or dismiss a case complaint. However, the protocols of the U.S. Air Force (USAF) have had success in early intervention. The protocols used by the USAF require that all patients presenting for care in a military hospital or dental clinic be screened by asking the patient, guardian, or caregiver if there has been any abuse or neglect within the past year. If the answer is "yes" or if the health-care provider has a reasonable suspicion that abuse or neglect is occurring, then further investigation is initiated.

The USAF program emphasizes the importance of health-care providers' education in the identification of maltreatment and appropriate treatment options. Dental professionals in particular can be helpful in identifying maltreatment since 60% of abuse injuries occur in the head region. Also, abusers may "doctor shop" to avoid detection, but they often overlook dental professionals as identifiers and mandated reporters of abuse.

Protocols and procedures call for social service consultation to examine the psychosocial aspects of the patient's living environment. Relationships and history of interpersonal or domestic violence are also discussed. An investigational team effort facilitates the process, eliminates redundancy, and yields a comprehensive evaluation.

In the presence of physical signs or symptoms, the health-care provider performs a physical examination that provides the basis of diagnostic testing for further identification, intervention, and treatment. The examination should be performed by a health-care provider using a standardized approach. Standardized procedures for assessment and documentation will minimize repetition and embarrassment for patients during the health-care visit, while paying special attention to injuries that may be found.

INTAKE AND PROCESSING OF ADULT MALTREATMENT COMPLAINTS

The literature, along with surveys to 12 states, revealed that the procedure for reporting elder maltreatment is fairly universal. A universal reporting mechanism is often initiated by an anonymous complaint called in to a toll-free number designated as the "elder abuse hotline." Complaints are taken using a set of standardized basic questions about the individual suspected of being abused, details of the situation, where the person resides, who resides with him or her, who the suspected perpetrator is, and how a follow-up investigator can locate the alleged victim and suspected perpetrator. Self-neglect reports are also called into the abuse hotline, despite being self-induced, and are still considered a reportable event. Suspected abuse or neglect of any kind warrants investigation that is overseen by state agencies under the Department of Health and Human Services. However, despite regulatory guidance and mandated reporting, there continues to be a gap in a standardized tool for investigation. Thus, each state conducts investigations, documentation, and follow-up according to their own set of protocols. Creating standardization across U.S. agencies investigating elder neglect and abuse cases would provide a consistent and reliable method of investigating reports, prosecuting perpetrators, and enhancing safety for elders.

The second step in the process involves assigning an investigator to the complaint that comes through the hotline. The investigator will follow up and inquire further into the nature of the maltreatment, safety issues, and the potential for violence or life-threatening living conditions for the elderly person. As part of their inquiry, investigators make home visits to evaluate the living quarters of the elderly person and interview caregivers suspected of abuse. Complaints originating in a long-term care facility or skilled nursing facility are referred to a surveyor from the state's department of public health in the nursing home investigation division for follow-up.

When a caregiver is suspected of maltreatment of or violence against a senior, the investigator may be met with hostility, threats, and possibly violent behavior. It is also common for a caregiver to deny the investigator access to the residence or an opportunity to interview the elderly person.

Case Study

FINANCIAL ABUSE AND NEGLECT LEADING TO DEATH

Maria is an 88-year-old female who is being "cared for" by her 52-year-old son. Maria and her deceased husband were retired and had accrued a comfortable and ample retirement savings and pensions. The couple had also invested in property that was valued at $1.5 million. Neighbors were concerned about her and discussed their concerns over coffee at the parish that Maria had previously attended. The concerned parties called into the elder abuse hotline to report that Maria had not been seen for several months. Her usual activities included walking around her flower garden and also out to the street to get the mail. James was an unmarried son who had lived several miles from Maria but who recently had lost his job, home, and car. He had moved in with his mother "to care for and look after her" approximately 5 months earlier. When neighbors attempted to visit or bring food to Maria, they were met with hostility and aggressive behaviors by James, including denial of visitation with his mother. Upon the initial visit to the home, the investigator was met with hostility to his introduction and reason for the home visit. The investigator could see Maria sitting on the couch looking thin and frail, but watching the television. The house was in disarray,

(case study continued on page 336)

Case Study

FINANCIAL ABUSE AND NEGLECT LEADING TO DEATH (continued)

with trash, soiled dishes, and clothes laying on the floor and on chairs in the living room. The investigator left, but told James that he would visit again. Several weeks later the investigator called on Maria at home. James again refused him entry or permission to talk with Maria. During this visit, it was noted that Maria was not sitting on the couch, but seemed to be slouched over and partly hanging over the side of the seat cushions. The house had a peculiar odor that permeated through the open door. The investigator noted seven kittens and two large cats. The investigator felt that his observation of Maria showed a decline, and the living conditions had also deteriorated. The odor from the house was also of a putrid nature. Law enforcement was called and met the investigator at the home of Maria. When James opened the door, he was abusive and then became violent and threatened to kill the police and the investigator. This was the key to legally obtaining entrance into the home. James was arrested for threatening the police and investigator. Maria was found on the couch in a febrile state, delirious and lacking in hygiene for an undetermined amount of time. Maria's skin turgor revealed severe dehydration. EMS was called to the scene. The paramedics attempted to move Maria from the couch to the stretcher and were taken aback by finding that the

couch cushions were imbedded into her back and buttocks. Human excrement, along with a pressure ulcer, complicated removal of the cushions. Once Maria had been fluid rescued in the ED, she was taken to surgery for surgical excision of the cushions and extensive wound débridement. Maria weighed 72 pounds; her hospital admission weight was 136 pounds approximately 1 year earlier for hip replacement surgery. Maria presented with a 64-pound weight loss, which calculates to a 47% decrease in body weight. (The American Society of Parenteral and Enteral Nutrition [ASPEN] definition of malnutrition is greater than 10% unplanned weight loss during a 6-month period.) Maria was severely malnourished and in a septic state. Despite an extensive surgical débridement, antibiotic administration, and fluid rescue, she expired 9 days after the admission. James was confined to the county jail and was charged with elder endangerment. Further investigation revealed that James had sold the property for a fraction of its actual value. All of Maria's savings were gone, as were her silver service, wedding band, engagement ring, and a diamond earring set that had been a gift to Maria from her late husband. James was sentenced to a 10-month jail term and 2 years probation. Fifty-six cats were removed from the premises and the house was condemned.

As part of the investigation, detailed documentation is compiled on the complaint and physical and contextual findings, as well as subjective and objective data that are more measurable. Narrative and subjective reports may be summative reports of findings that list generic references to skin lesions, bruises, unstable gait, frailty of the elder, and other nonspecific terms. This may contribute to the information that is needed for prosecution of an abuse case. However, the tendency toward use of ambiguous terminology makes the information being reported, investigated, and recorded less credible. For this reason, the use of valid and reliable instruments to assess and measure parameters that are observed and may be related to maltreatment is essential to the investigation. Clarity, credibility, and validity of documentation are critical components of investigation of elder maltreatment. Color and black-and-white photographs, with and without measurement scales, use special techniques of infrared or alternate light sources

to aid the visualization of findings that are suspected of being intentional injuries.

INTERVENTIONS TO IMPROVE OUTCOMES

Early intervention services (EISs) incorporate the promotion of healthy aging and the maintenance of independence and self-care. EIS is provided to individuals, elders, family and friends of elders, as well as general consumers. These services may be offered by health-care providers, health educators, hospitals, senior programs and centers, and community colleges. The Area Agency on Aging, a national program, provides "Answers on Aging," which connects individuals with appropriate community social service organizations. Early intervention is also vital to implementation of awareness and education regarding indicators of maltreatment, which may be overlooked and discounted because of its simplicity. This educational program provides critical assessment skills and links possible causes with presenting symptoms. Once indicators of maltreatment are identified, a plan for addressing the root causes and reducing risks can be developed and resources contacted.

Assessment and documentation procedures are put forth as guidelines for health-care institutions by the Joint Commission Accreditation of Health Care Organizations. Screening for abuse is a standard procedure in health-care settings and hospitals. While the requirement is specific, it has not been validated. Required screening for elder abuse is incorporated into the Minimum Data Set (MDS) used in long-term care facilitates and by home health agencies in the Outcome Assessment Information Set (OASIS). Both the MDS and OASIS have limited reliability, as objective measurement is lacking. The MDS is used to document the resident's health status and individualized needs for long-term care. The resident information is used as a mechanism for determining the reimbursement rate for that individual as well as for data collection for research purposes.

Prevention of negative health outcomes is the goal of quality patient care, but due to the nature of abuse and its recognition after the fact, other approaches must also be addressed. Patient self-reports of abuse or neglect or caregiver reports may not be reliable sources of information. The need for specificity in descriptive documentation would provide validity to examination findings. The application of forensic science methods and pathology would provide a solid basis to explain findings that are measurable and lead to the development of evidence-based interventions for prevention and intervention in adult maltreatment cases.

The use of valid and reliable tools as standard practice to record and identify the risks associated with conditions or the status of a condition should be based on a scoring rubric. Two examples of such tools that are relatively familiar to nurses are the Braden Assessment Tool for Measuring Risk for Skin Breakdown, which is used to evaluate pressure ulcers, and the Glasgow Coma Scale (GCS), which is used to document measurement of severity of unconsciousness. The Elder and Dependant Adult Abuse Education division of the California Medical Training Center at the University of California Davis developed a tool for forensic examination of the multiple forms of abuse. The tool was created by a multidiscipline task force in response to a law passed (Senate Bill 502) to add Section 11161.2 to the Penal Code. This act relates to domestic violence, dependent adult abuse and neglect, and elder abuse cases.

Another tool discussed by Sandmore described two instruments used in detecting abuse. The Indicators of Abuse (IOA) is a 29-item tool focused on the caregiver and the care recipient. In studies, the IOA identified 80% of abuse cases. The second instrument, Vulnerability to Abuse Screening Scale (VASS), is a self-reporting questionnaire. Outcome from a longitudinal study by Women's Health Australia of 10,500 women aged 73 to 78 years showed validity. However, the tool was recognized as needing additional study to determine the sensitivity and specificity of the VASS.

ELDER NEGLECT

Risk Factors for Elder Neglect

The maltreated elderly population has a 3.1 times greater risk of dying than do those with no reported maltreatment. Living with another person and experiencing social isolation have been associated with higher elder abuse rates. Spouses are frequently the source of abuse and carry out emotional abuse, physical violence, threats, and forced social isolation from family and members of the community.

The Elder Assessment Instrument (EAI) is a 41-item Likert scale instrument developed in 1984. The EAI has been shown to correlate higher with neglect than other types of elder mistreatment. The EAI items consist of evaluations of nutritional deficits, altered skin integrity, and changes in elimination, which relate to the increased need for assistance in activities of daily living—identified as a risk for elder neglect.

Critical appraisal of evidence regarding early recognition and intervention strategies is needed because the use of a proactive approach limits further maltreatment. Increased stress on caregivers is a precursor to caregiver burnout as well as mounting frustrations when caregivers are overwhelmed or succumb to exhaustion. Expectations within families may be diverse, and responsibilities may place obligations for care of elders on already burdened family members, placing the elderly family member at additional risk. Health-care professionals need to readily provide resources for caregivers that can be used to decrease caregiver stress.

Social expectations affect what is considered abusive behavior and neglectful care, requiring extra sensitivity and understanding to encourage disclosure of problematic situations. Differentiation of abuse from nonabuse and from neglect necessitates clinician recognition of elements that mimic neglect. A comprehensive physical examination, diagnostic evaluation, and history of incidents being investigated can expose the truth. Forensic nursing experts with knowledge and experience in assessment and investigative techniques are needed in geriatric settings to recognize injury patterns and their causes.

Identification and Assessment of At-Risk Elders

Relevant research reveals that lower Mini-Mental Status Exam scores and the need for assistance with activities of daily living were linked to neglect more frequently than other types of elder abuse. The American Medical Association (AMA) recommends that practitioners routinely ask geriatric patients about abuse, even if signs are absent. The red flags that may bring to light elder neglect include a shared living situation with an abuser, dementia, social isolation, and perpetrator pathology, such as alcohol misuse and mental illness. The presence of these criteria indicates the need for a course of action that will provide safety for the elderly to reduce the likelihood of elder maltreatment.

Elders who rely on caregivers to meet their needs will show declines in physical status if their basic physical needs are not met. Weight loss, malnutrition, low protein and albumin levels, and dehydration can result when assistance with daily intake and feedings is not provided. Additionally, lack of appropriate medical care is a common sign of neglect, evidenced by unfilled prescriptions, missed appointments, untreated chronic conditions, and decubitus ulcers. Patients who experience neglect are not always easy to identify because they may not have a primary care provider. As stated earlier, caregivers may "doctor shop," visiting different emergency departments, specialists, and clinics for care when seeking medical attention, rather than accessing routine and regular care and follow-up with one provider. Screening elderly patients for abuse and neglect should be done in a private respectful setting, using a valid tool. Every effort should be made to decrease the fear of institutionalization that many elders have, thereby allowing for improved care and appropriate case finding.

Palliative care teams and multidisciplinary teams are ideal groups for recognizing the various aspects of abuse. In most states, health-care providers are mandatory reporters of elder maltreatment. Knowledge of the laws and reporting procedures in one's state of practice is necessary to comply with mandates. Adult Protective Services (APS) and social service agencies can be used to investigate claims of abuse or suspected abuse. Also, medical case management systems, public health home visits, law enforcement, and the court system can all be used in a multidisciplinary process to promote elder safety. All 50 states have APS programs, with each state having unique laws

for reporting elder abuse. Completion of a thorough history and a comprehensive physical examination provide a means of ascertaining relevant information necessary to detect elder abuse. Probing questions that detail coping skills, stress, and social support systems can reveal the level of dependence of elderly patients and the relationships between them and their caregivers. Challenges include discrepancies in information or rehearsed stories, language barriers, and sometimes, functional status.

Understanding Self-Neglect

Self-neglect is a subgroup in the elder neglect category. With self-neglect there is no caregiver at fault, and the elder is thought to be physically and mentally competent enough to live without assistance. Self-neglect was found to be the leading type of elder maltreatment in the 1998 incidence study by NCEA. Self-neglect patients are less likely to need assistance with activities of daily living and more likely to suffer from psychiatric disorders and alcoholism. Patients with self-neglect identified as a problem have a significantly greater risk of mortality, which is increased with acute hospitalization. Conversely, they have improved outcomes within long-term care facilities, and self-neglect subsequently decreases after placement. Identification of self-neglect patients often is the responsibility of the APS worker, or they may be identified by community members. However, health-care providers may be asked to identify health risks or assess cognitive functioning while attempting to intervene.

Self-neglect by elders endangers their own health and safety. Comorbidities such as depression reduce the will to maintain personal cleanliness within societal standards. Malnutrition is often used as a marker for self-neglect and results from a poor intake of nutrients. In long-term care facilities, the most frequent cause of neglect is inadequate staffing to help individuals who need assistance with feeding.

Human rights advocacy efforts, along with federal regulations in long-term care, have led to changes in how society cares for those who cannot make decisions or speak for themselves. The regulations of the Omnibus Budget Reconciliation Act (OBRA) of 1987 granted the right of self-determination along with laws addressing advocacy and safety for vulnerable populations. In the early 1990s the regulations were heavily debated. Queries arose as to whether an impaired person has the right to live in squalor; go without eating, drinking, or taking prescribed medication; or having good personal hygiene.

Health-care system data show that senior populations are prescribed more treatments and pharmacological interventions than any other segment of the population, according to the American Hospital Association (AHA) *Report on Utilization 2005*. Multiple prescriptions and interventions occur frequently without discussion with the patient regarding available options and explanations of benefits and risks. The basis for this type of interaction or relationship has been studied in many conditions, symptoms, and disorders. The foundational work set forth by Gatz and Pearson was further confirmed by Gagliese and Melzack. Advocates of health reform and of senior care have suggested that reimbursement mechanisms and stereotyping hinder provider-patient interaction. For example, health-care provider reimbursement schedules seldom include coverage for education and counseling on options for care and treatment regimens. Additionally, health-care providers' ageist behavior/beliefs may surface early in a medical encounter with a patient over the age of 60, hindering care.

Perpetrators of Neglect

Perpetrators of elder neglect are often family members acting as primary caregivers, or professional health-care workers in various types of health-care institutions working with the elderly population. Understaffed and poorly managed care organizations had a higher potential for maltreatment of frail and dependent individuals. In one study, 20% of employees surveyed stated that they had witnessed elder abuse but had not reported it to authorities. Staff training and education must include ongoing and contemporary information, skills, and techniques for recognizing abusive behaviors, precipitating factors, and alternate, appropriate ways of responding to patients to provide ethical, respectful, nonabusive care that is patient specific and safe for both patient and provider.

Several factors increase the risk of a person perpetrating neglect of an elderly patient. The risk of carrying out abusive and neglectful behaviors with a patient is increased when the caregiver has experienced such treatment in his or her own personal history. Such findings are similar to the findings regarding child abuse and intimate partner violence patterns of abuse: one's personal history of abuse can increase the risk of carrying forward the abuse on another person. Awareness of the repetitive nature of abuse can help practitioners in the identification of potential abuse and neglect. Caregiver age and declining health status are also related to an increased incidence of neglect. Declining health status is a signal of increased stress and higher risk of abuse from an adult spouse caregiver or with siblings or children who take on the caregiver role. Furthermore, paid caregivers in the home carry out abusive and neglectful behaviors at a rate higher than nonpaid family caregivers, dispelling the myth that paid nonfamily caregivers offer better outcomes.

There is no specific appearance, socioeconomic level, ethnicity, religious preference, or gender common to abusive caregivers. A clear definitive profile of an abuser does not exist and may be male or female, but the abuser is more likely to be a family member than any other group. Children of seniors are the most common offenders, while the most common type of maltreatment stems from neglect. Reports indicate that spouse abusers are of growing concern in the elder caregiver roles. One of the reasons for this is the extended life span for elders and their desire to live as independently as possible.

Many seniors have outlived their children in recent generations, and caregiver stress may consequently be shared among multiple family members who are involved in care. Caregiver stress presents as an overreaction, with physical or verbal violence that escalates as the senior declines or if the need for care extends over a prolonged period. **Respite care** is short-term, temporary care of the elder to provide relief or a break for the caregiver. It is much needed, but limited in availability and unaffordable for many families. For other families, respite care may represent a failure to endure and give the appearance that the family cannot "take care of its own" or cannot "do the right thing." Caregiver burdens mount as the caregiver's personal sense of self and self-worth blurs with continued or mounting needs of the ailing elder for whom he or she is responsible. Many families perceive that they can provide the best care possible and would never consider a facility placement for their loved one. For some caregivers, the feeling of being trapped in a 24-hour-a-day, 7-day-a-week commitment, with no relief, was elucidated in the book, *The 36 Hour Day*. Often referred to as the "Dementia Bible," the book explained the tremendous stress and demands of being a caregiver and brought guilt-relief and comfort to many who thought that they were alone and ashamed of their feelings of being inadequate caregivers.

Provision of care is a complicated role to fulfill. Nursing students spend many hours learning appropriate safe techniques for bathing, hygiene, assisting others with activities of daily living, dressing, toileting, transfer, and ambulation. Time is spent in simulation before techniques and skills are used with patients. Safe and high-quality education, training, and patient care requires performance at a certain professional standard while meeting professional competencies. Caregivers are often unskilled and minimally prepared for the responsibility they assume. They may have no education or training for the performance of the same procedures and skills that nurses spend years learning, which places both caregiver and elder at great risk.

Case Study

Parental Abuse of Disabled Man Leading to Death

Barry is a 43-year-old man with a 23-year history of paraplegia resulting from a motor vehicle accident. Barry is homebound, bedfast, and completely dependent on his mother, Peggy, to care for his every need. He was being followed by a home care agency for care and treatment of a Stage IV pressure ulcer and for urinary catheter changes once per month due to recurrent urinary tract infections (UTIs). Peggy was very anxious about caregivers coming into the home. She closely guarded Barry's medications, did his wound care, would not let him up out of bed, and kept all sunlight out of the room with black drapes covering the windows. The home health nurse was tracking his UTIs, and within 5 days of every catheter change done by Peggy, Barry was running a temperature, had milky urine, and was somewhat disoriented. The nurse began inquiring into how the catheter changes were performed by Peggy. She offered to show her how she inserted a new indwelling catheter. The observation revealed that Peggy had never been taught how to maintain sterility of all of the supplies being used. She also was trying to save money and ordered supplies in separate pieces rather than as a kit. Cross-contamination and ineffective cleansing and preparation prior to inserting the catheter were factors that increased contamination and seeded the catheter with bacteria that caused the UTIs. Peggy became resistant to recommendations and protocols to preserve sterility during catheter changes as well as following instructions to aid the pressure ulcer wound in healing. She indicated that she would continue to do it her way as she knew what she was doing. Six months after Peggy dismissed the home care nurses, Barry was hospitalized with osteomyelitis. Osteomyelitis occurring in an immune-suppressed person gives a poor prognosis. Despite intravenous antibiotics and various interventions, Barry died 2 months later.

SEXUAL ABUSE OF THE ELDERLY

Sexual abuse is a global health concern that impacts people of every age, ethnicity, education level, and socioeconomic status. It is described as any nonconsensual sexual contact, which includes behaviors such as fondling, battery, penetration, as well as unwanted attention to one's body. Statistics indicate that 1 in 6 women and 1 in 33 men will experience sexual abuse at some point in their lives. However, these values are likely to be underestimated due to the low rate of reporting sexual abuse to law enforcement. Unreported cases of sexual abuse are projected to be up to 10 times those reported.

The majority of sexual abuse victims are female (93.5%), yet males can still be affected according to a meta-analysis by Burgess and colleagues (2006; 2008). The male victim may be more hesitant to report sexual abuse or seek medical assistance due to the social stigma associated with male sexuality and sexual behaviors and socialized expectations of the male. Males may also be resistant to report because feelings of vulnerability, humiliation, weakness, powerlessness, and loss of masculinity.

Although sexual abuse occurs more commonly in younger women, it also impacts the elderly. Societal attitudes may be dissolute and immoral regarding sexual behavior, however there is a distinct attitude that the elderly are asexual, less provocative, and unable to be abused.

The misconception is in the lack of understanding of rape, which is not a crime of passion or sexual desire based on physical attractiveness. Rape is a crime of violence, and victims are often the most vulnerable members of society.

Risk Factors for Sexual Abuse

Evidence informs us that there are several factors that contribute to an elderly person's risk of becoming a victim of sexual abuse. The majority of sexual assaults against the elderly occur within their own home. Elderly persons are more likely to be living alone than any other age group, and yet they are accessible to perpetrators in health-care settings as well. Also, the majority of sexual abuse perpetrators are the victim's husband, adult son, or caregiver. Dependency on others for safety, security, and care increases with age, but so also does the likelihood of sexual abuse. Most elderly victims are small and frail in stature. Moreover, they may suffer one or more physical or mental disabilities. The majority of sexual abuse perpetrators are male. Unlike other age groups, control of the elderly victim is easily attained by the mere presence of or threat of force from a perpetrator.

Elderly victims of sexual abuse are more likely than younger victims to sustain injuries that require medical treatment. Health-care providers play a key role in prevention of sexual abuse of the elderly when they are educated to be aware of the need for appropriate, timely, and accurate recognition, interventions, and treatment. However, many obstacles prevent providers from completion of a proper forensic nursing assessment.

Cognitive impairment of the elderly patient is one of the main barriers to accurate assessment. Impaired memory impedes the patient's ability to recall events and sequential timelines of events, and also limits his or her ability to understand the forensic assessment process. Elderly patients may believe unfamiliar providers are going to harm them, which can create resistance and combative behavior when attempting a physical examination. Secondly, elders often have one or more chronic conditions coexisting alongside the signs and symptoms of sexual abuse. As a result, abnormal behaviors and physical cues of sexual abuse may be misdiagnosed as part of another disease process.

Post-traumatic stress disorder (PTSD) can be disguised and diagnosed as depression or anxiety, which are common diagnoses in all age groups. Genital bruising can be misinterpreted as rough catheterization or perineal care. Erythematous genitalia or a rash in the perineal area may be from chemicals or urine leakage that can chafe the area and make the tissue more easily damaged or excoriated. An assessment of abuse or neglect must be based on first obtaining a full understanding the patient's lifestyle and medical history, including medications, which may contribute to or alter findings. The physical condition of the elder can also hinder proper examination. Bodily malformations such as leg contractures can obstruct the provider's view of the pelvic area, as can limited mobility or adipose tissue. Genital bruising, abrasions, or edema may be overlooked due to this limitation.

Lastly, there are variations of sexual abuse symptoms dependent on the victim's age. Postmenopausal women experience biological changes that increase the risk for injury and delayed healing. Women 40 years of age and older suffer from genital injury during sexual contact at a rate of five times that of the younger population. Also, it is common for elderly persons to experience dyspareunia and bleeding after sexual intercourse. Normal physiological factors that occur may be masking or misdiagnosed as abuse. Patience and careful attention to detail during the examination process will allow the provider to correctly diagnosis and recognize elder sexual abuse, but the diagnosis must be based on the understanding of current health conditions and medications.

COMPARISON INTERVENTION

A literature search reveals a plethora of interventions for abused children, parents who abuse their children, or partners who abuse their spouses. Yet, successful interventions that may be used in other populations may not be successful in the elderly. There are seven common interventions: (1) prevention: sharpen the abilities to detect abuse; (2) screening: carefully evaluate potential caregivers to identify instances of abuse in their background; (3) identifying: create and maintain a proactive approach to identify issues of abuse; (4) training: provide orientation and ongoing training programs regarding abuse; (5) protection: support and protect both accusers and the accused; (6) reporting and Investigating: ensure follow-up on any complaint being reported; and (7) responding: respond appropriately and in a timely fashion to put corrective measures in place, remediate, or discipline in accordance with governing laws. When intervening and treating sexual abuse in the elderly, each situation should be individualized based on the victim's cognitive status and specific needs. Cognitively impaired elders often cannot verbalize their needs. They will not benefit from support groups that focus on discussion of sexual abuse events. However, music therapy, removal of stressful stimuli, and providing care at a consistent time and place can be beneficial for these elders. Family members may be part of the problem or even the person through whom an abusive or neglectful situation is revealed. Nurses who work with the senile dementia patients and those with Alzheimer's disease have reported that spouses may withhold specific medications, for example, because antidepressants can reduce sexual desire in their partner.

Noncognitively impaired elderly victims can be treated similarly to younger adult victims. Support groups allow verbalization, recognition, and coping with abuse, which can be a positive intervention for this population. Also, providing patient care and treatment with specific, clear explanations can allow less cognitively impaired elders to regain a sense of control over their bodies. All people cope in different ways and have varying levels of need that must be taken into consideration when treating elderly patients with a history of sexual assault or abuse. In addition, the inner resources and strengths that elderly individuals have developed over time should be explored, emphasized, and applied in cases of sexual abuse.

Reporting of Elder Sexual Abuse

Elder sexual abuse is one of the most underreported crimes in the United States. It is estimated that only 30% of cases are reported to police. Continued research indicates that there are two reporting mechanisms, formal and informal. Formal measures of reporting include law enforcement and health-care providers; informal measures are family, friends, and clergy.

Cognitive disparities related to aging, comorbidities, and prescription medication may prevent elders from being reliable historians. Cognitively impaired elders may become socially withdrawn, isolated, or become combative following an episode of abuse. Their physical, cognitive, and psychological health can quickly deteriorate and hinder further police investigation. Furthermore, dependency on others creates a fear of retaliation, isolation, or institutional admission if the elder's behavior does not reflect the perpetrator's demands. In fact, many elderly victims, who live with their perpetrator, may actually fear separation or loneliness if separated from the caregiver on whom they have learned to depend. Exhibiting such behaviors can make elders appear to be resistant to assisting police. The role of the forensic nurse includes explaining the behavior and needs of the elderly to law enforcement and vice versa, thereby helping to close the communication gap.

Generational differences exist regarding marital behavior and gender role expectations. Older generations may accept abusive behaviors as normal or expected in marital relationships. As a result, differences in individual definitions of what constitutes sexual abuse exist. Feelings of humiliation and self-blame related to these generational differences can impede elders from reporting abuse and seeking medical and/or legal assistance. Prior negative interactions with medicolegal systems can also produce distrust and hesitance to initiate disclosure or totally block further contact and prolong treatment of sexual abuse. Such barriers create challenges for examiners and other professionals who seek to encourage reporting of elder sexual abuse cases to law enforcement and expand the availability of treatment options to all who need them.

Clinical Identification of Elder Sexual Abuse

Clinical intervention includes clinician identification and recognition of physical and psychiatric symptoms of abuse as two important aspects that precede intervention and treatment. Often, elderly victims do not report sexual abuse to law enforcement themselves, but rely on others to pick up on verbal and nonverbal cues that sexual abuse has occurred. It is important to note that blunt statements regarding the abuse are rarely offered by elderly victims. More commonly, fragmented statements within unrelated discussion are offered to family or caregivers when disclosing this sensitive information. Cognitively impaired elders need to rely on other methods to communicate that sexual assault has occurred. Abnormal behaviors or nonverbal cues can alert family and caregivers that an unusual event has occurred. Elderly patients who have experienced sexual abuse may present as withdrawn, isolated,

combative, or with a diminished level of consciousness. Physical, cognitive, and psychological health may quickly deteriorate. Elder sexual abuse victims may also participate in avoidance or reenactment behaviors. Reenactment behaviors involve repeating statements or acts completed by the perpetrator such as shouting threats and/or abusing others. Sexual abuse may also be discovered and reported through direct observation of abuse by a family member or caregiver. Elders should not be questioned further about abusive actions that have been witnessed firsthand, as the information may be embarrassing and humiliating to disclose. Recognition of sexual abuse can be difficult, yet careful attention to details and conversations will allow an increased chance of discovery.

Prosecution of Elder Sexual Abuse

Many professionals consider an additional intervention to be the successful prosecution of sexual abuse perpetrators, which can differ with age and presentation of the victim. Younger victims with cognitive orientation and ambulatory ability who are living within the community are more likely to be medically treated and have successful police investigations. Therefore, the likelihood of the perpetrator's successful prosecution increases with the elderly patient's cognitive status. Cognitively impaired elderly victims have multiple factors that impede their ability to contribute to successful police investigations. For example, physical and mental limitations may inhibit the elder from being a reliable historian. Failure to recognize abuse delays medical treatment and evidentiary collection. The success of elder sexual abuse prosecution is rare in cases that initiate with unclear histories from impaired individuals in whom an investigator has little confidence.

ELDER HOMICIDE

Consistent with all other types of abuse, elder abuse remains one of the most underreported health concerns. Factors associated with fatalities for persons 65 years of age and older include the relationship of the victim to the perpetrator, motive, location of death, and cause of death, as well as age, sex, and race. Evidence significant to these cases is exposed by a thorough evaluation of the elderly patient by using a multidisciplinary team approach. Abuse may contribute to little-known causes of death in persons 85 years of age and older, since most studies focus on persons 65 to 85 years of age. Low autopsy rates with deceased persons of older ages are related to regulations and the lack of investigations, particularly since the majority of deaths occur in private homes.

Case Study

MEDICAL SEDATION BY HEALTH PROFESSIONALS LEADING TO DEATH

Ken is an 87-year-old male. He was admitted to a nursing home due to ambulation difficulties and depression. His primary care provider's last visit was 1 week prior to his death. The last progress note indicated that Ken's depression had improved on the medication regimen instituted 6 weeks earlier. The note also indicated that Ken was ambulating without assistance, using a walker. Ken was found dead in his room at 2:00 a.m. The health-care provider was not comfortable signing the death certificate as Ken was in exceptionally good health in spite of the admitting diagnoses. The case then became a suspicious death, and subsequently a death investigation was performed. The protocol for a death investigation work-up includes a toxicology screen prior to autopsy. The report for toxicology revealed a lethal level of Dilaudid in the blood. The autopsy was then performed. Postmortem examination did not reveal any significant cause of death; however, the toxicology results pointed to overdosing with a narcotic. The medical record review reported that Ken was on aspirin therapy, non-steroidal anti-inflammatory medication, and antidepressants. There was no order for Dilaudid and no documentation that he had received that medication. Further investigation of the medication sign-out system revealed that in addition to Dilaudid being removed from stock, morphine and Vicodin were also being removed on a routine basis during the evening shift. Three additional residents were tested and found to have elevated levels of narcotics in their blood, and none of them had any of those medications ordered by a care provider either. Elder abuse charges were eventually filed against an evening nurse. Upon additional investigation, other staff members admitted that they were knowledgeable about the nurse's use of narcotics to keep the residents fairly sedated in order to not have to "deal" with them on her shift. The staff, however, did not report or think to report the activity, stating they did not realize that it constituted abuse. The staff and nurse who were involved in the abuse were discharged from their jobs and had criminal charges filed against them.

Death Investigation and Reporting

The National Association of Medical Examiners (NAME) has standard operational guidelines that can be used to standardize death investigation procedures. Only a small percentage of deaths in those aged 65 and older are reported to medical examiners and coroners: unreported deaths are certified by primary care practitioners with little or no investigation. Critical elements that may determine a natural death from a homicide are thus lost and never documented. According to a study by Gruszecki, only 12% of all nursing home deaths are reported, with just 4% being actively investigated. Also, fewer than 1% of nursing home resident deaths are autopsied. The age of the decedent highly influences the decision for autopsy, and elders who die outside a nursing home are more likely to be autopsied than those dying in a long-term care facility.

The leading causes of death (COD) for elder homicides are gunshot wounds (GSW) and blunt force trauma (BFT). Cases of GSW that are reviewed accounted for as many as 50% of the mortalities: cases of BFT account for between 28% and 35%, with the head being the primary location of wounds and injury.

In addition to GSW and BFT, stabbings, asphyxia, and burns were identified as common COD. Elders are not immune to violence that necessitates an acute investigation to assess for indications of suspected maltreatment and sexual assault of elders. With increasing numbers in this aging population, the challenge is to meet the legal requirements based on local, regional, and state laws for death regulations. The role for forensic nursing in medical examiner's and coroner's offices is growing (see Chapter 11).

The NAME promotes thorough investigations of unnatural deaths in all populations and recognizes that elder deaths should merit the same level of inquiry and investigation as deaths of younger persons. Medical examiners and coroners follow the legislative regulations for the medicolegal reporting and investigation of death. The process may require an autopsy, inspection, and/or scene examination. Circumstances surrounding a person's death that require further information should lead to an autopsy to understand unexplained circumstances and establish the cause and manner of death. The comprehensive assessment of a death suspected to be unnatural is referred to as the **medical-legal autopsy.** Components include a specialized examination that integrates personal, social, and medical history; scene investigation; external examination, including clothing; internal examination of tissues; microscopic evaluation; well as toxicological, laboratory, and evidentiary data (see Chapter 10).

The NAME Executive Committee supports the general concept of a National Violent Death Reporting System (NVDRS). The system has defined public health and safety goals, measurable project outcomes, planned and tangible benefits at the local and state level, and necessary support of medical examiner and coroner systems participating in the process.

Elder abuse death review teams are relatively new to states investigating incidents of abuse toward elders. Their purpose is to examine known incidents of elder abuse occurrences. The investigative team advises changes in all systems' responses to elder deaths to prevent future elder abuse deaths and develops recommendations for coordinated community prevention and intervention initiatives. The manual describing how to establish an elder abuse-fatality review team (EA-FRT) is available online for public use (http://abanet.org/aging/publications/docs/fatalitymanual.pdf). The evidence for using the team approach in investigation of child fatalities is strong, and thus the application is thought to be ideal for elder death fatality review as well.

Outcomes

NAME constructed and disseminated practice standards during the 1970s in an effort to standardize operations and accreditation criteria. A model for the individual case investigation was developed with the principal objective being to provide a constructive framework that defines the fundamental services delivered by a professional forensic pathologist (NAME, 2006). These standards have consolidated best practices demonstrating evidence-based practice guidelines across the nation. Specific areas pertinent to elder abuse include the following:

A2.1 Deaths due to violence

A2.2 Known or suspected non-natural deaths

A2.3 Unexpected or unexplained deaths when in apparent good health

A2.5 Deaths occurring under unusual or suspicious circumstances

A2.6 Deaths of persons in custody

A2.8 Deaths of persons not under the care of a physician (NAME, 2006)

A significant portion of medicolegal death investigation is carried out by forensic nurse death investigators. The integrated and multidisciplinary team approach constitutes an evidence-based practice framework that demonstrates appropriate care for elders subject to violence.

LEGAL AND POLITICAL EFFORTS TO ADDRESS ELDER ABUSE

In the United States, the federal government has acknowledged and addressed protection of the elderly in a number of ways: through The Older Americans Act, which authorizes NCEA legal services for older persons; the Long-Term Care Ombudsman Program; state and local programs for elder abuse prevention; and other aging services. The Social Security Act, encompassing Social Security, Medicare, Medicaid, and Social Services Block Grant programs, conveys long-term care facility licensing and certification, Medicaid Fraud Control Units, and funding of state APS programs. The Violence Against Women Act supports services and training about abuse against older persons and persons with disabilities. The Family Violence Prevention and Services Act supports domestic violence programs and shelter services.

Law enforcement professionals investigate reported crimes and collect data on the offenses committed. Several federal agencies maintain a database of violent crimes, such as the FBI Uniform Crime Reports, the National Crime Victim Survey, and the FBI National Incident-Based Reporting System. However, the databases contain limited or no information on elder abuse. Such lack of data collection is evidence of the inadequate recognition of crimes against the elderly.

The Elder Justice Coalition is a national organization dedicated to promoting elder justice in America through education, advocacy, and support of federal initiatives to address the growing crisis of elder abuse, neglect, and exploitation. The introduction of the Elder Justice Act (S. 795) by Senators John Breaux and Orrin Hatch, and the later introduction of a House companion bill (H.R. 2006), served as the catalyst for the establishment of the Elder Justice Coalition. The coalition's focus is to increase public awareness of elder abuse, neglect, and exploitation at the local, state, and national levels using a comprehensive approach to address elder justice issues.

The noteworthy actions of politicians led to the United Nations highlighting the need to prioritize assistance to national governments, the international community, and the public at large to better assess abuse of older persons. The literature pertaining to elder abuse is lean and uses research that is out-of-date. The Department of Economic and Social Affairs of the U.N. Secretariat

Second World Assembly on Aging met to discuss the challenges and opportunities of aging in the 21st century. Innovative international policy documents were adopted, such as the *Political Declaration* and the *Madrid International Plan of Action on Ageing* (United Nations, 2008). The Madrid plan provided information on the dimensions of aging and changes in quality of life of older persons in all five U.N. regions of the world. Findings indicate that further research in primary prevention efforts is necessary to assess practice initiatives that support interventions to eradicate violence in the aging population. It is suggested that a rigorous analysis can provide for evidence-based policies aimed at building a safe society for all ages.

The use of existing or newly developed injury surveillance systems will improve the measurement and monitoring of trends in elder maltreatment. For example, the inclusion of violent elder deaths in a new National Violent Death Reporting System will provide more information than is currently available from existing data sources.

The Health Care Finance Administration designates steps to improve the outcomes of the elderly who have a potential risk for abuse or neglect. An Advocacy Intervention Model uses the framework of the ombudsman program in long-term care that serves as an objective set of eyes and ears to evaluate persons in such settings. Once an ombudsman is involved, the regulated setting (long-term care facility or home care agency) is notified. In the case of assisted or supportive living centers, regulations may not be enforceable due to the type of licensing of that particular site: hence, elder abuse investigators would be responsible for follow-up on complaints.

Guardians are court-appointed individuals who serve as advocates for fiduciary or health-care matters. A power of attorney may also be a mechanism that affords advocacy in the event of illness, cognitive impairment, or mental conditions. A power of attorney is designated by request of the party involved to have a specific individual serve on his or her behalf, if circumstances defined in the document warrant such designation.

Multidisciplinary teams provide a comprehensive approach to evaluating a spectrum of situations. The nurse should lead the team in thorough assessment of the person, including recall of an event, medical history, caregiver or guardian's account of the event, and the living situation. Social workers also play an important role in the discovery of long-term and deep-seated interpersonal aspects that may contribute to the differentiation between normal aging changes and maltreatment; therefore, the need for interdisciplinary approaches cannot be overstated. The investigation team would not be complete without law enforcement

and prosecutors to support the investigation with additional evidence collection and prosecution of perpetrators. The collaboration among the team strengthens the entire process.

Public awareness education exposes a wide audience to the issue of elder abuse. In Illinois in 2006, state funding and a grant from the Area Agency on Aging were directed toward the development of public service announcements to increase awareness of elder maltreatment. Radio and television segments and newspaper ads were implemented for a 6-month time period. During the first 90 days of the awareness campaign, the number of reported maltreatment cases rose by 20 cases when compared to the previous year. After 12 months, the campaign realized a 17% increase in the number of elder abuse reports.

PROTOCOLS, TOOLS, AND DOCUMENTATION

Current investigative procedures for alleged elder abuse vary state by state. Protocols related to screening and assessing reported cases include subjective findings, measurements of conditions, and assigning risk.

Documentation processes and forms currently used by abuse investigators include bodygrams (Fig. 17.1),

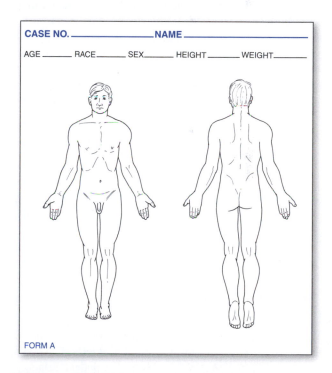

CASE NO. _____ NAME _____

AGE _____ RACE _____ SEX _____ HEIGHT _____ WEIGHT _____

FORM A

■ **FIGURE 17.1** Bodygram to document injuries and alterations.

photographs, and written documentation. Using a standardized, comprehensive, and descriptive assessment form of injury documentation will provide in-depth information and a degree of determinants that are viewed as valid and reliable in a court of law. Further documentation will assist in working up a case to identify the cause, age, and severity of injury as well as refining details to accurately determine if the findings are age-related physiological changes or the result of maltreatment.

A complete and thorough history and physical must be performed. During the history taking, questioning should be done in a nonthreatening, nonadversarial manner. Posing questions in an open-ended manner will preclude any potential for prejudicial "leading" of the responses, such as, "Mr. Jones what made you call EMS? Did you suspect that her home care aide had pushed her to the floor?" An open-ended inquiry may be, "Mr. Jones, how did you find your mother once you entered the house? Was anyone else in the home at that time? When you last saw your mother how did she seem to you?"

Any case report should also include a nutritional status assessment. This indicator is an underused marker of well-being and health status. When taking a history, ask current weight as well as weight 6 and 12 months ago, then obtain the actual weight. As stated previously, the American Society of Parenteral and Enteral Nutrition defines malnutrition as the unintentional loss of greater than 10% of body weight in 6 months or less. Findings of malnutrition can further be evaluated by laboratory testing of prealbumin, total protein, and urine for microalbuminuria. All of these laboratory results are determinants of protein body stores. Protein levels indicate muscle wasting and alterations in intake or metabolism. Also, hydration status must be reviewed and contrasted with the serum levels: blood urea nitrogen (BUN), creatine, and glomerular filtration rate (GFR) are indicators of hydration status.

Forensic medical examinations can determine area and depth of injuries as well as type of injury. Examples are penetration, type of object used to inflict the injury, and number of blows or times of penetration. Black eyes, commonly referred to as raccoon eyes, may have two causes: a fall involving head trauma or direct contact of an object with the orbital region.

Informed Treatment Option Communication

Work done by Hellebusch and colleagues (1989) examined the attitude of physicians toward the elderly. Gatz and Pearson reported that biased physician-patient relationships occur when the physician or nurse exerts control over the patient and in which the patient has very little if any

contribution to information, discussion of treatment pros and cons, or even the right to make the choice of treatment options. Their work further points out that physicians and nurses do not always consider that the elderly person's medication dosages may need to be modified due to age-related physiological changes in gastrointestinal motility, absorption, and liver function. Toon (2002) was the first to present data on the fact that many common medications create an anticholinergic effect in seniors that cause mistaken assumptions that the person is becoming demented. This anticholinergic effect creates a delirium that is reversible once the medication is appropriately withdrawn from the treatment regimen of the patient. Use of geriatric guidelines and considerations in prescribing are published and are accessible on a variety of Web sites such as The American Geriatric Society (http://americangeriatrics.org/) and the National Institutes of Health's Institute on Aging (http://www.nia.nih.gov/).

Education and Training

Specific training and education is needed for nurses to be able to identify high-risk indicators during a screening and assessment of elders presenting for all health or medical encounters. It is necessary to identify the need for early interventions as evidenced by physical and psychosocial indicators of an alteration that warrants follow-up. Protocols focused on differential exploration of a presenting or chief complaint would also aid in the distinctions between health conditions and signs of abuse.

The validity and importance of nurses' documentation of findings has been deemed more credible than that of other disciplines in many areas of litigation, primarily as evidenced in sexual assault cases treated by trained Sexual Assault Nurse Examiners (SANEs). Training and advanced education for nurses on the subject of elder maltreatment is necessary to decrease the incidence of cases that are not reported. Identifying and validating specific characteristics with scientific explanations and descriptions will advance the role of nursing by developing a conceptual framework and standards of practice related to elder maltreatment. Recommendations for educational curricula for the prevention, early identification, and assessment of elder maltreatment must include input from members of the health-care team, law enforcement, regulators, policy makers, and elder advocates.

Elder abuse identification data can be more robust with actual quantitative and qualitative documentation of comprehensive parameters of conditions and injuries, as well as physical and psychosocial findings of elderly patients presenting for medical care. Corelating symptoms, signs, and explanations of injuries or complaints increase early identification and interventions to create a safe environment and opportunities to advocate for the affected person.

The development of validated and reliable screening, assessment, and intervention tools and protocols in evidence-based practice, by nurses and for nurses, may be the first step in formalizing a strategic and standardized nursing approach to advocate for and intervene with vulnerable populations at risk. Nurses have the opportunity to identify, assess, document, and report suspicious and obvious indicators of senior maltreatment.

In situations where nurses are familiar with the routine and lifestyle characteristics of the senior's living environment, any unexplained withdrawal from normal activities, sudden change in alertness or orientation, and new or exacerbated depressive symptoms may be viewed as warning signs of elder maltreatment. Assessment findings that reveal bruising, marks, drainage, or unusual odors around the breasts or genital area that are not associated with any underlying medical conditions should be documented and reported as suspicious. Additionally, pressure sores, malnutrition, dehydration, poor hygiene, weight loss, or findings of foreign bodies embedded in tissue folds, skin, shoes, or clothing are telltale signs of willful or self-neglect.

Observations made during examinations, visits, or assessments of behaviors by caregivers perceived as belittling, threatening and intimidating, as well as other power plays or controlling tendencies, place the senior at risk for emotional and/or physical abuse. Additionally, tense or strained relationships, arguments, or unusual senior silence when caregiver or family is present serve as warning signs and indicate additional follow-up and examination may be warranted. Nurses must be alert to the signs of senior maltreatment—a silent, suffering, and painful life situation.

CONCLUSIONS

The experience of abuse places an elderly individual at risk for increased morbidity and mortality. Additional consequences of abuse are poor quality of life, emotional distress, and loss of property and security. Elder abuse is an extreme form of ageism and is recognized as a form of oppression. Additionally, neglect has been shown to be an independent risk factor for increased mortality. Critical attributes of elder abuse that appear in the literature demonstrate harm and intent to harm as characteristics leading to elder injury and mortality. Despite what is known about elderly adults as a vulnerable population, health-care providers do not routinely assess for abuse of the elderly. Health-care providers need to be aware of the physiological changes of the aging process and be able to distinguish normal change from injury or abuse. Signs of neglect may mimic the symptoms of commonly found acute or chronic medical conditions such as malnutrition, dehydration, wasting, anemias, skin breakdown, incontinence, falls, depression, mental illness, and conditions related to exposure and weather-associated temperature extremes. While general findings may trigger suspicion of abuse, the following signs are most likely indicators of physical abuse: multiple bruised areas, especially in well-protected areas (for example inner thigh), or bruising that is observed to be in different stages in resolution; burns, especially in unusual areas of the body; any injury that has a "pattern" of an object; unexplained fractures, especially when details are inconsistent; pressure ulcers or other untreated wounds; weight loss that is unexplained; and inappropriate use of medications, such as overdosing or drowsy and lethargic states.

Health-care professionals are some of the few contacts who maintain a moderately close connection between elders and the outside world. Understanding the consequences of reporting strengthens the process for risk reduction and ensuring the safety of the aging population. The education of health-care professionals across the nation regarding reporting requirements can support positive changes in the care of elders. Awareness of the risk factors associated with abuse (isolation, dependency on care) may lead to increased reporting of suspicious incidents that warrant investigation. Professional awareness and investigation of elder abuse, as well as the multidisciplinary team approach, are ideal early intervention efforts for the identification and documentation of morphological variations in suspected cases of elder abuse.

All health-care providers have a responsibility to recognize and identify injury and abuse. Performing a comprehensive medical examination and correlating the information with the noted findings will yield robust investigative data to increase recognition of and reduce the risk for elder abuse. The paucity of prosecution of elder abuse cases has sent a message that elders are disposable people, but it is through evidence-based practice that we can reverse this perception and recognize that elders are significant contributors to society.

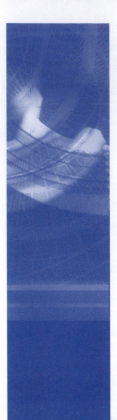

EVIDENCE-BASED PRACTICE

Reference Question: What is the role of forensic nurses in elder abuse cases?

Database(s) to Search: PubMed

Search Strategy: "Elder abuse" is a MeSH term so search "elder abuse" and then combine the results by using "AND" with the other subject, "forensic nursing."

Selected References From Search:

1. Burgess, A.W., Ramsey-Klawsnik, H., & Gregorian, S.B. (2008). Comparing routes of reporting in elder sexual abuse cases. *Journal of Elder Abuse Negligence, 20*(4): 336-352.
2. Cox, K. (2008). The application of crime science to the prevention of elder abuse. *British Journal of Nursing, 17*(13):850-854.
3. Baker, M.W., LaCroix, A.Z., et al. (2009). Mortality risk associated with physical and verbal abuse in women aged 50 to 79. *Journal of the American Geriatrics Society, 57*:1799-1809.

Questions Used to Discern Evidence:

From the studies listed, read about them, and answer the following questions:

1. What are the differences between the two studies in the design, methods, and results?
2. What are the similarities between the two studies in the number of subjects, measures used, and interventions, if any?
3. What skills do you need to learn in preventing elder abuse?

REVIEW QUESTIONS

1. Several theories of aging are suggested by theorists: biological aging, functional aging, sociological aging, and psychological aging. The theory of aging that involves the capacity of an individual to interact with others of the same age is:
   A. Functional theory of aging.
   B. Psychological theory of aging.
   C. Sociological theory of aging.
   D. Biological theory of aging.

2. Elder abuse or neglect is an extreme form of ageism and is recognized as a form of:
   A. Stereotyping.
   B. Oppression.
   C. Disrespect.
   D. Dishonor.

3. Immobility or inactivity results in:
   A. Increased production of growth factors.
   B. Decreased mental capacity.
   C. Decreased production of important growth factors.
   D. Increased production of chemical nutrients.

4. While general findings may trigger suspicion of abuse, one of the signs most likely to be an indicator of physical abuse is multiple bruised areas, especially in:
   A. Unprotected areas of the body.
   B. Face and mouth.
   C. Vital organs.
   D. Well-protected areas of the body.

REVIEW QUESTIONS—cont'd

5. Self-neglect is a subgroup in the elder neglect category for which there is no caregiver at fault for the lack of care because the elder is thought to be physically and mentally competent enough to live:

A. With assistance.

B. Without assistance.

C. Without medications.

D. With supervision.

6. Research indicates that there are two types of reporting mechanisms for elder abuse:

A. Formal and informal.

B. External and internal.

C. Direct and indirect.

D. Medical and legal.

7. Toon (2002) suggests that many common medications create an effect in seniors that causes mistaken assumptions that the person is becoming demented. This effect is called:

A. Antimanic effect.

B. Anticholinergic effect.

C. Antidelirium effect.

D. Antiemetic effect.

8. Black eyes, commonly referred to as raccoon eyes, may have two causes—direct contact of an object with the orbital region and a fall with:

A. Back trauma.

B. Internal organ trauma.

C. Head trauma.

D. Shoulder trauma.

9. High-risk indicators of abuse for clinicians to be aware of are social isolation of persons with or without short-term or permanent:

A. Behavioral impairment.

B. Affective impairment.

C. Social impairment.

D. Cognitive impairment.

10. Which of the following incorporates the promotion of healthy aging, the maintenance of independence and self-care, and implementation of awareness and education on indicators of maltreatment?

A. Early Intervention Services (EIS)

B. Health Education and Legal Program (HELP)

C. Informed Treatment Option Communication (ITOC)

D. National Center on Elder Abuse Services (NCEA)

References

Ayres, M. (2001). Concept analysis: Abuse of ageing caregivers by elderly care recipients. *Journal of Advanced Nursing, 35*(3)326-334.

Banaji, M.R. (1958). *Implicit attitudes can be measured. The nature of prejudice.* Garden City, NY: Doubleday Publications.

Basile, K.C., Hertz, M.F., & Back, S.E. (2007). Intimate partner violence and sexual violence victimization assessment instruments for use in healthcare settings: Version 1. Atlanta, GA: Center for Disease Control and Prevention, National Center for Injury Prevention and Control.

Bayer, A., & Tadd, W. (2000). Unjustified exclusion of elderly people from studies submitted to research ethics committee for approval: Descriptive study. *British Medical Journal, 3*(21):992-993.

Berzlanovich, A., Missliwetz, J., Sim, E., et al. (2003). Unexpected out-of-hospital deaths in persons aged 85 years or older: An autopsy study of 1886 patients. *American Journal of Medicine, 114*(5).

Blair, I.V., & Banaji, M.R. (1996). Automatic and controlled process in stereotype priming. *Journal of Personality and Social Psychology, 70*(6):1142-1163.

Bonnesen, J.L. & Hummert, M.L. (2002). Painful self-disclosures of older adults in relation to aging stereotypes and perceived motivations. *Journal of Language and Social Psychology, 21*(3):275-301.

Bonnie, R., & Wallace, R. (2003). *Elder mistreatment: Abuse, neglect and exploitation in an Aging America.* Washington, DC: National Academies Press, p. xiii.

Bove, G., Stermac, L., & Bainbridge, D. (2005). Comparisons of sexual assault among older and younger women. *Journal of Elder Abuse & Neglect, 17*:1-19.

Bowling, A. (1999). Ageism in cardiology. *British Medical Journal, 3*(19):1353-1355.

Brandl, B., & Cook-Daniels, L. (2002). Domestic abuse in later life. Retrieved June 5, 2009, from http://www.ncea.aoa.gov/NCEAroot/Main_Site/pdf/research/statistics.pdf

Brandl, B., Dyer, C.B., & Heisler, C. (2006). *Elder abuse detection and intervention.* New York: Springer.

Brewer, M.B., Duli, V., & Lui, L. (1981). Receptions of the elderly: Stereotypes as prototypes. *Journal of Personality and Social Psychology, 41*(4):656-670.

Burgess, A. & Clements, P. (2006). Information processing of sexual abuse in elders. *Journal of Forensic Nursing, 2*:113-120.

Burgess, A., Hanrahan, N., & Baker, T. (2005) Forensic markers in elder female sexual abuse cases. *Clinics in Geriatric Medicine, 21*:2.

Burgess, A., Ramsey-Klawsnik, H., & Gregorian, S. (2008). Comparing routes of reporting in elder sexual abuse cases. *Journal of Elder Abuse & Neglect, 20*:336-352.

Butler, R.N. (1975). *Why survive? Being old in America.* New York: Harper & Rowe.

Butler, R.N. (1980). Ageism: A forward. *Journal of Social Issues, 36*(2):8-11.

Buzgova, R., & Ivanova, K. (2009). Elder abuse and maltreatment in residential settings. *Nursing Ethics, 16*(1):10-126.

Cahan, V., & Feldman, C. (1998). Abuse associated with increased risk of death for older people. Retrieved June 7, 2009, from http://www.nia.nih.gov/NewsAndEvents/PressReleases/PR19980804Abuse.htm

Centers of Disease Control and Prevention. (2007) *Understanding sexual violence: Fact sheet.* Available from http://www.cdc.gov/ViolencePrevention/pdf/sv-factsheet-a.pdf

College of American Pathologists. (2003). Medical-legal death investigation and autopsy. Retrieved June 5, 2009 from

Cooper, C., Selwood, A., & Livingston, G. (2008). The prevalence of elder abuse and neglect: A systematic review. *Age and Aging, 37*:151-160.

Criddle, L. (2006). Outcome in the injured elderly: Where do we go from here? *Journal of Emergency Nursing, 32*:234-240.

Department of Health and Human Services. Health Care Finance Administration: Abuse and neglect detection and prevention curriculum, 42 CFR 488.301. Washington, DC.

Devine, P.G. (1989). Stereotypes and prototypes: The automatic and controlled components. *Journal of Personality and Social Psychology, 56*(1):5-18.

Eisenmenger, W. (1989). Zur Begutachtung von Decubitalulzera. *Beitr Gerichtl Med* 447:345-347. In Ortmann, C., Fechner, G., Bajanowski, & Brinkman, B. (2001). Fatal neglect of the elderly. *International Journal of Legal Medicine, 114*:191.

Erlingsson, C.L. (2007). Searching for elder abuse: A systematic review of database citations. *Journal of Elder Abuse & Neglect, 19*(3/4):59-78.

Folstein, M.F., Folstein, S.E., & McHugh, P.R. (1975). Mini-mental state. A practical method for grading the cognitive state of patients for the clinician. *J Psychiatric Research, 12*(3):189-198. PMID: 1202204.

Gruszecki, A., Edwards, J., Powers, R., et al. (2004). Investigation of elderly deaths in nursing homes by the medical examiner over a year. *The American Journal of Forensic Medicine and Pathology, 25*(3):209-212.

Hanrahan, N., Burgess, A., & Gerolamo, A. (2005). Core data elements tracking elder sexual abuse. *Clinics in Geriatric Medicine, 21*:2.

Hellbusch, J.S., Dixon, R.A., & Baltes, P.B. (1989). Physicians' attitude toward aging. *Gerontology and Geriatrics Education, 15*(2):55-65.

Hess, T.M., & Blanchard-Fields, F. (1999). *Social cognition and aging.* San Diego: Academic Press.

Hummert, M.L. (1990). Multiple stereotypes of elderly and young adults: A comparison of structure and evaluations. *Psychology and Aging, 5*(2):182-193.

Interagency Council on Child Abuse and Neglect. *Elder abuse fatality review.* Retrieved June 5, 2009, from http://ican-ncfr.org/hmElderAbuseFatality.asp

Jayawardenam, M. & Liao, S. (2005). Elder abuse at end of life. *Journal of Palliative Medicine, 9*(3):127-136.

Katz, P.R., & Seidel, G. (1990). Nursing home autopsies. *Archives of Pathology & Laboratory Medicine, 114*:145-147. In Gruszecki, A., Edwards, J., Powers, R., & Davis, G. (2004). Investigation of elderly deaths in nursing homes by the medical examiner over a year. *The American Journal of Forensic Medicine and Pathology, 25*(3):209-212.

Kite, M.M. & Johnson, B.T. (1988). Attitudes toward older and younger adults: A meta analysis. *Psychology of Aging, 3*(3):233-244.

Kleinschmidt, K.C. (1997). Elder abuse: A review. *Annals of Emergency Medicine, 30*:463-472. In Ortmann, C., Fechner, G., Bajanowski, & Brinkman, B. (2001). Fatal neglect of the elderly. *International Journal of Legal Medicine, 114*:191.

Lachs, M.S., Williams, C.S., O'Brien, S., et al. (1998). The mortality of elder mistreatment. *Journal of the American Medical Association, 280*:428-432. In Jayawardena, K., & Liao, S. (2006). Elder abuse at end of life. *Journal of Palliative Medicine, 9*(1),128.

Mace, N.L., & Rabins, P.V. (1981). *The 36 hour day: A family guide to caring for persons with Alzheimers disease, related to dementing illnesses, and memory loss in later life.* Baltimore: Johns Hopkins Press.

Morgenbesser, L., Burgess, A., Boersma, R., et al. (2006). Media surveillance of elder sexual abuse cases. *Journal of Forensic Nursing, 2*:121-126.

Mosqueda, L. (2001). *Elder maltreatment in long term care.* Presented at the Geriatric Institute Conference on Aging. University of California, Irvine School of Medicine.

National Association of Medical Examiners (NAME). (2006). *Forensic autopsy performance standards.*

National Association of Medical Examiners (NAME). (2007). *NAME position statement on National Violent Death Reporting System (NVDRS).* Retrieved June 5, 2009 from http://thename.org/index.php?option=com_docman&task=cat_view&gid=38&Itemid=26

National Center on Elder Abuse. (2007). *Risk factors for elder abuse.* Retrieved June 7, 2009, from http://www.ncea.aoa.gov/ncearoot/Main_Site/FAQ/Basics/Risk_Factors.aspx

Nelson, T.D. (2004). *Ageism: stereotyping and prejudice against older persons.* Cambridge, MA: MIT Press.

Neno, R., & Neno, M. (2005). Identifying abuse in older people. *Nursing Standard, 20*(3):43-47.

Palmore, E. (1977). Facts on aging. *The Gerontologist, 17*(4):315-320.

PAR. Mini-mental state examination. A practical method for grading the cognitive state of patients for the clinician. Retrieved from http://mmse.com/

Pearsall, C. (2005). Forensic biomarkers of elder abuse: What clinicians need to know. *Journal of Forensic Nursing, 1*(4):182-186.

Poulos, C., & Sheridan, D. (2008) Genital injuries in postmenopausal women after sexual assault. *Journal of Elder Abuse & Neglect, 20*:323-335.

Roberto, K., & Teaser, P. (2005). Sexual abuse of vulnerable young and old women. *Violence Against Women, 11*:473-504.

Roberto, K, Teaser, P., & Nikzad, K. (2007). Sexual abuse of vulnerable young and old men. *Journal of Interpersonal Violence, 22*:1009-1023.

Robinson, B. (1994). *Ageism.* Berkeley, California: American Geriatric Resource Program, University of California.

Sellas, M., & Krouse, L. (2006). Elder abuse. Retrieved April 20, 2009, from http://emedicine.medscape.com/article/805727-overview

Teaster, P.B., & Roberto, K.A. (2004). Sexual abuse of older adults: APS cases and outcomes. *The Gerontologist, 44*(6):788-796.

Tonks, A. (Ed). (1999). Medicine must change to survive an ageing society. *British Medical Journal, 3*(19):150-1451.

United Nations. (2006). Program on ageing. Issue 4. Retrieved from http://www.un.org/esa/socdev/ageing/un_network4.html

United Nations. (2008). *Regional dimensions of the ageing situation*. New York: United Nations Publications. Retrieved June 6, 2009, from http://www.un.org/ageing/documents/publications/cp-regional-dimension.pdf

World Health Organization (WHO). (2002). *Abuse of the elderly*. Retrieved June 4, 2009, from http://www.inpea.net/images/Elder_Abuse_Fact_Sheet.pdf

World Health Organization (WHO). (2008). A global response to elder abuse and neglect: Building primary health capacity to deal with the problem worldwide: Main report. Retrieved from http://www.who.int/ageing/publications/ELDER_DocAugust08.pdf

Woolf, L.M. (2001). *Elder abuse and neglect*. Webster University Gerontological Conference on Aging. Webster Groves, MO.

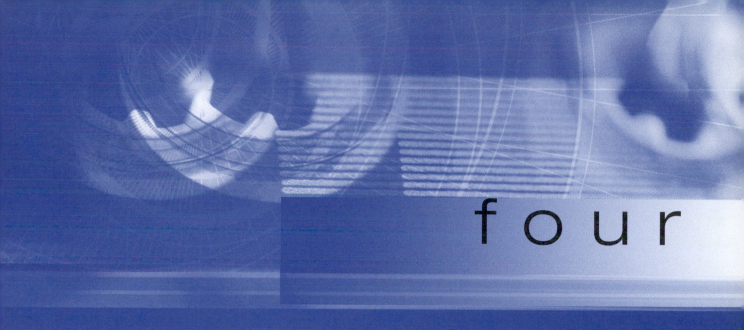

four

FORENSIC NURSING IN COLLECTIVE VIOLENCE

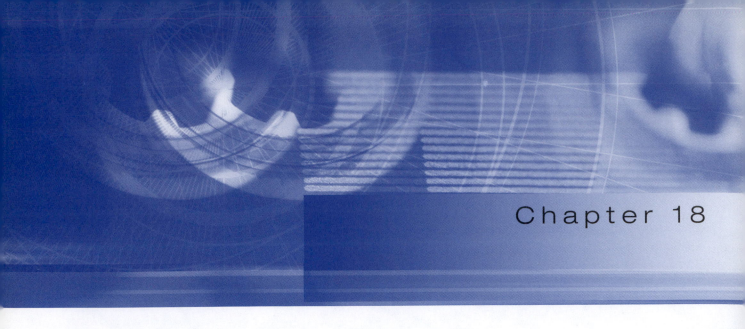

Chapter 18

THE FORENSIC NURSE AND HUMAN TRAFFICKING

Diane Kjervik and Tasha Venters

*"Ever since coming to this country people have taken advantage of us . . . .
We thought it would be different. You are the first people to really help us.
Thank you."*

Survivor of sex trafficking helped by the Polaris Project

Competencies

1. Defining the scope and significance of human trafficking.
2. Analyzing the challenges of identifying victims of human trafficking.
3. Describing resources and avenues for assistance for victims of trafficking.
4. Outlining current national and international initiatives and policies to address human trafficking.
5. Locating and using tools for screening and intervention related to human trafficking.

Key Terms

Human trafficking
Nongovernmental organizations (NGO)
Trafficking in persons
Trafficking in Persons (TIP) report
Sex trafficking
Victims of Trafficking and Violence Protection Act of 2000 (TVPA)
Voluntary migrant

INTRODUCTION

Trafficking in persons, or human trafficking, is a worldwide problem. As first responders, nurses and other health professionals must understand the issue so that they may provide the best care. The purpose of this chapter is to define human trafficking, review literature on the subject, and present approaches to best health-care practices for victims and survivors based on available evidence in order to increase awareness of the issue and ensure that nurses respond effectively and sensitively to trafficked persons.

BACKGROUND

The U.S. Department of State estimates that 17,500 women and children are trafficked annually to the United States as sex workers and another 20,000 people (men, women, and children) are trafficked across national and international borders for other forms of slave labor. Worldwide, approximately 600,000 to 800,000 men, women, and children are trafficked across international borders. Trafficking in persons is the third largest criminal industry in the world, after drugs and arms, and it is estimated that trafficking in persons generates US$9.5 billion in annual revenue. Trafficking is predicted to become the most lucrative business when compared to drugs and arms by the *Trafficking in Persons (TIP) report* (2006) within 10 years if left unchecked.

Nurses and other health professionals are often first responders to the initial reports and cries for help from persons in the midst of human trafficking or recent survivors. Persons being trafficked may present in emergency departments, public health departments and clinics, or other health-care institutions. Forensic nurses, such as Sexual Assault Nurse Examiners, working in clinical settings have helped victims of other crimes, and yet sex trafficking victims remain elusive and difficult to identify. After health professionals receive awareness training, trafficking victims may no longer be invisible to health professionals. Forensic nurses may be ideally situated in their clinical positions to be a consultant or referral resource for health-care institutions in meeting the needs of trafficked persons.

Trafficking Definitions

The United Nations' Protocol to Prevent, Suppress and Punish Trafficking in Persons, especially in Women and Children, defines **trafficking in persons** in two ways. Initially, the protocol defines **human trafficking** as "the recruitment, transportation, transfer, harboring or receipt of persons, by means of threat or use of force," in order to exploit a vulnerable person. The second definition is "exploitation for prostitution of others or any form of sexual exploitation of others, forced labor or services, slavery or practices similar to slavery or servitude or the removal of organs."

Various legislative acts prohibited commercial sexual exploitation of women and children, yet prior to 2000 no comprehensive law existed that addressed the illegality of all manner of offenses involved in the practice of human trafficking, domestically and internationally. Under the U.S. anti-trafficking legislation, the **Victims of Trafficking and Violence Protection Act of 2000 (TVPA),** all definitions of human trafficking were clarified. The most severe form of trafficking in persons is **sex trafficking,** which is defined as a sex act that is "induced by force, fraud, or coercion, or in which the person induced to perform such acts is under 18 years old." They further define trafficking as "the recruitment, harboring, transportation, provision or obtaining of a person for labor services, through the use of force, fraud or coercion, for the purpose of subjecting the person to involuntary servitude, peonage, debt bondage or slavery." Domestic sex traffickers target the most vulnerable youth, such as runaways and homeless adolescents. In the United States, the average age of entry into prostitution is 12 to 13 years old.

The U.S. Department of Labor expanded the definition of human trafficking to include persons who were

Case Study

A WOMAN'S SERVITUDE

A woman kept in domestic servitude in the United States for several years was rescued when a neighbor, noticing that she had a large tumor, offered to take the woman to the emergency health clinic. The nurse in the emergency department had been to a recent state-sponsored training on awareness of trafficking in the United States. The nurse asked the right questions and realized the woman was a victim of human trafficking. As a result, she was able to contact local resources and assist the woman in obtaining help. The woman escaped her situation and received the medical care she desperately needed. Her employers received 15 to 20 years in jail.

forced to work as domestic servants, laborers in factories, or migrant agricultural workers. Labor trafficking of U.S. citizens occurs in locations such as restaurants, the agricultural industry, traveling carnivals, peddling/begging rings, and in traveling sales crews.

There is no centralized U.S. or international entity systematically compiling data that is based on a consistent universal definition and interpretation of human trafficking. An ongoing debate exists regarding whether to include the coercion aspect as a necessary element of the definition of trafficking or if trafficking can actually occur with or without the consent of the survivor. Many **nongovernmental organizations (NGOs)** recommend that the definition and legislation developed from the definition be based on human rights. The definition should apply to trafficked persons both internationally and within the United States. A majority of the NGOs believe the legislation should follow the U.N. protocol and focus on the exploitation of the person and not the transport between borders.

Risks and Causes of Human Trafficking

The causes of human trafficking are varied and complex, often reinforcing one another. Human trafficking has become a global industry, and trafficked persons are supplied on demand for myriad international abusive employers. Many trafficked persons are merely trying to survive a lifetime of poverty and lack of education. They hope for a higher standard of living, vast employment opportunities, freedom from organized crime, and political stability. They long to live without armed conflicts, government corruption, and discrimination. Gender-based discrimination occurs in countries in which women and girls are considered to be of lower status than men, making them more vulnerable to traffickers who promise a hopeful future and enough money to support their families and loved ones they leave behind. Their hopes and dreams are further fueled by the dream of being able to share their good fortune and higher income with family and community members.

Economic causes (poverty, unemployment, lack of training, and employment opportunities) are widespread among women and children within the countries from which trafficking originates. Many countries burdened by overpopulation, extensive poverty, and scant resources cannot provide educational opportunities to meet the needs of their citizens. Even if the government could play a role in assisting with expanding educational opportunities, the country lacks the employment opportunities for those who do acquire higher education. There is rapid international growth of unregulated factory work for low wages that are inadequate to sustain family livelihood. Many countries

offer little in the way of affordable medical care. Urgent care needs or chronic health-care issues may lead the poor to seek employment for higher wages at a great distance, leaving behind family and support. The opportunities offered to them are distorted and based on prevarication, yet they seek to satisfy their needs and dreams. People who are desperate to leave their country in pursuit of survival will trust strangers indiscriminately to obtain a visa, airline ticket, or other transportation to the United States.

Migrant women from developing countries become domestic workers or entertainers in the sex industry, factory workers, or mail-order brides. Marriage may be seen as the only way to obtain legal status and live in a foreign country where there is abundant opportunity for employment. Women who leave their country of origin commonly have the equivalent of a middle-school education, or at most a community college education. Raymond and colleagues (2002) reported that the majority of the women trafficked into the United States were forced into the sex industry between the ages of 13 and 18.

Globalization, while not necessarily a direct cause of trafficking, has made it easier to move people, goods, and money around the world. People move to maximize their individual utility, usually through higher income. Impoverished individuals who wish to move where there is employment opportunity and likelihood of financial success may be faced with more stringent restrictions if migration were legal. The demand for migrant work in the low-paid, undesirable jobs continues to grow, but immigration laws prevent employers from satisfying the demands. The buying and selling of people has become a profitable business. Inevitably, individuals who cannot migrate legally or pay fees in advance for being smuggled across borders are at high risk for falling into the hands of traffickers, with their alluring promises and past history of success.

Economists argue that the North American Free Trade Agreement (NAFTA) has made a significant contribution to the flood of migration, particularly with movement from the south into the United States. Economists further maintain that low-quality U.S. corn imported into Mexico has driven millions of Mexican peasant corn farmers out of business and off their land. It is estimated that for every ton of corn imported into Mexico, two Mexicans migrate to the United States. Heightened border security since September 11, 2001, has made the crossing from Mexico into the United States a far more strenuous obstacle than it was in the past for the Mexican migrants. Heightened border security, as a need to increase control, has resulted in a doubling of the cost for being smuggled across the U.S. border. Prices that were once from $1000 to $2000 per person have been reported to now be as high as $50,000. In one trafficking case, a woman revealed that she had to re-pay $60,000 for airline tickets and travel arrangements. Re-payment of this debt was to be achieved by dancing nude in strip bars. The woman arrived indebted and was forced into modern-day slavery to repay the debt. Portrayal of the United States as a country with myriad opportunities makes individuals in need of work more vulnerable to traffickers' false promises of easy money and glamorous lifestyles.

Traffickers and Their Operation

There is no standard profile of traffickers. Business per-sons know of a need and seek vulnerable persons to meet that need. Trafficked persons are meeting an unmet need in the work market. However, organized businesses and crime networks, such as the Mafia, escort services, bars, brothels, strip clubs, and massage parlors play a role in in-ternational and domestic trafficking of women for domes-tic work and the sex industry. Local legitimate businesses, farms, and U.S. military servicemen also are major forces in sustaining the transport of women to meet their needs.

The FBI estimates that approximately a dozen Russian dance and modeling agencies have supplied 60 to 200 Eastern European women for strip bars and peep shows that are run by the Italian and Russian mobs in New York and New Jersey. International traffickers use tourist, training and education visas, and work permits initially to lure the vulnerable women into the United States. With one program, the Visa Waiver Pilot Program, the women are transported into the United States with their legal doc-uments. This action may be the first link in the chain of slavery. However, the women are kept beyond their visa expiration date, which adds another link to the chain of slavery. Thriving on the women's vulnerability, the chain is strengthened further by traffickers' threats to report the women to legal authorities, who would arrest them and deport them. Recruiters and traffickers are reported to use exceptions to the visa process to their advantage.

Smuggling networks are another method by which women are trafficked into the United States. Affiliation networks exist in both the originating country and the country of arrival. Both have investment in and seek profit from smuggling women. One example is the Chinese "snakeheads," which traffic persons for a high fee. The kinship affiliation networks in the United States and China are used to keep individual workers under control so that debts are repaid.

Trafficked Persons

People are trafficked for a variety or reasons. These in-clude but are not limited to domestic service, commercial sexual exploitation, servile marriage, factory work, agri-cultural work, and criminal activity.

Trafficking routes exist into or out of almost every country in the world. The *TIP Report* created by the U.S. State Department lists 149 countries that are ranked ac-cording to their efforts to eradicate human trafficking, in-cluding Colombia, France, Morocco, South Korea, and the Philippines, to name a few. A report from the United Nations Center for International Crime Prevention (2004) stated that more trafficked women came from Russia than any other country and that the United States was rated second in the list of top destinations to which women are trafficked.

Nearly half of all trafficked persons are children, and 80% are females. These women in the adolescent group may be as young as 14 years old, or even younger, and most are forced into the sex industry.

Another category of persons vulnerable to traf-ficking is the **voluntary migrant.** Based on unmet labor needs within a country, persons in need of work mi-grate, often illegally, to help meet the labor needs of the receiving country. Migrants are dependent on the person coordinating their migration, and they are vulnerable to further exploitation when they do not have legal papers. Ethnic, religious, and language discrimination are barri-ers. The barriers increase their dependence on others for information about the laws in general, but specifically workers rights, local legal rights, government systems, and cultural practices.

Individuals who are trafficked are victimized by co-ercion, threats of violence against them, and often threats to harm family members or loved ones in their home coun-try. The chain of slavery is strengthened further by other

A Bill of Rights for Victims of Trafficking

Victims of trafficking in persons are entitled to:

- The right to safety
- The right to privacy
- The right to information
- The right to legal representation
- The right to be heard in court
- The right to compensation for damages
- The right to medical assistance
- The right to social assistance
- The right to seek residence
- The right to return

inhumane and illegal acts severe enough to tighten the traffickers' control. Traffickers rely on the fact that they can intimidate their victims with threats of arrest, detention, and removal from the United States by government authorities. The removal of survivors of trafficking as illegal migrants can result in favorable outcomes for the traffickers, such as forcing survivors back into the country where the coercion continues and left unchecked. The business of buying and selling people to be trafficked is comparable to slavery in the 17th and 18th centuries, although slightly different and perhaps easier to initiate and maintain. In 1850, slaves in Alabama cost $1000 to $1200, the equivalent of $40,000 today. However, today one can buy two young male farm workers in Mali for $40 each. It becomes easy to replace women and children who have been trafficked when they are objectified. The product (human beings) is readily reproducible, ensuring an endless supply to meet market need. The market is boundless, with an insatiable demand. Meeting the market demand is sustained further by the driving force of the needs of the vulnerable persons living in economic distress and desperation.

Identification of Trafficked Persons

One study identified nurses' work with survivors of sex trafficking. A report on human trafficking in Minnesota found several nurses who reported working with survivors of trafficking, two nurses who treated survivors of labor trafficking, and three who treated survivors of sex trafficking. The nurses reported that survivors of sex trafficking suffered from "injuries associated with battering and maltreatment, rape, and being struck by or against an object." No other details were provided about the types of intervention employed by nurses as they worked with the women. However, people who experience interpersonal violence are commonly seen in health-care facilities nationwide. The development of screening and prevention and intervention strategies for crime victims must begin to include the unique posttrauma needs of the marginalized and disconnected individuals who have been trafficked and who have limited or no resources in the United States. Until high-level research studies are completed that help clinicians improve practice based on scientific evidence, the evidence-based interventions in health care must draw on associated literature about persons who have experienced other types of trauma.

Assessment begins with the identification of a community in which trafficked persons are suspected to reside or clinical setting in which they are seen. Those who remain enslaved by the trafficker may exhibit unique symptoms. They may have feelings of fear associated with loss of freedom of movement. The abuse they suffered may lead to psychological, physical, and sexual responses similar to other sexual abuse and assault victims. They may experience disorientation to place and time or have a poor recollection of facts of what happened to them. Many victims are in the "pipeline" and after entry into the United States are transported from city to city using fake business names. Often they are not aware of the city or state to which they are going or from which they are coming. Even more challenging is that they may lack awareness and judgment regarding the severity of their situation and all the health and legal ramifications.

Conversely, those who have left the trafficking situation may continue to suffer with fear for themselves or their family, friends they have made during transport, or family members in their home country. Diseases they suffer and beatings they endured leave many in poor health. Traffickers are also reputed to retaliate against their families and loved ones. Escaping a trafficker does not always equate with survival, and the mental and physical scars associated with the experience can be highly morbid and mortal conditions. The social stigmatization and general negative attitudes of others who judge them are long-term burdens as well. The experiences they had with slavery and the sex work they were forced to endure result in feelings of low self-worth, which increase stress. The use of adaptive coping mechanisms that were helpful in the past may no longer be available or helpful, and they are at a loss as how to cope with the current feelings. There are often unique features exhibited by trafficked persons that may assist the nurse or health-care provider in identifying them (Box 18.1).

Health Problems

Health problems faced by survivors of trafficking fall into several categories: substance abuse (cocaine and

---

Box 18.1   Identification of Trafficking Victims

- Evidence of being controlled
- Evidence of an inability to move or leave job
- Bruises or other signs of battering
- Fear or depression
- Non-English speaking
- Recently brought to this country from Eastern Europe, Asia, Latin America, Canada, Africa, or India
- Lack of passport, immigration, or identification documentation

(Data taken from U.S. Department of Health and Human Services, Campaign to Rescue and Restore Victims of Human Trafficking, retrieved January 19, 2007, from www.acf.hhs.gov/trafficking/campaign_kits/tool_kit_health/identify_victims.html)

methamphetamine are common), intimate partner violence across the continuum from verbal to physical abuse, sexual abuse and murder, HIV/AIDS, sexually transmitted diseases (STDs), fertility problems, and mental health concerns, such as post-traumatic stress syndrome. Public health systems have focused primarily on the spread of HIV. An expanded list of health problems can be seen in Figure 18.1.

Health problems in trafficking victims may require evaluation of a variety of research categories due to the co-occurring health problems and long-term lack of health care. All areas should be evaluated in a holistic and comprehensive health assessment initially, prioritizing the most imminent threat to the person's overall health status and quality of life (Box 18.2).

In one study of women trafficked in Europe ($n = 207$) 60% had a history of interpersonal violence in their life prior to being trafficked; 11% were married, and 40% reported that they had children. While in the trafficking situation, 95% reported being treated violently, and 77% were not allowed to move about freely. Physical injuries of all parts of the body were reported, and 90% reported being forced to perform sexually.

The most common physical symptoms were fatigue, weight loss, and neurological and gastrointestinal problems. Trafficking victims (89%) reported threats of harm to themselves or their families, and most of these persons reported that the threats were actualized. Zimmerman and colleagues (2006) compared the type of violence suffered by trafficking victims to that received by victims of torture and noted that the trafficking victims reported receiving the same or worse treatment. Women in the sex industry in the

| Box 18.2 | Health Concerns of Trafficking Victims |

- Sexually transmitted diseases, HIV/AIDS, pelvic pain, rectal trauma, and urinary difficulties from working in the sex industry.
- Pregnancy resulting from rape or prostitution.
- Infertility from chronic untreated sexually transmitted infections or botched or unsafe abortions.
- Infections or mutilations caused by unsanitary and dangerous medical procedures performed by the trafficker's so-called doctor.
- Chronic back, hearing, cardiovascular, or respiratory problems from endless days toiling in dangerous agriculture, sweatshop, or construction conditions.
- Weak eyes and other eye problems from working in dimly lit sweatshops.
- Malnourishment and serious dental problems. These are especially acute with child trafficking victims who often suffer from retarded growth and poorly formed or rotted teeth.
- Infectious diseases such as tuberculosis.
- Undetected or untreated diseases, such as diabetes or cancer.
- Bruises, scars, and other signs of physical abuse and torture. Sex-industry victims are often beaten in areas that won't damage their outward appearance, such as their lower back.
- Substance abuse problems or addictions either from being coerced into drug use by their traffickers or by turning to substance abuse to help cope with or mentally escape from their desperate situations.
- Psychological trauma from daily mental abuse and torture, including depression, stress-related disorders, disorientation, confusion, phobias, and panic attacks.
- Feelings of helplessness, shame, humiliation, shock, denial, or disbelief.
- Cultural shock from finding themselves in a strange country.

(Data taken from U.S. Department of Health and Human Services, Campaign to Rescue and Restore Victims of Human Trafficking, retrieved January 19, 2007, from www.acf.hhs.gov/trafficking/campaign_kits/tool_kit_health/health_problems.html)

United States, South Africa, Thailand, Turkey, and Zambia reported the same trauma experiences as do soldiers in war.

Within the United States, trafficked persons are reported to suffer high rates (85% to 100%) of physical violence, sexual assault, emotional abuse, and sadistic sex acts. The women reported sustaining physical injuries such as bruises from being beaten, vaginal bleeding, head trauma, and internal pain. Most of them stated that their health status became worse. They developed drug

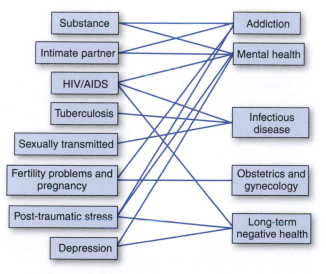

■ **FIGURE 18.1** Health problems of trafficking victims.

and alcohol dependencies, depression, and HIV/AIDS. Feelings of depression, anger, and rage were reported by 85% of the women. A majority of them were unable to feel anything and experienced total emotional and mental numbness. The U.S. Department of Health and Human Services provides a list of agencies that are available to help victims of human trafficking, including health departments and private agencies and organizations (www.acf.hhs.gov/trafficking/about/coalition_list.html).

PLANNING INTERVENTION

Planning care must take both personal and contextual details into consideration. Nurses may identify patients who are victims of sex trafficking in such settings as emergency rooms, child protective agencies, domestic violence centers, homeless shelters, churches or other religious centers, school counselors' offices, and refugee services centers. One of the greatest challenges for the nurse or health-care provider to overcome is that victims of sexual trafficking fear that others mean to harm them just as they were harmed in the past. Young victims who have been prostituted may appear not to want help, or they are too scared to seek or accept help. Many trafficking victims have been groomed to accommodate their victimization. They may have been threatened, blackmailed, beaten, mutilated, and tortured. Nurses are considered to be honest and trustworthy by the public in general. Despite the overall positive attitude toward nurses, trafficking victims may need evidence that the nurse is trustworthy and honestly cares about them. Without trust, the health assessment is jeopardized. Planning effective focused intervention strategies may be inhibited, and trafficking-related mental and physical health symptoms prolonged.

INTERVENTIONS

Models of best practices for health professionals working with survivors of trafficking are lacking due to the dearth of research and intervention studies with this population. Zimmerman et al (2006) recommended that models be developed based on similar models for other survivors of violence and for care of migrants and refugees. Information on sensitization, common morbidities, treatment approaches, confidentiality issues, and referral possibilities are recommended content.

Evidence-based care for trafficking victims ultimately will offer the highest standard of care that is maximally effective and acceptable to the patient. Evidence-based practice stems from the identification of the clinical question and appraisal of the identified surveys, guidelines, and treatment intervention literature addressing that issue. Literature should be critically appraised in areas of best outcomes, acceptability to the patient, and clinical factors. Based on the appraisals, interventions can be planned and tested. Positive outcomes can then be used to institute practice changes for trafficking victims and education of all providers who care for them. Symptoms identified in trafficking victims are similar to those of other patients who experience interpersonal violence: STD, HIV/AIDS, post-traumatic stress, etc. The evidence-based literature addressing similar identified problems in other populations will guide the initial clinical questions to be investigated and the development of interventions and practice changes in the care of trafficking victims as patients.

Health concerns in four stages of the trafficking process have been described by the International Organization for Migration (IOM). The health concerns vary according to the context of the person in the trafficking process: (1) origin (recruitment); (2) transit (travel); (3) destination (detention and exploitation); and (4) return (rescue). The IOM studied trafficking of women from Ethiopia to the Middle East for domestic servitude and from Mozambique to South Africa and from Thailand to South Africa for sexual exploitation.

In the origin phase, the causes of a woman's vulnerability (such as poverty) to trafficking must be considered. Interventions must address the possibility for legitimate employment, improving self-care strategies, and maximizing women's access to health care. A personal history of interpersonal violence and the socioeconomic conditions of the country of origin affect the vulnerability in this beginning stage.

In transit, preexisting symptoms related to past violence, such as rape, and the more recent victimization experiences will need to be addressed. For some victims, the legal barriers, such as immigration laws, represent a much greater threat and must be ascertained. Debt bondage and the associated fear-inducing factors may also appear while in transit. Difficult travel conditions may pose health consequences, such as those related to communicable diseases for groups of people, weather extremes, inadequate shelter, and more. At the point of destination, issues include financial vulnerability, health deterioration, and poor access to health care. Substance abuse and fear of isolation may be experienced at this point. Upon return to the country of origin, issues of stigmatization, accessing employment opportunities, and threats from past traffickers should be evaluated. Repatriated Nepalese women and girls who have been involved in sex trafficking returned with high rates of HIV infection (38% and 60.6%, respectively). Longer-term mental health problems such as chronic post-traumatic distress disorder (PTSD), chronic depression, and anxiety may surface during this time as well.

Vulnerability to trafficking includes poverty and a past history of personal violence. The previous issues are likely to be unchanged after the return home. However, the trauma experience was increased while they were away. Past abusers may spring back into heightened levels of violence toward the victims.

The stages that trafficked women experience fall logically into public health models of prevention. The origin or predeparture and recruitment stage and transit or travel stage are the initial two trafficking stages in which primary prevention efforts may best address the issues that make individuals vulnerable to trafficking and efforts aimed at developing problems can be addressed. The destination and detention stage is the stage in which secondary prevention of legal and health-care interventions may be most focused and forceful. Problems are in full process; interventions may prevent further harm, and long-term health issues can be prevented. The final stage of return or rescue, when survivors may be attempting reintegration, will be the stage in which tertiary prevention efforts will address the problems once the harm has occurred.

IMPLICATIONS FOR NURSES AS FIRST RESPONDERS

Interviewing is part of the nursing assessment and includes the collection of subjective data about victims and their circumstances. The interview must be culturally sensitive, maintain confidentiality, and be conducted in a nonjudgmental manner. Questions about the culture and values of the country of origin may be of value during interviews at this point. Cognitive function is often reduced after the trauma of a trafficking incident, and participation in the interview process may be impaired as in subsequent legal proceedings. Moynihan (2006, p. 101) suggests the following three questions are key for the forensic nurse to ask a suspected victim of trafficking:

1. What type of work to you do?
2. Can you leave your job if you wanted to?
3. Can you come and go as you please?

A complete set of screening questions is offered by the Campaign to Rescue & Restore Victims of Human Trafficking of the U. S. Department of Health and Human Services (Box 18.3).

An ethical perspective must always be considered when the nurse conducts interviews with known or potential victims of trafficking. The ethical principle of self-determination or autonomy is less likely to be exercised when the survivor of trafficking is marginalized by culture change, inability to communicate, and isolation. When there is inadequate information about the possible choices, low self-worth and value do not allow victims to make decisions or participate in making decisions about their own care or their future. Justice is more likely to be exercised in a society or family when there is a balance in power and a differential power level is not exploited through abusive relations. The nurse can provide this balance in a relationship with the victim. Beneficence is demonstrated through holistic consideration and cultural respect. The nurse should be a source of empathy and support. Zimmerman and Watts (2003) suggest several questions that can be asked to help a known trafficking victim feel safe during the interview process:

1. Do you have any concerns about carrying out this interview with me?

Box 18.3   Recommended Screening Questions

- Can you leave your job or situation if you want?
- Can you come and go as you please?
- Have you been threatened if you try to leave?
- Have you been physically harmed in any way?
- What are your working or living conditions like?
- Where do you sleep and eat?
- Do you sleep in a bed, on a cot, or on the floor?
- Have you ever been deprived of food, water, sleep, or medical care?
- Do you have to ask permission to eat, sleep, or go to the bathroom?
- Are there locks on your doors and windows so you cannot get out?
- Has anyone threatened your family?
- Has your identification or documentation been taken from you?
- Is anyone forcing you to do anything that you do not want to do?

(Data taken from U. S. Department of Health and Human Services, Campaign to Rescue and Restore Victims of Human Trafficking, retrieved January 19, 2007, from www.acf.hhs.gov/trafficking/campaign_kits/tool_kit_health/identify_victims.html)

2. Do you think that talking to me could pose any problems for you, for example, with those who trafficked you, your family, friends, or anyone who is assisting you?
3. Have you ever spoken with someone in (interviewer's profession) before? How was that experience?
4. Do you feel this is a good time and place to discuss your experience? If not, is there a better place and time?

Initiating the patient interview from a culturally competent and ethical position will demonstrate respect by the nurse and promote a feeling of safety for vulnerable survivors of trafficking. Often nongovernmental or social support agencies are the safest place for interviews to be held. The screening questions for assessment do not prevent or resolve the survivor's problems and do not constitute primary prevention. Sensitive, culturally appropriate questions are a form of intervention, however, that may increase survivor awareness and enhance self-worth.

The nurse should find a staff interpreter rather than rely on the person accompanying the survivor, who might be the trafficker. Interpreters should be screened carefully to ensure that they have no connection to the survivor or have a conflict of interest. If another person accompanies the survivor to the interview and interacts in a controlling manner with the survivor, the nurse should remove that person from the interview.

Another therapeutic intervention is offering unconditional support and praising the survivor's strength and coping ability during the ordeal. Building trust is critically important to trafficking survivors of abuse and entrapment and is instrumental to their growth and progress. They will need to establish trust when being referred to other resource services. Care should be used to maintain the survivor's confidentiality. A small card in the survivor's language with addresses and numbers for future use is one way to ensure contact and outreach for help for survivors. The card does not need to specify the type of service, which may help keep the information anonymous and not expose the survivor to additional risk from traffickers. The long-term goal for survivors of trafficking includes placement in a safe environment where they can achieve goals of recovery, restoring resilience, and control over their lives.

When the trafficking survivors are children, special protocols are required. Kellogg (2005) presents detailed protocols for interviewing child and adolescent abuse survivors who suffer from substance abuse, sexual exploitation, STDs, genital injury, and nongenital injuries such as those from hand restraint, choking, biting, hair pulling, and hitting. In addition to diagnostic evaluation, Kellogg (2005) recommends medications that can be used to treat injuries and illnesses as well as follow-up considerations at 2 weeks and 2 to 3 months after injury. Watkins (2005) reviews types of genital injuries in children who have been sexually exploited, such as straddle injury and female circumcision, and recommends medical treatments. A detailed conceptual framework that highlights risks, abuse, and health consequences for physical, sexual, psychological, and substance abuse; social restrictions; economic exploitation; legal insecurity; living conditions; and marginalization may be helpful. One example of risks for the category of physical abuse includes sleep deprivation, restraints, and withholding care. The health consequences are listed as injuries, fatigue, poor nutrition, and worsening of preexisting conditions. The intervention plan can be developed for each child survivor individually and be based on the evidence for similarly traumatized children. The plan must address both the mental and physical health issues and the types of abuse that were most severe and damaging to the child to prevent the associated consequences.

Attending to the survivor's safety and intervention and prevention goals, the forensic nurse must exercise self-care as well during the process of helping sexual trafficking survivors. A personal history of abuse or other form of trauma may result in a resurgence of negative feelings for the nurse. Managing one's own symptoms must be undertaken and is not an abnormal occurrence. The nurse may also need to reflect on and address personal biases about persons who have been prostituted. Moreover, Zimmerman and Watts (2003) warn that self-care and survivor care include avoidance of the following actions:

1. Making a "run for it" with the survivor
2. Taking a trafficking survivor into the interviewer's home
3. Escorting the survivor back to her home or place of work to pick up her belongings
4. Assisting the survivor to discuss matters with an employer, boyfriend, agent, coworker, etc., or acting as an intermediary in any way

EVALUATION OF THE EFFECTIVENESS OF INTERVENTIONS

Evaluation of the effectiveness of interventions is multifaceted. Safety considerations are foremost. Mental, physical, and emotional health of survivors and their families must be evaluated. Supportive actions taken to activate the legal process and to charge perpetrators with crimes may be appropriate and related to safety, financial resolution, and mental wellness. Forensic nurses who witness sexual trafficking may be asked to testify in court about observed facts or opinions. As Cooper (2005) notes, there are three types of witnesses in criminal trials. The background witnesses speak to the scientific findings that place the act of violence in context. Case witnesses review specific information about a case before the court as an expert. Evaluating witnesses review records and interview and evaluate survivors of trafficking. Forensic nurses may serve adequately in any one of these three roles.

Evaluating the effectiveness of interventions is most informative when compared to best practice guidelines. The North Carolina Chapter of the International Association of Forensic Nurses and the North Carolina Pediatrics Society have collaboratively developed and recommended guidelines for Sexual Assault Nurse Examiners (SANE) who perform examinations on children suspected of being survivors of child abuse and neglect. Similar guidelines for North Carolina physicians exist to serve as a resource for emergency department medical professionals. The guidelines can be the basis for developing the clinical questions and intervention testing for trafficking survivors. The recommendations outline the interview process, record keeping, physical examination, and reporting requirements to child protection agencies. A list of resource centers is provided that specializes in various types of treatments for children who have been maltreated.

EFFECTS ON SOCIETY AND HEALTH

Human trafficking violates universal human rights to life, liberty, and freedom from slavery. Trafficking promotes social breakdown in multiple essential categories. In the area of human development, trafficking weakens parental authority, undermines family ties, and prevents nurturing and moral development of children. Trafficking tears families apart and interrupts the passage of cultural values from parent to child, further weakening a core value within the societal groups. The inability to benefit from the necessary educational opportunities reduces survivors' future economic opportunities and increases their vulnerability to continued trafficking. Trafficking survivors have depressed wages. The effects of trafficking help to maintain the status of depressed wages and loss of future productivity and

earning power. Trafficking also undermines public health conditions. Persons involved in the sex industry are likely to be infected with sexually transmitted diseases and HIV/AIDS. Groups of trafficked people live in unsanitary, overcrowded living conditions coupled with poor nutrition. Such conditions can foster diseases such as scabies, tuberculosis, and multiple other communicable diseases. Offenders and survivors of trafficking bring a variety of health issues to the receiving country. Ultimately, all health issues of the trafficking groups may not be dealt with effectively in the receiving country during the trafficking experience. If the trafficking experience is interrupted and they are returned and attempt reintegration in the country of origin, their health issues have worsened considerably so they may be a burden within their own country and a danger to the health of all around them.

Transnational crime has an impact on health in correctional settings also. The health officials at the Centers for Disease Control and Prevention and the American Medical Association reported that immigrants accounted for nearly 42% of the tuberculosis cases reported nationwide. As the immigrant population increases and repeated exposure to crime may result in involvement in criminal activity, the possibility that immigrants will carry their health problems into correctional facilities increases as well. Despite all efforts to prevent the spread of disease, immigrants and trafficking victims will carry their communicable diseases into the correctional facilities and back into communities with large immigrant populations.

CONCLUSIONS

As Moynihan (2006) points out, the forensic nurse can be the "link to freedom" for survivors of human trafficking in the public health, pediatric, women's health, and psychiatric settings. Nurses who care for women and children in primary, secondary, or tertiary care settings may hold the well-being of the survivors of trafficking and be the key that releases the chains of slavery.

Nurses have the professional responsibility to promote policy that provides for the safety and health care of trafficking survivors. A recent report by the Center for Women Policy Studies stated that 11 states in the United States have enacted laws that assist trafficking survivors with their physical and emotional recovery. However, the best practices for identification and methods to assist current victims and recent survivors with medical and legal problems are scarce. It is unclear what the actual number of trafficked persons is, how reports arrived at an estimate, and if estimates are verifiable.

Nurses who work in institutions around the world can be instrumental in policy development and improved services by conducting and participating in research on various aspects of human trafficking. Nurses are oriented toward action-based approaches in patient care and in general want to use best practices that are recommended by research. However, there are few studies that compare aspects of care to apply to practice. In general, care providers focus on special vulnerable populations, such as women and children, who have been used for sexual exploitation, and other forms of trafficking get neglected. There is little independent evaluation of trafficking policies and programs to assess the beneficial impact and effectiveness. Furthermore, due to lack of awareness and education, health-care providers and policy makers often focus on international trafficking and less on domestic trafficking or the connection between the two.

To advance the research and ability to improve identification and health care of trafficked persons and advance policy development, there must be agreement on definition of terms and what actually needs to be studied. Programs and training materials address the invisibility of trafficking victims. They are difficult to identify, and interviewing victims of trafficking is even more challenging. Much time is required to elicit the histories, and few resources may be available in the community.

Nurses need evidence-based practice protocols that focus on the individual person's trafficking experience, the perceived threat to the person, and at what stage of the process the person is in to best assess health needs. The following key points are recommended to nurses who suspect human trafficking involves a patient:

1. Conduct an ethical interview and demonstrate care and a nonjudgmental sensitivity to cultural values.
2. Maintain confidentiality of personal information.
3. Recognize and assess the health problems associated with each of the phases of trafficking: origin (recruitment); transit (travel); destination (detention and exploitation); and return (rescue).
4. Promote safe interaction in a safe environment.
5. Refer to trustworthy sources in health care, social work, and criminal justice fields.
6. Find reliable translators who understand that the legal and health-care implications of human trafficking are very diverse for each individual.
7. Listen to and follow the preferences of the person who experiences trafficking to the extent possible, since that is the only way to comprehend and develop policy and health-care practices that will be most effective.
8. Self-care and safety for interviewers and health-care providers should include debriefing with others who can provide support and reduce secondary traumatization.
9. Keep careful records of mental and physical health-care issues with patient quotes if possible, as nursing records may be key forensic documentation in criminal prosecutions.
10. Develop protocols for assessment and intervention that are posted in emergency departments and other agencies where trafficking victims may be identified and assisted toward survival.

Case Study

CARLOS

Carlos lived in Mexico and wanted to come to the United States to work, so he paid a coyote to be brought into the United States. Once he crossed the border, he was taken to a safe house and then transported to a peanut farm in Georgia to work. Carlos was told that the cost of being brought into the United States and transported to the farm was $2500.

Once at the farm, it was explained to Carlos that he could not leave and that he would be beaten if he attempted to flee.

Carlos was paid for his work but was also charged for rent and food costs, which were subtracted from his pay. Carlos was moved to other farms throughout the East Coast, depending on the season.

Discussion Questions

1. Is Carlos a victim of trafficking?
2. Did he choose to come into the United States?
3. How and when might Carlos be identified?

Case Study

TINA

Tina, who is 15 years old, has been prostituting in several businesses for the past 6 months, moving from Houston to Dallas to Atlanta for several weeks at a time. She works for her pimp-boyfriend, Bobby. Tina has a $1000 quota per night that she must earn for Bobby, who says he is saving the money for them to buy a house in whichever city she likes the best. Tina is often scared while out on the streets, but Bobby reminds her that she is making money for their future and that the situation is only temporary. Bobby has other girls who work for him, but Tina knows that she is special to him because Bobby does not hit her like he does the others. Tina is picked up one night by an undercover officer.

Angry and defensive, Tina does not cooperate with the officer. She admits that Bobby is her pimp, but swears that prostitution was her choice and that Bobby has never forced her to do anything.

Discussion Questions

1. Is Tina a victim of trafficking?
2. Did she choose to live the life she leads?
3. What are ways to help her understand the legal aspects of her activities?
4. Compare critical aspects of the cases of Tina and Carlos.

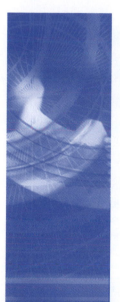

EVIDENCE-BASED PRACTICE

Reference Question: What are the current opinions or stances regarding using advocacy interventions with human trafficking?

Database(s) to Search: LexisNexis

Search Strategy: Due to the narrowness of this question, search only the term "advocacy" and then use it with "AND" and the phrase "human trafficking." To get the most appropriate results for research, make sure to select the "legal" source option.

Selected References From Search:

1. Sidel, M., & Richard, B. (2008). Lillich Memorial Lecture: New directions in the struggle against human trafficking. *Journal of Transnational Law & Policy, 17*(187).
2. Cianciarulo, M.S. (2008). The trafficking and exploitation victims assistance program: A proposed early response plan for victims of international human trafficking in the United States. *New Mexico Law Review, 38*(373).
3. Payne, V.S. (2008/2009). National Security Symposium: The battle between Congress & the courts in the face of an unprecedented global threat: Note: On the road to victory in America's war on human trafficking: Landmarks, landmines, and the need for centralized strategy. *Regent University Law Review, 21*(435).

Questions Used to Discern Evidence:

Choose two studies among the studies listed, read about them, and answer the following questions:

1. What are the differences between the two studies in the design, methods, and results?
2. What are the similarities between the two studies in the number of subjects, measures used, and interventions, if any?
3. What skills do you need to learn to prepare for forensic nursing practice with this population?

REVIEW QUESTIONS

1. Persons who experience trafficking are at risk for physical abuse due to:
   A. Sleep deprivation, restraints, withholding care.
   B. Poor memory and poor judgment.
   C. Lack of health-care knowledge and inability to provide information to law enforcement.
   D. Desire to go home and no place to go.

2. Detention and exploitation are more likely to take place in which stage of human trafficking?
   A. Origin
   B. Transit
   C. Destination
   D. Return

3. The forensic nurse may be called to testify in court as a witness in a human trafficking trial. When speaking about the scientific findings that place the act of human trafficking in context, the nurse is a/n:
   A. Case witness.
   B. Background witness.
   C. Fact witness.
   D. Eye witness.

4. The forensic nurse may be called as a witness to review specific information about a case as an expert so is therefore a/n:
   A. Case witness.
   B. Background witness.
   C. Fact witness.
   D. Evaluating witness.

5. How many states have enacted laws that assist persons who have been trafficked?
   A. Fifty states
   B. Forty states
   C. Twenty states
   D. Eleven states

6. Which of the following questions should the nurse ask to help the person feel safe prior to an interview?
   A. Do you have any concerns about carrying out this interview?
   B. Have you ever spoken with someone in law enforcement before?
   C. How is this experience making you feel?
   D. When did you realize you are a victim of human trafficking?

7. Unique features often exhibited by persons who are being trafficked may assist the forensic nurse in identification of their health and safety needs and include:
   A. Inability to move or leave their job.
   B. Lack of social support system.
   C. Inability to speak English.
   D. Presents in the clinical setting alone.

8. The ethical principle of _____is not likely to be exercised when the trafficking victim is marginalized by culture change, inability to communicate, and isolation.
   A. Justice
   B. Autonomy
   C. Beneficence
   D. Isolation

9. Self-care for forensic nurses who care for survivors of trafficking include:
   A. Making a "run for it" to a safe place with the survivor.
   B. Taking the person home where it is safe.
   C. Reflecting on personal biases.
   D. Assisting the survivor to discuss matters with an employer/trafficker.

10. Moynihan (2006) suggests the following three questions are key for the forensic nurse to ask a suspected survivor of trafficking: (1) What type of work to you do? (2) Can you leave your job if you wanted to? and (3):
    A. Where were you born?
    B. Can you come and go as you please?
    C. Did you finish high school?
    D. When did you arrive in this country?

References

Alexander, M., Kellogg, N., & Thompson, P. (2005). Community and mental health support of juvenile victims of prostitution. In S. Cooper, R. Estes, A. Giardino, et al (eds.). *Medical, legal, & social science aspects of child sexual exploitation: A comprehensive review of pornography, prostitution, and internet crimes (Vol. 2)*. St. Louis: G.W. Medical Publishing.

Bales, K. (1999). Disposable people: New slavery in the global economy. Berkley, CA: University of California Press.

Basch, L. (2004). Human security, globalizations, and feminist visions. *Peace Review,16*:5.

Campion, M. (2007). *Human trafficking in Minnesota: A report to the Minnesota legislature.* Minnesota Department of Public Safety Office of Justice Programs, St. Paul, Minnesota.

Castles, S. (2004). The factors that make and unmake migration policies. *International Migration Review, 38*:852.

Center for Women Policy Studies. (2007). *Report card on state action to combat international trafficking.* Washington, DC: Center for Women Policy Studies.

Cockburn, A. (2003). 21st century slaves. *National Geographic, 204*:2.

Cooper, S. (2005). The medical expert and child sexual exploitation. In S. Cooper, R. Estes, A. Giardino, et al. (eds.). *Medical, legal, & social science aspects of child sexual exploitation: A comprehensive review of pornography, prostitution, and internet crimes (Vol. 2)*. St. Louis: G.W. Medical Publishing.

Cooper, S. (2006). Personal communication.

Farley, M. (Ed.). (2003). *Prostitution, trafficking, and traumatic stress (Vol. 2)*. New York: Hawthorne Press.

Farley, M., Baral, I., Kiremire, M., et al. (1998). Prostitution in five countries: Violence and post traumatic stress disorder. *Feminine Psychology, 8*(4):405-425.

Florida Department of Children and Families. Office of Refugee Services. Florida State University Center for the Advancement of Human Rights. *Florida responds to human trafficking.* Retrieved January 24, 2006, from www.cahr.fsu.edu/the%20report.pdf

Germany, U.S. receive most sex trafficked women. (July-August 2003). *Off our backs, 33,* (4).

Helton, A., & Jacobs, E. (2000). Combating human smuggling by enlisting the victims. *Migration World Magazine, 28*:12.

Hughes, D., & Raymond, J. (2001). Sex trafficking of women in the United States: International and domestic trends. Retrieved January 24, 2006, from action.web.ca/home/catw/attach/sex_traff_us.pdf

International Organization for Migration (IOM). (2006). *Breaking the cycle of vulnerability: Responding to the health needs of trafficked women in East & southern Africa.* Pretoria, South Africa: International Organization for Migration.

Kellogg, N. (2005). Medical care of the children of the night. In S. Cooper, R. Estes, A. Giardino, N. Kellogg, & V. Vieth. (Eds.). *Medical, legal, & social science aspects of child sexual exploitation: A comprehensive review of pornography, prostitution, and internet crimes (Vol. 1)*. St. Louis: G.W. Medical Publishing.

Malarek, V. (2003). *The Natashas.* New York: Arcade Publishing.

McKelvey, T. (2004). Of human bondage: A coalition against human trafficking worked well until a prostitution litmus test was imposed. Now, groups are losing funding and the women aren't necessarily better off. *The American Prospect, 15*:17.

Miller, E., Decker, M., Silverman, J., et al. (2007). Migration, sexual exploitation and women's health. *Violence Against Women, 13*(5):486-497.

Moynihan, B. (2006). The high cost of human trafficking. *Journal of Forensic Nursing, 2*(2):100-101.

Orlova, A. (2004). From social dislocation to human trafficking. *Problems of post-Communism, 51*:14.

O'Rourke, M. (2002). Transnational crime: A new health threat for corrections. *Corrections Today, 64*:86.

Polaris Project. *Law enforcement toolkit on trafficking in persons.* Polaris Project. Retrieved February 15, 2006, from www.polarisproject.com

Raymond, J., D'Cunha, J., Dzuhayatin, S., et al. (2002). *A comparative study of women trafficked in the migration process: Patterns, profiles, and health consequences in five countries, Indonesia, the Philippines, Thailand, Venezuela and the United States.* Retrieved March 9, 2008, from action.web.ca/home/catw/readingroom.shtml?x=17062

Sage, J. (2000). Guarding America's first right: Freedom from bondage: The civil rights community must respond to the disturbing rise in cases of involuntary servitude in the United States. *Civil Rights Journal, 5*:4.

Silverman, J., Decker, M., Gupta, J., et al. (2007). Experiences of sex trafficking victims in Mumbai, India. *International Journal of Gynecology and Obstetrics, 97*:221-226.

Silverman, J., Decker, M., Gupta, J., et al. (2007). HIV prevalence and predictors of infection in sex-trafficked Nepalese girls and women. *Journal of the American Medical Association, 298*(5):536-542.

U.S. Department of Justice, Civil Rights Division. (2004). Recent notable prosecutions. *Anti-Trafficking News Bulletin, 1.*

U.S. Department of Justice (USDOJ). (2006). *Report on activities to combat human trafficking fiscal years 2001-2005.* United States Department of Justice. Retrieved July, 2006, from www.usdoj.gov

U.S. Department of State. (2002). Off our backs. State Department releases problematic report on trafficking, *7.*

U.S. Department of State. (2005). *The Trafficking in Persons (TIP) Report.* Retrieved July, 2005, from www.state.gov/g/tip

U.S. Department of State. (2006). *The Trafficking in Persons (TIP) Report.* The United States Department of State. Retrieved July, 2006 from www.state.gov/g/tip

The U.S. 9/11 Commission on Border Patrol. (2004). *Population and Development Review, 30*:569.

Venkatraman, B., Jacob, E., & Henley, D. (2005). The hidden truth of involuntary servitude and slavery. In S. Cooper, R. Estes, A. Giardino, N. Kellogg, & V. Vieth (Eds.). *Medical, legal, & social science aspects of child sexual exploitation: A comprehensive review of pornography, prostitution, and internet crimes (Vol. 2)*. St. Louis: G.W. Medical Publishing.

Watkins, F.B. (2005). The medical implications of anogenital trauma in child sexual exploitation. In S. Cooper, R. Estes,

A. Giardino, N. Kellogg, & V. Vieth (Eds.). *Medical, legal, & social science aspects of child sexual exploitation: A comprehensive review of pornography, prostitution, and internet crimes (Vol. 1).* St. Louis: G.W. Medical Publishing.

Wells, M. (2004). The grassroots reconfiguration of U.S. immigration policy. *International Migration Review, 38*:1308.

Zimmerman, C., Hossain, M., Yun, K., et al. (2006). *Stolen smiles: A summary report on the physical and psychological health consequences of women and adolescents trafficked in Europe.* London: London School of Hygiene & Tropical Medicine.

Zimmerman, C. & Watts, C. (2003). *WHO ethical and safety recommendations for interviewing trafficked women.* London: World Health Organization.

Zimmerman, C., Yun, K., Shvab, I., Watts, C., et al. (2003). *The health risks and consequences of trafficking in women and adolescents: Findings from a European study.* London: London School of Hygiene & Tropical Medicine.

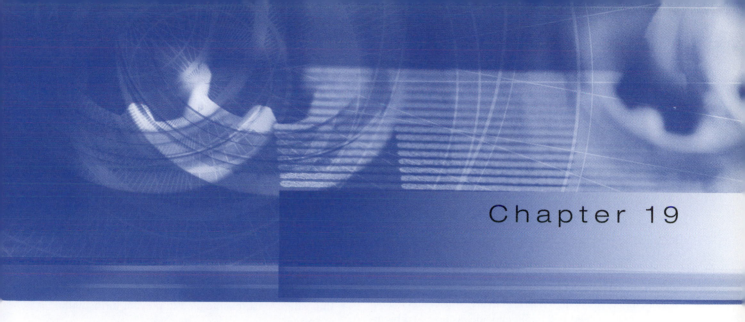

Chapter 19

FORENSIC EXPLORATION OF GLOBAL HUMAN RIGHTS VIOLATIONS AND GENOCIDE

Cheyenne Martin

"Silence lost its way when a hand opened the doors to the voice."
Francisco Morales Santos, Guatemalan Poet

Competencies

1. Describing the primary components of genocide as defined by the United Nations in 1948.
2. Analyzing key sociopolitical, economic, and cultural variables that have contributed to the origins of massive human rights violations and genocide during the 20th century and first decade of the 21st century.
3. Describing specific forensic roles of nurses and other health professionals related to the identification of victims of violence in war and genocide, collection of forensic evidence, documentation of findings, and provision of legal testimony.
4. Analyzing evidence-based strategies that can be used in primary, secondary, and tertiary prevention of mass violence and genocide.
5. Analyzing relevant ethical and legal dimensions of using forensic science to examine and document mass violence and genocide.
6. Examining potential threats to nurses and other health-care providers who participate in forensic studies during and after civil war and genocide.

Key Terms

Ethnic cleansing
Genocide
Mass grave excavation
Minimum number of individuals (MNIs)
Nuremberg Trials
War crimes

INTRODUCTION

One of the tragic legacies of the 20th century is the staggering upward spiral in genocide across the globe. The extent of violence and mass murder of civilians based on ethnicity, religion, or political beliefs that occurred during the Holocaust and in the Soviet Union, Cambodia, and the more recent conflicts in Bosnia, Rwanda, and Darfur is unparalleled. An estimated 40 million people perished in those genocides as reflected in the group-specific data cited in Box 19.1.

Unfortunately, numerous other areas around the world, including the Congo and Somalia, are currently experiencing, or are at high risk for having, substantial human rights violations and potential genocide, as assessed by international humanitarian groups and genocide researchers.

DEFINITION AND SCOPE OF GENOCIDE

The term **genocid**e was originally conceived by Raphael Lemkin, a Polish Jewish attorney who escaped Poland after the Nazi invasion. In an effort to describe the mass killing of Jews and others that was occurring under Hitler,

Box 19.1 Genocide in the 20th Century

- Ottoman Turks' killing of Armenians in Turkey, 1915–1918: 1,500,000 deaths (Dadrian, 1995)
- Stalin's forced famine and starvation of Soviet citizens living in the Ukraine and Kazakhstan, 1932–1933: 4,000,000 deaths (Werth, 2009)
- Stalin's murder of political opponents during the Great Terror, 1937–1938: 5,000,000 deaths (Werth, 2006)
- Nazi Holocaust, 1938–1945: 6,000,000 Jewish deaths and 10,000,000 deaths of other minority groups, including Gypsies, Christian Scientists, homosexuals, and political prisoners (International Military Tribunal, 1946)
- Pol Pot regime's murder of Cambodians, 1975–1979: 2,000,000 deaths (Kissi, 2006)
- Guatemalan army's massacre of Mayan Indians and Ladinos, 1982–1985: 200,000 deaths (Commission for Historical Clarification, 1998)
- Bosnia-Herzegovinan Serbian's killing of Muslim Bosniaks, 1991–1995: 200,000 deaths (Tribunal for War Crimes in Bosnia, 2005)
- Rwandan Hutu's killing of Tutsis, 1994: 800,000 deaths (UN, 2002)
- Darfurian government-sponsored militia's (Janjawiid's) murder of civilians, 2003–2006: 200,000 deaths (UN, 2008)

Lemkin (1994) combined the Greek word for race, *genos,* with the Latin term for killing, *cide*. Lemkin's work and the results of the **Nuremberg Trials,** persuaded the United Nations to officially define genocide in 1948 to include any of the following acts that are committed with the intent to destroy, either wholly or in part, a national, ethnic, racial, or religious group:

- Killing members of the group
- Causing serious bodily or mental harm to members of the group
- Deliberately inflicting on the group conditions of life calculated to bring about its physical destruction in whole or in part
- Imposing measures intended to prevent births within the group
- Forcibly transferring children of the group to another group

Acts of genocide not only destroy members of targeted groups, but also often have devastating effects on surviving populations. Many survivors endure severe and often long-lasting physical and emotional injuries, forced evacuations away from homelands, and separations from family and community support systems. At a societal level, genocide often leads to overall destabilization of existing governments, community structures, and economies. That level of destabilization can in turn lead to further power struggles and violence in war-torn societies that seriously impede possible reconstruction and reconciliation.

THE GENEVA CONVENTIONS

The Geneva Conventions of 1949 not only provide for the humanitarian treatment of combatants but also prohibit the use of violence toward civilians. In 1977, the provisions of the Geneva Conventions were expanded to include noninternational wars and conflicts. One of the most significant features of the Geneva Conventions is that they provide a standard for examining and prosecuting **war crimes** that may occur during wars and civil conflicts. Other United Nations resolutions on human rights and war crimes can be seen in Box 19.2.

SIGNIFICANCE OF FORENSIC SCIENCE IN EXPLORING AND DOCUMENTING HUMAN RIGHTS VIOLATIONS AND GENOCIDE

In the midst of continuing civil wars and escalating acts of genocide, the use of forensic science to explore and

Box 19.2   United Nations Resolutions on Human Rights and War Crimes Tribunals

- UN Resolution on Genocide (1948)
- Geneva Conventions of 1949
- International Military Tribunal at Nuremberg (1945–1949)
- International Criminal Tribunal for the Former Yugoslavia (1993–2011)
- International Criminal Tribunal for Rwanda (1994)
- International Commission on Missing Persons (1996)
- International Criminal Court (2002)
- UN Resolution on Trafficking in Women and Girls (2008)

document these events has become pivotal. It provides an evidenced-based, systematic process for examining and helping to establish the extent and nature of massive violence directed at selected populations in varying geographic locations.

This chapter examines the historical evolution of forensic science as a tool for exploring and documenting global violence and genocide during the past 60 years as well as the important, multifaceted roles of nurses, physicians, and other health providers in forensic investigations of mass torture and murder of civilians. It also addresses some of the inherent ethical-legal and political issues that often arise in conducting forensic investigations of massive crimes that occur during civil wars and regional conflicts.

Specifically examined is the use of forensic science to explore mass violence and genocide during the Holocaust as well as civil wars in Argentina and the former Yugoslavia. Those seminal events in the history of genocide provide a unique backdrop for analyzing the relevance and significance of forensic science as a tool for exposing and documenting large-scale violations of human rights. The use of forensic science by the investigative team of the International Military Tribunal in preparation for indicting and trying Nazi perpetrators for war crimes stands as one of the first and most extensive global forensic efforts of the past century.

OVERVIEW OF HEALTH PROFESSIONALS' PARTICIPATION IN GLOBAL FORENSIC MISSIONS

International human rights groups, forensic organizations, and international courts have increasingly recognized the crucial contributions that multidisciplinary teams including nurses, physicians, forensic anthropologists, and archaeologists can make to complex forensic investigations during or after civil war and genocide. These team members play key roles at all levels of forensic exploration, including as material witnesses, as forensic investigators, and as expert witnesses and consultants. Health providers who have been primary witnesses to and/or targets of violence and genocide can often provide critical first-person documentation and testimonies regarding the context, nature, and location of specific violations of human rights as well as identification of both victims and perpetrators. This eyewitness role is exemplified by Christina Schmitz, a German nurse, and Daniel O'Brien, an Australian physician, who were working for Médecins Sans Frontières (MSF) in Srebrenica when it was attacked by Serbian troops in July 1995. They were able to provide first-person accounts of the roundup and massacre of an estimated 8000 male civilians over a several-day period to local authorities and later testified to the French government on behalf of MSF.

Additionally, health professionals who have specific forensic expertise have been instrumental in helping forensic teams document and verify the nature, extent, causes, and patterns of injuries and death. They have also played a crucial role in helping to identify individual victims of violence as well as in helping establish demographic profiles of the collective victims. Forensic teams have provided evidence-based expert testimony to appropriate legal bodies at local, national, and international levels, including officially convened tribunals and special investigative or truth commissions.

Health professionals' documentation and legal testimonies are a critical part of collaborative efforts to bring perpetrators to justice and punish their crimes. For example, numerous nurses, physicians, and other health professionals who had been imprisoned in Nazi concentration camps provided key testimonies about the atrocities they witnessed or had been subjected to at the Doctors' Trial at Nuremberg (*United States v. Karl Brandt, et al*) as well as other war crimes trials. More recently, the in-depth investigations and expert testimonies provided by members of the forensic teams from Physicians for Human Rights International, such as Dr. Bill Haglund, were instrumental in helping document violations of human rights for tribunals in both the Rwandan and Bosnian conflicts. Physicians for Human Rights continues to be involved in forensic missions in Darfur and the Congo.

Forensic Science and Reconciliation

In addition to the contributions of forensic science to prosecutorial efforts, there has been a growing recognition during the past several decades that forensic science can possibly play an equally important role in reconciliation efforts following war and mass violence. Finding and identifying persons who have "disappeared" during mass killing campaigns and returning the remains of those victims to their families has been reported as a major factor in many families finding some degree of comfort and closure that may then allow them to rebuild their lives and communities.

Similarly, many experienced forensic experts and legal scholars believe that documenting and exposing the truth about perpetrators' crimes and holding them accountable through the justice system may contribute to reconciliation efforts in war-torn communities as well as potentially help prevent, mitigate, or deter future violence and genocide. Totten, a widely respected genocide scholar, believes, however, that the tools of forensic science and international criminal justice cannot by themselves prevent or deter mass hatred and violence. He emphasizes that global communities and leaders must engage more directly in dialogue and programs to prevent and respond to genocide, as well as to exercise moral and political will to stop it (Totten & Parsons, 2009).

Although it is beyond the scope of this chapter to provide an in-depth analysis of mass violence and genocide, it is vitally important that health professionals who engage in global forensic missions have a substantial understanding of the historical, sociopolitical, and cultural factors that contribute to human rights violations and genocide. That knowledge can help inform forensic investigations and analysis of violent events and their outcomes. Many of those issues will be examined in the following discussion of genocide and war crimes that occurred during the Nazi era and in Argentina and the former Yugoslavia.

WAR CRIMES AND GENOCIDE DURING THE NAZI ERA

The Holocaust remains the single largest state-sponsored genocide in history. It also has the distinction of being the first forensic investigation of massive global human rights violations. An estimated 6 million Jews and 8 to 10 million other persons who were deemed undesirable by the Third Reich, including Gypsies (Roma), homosexuals, Christian Scientists, disabled children and adults, and political dissidents, were murdered during the Nazi era. Hundreds of thousands of others who survived the brutality of ghettos and concentration camps sustained long-lasting illness and injuries.

Forensic Evidence of War Crimes

As evidence of Nazi atrocities began to filter out during the war, Allied leaders entered into an agreement to establish war crimes trials of major war criminals once the war was over. In an effort to gather ample forensic evidence of

"crimes against humanity," special teams of Allied troops were deployed across Germany and other parts of occupied Europe in the last days of the war to seek out important documentation and to gather important eyewitness testimonies. It was a massive undertaking because of the sheer number of crime scenes—hundreds of labor and death camps that were sites of mass atrocities and murder as well as large numbers of mass graves that had been constructed to hide the bodies of victims spread across Poland, Russia, and most of the countries that had been occupied by the Third Reich.

Although Nazi officials were able to destroy some evidence incriminating them for alleged war crimes as Allied troops advanced, investigators were still able to capture significant documents, photos, and films in government buildings, Nazi headquarters, and concentration camp administrative offices throughout Germany and occupied Europe. Many of these documents, for example, the personal files of Gestapo chief Himmler, provided detailed evidence of the Third Reich's war of aggression against most of Europe and their extensive plans to systematically murder Jews and other groups they deemed undesirable. The documentary evidence, coupled with eyewitness testimonies and selected physical evidence of experimentation, torture, and murder formed the backbone of the forensic evidence.

Eyewitness Testimonies as Forensic Evidence

In addition to significant Nazi documents, one of the most crucial and potent sources of forensic evidence of war crimes came from eyewitness accounts and testimonies of Holocaust survivors, including nurses and physicians, who had been imprisoned in ghettos and labor and death camps in Germany, Poland, Czechoslovakia, and other occupied countries. Their personal testimonies at the first and subsequent Nuremberg Trials and other postwar trials provided powerful evidence of deliberate starvation, forced labor, and medical experiments on and systematic murder of prisoners. Those testimonies were pivotal to prosecutions of alleged Nazi war criminals and will be discussed further in the Nuremberg Doctors' Trials section below.

Liberator Testimonies

Additional forensic evidence of war crimes was provided by members of armed forces from the United States, Great Britain, the Soviet Union, and other Allied countries who helped liberate the camps in the winter and spring of 1945. There were a number of nurses and physicians among the various Allied troop liberators who bore witness to prisoners' emaciated state and extreme medical conditions as they attempted to provide the survivors with medical care and food. As an example, Dr. Marcus Smith, a young U.S. Army physician, was one of the first military physicians to reach Dachau after it was liberated by American troops on April 29, 1945, and he stayed on to command the medical team in the Displaced Persons' camp. He took extensive notes about the emaciated conditions of prisoners and their many injuries from both hard labor and Nazi medical experiments. He shared those observations with senior military commanders and forensic investigators and later chronicled his experiences in a poignant and revealing book about Dachau.

Photographic Evidence of Atrocities and Mass Killing

Photographic evidence of the deplorable conditions found in both slave labor and death camps after liberation played a central role in the documentation of Nazi atrocities and murder of Jews, Gypsies, political prisoners, and others who had been imprisoned there. Many of the graphic photos and films of emaciated and dead prisoners that are so symbolic of Nazi brutality were originally taken by the U.S. Army Signal Corps photographers, as well as by newspaper photographers and liberating soldiers.

Many of the photos and films were later admitted as forensic evidence of Nazi war crimes at the Nuremberg Trials and other war crimes trials held across Europe after the war.

International Military Tribunal (Nuremberg War Trials)

The substantial documentary evidence of widespread atrocities coupled with prisoner testimonies and expert medical evidence of torture and deliberate injuries of prisoners were used to support the indictments and prosecutions of Nazi defendants at the International Military Tribunal (IMT) at Nuremberg. This series of trials, held between November 1945 and April 1949, were highly significant since they were the first tribunals in history to specifically prosecute war crimes. This section briefly describes the initial Nuremberg Trial but also focuses more extensively on the forensic evidence presented at the subsequent Doctors' Trials.

The first and most publicized of the trials, the International Military Tribunal, largely focused on prosecution of leading officials in the Third Reich. Although Adolf Hitler and two other key Nazi figures, Heinrich Himmler, head of the notorious SS, and Joseph Goebbels, minister of propaganda, had eluded capture by committing suicide as the Reich collapsed, the IMT indicted 22 other major leaders in the Nazi party. These included Hermann Goering, Rudolf Hess, Albert Speer, and Martin Bormann (tried in absentia), who were charged with violating the existing laws of war and committing crimes against humanity.

In total, 19 of the 22 defendants were found guilty of war crimes, with 12 of them sentenced to death by hanging and 7 sentenced to imprisonment. Three other defendants were acquitted. Goering was one of the most high-profile Nazi officers sentenced to die, but he committed suicide by swallowing a cyanide capsule several hours before he was to be hanged.

The convictions of major Nazi officials at the first Nuremberg Trial established a powerful legal precedent for holding individuals culpable for their own independent actions in committing war crimes. It also set the stage for 12 additional separate trials known as the Subsequent Proceedings, which included the infamous Doctors' Trials.

Doctors' Trials at Nuremberg—Unmasking Medical Crimes and "Mad Science"

The Doctors' Trials, officially entitled Medical Case No. 1, *United States v. Karl Brandt, et al*, convened in Nuremberg on December 9,1946. The defendants included 20 physicians and three top level administrative assistants who were charged with engaging in medical experiments on concentration camp prisoners without their consent in Auschwitz, Dachau, Ravensbruck, Buchenwald, and other camps. Several of the defendants were also charged with participating in euthanasia programs to murder German children and adults with mental and physical disabilities or participating in deliberate murder of forced laborers from Eastern Europe.

Although there were no nurses specifically indicted for war crimes as part of the Doctors' Trials at Nuremberg, a number of nurses who participated in experiments on prisoners and euthanasia of disabled children and adults were charged and tried at separate trials in Germany, Poland, and other previously occupied countries. Their involvement in those trials will be discussed later in this chapter.

Many of the defendants at the Doctors' Trials were leading German physicians who were high-ranking military officers and members of the Nazi Party. Dr. Karl Brandt was Hitler's personal physician and commissioner for health, the highest ranking health official in the Reich. He was also a major general in the Waffen SS (the Schutzstaffel, a special armed division of the Nazi Party). Dr. Gerhard Rose, a brigadier general in the Luftwaffe (German Air Force), headed the prestigious Koch Institute for Tropical Medicine in Berlin. Dr. Karl Gebhardt was chief surgeon of the SS and president of the German Red

Cross. Dr. Paul Rostock was chief of the Reich's Office for Medical Science and Research and had served as the dean of the School of Medicine at the University of Berlin.

The magnitude of the alleged crimes by these doctors is reflected in a brief excerpt of the prosecution's opening statement at the Doctors' Trials, delivered by General Telford Taylor, chief of counsel for the war crimes trials, on December 9, 1946:

> The defendants in this case are charged with murders, tortures, and other atrocities committed in the name of medical science. The victims of these crimes are numbered in the hundreds of thousands. A handful only are still alive; a few of the survivors will appear in this courtroom. But most of these miserable victims were slaughtered outright or died in the course of the tortures to which they were subjected. (International Military Tribunal, p. 27)

In a later statement, Taylor calls attention to the significance of the trial for future forensic medicine and international law:

> The tribunal judgment will be of profound and enduring value in the field of medical jurisprudence; and the trial as a whole is an epochal step in the evolution of forensic medicine. The trial illustrates, furthermore, how rapidly the focus of international law has moved from the academic lecture hall and toward the courtroom. The Nuremberg proceedings are among the outstanding examples of modern international law in action. (Mitscherlich & Mielk, 1949, p.140)

Forensic Evidence of Medical War Crimes

Experiments on Prisoners

Much of the compelling evidence of war crimes at the Doctors' Trials was linked to medical experiments on prisoners. Both documentary and eyewitness evidence established that many of the defendant physicians had knowingly directed and participated in a wide range of horrific medical experiments on nonconsenting camp prisoners. These included sterilization studies on Jewish women inmates and a series of studies in collaboration with the German Air Force to test experimental vaccines for malaria as well as testing of experimental bone regeneration and transplant techniques.

The collaboration between the Nazi party and the scientific and medical community was seen as beneficial for both groups—furthering the military objectives of the party by supposedly improving medical care of soldiers while also enhancing the reputation of medical

researchers who were often affiliated with medical schools in Germany.

Freezing Experiments at Dachau

Some of the most brutal experiments detailed at the Doctors' Trials occurred at Dachau and Buchenwald Camps in Germany. Many of the studies were allegedly focused on finding effective treatments for Air Force pilots and crews' high-altitude sickness and exposure to freezing water following airplane crashes, as well as testing various methods that could help navy seamen survive in seawater. Under the direction of Drs. Weitz and Rascher, numerous camp prisoners at Dachau were forced to stay outdoors in freezing weather without any clothing for up to 14 hours, or they were submerged in freezing water for long periods of time in order for researchers to study the most effective methods of "rewarming" frozen limbs. The freezing experiments at Dachau were carried out between August 1942 and May 1943.

The experiments were detailed in camp records and reflect that an estimated 300 prisoners at Dachau were used in these freezing experiments and approximately 80 to 90 of them died as a result of the tests. Additional evidence included dozens of letters between the teams of research physicians as well as direct correspondence with Himmler and other Nazi leaders. For example, Dr. Rascher, a coinvestigator in the studies, described some of the effects of the freezing experiments on his prisoner subjects at Dachau in a letter to Himmler in August 1942:

> Electrical measurements gave low temperature readings of 26.4 degrees in the stomach and 26.5 degrees in the rectum. Fatalities occurred only when the brain stem and the back of the head were also chilled. Autopsies of such fatal cases always revealed large amounts of free blood, up to ½ liter, in the cranial cavity. The heart invariably showed extreme dilation of the right chamber. As soon as the temperature in those experiments reached 28 degrees, the experimental subjects died invariably despite all attempts at resuscitation. (Taylor, 1995)

Additional correspondence between the research team revealed that the freezing victims' organs were frequently removed and sent to the Pathological Institute at Munich for further examination and study by academic scientists.

Forensic evidence was also provided by several prisoner survivors who testified that they were forced to undergo the freezing experiments. One of those included Father Leo Miechalowski, a Polish priest who was among an estimated 2000 clergymen imprisoned at Dachau for opposing the policies of the Third Reich. Testifying for the prosecution, in this excerpted statement Father

Miechalowski related his experience of being placed in freezing water for a long period of time:

> I was freezing very much in this water. Now my feet were becoming rigid as iron, and the same thing applied to my hands, and later on my breathing became very short. I once again began to tremble, and afterwards cold sweat appeared on my forehead. I felt as if I was just about to die, and then I was still asking them to pull me out because I could not stand this much longer. (Taylor, 1995)

He later lost consciousness and awoke to find himself in a bed being warmed by blankets and heat lamps. He testified that he had been told by one of the doctors to never reveal what had happened because it was a military secret. He survived the ordeal, but experienced heart and mobility problems which persisted after he was liberated from the camp.

Bone Transplant Experiments at Ravensbruck Camp

In addition to the Dachau studies, the trial highlighted a series of painful and often lethal bone regeneration experiments performed on a group of 75 Polish women prisoners at Ravensbruck Camp for women in Germany. Among those physicians charged with inhumane experiments on prisoners without their permission were Dr. Karl Gebhardt, chief surgeon of the SS; Dr. Fritz Fischer, assistant to Dr. Gebhardt; and Dr. Herta Oberheuser, a German physician at the camp as well as at nearby Hohenlychen hospital. She was the only woman defendant at the Doctors' Trials. According to camp records and the defendant doctors' testimonies, the bone experiments were apparently carried out in an attempt to regenerate bone and/or test bone transplant procedures for German soldiers who had lost limbs in combat. Camp prisoners, including health professionals, who had been subjected to torturous experiments or who witnessed those experiments, provided riveting testimonies about the physician defendants' complicity in these bizarre studies.

One of the most impressive witnesses at the trials was Ms. Jadwiga Dzido, who had been a graduate student in pharmacy in Poland before the war and a member of the Polish resistance. She had been captured and sent to Ravensbruck to die, but was offered the chance to live by the Gestapo if she would participate in the experimental studies. She provided personal testimony about the sulfanilamide and bone experiments she endured while at Ravensbruck. Dr. Leo Alexander, a Boston physician, testified for the prosecution about the extent of her injuries. He concluded that her injuries had been caused initially by an infectious agent injected into her leg and that she was later given a high does of sulfa, which caused extensive injures to her nerves and tibia. Ms. Dzido became one of the most visible survivors and symbols of the massive experimental trials.

Physician Prisoners' Testimonies Corroborate Bone Transplantation Experiments

Two former physician prisoners at the Ravensbruck camp, Dr. Zofia Maczka from Krakow, Poland, and Dr. Zdenka Nedvedoca-Nejedla from Prague, Czechoslovakia, provided affidavits attesting to the atrocities committed by Drs. Gebhardt, Fischer, and Oberheuser in the bone regeneration and transplantation experiments.

The tragic outcome of these bone experiments at Ravensbruck is that most of the 75 women prisoner subjects died due to blood loss and infection. The few who survived, such as Ms. Dzido and Ms. Karolewska, were left with substantial injuries, pain, and difficulty in walking that endured throughout their lives. In a double tragedy, most of the German soldiers who were given the bone implants also died due to the inferior surgical techniques used during transplantation.

Euthanasia Programs—Murder of Disabled Children and Adults

In addition to the charges of experimenting on nonconsenting camp prisoners, several of the defendants were also charged with participating in a series of euthanasia programs of mentally and physically disabled patients, political dissidents, and prisoners of war during the Nazi era. The euthanasia programs were an outgrowth of eugenics or racial hygiene policies adopted by Hitler and the National Socialists Party to "cleanse" Germany of lives that were "not worth living" or deemed useless to the "Volk" or the German State.

Children's Euthanasia Program

Initial euthanasia programs were developed to murder German infants and children who were severely disabled, and an estimated 5000 of those children were killed between 1939 and 1945 in 22 different state psychiatric institutions and clinics across Germany. To keep the intent of the euthanasia programs secret from parents and the public, the killing centers were disguised and promoted as expert treatment wards for disabled infants and children. Pediatric physicians and midwives were directed to encourage parents of children with disabilities to have them admitted to the Centers (McFarland-Icke, 1999). Once on the wards, the children were given lethal injections of luminal or suppositories with high-dose morphine.

Euthanasia of Adults with Mental Illness and Senility

The children's program was expanded to the larger T4 Euthanasia Program in 1939 to include murder of adult patients with mental illness or senility residing in psychiatric hospitals or nursing homes. Patients were transported to one of six institutions across Germany, including Grafeneck, Brandenburg, Hartheim, Sonnenstein, Bernberg, and Hadamar, where they were killed with carbon monoxide in specially constructed gas chambers. An estimated 70,273 patients were killed in these institutions. These same institutions were later used in Operation 14f13 to murder inmates from some of the concentration camps as well as slave laborers from several Nazi-occupied countries.

In many respects, these early euthanasia programs laid the groundwork for the large-scale murder of Jewish and other prisoners who had been sent to labor and death camps across Europe. Numerous scholars and researchers have noted that the killing machinery and technical know-how that was used to euthanize disabled and mentally ill children and adults in Germany was exported to the death camps.

Forensic Evidence of Euthanasia

Evidence of physicians' and nurses' involvement in the euthanasia programs at the six killing institutions as well as at other sites was found in records of the various institutions, in official SS memos, and letters between supervisory personnel and high-ranking Nazi leaders, including Dr. Karl Brandt. Similar to evidence presented about the experimental studies, testimonies of nurses, physicians, and other personnel who had assisted in the euthanasia programs as well as prisoners who observed the euthanasia episodes played a powerful role in establishing the scope and nature of the euthanasia programs.

For example, Viktor Brack, who had been one of Hitler's chief administrative officers, was indicted for his major role in organizing the euthanasia programs. He testified that these killing programs were intended to eliminate all of those persons considered to be "superfluous eaters" and useless to the Reich. He noted that Hitler believed that eliminating these unfit persons would free up doctors and nurses, bed space, and money that could be directed toward the war effort.

Sentencing of Physicians at Nuremberg Doctor's Trials

The Doctors' Trials at Nuremberg officially concluded on August 20, 1947, after 139 days of testimony and a total of 1471 documents entered into the record as evidence. Overall, 15 of the 23 defendants charged were found guilty of war crimes. Four of the physicians, including Brandt, Gebhardt, Hoven, and Mrugowski, were sentenced to hang, along with three administrative assistants. Five of the defendants were sentenced to imprisonment, and three received sentences varying from 10 to 20 years in prison. Seven doctors were acquitted of all charges.

Other Medical Trials

In addition to the Doctors' Trials at Nuremberg, there were a series of other, less well-known trials across Germany, Poland, and other formerly occupied countries. These trials were under the jurisdiction of individual Allied countries rather than the International Tribunal. Eventually, cases were heard in the reconstituted courts of formerly occupied countries. What is significant about this series of trials is that they included nurse and physician defendants who had been caretakers at many of the institutions for the mentally ill and disabled across Germany and who were rank and file members of the Nazi party. For example, several nurses and attendants at the Hadamar Institution were tried for murder of children with mental disabilities, and their own testimonies reflect compliance with orders to kill and justifications of their actions as being in the best interest of the children.

In reality, the defendants at the Doctors' Trials at Nuremberg, as well as at the Hadamar Trial and others, represented only a small fraction of the hundreds of health professionals who had been involved in committing atrocities against camp prisoners and institutionalized patients with mental and physical disabilities.

After the war, many of those medical and nursing professionals who were convicted of war crimes and sentenced to imprisonment eventually had their sentences reduced, returned to clinical practice in Germany or other European countries, and faded back into private life. For example, Dr. Herta Oberheuser's 20-year sentence was eventually reduced to 4 years and she resumed her practice, although she was forced to relocate to another town due to hostility from the community.

Postwar Outcomes of Forensic Data Used at Nuremberg Trials

In spite of the limited number of health professionals who were prosecuted, the IMT and various other medically related trials established a significant precedent that individual physicians, nurses, and other caregivers can be held accountable for crimes against humanity. The trials also established the significance of forensic science as a critical tool in documenting and tracing crimes against humanity and genocide and highlighted the significance of using first-person witness testimonies as well as perpetrator testimonies.

Contemporary Forensic Study of Nazi Genocide

In the decades since the Nuremberg Trials, there have been continued efforts by Israeli intelligence, Holocaust survivor organizations, the U.S. Department of Justice, and others to locate and prosecute additional Nazi officers, soldiers, and medical professionals who were alleged to have committed war crimes. This search has been aided by advanced developments in forensic tools and methodologies, including DNA testing, as well as more sophisticated surveillance technologies and enhanced communications between international criminal justice agencies.

The Search for Josef Mengele, "The Angel of Death"

One of the most fascinating uses of contemporary forensic technology was used in the tracking of Dr. Josef Mengele and the eventual identification of his remains. Mengele was the most notorious and visible of the Nazi physicians who had been implicated in selecting prisoners for death at their arrival in Auschwitz as well as overseeing some of the inhumane experiments on prisoners at Auschwitz (Fig. 19.1).

He had been especially interested in research on twins and established a series of experiments that focused on genetics and germ warfare. His "experiments" were based on faulty science and frequently involved painful and lethal treatments for the twins. Eva Kor and her sister Miriam were forced to participate in the studies. She described one chilling study in which Mengele surgically attached a set of Gypsy twins back-to-back and returned them to the barracks (Fig. 19.2). "Mengele had attempted to create a Siamese twin by connecting blood vessels and organs. The twins screamed day and night until gangrene set in and after 3 days they died." (Kor, 1992, p. 57) In some cases, he killed one twin to examine anatomical differences in organs and disease progression between the pair.

Mengele had been able to avoid capture by Allied troops after the liberation of Auschwitz and eventually made his way to South America, where he was protected for decades by Nazi sympathizers in Argentina, Paraguay, and Brazil. There were intensive efforts to find Mengele in South America for several decades and repeated sightings that could never be confirmed.

Mengele was alleged to have drowned in Bertioga, Brazil, in 1979, and his remains were located and exhumed in 1985 by a Brazilian team led by the police chief

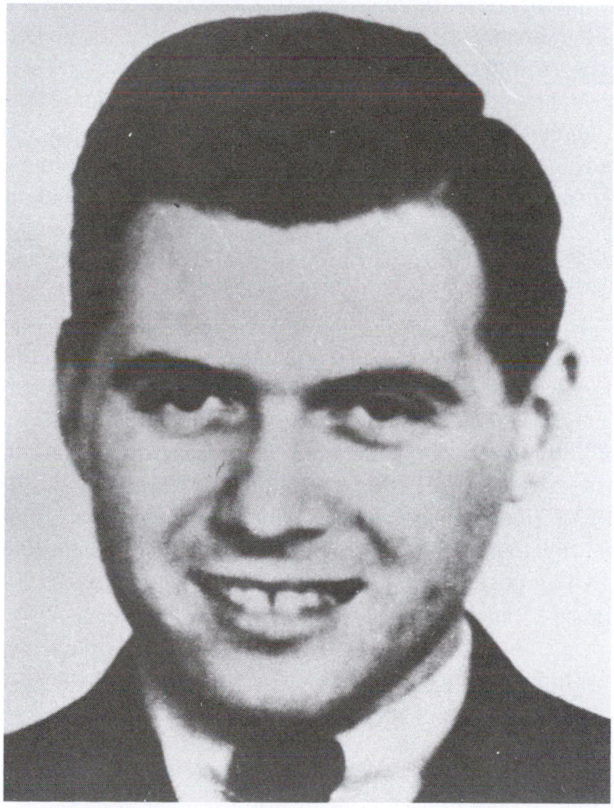

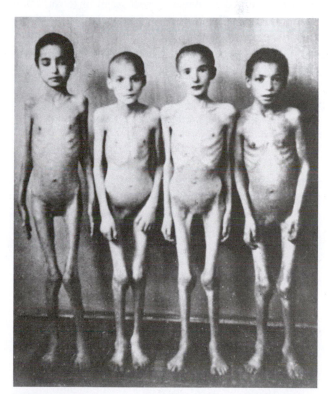

■ **FIGURE 19.1** Dr. Josef Mengele. *(United States Holocaust Museum.)*

■ **FIGURE 19.2** Gypsy twins who were victims of Mengele's experiments in Auschwitz. *(United States Holocaust Museum.)*

of São Paulo. A group of leading American forensic pathologists and anthropologists, including several from the U.S. Department of Justice, also conducted a series of examinations of the badly decomposed body. Based on their extensive reconstruction of bone fragments and dental work, the American team concluded that the remains seemed to match the profile of Mengele. However, there remained great skepticism in the international community, and eventually Dr. Alec Jeffreys, internationally respected geneticist, was asked to conduct DNA analyses on the remains. He was able to acquire blood samples from Mengele's wife and son, Rolf, and used a process of PCR-based DNA typing to confirm that there was a 99% certainty that the remains were those of Mengele.

Use of Forensic Science to Locate and Identify the "Disappeared" of Argentina

The use of advanced forensic science techniques and multidisciplinary teams to investigate and document contemporary human rights violations originated in Argentina. The military junta that overthrew Eva Peron's government in 1976 instituted a ruthless 7-year reign of terror, often referred to as the "Dirty War," which resulted in the disappearance of an estimated 10,000 to 30,000 people, including hundreds of children abducted with their parents. Citing security concerns, the military government began a campaign of kidnapping, imprisoning, and torturing suspected communists, Peron supporters, university students, Jews, journalists, and other citizens suspected of opposing the dictatorship. They were imprisoned in one or more of the 300 secret detention centers located across the country. The vast majority of the *desaparecidos,* victims who went "missing," were eventually murdered, and their bodies were buried in unmarked graves in cemeteries or in mass graves that were located on military bases throughout Argentina. Additionally, many infants who had been born to women prisoners were forcibly taken from their mothers and given up for adoption to military families and other influential civilians. The biological mothers of the infants were later murdered.

In response to the disappearances of their sons, daughters, and grandchildren, in 1977 a group of mothers and grandmothers formed the Mothers of Plaza de Mayo, a human rights organization, to protest the practices of the military and to demand that their children be returned. The group held daily vigils to call attention to the plight of the missing, and upon the return to a democratic government under President Alfonsin in 1984, they were instrumental in lobbying for the formation of a National Commission on Disappeared Persons.

The commission was charged with investigating violations of human rights and disappearances by the military and with bringing criminals to justice. In an effort to establish forensic evidence of mass crimes and to help locate and identify the victims, the commission requested assistance from Dr. Eric Stover at the American Association for the Advancement of Science in 1984 in creating a delegation of forensic scientists to help train and direct forensic teams in Argentina. Under the leadership of Dr. Clyde Snow, an international expert in forensic anthropology, the Argentine Forensic Anthropology Team (EAAF) was created and assumed major responsibility for excavations and exhumations of mass graves of disappeared victims.

The Creation of a Global Multidisciplinary Forensic Team Model

The EAAF pioneered the use of multidisciplinary teams to examine and document mass murders and other atrocities in Argentina and to present evidence of violations to courts and other relevant government entities, as well as to international tribunals and truth commissions. The use of the forensic team model, including pathologists, geneticists, radiologists, nurses, anthropologists, and archaeologists, proved to be very effective in the location and identification of thousands of mass graves and skeletal remains of victims through dental and medical records, human leukocyte antigen (HLA) and DNA testing, and interviews with remaining family members. The teams also used forensic techniques to determine signs of torture and execution style murders. The evidence generated from those investigations was instrumental in the initial and subsequent indictments and convictions of numerous military leaders and soldiers who had perpetrated the crimes against Argentinean civilians. This included two leading military figures, General Jorge Videla and Admiral Emilio Massera, who were implicated in the kidnapping and selling of infants of female prisoners and the murders of approximately 50 prisoners. The convictions were based on EAAF's positive identification of skeletal remains of victims exhumed from 10 cemeteries in Buenos Aires.

Unfortunately, many of the initial convictions were overturned or dismissed due to a series of controversial amnesty laws adopted by the government between 1989 and 1999 in an effort to appease the military. These amnesty laws were later repealed in 2003 under President Kirchner, and prosecutions of war criminals resumed. As of October 2009, 625 people have been charged with human rights violations in Argentina, with 62 convictions and approximately 279 currently on trial (International Center for Transitional Justice, 2009). Most recently, General Bignone, who had served as Argentina's last military dictator, was convicted of the detention and torture of 56 people held at the infamous Campo de Mayo military base where some of the worst atrocities are alleged to have been committed.

While forensic science has played and will continue to play a major role in the conviction of war crimes in Argentina and other areas of the world, Mercedes Doretti, a founding member of the Argentine Forensic Team, has emphasized that the team's ability to give back identities to the victims and to give some sense of closure to their families is equally significant to the cause of justice.

Importantly, the Argentina Forensic Team as well as teams from Physicians for Human Rights established a normative forensic process for examining and documenting global human rights violations that has continued to be used in investigating abuses and mass murder in Guatemala, Brazil, and more recently in Bosnia and sub-Saharan Africa. The use of forensic science in Guatemala and Bosnia is detailed in the following discussions.

FORENSIC EXPLORATION OF MASS MURDER AND HUMAN RIGHTS VIOLATIONS IN GUATEMALA

Similar patterns of political oppression and government-directed abuse and murder occurred in Guatemala during the civil wars that raged between 1980 and 1996. The series of insurgencies and counterinsurgencies were one of the longest and most brutal civil wars in Latin America. Largely driven by military dictators Garcia and Montt, an estimated 200,000 people were killed by the army or "disappeared," including many urban-area intellectuals and political opponents of the government. In addition to those groups, from 1980 to 1983 government forces specifically targeted thousands of indigenous Mayan Indians living in the countryside. In some instances whole villages were massacred, such as the jungle town of Cuarto Pueblo.

A Peace Accords agreement between the military government and the major resistance organization brought the war to an end in 1996. One of the conditions of the peace settlement brokered by the United Nations was the establishment of the Guatemalan Historical Commission charged with investigating the scope and nature of the apparent genocide. The commission relied heavily on the data collected by the Guatemalan Forensic Anthropology Team (FAFG), which had been founded during the war in 1994. The FAFG is one of several nongovernmental organizations that has examined mass murder and torture of victims during the past two decades. FAFG adopted the forensic model pioneered by the Argentine forensic team to document the extent and nature of atrocities. Teams of forensic anthropologists, archaeologists, pathologists, and other medical and nurse professionals, including numerous professionals from Physicians for Human Rights, have excavated mass burial sites across Guatemala, especially in rural areas of the country where many of the massacres occurred.

Similar to the forensic explorations in Argentina, forensic teams have attempted to recover and reconstruct disarticulated and conjoined remains of victims and determine the primary cause of injury and death. The process of determining the identity of victims has been aided by the 2008 opening of the first DNA laboratory in Guatemala. The laboratory is in the process of comparing DNA taken from bone fragments of recovered murder victims with DNA samples from hundreds of victims' family members. Dr. Fredy Peccerelli, a forensic anthropologist and current executive director of FAFG, has expressed hope that the use of DNA to identify victims will play a major role in the indictment and criminal prosecution of Guatemalan soldiers and police who were involved in the killings, as well as the government leaders who directed the slaughter of dissidents and indigenous groups. Unfortunately, only a handful of low-ranking soldiers and police officers have been charged and tried with murdering civilian victims to date, while forensic workers and victims' families continue to be the target of intimidation and assault by persons who are believed to be linked to those who committed murders and atrocities during the war. In spite of threats to their personal safety and that of their families, members of the forensic teams have continued their important work in returning identities to the victims and aiding in the potential prosecutions of war crimes.

CONFLICTS AND GENOCIDE IN THE FORMER YUGOSLAVIA

This section explores the use of forensic investigation to document the extent of human rights violations and mass killing that occurred during the civil wars in the former Yugoslav republics of Croatia, Bosnia-Herzegovina, and Kosovo during the 1990s. It is important that health professionals who are involved in forensic missions in war-torn countries understand the history and context of massive human rights violations and mass murder in the regions they are examining. Historical context provides forensic teams with a framework for examining, processing, and interpreting forensic data that is grounded in the reality of historical events. The civil wars in Yugoslavia were an outgrowth of centuries-old ethnic divisions and conflicts between Serbians, Croatians, and Muslims in the Balkans. Although Marshall Tito had forged these factions into a unified Yugoslavia after World War II, with varying degrees of peace, the union eventually collapsed after his death in 1980, and the country was plunged once again into conflict and chaos. There were three separate, but related, civil conflicts with massive civilian murders in the Yugoslavian republics of Croatia, Bosnia-Herzegovina, and Kosovo from 1991 to 1999.

Slovenia and Croatia

In 1991 two of the Yugoslavian republics, Slovenia and Croatia, declared independence from Yugoslavia, an act that provoked a swift military response from the leaders in the Serbian Republic, in part due to ardent nationalism and in part due to the vast territory that would be lost to Yugoslavia. Under the leadership of Serbian President Slobodan Milosevic, the Serbian army invaded both of these republics in July 1991 with the stated goal of protecting the Serbian minorities who lived there. After an initial short skirmish in Slovenia, Serbian forces moved on to a larger and more deadly war in Croatia.

Ethnic Cleansing

In one of the most brutal episodes of the war in Croatia, Serbian troops overran the town of Vukovar and massacred hundreds of Croatian men, burying them in mass graves. These mass murders became the first in a series of genocidal actions that would occur during the next decade in the former Yugoslavia. Since the Serbian army had previously declared their intention to "cleanse" the area of undesirable people, the term **ethnic cleansing** emerged as part of the language of war. Semelin, who has long studied mass violence, notes that ethnic cleansing of a territory with forced mass relocations and selected murders of targeted groups is often the first stage in creating a severe climate of fear that may escalate to genocide and the complete annihilation of a group. Although a peace agreement between Serbia and Croatia was brokered by the United Nations in late 1991, ethnic tensions continued and other republics attempted to break away from Yugoslavia.

Bosnia-Herzegovina—Mass Graves and "Rape Camps"

Bosnia-Herzegovina, a largely Muslim republic, also declared its independence from Yugoslavia in October 1991, and its status was recognized by the United States and Europe. This move further aggravated the fears of the Serbian government about the breakup of Yugoslavia and the rise of a Muslim republic. In response, Serbian President Milosevic launched a massive attack on Sarajevo, the Bosnian capital, in April 1992. Serbian forces continuously bombarded the city in an effort to overpower the Bosnian army, but they also deliberately targeted civilian neighborhoods, schools, marketplaces, as well as hospitals and clinics, and set up a blockade around the city to prevent food and medical supplies from getting into citizens.

The Serbian army set up a series of notorious detention camps for civilians, including those at Prijedor, Omarska, and Konjc where prisoners were starved and tortured. The army also launched a "new weapon" in the Balkan wars—massive acts of sexual violence and rape of Bosnian Muslim women and often young girls. Rapes occurred in homes and other sites, but more ominously, in a series of special "rape camps" set up specifically for the purpose of enslaving the women and subjecting them to repeated sexual abuse and rapes by Serbian soldiers. Some of the women were also "sold" into slavery as prostitutes. An estimated 20,000 women and young girls were raped during the Bosnian conflict, although the United Nations and Amnesty International researchers believe that estimate may be extremely low. They note that the stigma and fear of reporting sexual assault to officials, as well as the extended displacement of many of these women during and after the war, may have prevented many women from coming forward.

Sexual violence became a major piece of the war "machinery" calculated to induce fear and degradation among women and their families to force them to leave their homelands and relocate. Rehn and Sirleaf (2002) captured the disturbing nature of rape as a weapon in the Balkan wars as well as Rwanda and Darfur in a statement from their definitive research report to the United Nations entitled *Women, War, and Peace:*

> Clearly the nature of war has changed. It is being fought in homes and communities—*and on women's bodies*—in a battle for resources and in the name of religion and ethnicity. Violence against women is used to break and humiliate women, men, families, and communities, no matter which side they are on. Women have become the great victims of war—and the biggest stakeholders of peace. (2002, p. 1)

Massacre at Srebrenica

Some of the worst atrocities of the Bosnian war occurred in the city of Srebrenica, which had been deemed a "Safe Haven" for Muslims by the United Nations. In spite of that designation, however, the Serbian army, under the direction of General Ratko Mladic, launched an attack on the town. The army rounded up an estimated 8000 civilian Muslim men and boys over age 12 and slaughtered them in a field over several days in July 1992. Victims were hastily buried in mass graves. Many of these massacre victims' wives, daughters, and mothers were beaten and raped and many of them sent to rape camps, but thousands fled to neighboring republics, creating a huge wave of refugees.

In response to the Srebrenica tragedy, NATO forces bombed Serbian military positions and eventually forced Milosevic into a series of peace talks. Those negotiations resulted in the Dayton Agreement in December 1995, which divided the region into largely separate Serbian and Muslim states. By the end of the 3-year conflict in Bosnia-Herzegovina, an estimated 100,000 people had been killed and at least two million had become refugees.

Kosovo—Mass Murders and Refugees

In spite of the Dayton Agreement, there continued to be political instability in the region. The ethnic Albanian population of Kosovo, a province in Serbia, declared its independence from Serbia, citing long-standing discrimination and oppression by the Serbian government. Although many leaders in Kosovo had pursued a course of passive, nonviolent resistance against Serbian repression, the Kosovo Liberation Army (KLA) openly supported armed rebellion, and the Serbian army was sent in to counter the resistance forces. In a pattern similar to the earlier conflicts in Bosnia, the Serbian army systematically targeted civilians, shelling and burning homes, schools, medical centers, and religious sites. The use of rape as a terrorist weapon also reappeared as Serbian forces sexually abused and raped thousands of Albanian women in Kosovo.

The violence escalated in spite of intense diplomatic attempts to negotiate a ceasefire between KLA and Serbian forces by NATO-aligned countries. By spring of 1999, an estimated 1.5 million Kosovo Albanians had been driven from their homes and approximately 6000 were murdered and buried in mass graves (Ronayne, 2004). In view of what appeared to be a growing genocide, NATO engaged in air strikes for 3 months, eventually forcing Milosevic and the Serbian government to withdraw its troops in June 1999. The peace agreement kept Kosovo within the Serbian republic but provided that Kosovars would be protected by UN and NATO troops stationed in the region. Thousands of Kosovar Albanian refugees eventually returned home, but unfortunately strife continued as many of them sought retribution on Serbs living in the area. Many Serbian civilians were shot by Kosovo Muslims, and thousands of Serbs fled the area.

The International Criminal Tribunal of the Former Yugoslavia

In response to the apparent massive human rights violations and mass murders in the Croatian and Bosnia-Herzegovina conflicts, the United Nations established the International Criminal Tribunal for the former Yugoslavia (ICTY) in 1993 to prosecute war crimes. The creation of this tribunal was significant in that it was the first international court convened in the almost 50 years after Nuremberg to address human rights violations.

The tribunal was charged with prosecuting those who had engaged in murder, torture, enslavement, and destruction of property during the conflict, as well as those who had participated in sexual violence and rape. The United Nation's decision to include rape and sexual violence as a war crime that could be prosecuted in the tribunal was a major breakthrough in international law. It was due in large measure to the lobbying efforts of women victims of rape during the war and support from many humanitarian groups who had interviewed and provided care to these women after the wars had ended. Those efforts helped the United Nations recognize that sexual violence toward women and girls in wartime had increasingly become part of the weapons of war.

Part of the mandate and the challenge for the International Criminal Tribunal was to investigate allegations of war crimes and genocide and to secure forensic evidence that would allow indictments and prosecutions to go forward. To accomplish this task, the ICTY Office of the Chief Prosecutor contracted with nongovernmental organizations (NGOs) with forensic experience, such as Physicians for Human Rights and the International Commission for Missing Persons, to bring in teams of forensic experts who could gather and analyze crucial forensic data.

Forensic Evidence of War Crimes and Genocide

The search for and analysis of forensic evidence in the former Yugoslavia was complex and lengthy due to the multiple civil wars that occurred during the 1990s, resulting in an estimated 200,000 deaths overall, with thousands of victims buried in multiple mass graves throughout the region and thousands more reported to have disappeared. There were an estimated 40,000 persons reported as missing by the end of all of the civil wars in 1999. There were also thousands of civilian survivors who had been injured as the result of beatings and torture by soldiers and others, including large numbers of women who had been sexually abused and raped. The process of gathering forensic evidence from both living and deceased victims was daunting, as reflected in the writing and testimonies of forensic specialists in the field. It was multifaceted and involved numerous teams gathering data from interviews with eyewitnesses and survivors, families of missing persons and those believed to have been murdered, as well as searching for and excavating individual and mass graves of possible victims.

ICTY Objectives of Forensic Exploration and Analysis

The chief investigator for the International Criminal Tribunal outlined the following basic objectives of the exhumations and forensic examinations in his testimony to the ICT during the trial of President Milosevic in 2003:

- To corroborate victim and witness accounts of the massacres
- To determine an accurate count of victims
- To determine cause of death and time of death
- To determine the identity of the victims and any link to the missing from Srebrenica
- To determine the gender of the victims
- To identify any links between primary mass graves and secondary mass grave sites
- To identify links to the perpetrators

Mass Grave Excavations

Much of the early forensic investigative work in the former Yugoslavia involved **mass grave excavations,** first locating mass grave sites scattered throughout the country and then excavating bodies from those sites in an effort to identify the victims and determine the cause of death. Although surviving witnesses were aware of some mass graves (e.g., the site of the Vukovar massacres in Croatia), many of the burial sites were hidden in obscure and remote areas that were hard to find and excavate. Forensic teams gathered information about possible sites from witnesses and family members of those missing, as well as from interviews with and testimonies from suspected perpetrators.

Aerial Photos from U.S. Reconnaissance

The forensic teams' efforts to locate mass grave sites in Srebrenica were given a major assist from classified aerial photographs of the area that had been gathered by U.S. reconnaissance. Ambassador Madeline Albright informed the United Nations Security Council that the series of photos were available, and they were released to the tribunal investigative team in March 1996. The photos indicated that there were numerous areas of disturbed soil and anomalies in certain geological features that indicated the presence of several mass graves in specific locations around Srebrenica.

Minimum Number of Individuals (MNI)

In addition to problems locating graves, some of the most difficult challenges for the forensic teams were not only that the grave sites often contained hundreds of decomposed bodies that had been buried for years, but also that many of the remains, especially those from the Srebrenica massacres, had been relocated from previous gravesites. The relocations were carried out by perpetrators who were concerned that they might be investigated. Moving the bodies resulted in significant disarticulation of skeletons as well as comingling of different victims' remains in the same site. In addition to relocation, many of the bodies had been mutilated or burned in order to disguise the cause of death.

Teams of forensic anthropologists and archaeologists helped excavate the bodies and reassemble the skeletons, trying to ascertain the MNIs in each grave site. Huffines (2008) and Hagland (2006) have discussed the tedious and complex procedures used by forensic teams to capture the MNIs at gravesites across each of the war zones. They performed detailed analysis of the skeletons, including estimates of age, ethnicity, gender, and any unusual or identifying features, clothing, or possessions.

Probable Causes of Death

Many of the same issues that complicated the reassembling of individual skeletons of victims and determining the MNIs in each grave site also presented challenges to forensic pathologists and biologists attempting to identify types of injuries sustained and possible causes and manner of death from hundreds of disarticulated body parts. A study by one team of forensic pathologists and anthropologists reported the methods they developed to ascertain types of trauma and causes of death of an estimated 298 individuals recovered from a mine shaft near Prijedor in northwestern Bosnia in 2001. These civilian victims were reported to have been killed in 1993 by Serbian troops during the Serbian war with Bosnia-Herzegovina and initially buried at one site, then later relocated to the mine at Jakarina Kosa. There had also been an attempt to blow up the mine shaft with explosives after the bodies were buried there, causing the remains to be covered with rubble and rocks.

In their analysis, team members explored types of trauma, including blunt force trauma, sharp force trauma, and gunshot wounds. These traumatic injuries, especially gunshot wounds, were further classified into "lethal," including shots to the head and chest, as well as "lethal if untreated," including trauma to the abdomen and gunshot fractures of the humerus and femur that would have caused severe blood loss. Since the bodies were often disarticulated, the scientists calculated the number of injuries for each anatomical section as well as the combined number of injuries from each section. This protocol linking pathological evidence with clinical correlates such as survival times allowed the team to determine the "most probable cause of death."

Based on their data analysis, the team concluded that the majority of victims died from gunshot wounds rather than shrapnel-related injuries from bombs or long-range shelling and that most of the gunshots were fired into the back of the victims' heads, chests, or torsos, indicating that these injuries were deliberate wound inflictions at close range rather than battle-related injuries. Their conclusion that these deaths resulted from an intentional mass killing, rather than battle-inflicted wounds, was significant and was further supported by the attempts of soldiers and others to relocate and hide the remains. These results were presented to the prosecutor for the International Tribunal in the indictment and prosecution of Radoslav Brdjanin.

DNA Testing and Identification of Human Remains

Although some of the recovered victims' bodies were identified through skeletal remains, dental records, and clothing and possessions found at the burial sites, it was not possible to identify the thousands of remaining victims without the widespread use of DNA analysis. Forensic teams in Croatia began in 1995 to conduct standard DNA testing of material extracted from teeth and bones of victims' remains that had been recovered in various sites. While Croatia was successful in identifying many victims of its war with Serbia in 1991, it proved difficult to duplicate the same DNA-testing process in Bosnia-Herzegovina due to the much larger volume of remains, the slowness in obtaining samples from possible family members of victims, and the need to ship large numbers of samples overseas for analysis. This cumbersome process led to long lag times in identifying human remains of victims recovered at the gravesites as well as frequent false identifications of remains.

The inability to recover and reliably identify the mortal remains of so many victims from the various mass grave sites across the former Yugoslavia not only delayed the indicting and prosecuting of alleged war criminals by the International Criminal Tribunal, but also created a furor among families of missing persons who wanted to recover their loved ones and see justice done.

International Commission on Missing Persons (ICMP)

In an effort to help promote a more systematic, rapid, and reliable process for mass victim identification, the International Commission on Missing Persons (ICMP) was established in 1996 by the G7 Summit, an alliance of leading industrialized nations, including the United States, France, and Great Britain. The ICMP helped establish on-site DNA laboratories and trained scientists and other personnel in the process of DNA testing and analysis in Bosnia and Kosovo. Beginning in 2000, the laboratories developed a system for mass grave DNA identification that used blind DNA matching in which DNA recovered from victims was compared to an integrated database of blood samples derived from family members whose relatives had been reported missing.

The director of the Commission on Missing Persons' DNA program estimated that by the end of 2003, the collective laboratories in Bosnia-Herzegovina were testing more than 500 bodies and thousands of reference samples per month. To date, the laboratories have collected 88,000 reference samples from family members of the missing and have assisted in the identification of the remains of 15,462 persons who had been reported missing during the various conflicts. The commission is hopeful that the estimated 14,000 additional victims who disappeared during the wars can eventually be identified if their remains are located.

Prosecutions of War Crimes at the International Criminal Tribunal

The volume of forensic evidence gathered by teams of forensic specialists across the former Yugoslavia, including eyewitness testimonies, mass graves exploration, and DNA testing of victims' remains, was instrumental in the tribunal's ability to indict and prosecute persons who were accused of committing war crimes during the various conflicts. At this writing, the tribunal has indicted 160 persons for war crimes, including the former President of Serbia, Slobodan Milosevic, who recently died in prison before his trial could be completed, as well as numerous high-level officials and political leaders in the various republics and high-ranking members of the Serbian military.

The ICTY has tried and convicted more than 60 individuals, including General Radislav Kristic, who ordered and oversaw the massacre of Bosnian civilian men at Srebrenica. An additional 40 persons are currently in trial proceedings before the tribunal, including Dr. Radovan Karadzic, a psychiatrist who had been the leader of the

Bosnian Serb Republic during the war. While the vast majority of indictments and convictions have been related to crimes committed by Serbians against Muslims, there have been a number of convictions of Muslims for crimes against Serbian citizens.

Selected Cases from the International Criminal Tribunal

Several significant cases prosecuted by the ICTY included physicians Dr. Milomir Stakic and Dr. Milan Kovacevic, who were charged with war crimes committed while they held high-level government positions in the municipality of Prijedor in the Republic of Bosnia-Herzegovina. Drs. Stakic and Kovacevic helped set up detention camps for Muslim prisoners and oversaw the torture and murder of camp prisoners both within the camps and at other locations.

Some of the key forensic evidence related to their crimes was presented in testimonies provided by several physician eyewitnesses who were either imprisoned by Serbian military or whose family members disappeared during the war. For example, Dr. Idriz Merdzanic, a Bosnian doctor testified for the prosecution in the Stakic case in 2002. Dr. Merdzanic was working in a clinic in the town of Korzarac when it was attacked by Serbian military, and he described his agonizing experiences in trying to treat a child who had been severely injured by gunfire:

> There was a little girl there whose lower legs, both of them were completely shattered. She was dying. And then we had another child . . . I couldn't evacuate the children or others who were wounded. The only thing they (soldiers) told us was "Let all of you balija, derogatory for Muslims, die there. We'll kill you anyway." (ICTY, Case 97-24, p. 7737)

Dr. Merdzanic was captured by Serb soldiers several days later and transported with hundreds of other Bosnians to the notorious Trnopolje Camp. He described for the court the inhumane conditions at the camp and the severe beatings of male prisoners, including several who died as a result of their injuries. He had personally heard the screams of many of the men being beaten and later treated many of them. He estimated that at least 200 prisoners had been killed at Trnopolje Camp. He also noted the frequent rape of women in the camp and his attempts to treat their rape-related injuries as best he could and to document the extent of their injuries, even though he was warned that he was putting himself at risk for trying to give these women medical attention.

In one of the most dramatic moments in the trial, Dr. Merdzanic described secretly taking photos of the prisoners who had been beaten and starved. He and a colleague had managed to smuggle the photos to a British film crew who visited the camp in August 1992. One of the journalists asked Dr. Merdzanic about conditions in the camp, and he quite honestly described the lack of food and medicines. That interview and several of his photos were featured in a documentary shown in England and the United States. That film, depicting the severe conditions in the camp, forced the military to provide at least some food and medicines to prisoners through the Red Cross. Dr. Merdzanic recounted that he had received several death threats from guards regarding his actions, but he managed to survive that camp and was eventually transferred to another camp. Several of his photos of prisoners were used as prosecution exhibits in the Stakic case.

Both Dr. Merdezanic's testimony and positive DNA results of at least 64 murdered camp prisoners were instrumental in Dr. Stakic's conviction for murder, persecution, forced expulsion, and extermination of prisoners and other citizens in the Prijedor region. He was sentenced to life in prison in July 2003 by the International Criminal Tribunal in the Hague. His sentence was reduced to 40 years in prison on appeal in 2006. Dr. Kovacevic was being tried on similar charges in July 1998, but died in prison before his trial had been completed.

Prosecution of Sexual Violations and Rape

As noted previously, the tribunal elected to prosecute persons who were accused of committing sexual violations and rape during the civil wars in response to widespread reports of vicious assaults on an estimated 20,000 women and young girls. It was an unprecedented recognition by an international court that sexual violence had increasingly become a weapon of war. Many human rights groups believed this judicial step was long overdue.

Currently, 18 cases including charges of rape and other types of sexual violence that occurred during the war in Bosnia-Herzegovina have been prosecuted by the ICTY. A number of pending cases include similar charges. One of the important precedents established by several of these cases is that rape was defined as a specific crime under international law, therefore providing that it be prosecuted under one of three categories: as a crime against humanity, a war crime, or genocide, depending on the unique circumstances under which it occurred.

One of the most egregious cases involved three officers in the Bosnian Serb Army who were charged with torture, rape, and enslavement of Muslim women in the town of Foca, in southeastern Bosnia, while they were deployed in the ongoing war there during 1992 to 1993. These defendants were Dragoljub Kunarac, Radomir Kovac, and Zorran Vukovic. For purposes of prosecution, the tribunal merged all of their trials into one case under Kunarac's name due to the related nature of their offenses in the Foca area. Testimonies presented to the tribunal by victims of the assaults as well as eyewitnesses established that each of these men had deliberately detained many Bosnian women in a series of detention centers and regularly took selected ones to private houses and other locations known as rape camps where they were repeatedly and forcibly raped. Kovac enslaved four girls in his apartment for months at a time and arranged for gang rapes by other soldiers. He also sold three of the women to other soldiers for purposes of prostitution. One of the girls was only 14 years old. The women were also forced to do household duties and were constantly beaten and assaulted.

Several of the survivor witnesses discussed their personal humiliation, as Muslim women, at being raped, especially in front of other soldiers. They also expressed the significant and often painful aftereffects of being raped on relationships with their families, especially male members. It was clear from these witnesses' testimonies that they believed the soldiers' actions were intended to not only satisfy their own sexual desires, but also to humiliate, degrade, and terrify them. One witness recounted that Kunarac and two other soldiers under his command raped her in succession and then threatened to kill her and her young son if she ever discussed the incidents with others. In rendering judgment about their crimes, the Trial Chamber made the following statement:

> The evidence showed how Muslim women and girls, mothers and daughters together, were robbed of the last vestiges of human dignity; how women and girls were treated like chattels, pieces of property at the arbitrary disposal of the Serb occupation forces and more specifically, at the beck and call of the three accused. (*Prosecution vs. Kunarac,* Case Nos. IT-96-23)

All three defendants were convicted of the charges of rape and torture, while Kunarac and Kovac were also convicted of enslavement. Kunarac was sentenced to 28 years of imprisonment, Kovac to 20 years, and Vukovic to 12 years on February 22, 2001. Their convictions were upheld by the Appeals Chamber in 2002.

A series of other cases involving sexual violations and rape were transferred by the International Criminal Tribunal to the War Crimes Chamber (WCC) of the State Court of Bosnia-Herzegovina as well as to other courts in local jurisdictions. Two cases at the WCC, Samardzic and Stankovic, also addressed the issue of enslavement and rape of women prisoners through "ownership" and coercion, but further noted that coercion could be even more extreme when soldiers and police were present at and or participated in the rapes (*Prosecutor v. Samardzio* No.

KT-RZ89/05 and *Prosecutor v. Stankovic,* No.X-K-R-o5/70). The court also found that the age of the rape victims was a very important mitigating factor in evaluating the gravity of the crime, especially for girls under the age of 16. This was a critical finding in view of the numerous rapes of young girls by Serbian troops throughout Bosnia-Herzegovina.

Although the ICTY, WCC, and other local courts have continued to prosecute sexual violence, many human rights organizations and legal scholars have expressed concerns regarding the following issues:

- The small ratio of cases involving sexual violence and rape that have been prosecuted in proportion to the actual number of rapes that were allegedly committed throughout the former Yugoslavia
- The ability of the state and regional courts to assume full responsibility from the ICTR for prosecution of war crimes of a sexual nature due to limited legal and investigative personnel and limited judicial experience in the prosecution of such crimes
- The lack of protections and support for many of the women victims who have previously testified or will testify in the future about their sexual assaults, particularly in cases where the alleged perpetrators live in the same areas as the victims
- The overall lack of court-ordered restitution and reparations for the victims of violent sexual crimes. Many of these women have been left with both long-term physical and psychological injuries and have very limited resources for treatment and subsistence for housing and food.

ETHICAL ISSUES IN FORENSIC EXPLORATION OF WAR AND GENOCIDE

As reflected in this chapter's overall discussion of the use of forensic science in exploring war crimes committed during the Nazi era, in Argentina, and the former Yugoslavia, there are often substantial and complex ethical, legal, and political issues that can arise during that process. Some of these issues include the following:

- Differential perspective of forensic work as prosecutorial versus victim identification and reconciliation
- Lack of international codes governing forensic work, especially related to excavation of mass grave sites
- Need for clearer delineation of multiple forensic team members' scope of work, methodologies, ownership of work products, and reporting mechanisms

- Competing interests of both forensic teams and political groups regarding methods, outcomes, and reporting of forensic findings
- Need for all forensic team members to have better understanding of cultural norms and practices of victims' families and communities relative to disinterring victims in mass graves, identification of remains, confirmation of death, and reporting rape or other sexually induced trauma
- Need for more systematic protection of forensic teams working in war zones during or after civil war and genocide
- Need for more extensive support and protection of local witnesses who testify at international or local courts regarding genocide

CONCLUSIONS

It is clear from the preceding discussion of forensic investigations of war crimes in the Nazi era and in the civil wars in Argentina and the former Yugoslavia that health professionals have played important, strategic roles in helping to examine and document human rights violations through the use of forensic science. They have made major contributions to the successful prosecution of persons who committed those crimes. Those prosecutions have in some instances served to help prevent or deter mass violence and genocide and may serve that purpose in the future.

It is equally clear, however, that the use of forensic science and the involvement of nurses and other health professionals in that process has a purpose that extends beyond the prosecution of war criminals. It has the potential for helping achieve greater social justice through restoring identities of those who have been murdered and "disappeared" by returning these victims to their families and communities and by helping to create a climate for reconciliation. This unique role of forensic science is expressed in Clea Koff's statement about her own work as a forensic anthropologist in both Rwanda and Bosnia:

> I have come to understand that the global role of forensic science is not only to deter killing, but also to contribute, in a post-conflict setting, to improved and real communication between "opposing" parties. This is done by helping to establish the truth about the past—what happened and to whom—which in turn strengthens ties between people in their own communities. Despite the facts—whether religious, ethnic, or historical—that are supposed to differentiate places like Rwanda and Kosovo, their dead reveal their common humanity, one that we all share. (Koff, 2004, pp. 16-17)

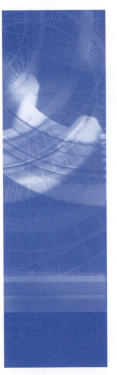

EVIDENCE-BASED PRACTICE

Reference Question: What are the mental health consequences of terrorism, torture, and wars?

Database(s) to Search: PsychINFO

Search Strategy: Each subject in this question happens to be a MeSH term, so search each term individually. Using "OR" with "terrorism," "torture," and "war," will collect all articles published on those three subjects. Add "AND" the OR set with "mental health," and then limit to the years of interest.

Selected References from Search:

1. Marmar, C.R. (2009). Mental health impact of Afghanistan and Iraq deployment: Meeting the challenge of a new generation of veterans. *Depression and Anxiety* 26:493–497.
2. Tol, W.A., Komproe, I.H., Jordans, M.J.D., Thapa, S.B., Sharma, B., & De Jong, J.T.V.M. (2009). Brief multi-disciplinary treatment for torture survivors in Nepal: A naturalistic comparative study. *International Journal of Social Psychiatry, 55* (1):39-56.
3. Neria, Y., Olfson, M., Gameroff, M.J., Wickramaratne, P., et al. (2008). The mental health consequences of disaster-related loss: Findings from primary care one year after the 9/11 terrorist attacks. *Psychiatry: Interpersonal and Biological Processes, 7*(4):339–348.

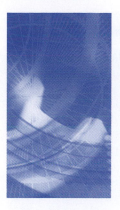

EVIDENCE-BASED PRACTICE (continued)

Questions Used to Discern Evidence:

Choose two studies among the studies listed, read about them, and answer the following questions:

1. What are the differences between the two studies in the design, methods, and results?
2. What are the similarities between the two studies in the number of subjects, measures used, and interventions, if any?
3. What skills do you think you need to learn to practice forensic nursing with survivors of terrorism, torture, or war?

REVIEW QUESTIONS

1. Lemkin's work and the results of the Nuremberg Trials persuaded the United Nations to officially define genocide as:
   A. Killing a group or members of a group with the intent to destroy, either wholly or in part, a national, ethnic, racial, or religious heritage.
   B. Causing bodily or mental harm to a member of a group to save life.
   C. Deliberately planning to inflict on group members conditions of life calculated to bring about racial profiling.
   D. Forcibly transferring children of the group to another group to protect them from starvation.

2. One of the most significant features of the Geneva Convention is that it provides a/an:
   A. Standard for examining and prosecuting crimes that may occur during wars and civil conflicts.
   B. Avenue for war criminals to choose a tribunal to try war crimes.
   C. Guideline for prosecution and defense attorneys to settle cases without a trial.
   D. Declaration of war or peace.

3. The Holocaust remains the single largest state-sponsored genocide in history. It also has the distinction of being the:
   A. First genocide in the history of the world.
   B. First forensic investigation of massive global human rights violations.
   C. First trial where prosecution and defense were not represented by lawyers.
   D. Most disorganized trial in the history of the world.

4. Much of the compelling evidence of war crimes at the Doctors' Trials of the Nuremberg Trials was linked to:
   A. Physical evidence of starvation in prisoners.
   B. Emotional evidence of torture and mental illness.
   C. Medical experiments on prisoners.
   D. Looting of prisoners' fine art and jewelry.

5. The Geneva Convention of 1949 provide for the humanitarian treatment of combatants but also prohibit the use of violence toward civilians. In 1977, the provisions of the Geneva Conventions were expanded to include noninternational wars and conflicts (International Red Cross, 2010). One of the most significant features of the Geneva Conventions is that they provide:
   A. Restitution to victims.
   B. Sanctuary to accused war criminals before the trial.
   C. Health and legal referrals to accused criminals.
   D. A standard for examining and prosecuting war crimes that may occur during wars and civil conflicts.

6. The International Commission on Missing Persons (ICMP) was established in 1996 by the G7 Summit, an alliance of leading industrialized nations, including the United States, France, and Great Britain. The ICMP helped establish a/an:
   A. On-site DNA laboratories and training for scientists and other personnel in the process of DNA testing and analysis.
   B. Procedure for mass grave identification.
   C. Blood typing and matching training program for laboratory technicians.
   D. Bone morrow typing and matching training program for laboratory technicians.

(review questions continued on page 388)

REVIEW QUESTIONS—cont'd

7. The use of forensic science and the involvement of nurses and other health professionals in DNA testing and analysis has a purpose that extends beyond the prosecution of war criminals. It has the potential for helping achieve a/an:

A. More useful evidence of the suffering of victims.

B. Equitable distribution of punishment to those who are found guilty of war crimes.

C. Greater social justice through restoring identities of those who have been murdered and "disappeared."

D. Return of victims' remains to their families and communities.

8. Although the role of forensic nurses in assessing and examining war crime victims is not direct or proximate, it is suggested that nurses and health-care providers help create a climate of:

A. Peace.

B. Repudiation.

C. Retribution.

D. Reconciliation.

9. In discussing the ethical issues related to global human rights violations and genocide, it is suggested that there is a need for more:

A. Systematic protection of forensic teams working in war zones during or after civil war and genocide.

B. Systematic provision of food, clothing, and shelter to health-care providers in war zones.

C. Systematic identification of "disappeared" children and their parents.

D. DNA collection and analysis for all health-care providers in war zones.

References

Ainsworth, C. (2006). Disasters drive DNA to reunite families. *Nature, 441*:673.

Amnesty International. (2008). *Uncovereing the truth: The Guatemalan Forensic Anthropology Foundation,* pp. 1-4. Retrieved from www.amnesty.org

Amnesty International. (2009). *Whose justice? The women of Bosnia-Herzegovina are still waiting.* London: Amnesty International Publications.

Amnesty International. (2010). *World by region:Global update.* London: Amnesty International Publications.

Annas, G.J., & Grodin, M.A. (1992). *The Nazi doctors and the Nuremberg Code.* New York: Oxford University Press.

Baraybar, J., & Gasior, M. (2006). Forensic anthroplogy and the most probable cause of death in cases of violations against international law: An example from Bosnia and Herzegovina. *Journal of Forensic Science, 51*(1):103-108.

Benedict, S. (2003). Killing while caring: The nurses of Hadamar. *Issues in Mental Health Nursing, 24*:59-79.

Benedict, S., & Georges, J.M. (2006). Nurses and the sterilization experiments of Auschwitz: A postmodernist perspective. *Nursing Inquiry, 13*(4):277-288.

Blewitt, G. (1997). The role of forensic investigations in genocide prosecutions before an international tribunal. *Medical Science Law, 37*:286-287.

Bloom, J., Hoxha, I., Sambunjak, D., et al. (2006). Ethnic segregation in Kosovo's post-war health care system. *European Journal of Public Health, 17*(5):430-436.

Campbell, K. (2007). The gender of transitional justice: Law, sexual violence and the International Criminal Tribunal for the former Yugoslavia. *The International Journal of Transitional Justice, 1*:411-432.

Commission for Historical Clarification. (1999). *Guatemala: Memory of silence.* Guatemala City: United Nations Office for Project Services.

Cordner, S., & McKelvie, H. (2002). Developing standards in international forensic work to identify missing persons. *IRRC, 848*:867-883.

Cox, M., Flavel, A., Hanson, J., et al, (eds.). (2007). *The scientific investigation of mass graves: Toward protocols and standard operating procedures.* Cambridge: Cambridge University Press.

Czech, D. (1990). *Auschwitz chronicle 1939-1945.* New York: Henry Holt.

Dadrian, V.N. (1995). *The history of the armenian genocide.* Providence: Berghahn Books.

Doretti, M.M. & Snow, C. (2002). Forensic anthropology and human rights: The Argentine experience. In D. Steadman (Ed.), *Hard evidence: Case studies in forensic anthropology.*

Edman, A. (2008). Crimes of sexual violence in the War Crimes Chamber of the state court of Bosnia and Herzegovina: Successes and challenges. *Human Rights Brie*f, *16*(1):21-28.

Friedlander, H. (1995). *Origins of Nazi genocide: From euthnasia to the final solution.* Chapel Hill: University of North Carolina Press.

Funari, P., Zarankin, A., & Salerno, M. (2009). *Memories from darkness: Archaeology of repression and resistance in Latin America.* New York: Springer.

Gellately, R., & Kiernan, B. (eds.). (2006). *The spector of genocide: Mass murder in historical perspective.* New York: Cambridge University Press.

Genocide Watch. (2010). Countries at risk of genocide, politi-cide, or mass atrocities in 2010. Retrieved from www. genocide watch.org

Gering-Munzel, U., Dallas, M., & Perrry, I. (eds). 2007. *How healing becomes killing.* Houston: Holocaust Museum Houston.

Haas, A. (1985). *The doctor and the damned.* London: Granada Publishing.

Hadamar Trial. Alfonso Klein et al. (1945). *Law reports of trials of war criminals,* Vol.1. London: UN War Crimes Commission.

Haglund, W., & Sorg, W. (2002). *Advances in forensic taphon-omy: Method, theory, and archaeological perpsectives.* Boca Raton: CRC Press.

Harrowing, J., Mill, J., Spiers, J., et al. (2010). Culture, context, and community: Ethical considerations for global nursing research. *International Nursing Review,* pp.70-77.

Huffine, E. (2008). International impact of forensic data tech-nology. *Forensic Magazine,* 10/11:1-4. Retrieved from www.forensicmag.com/Article_Print.asp?pid=230

Huffine, E., Crews, J., & Davoren, J. (2007). Developing role of forensics in deterring violence and genocide. *Croatian Medical Journal,* 48:431-436.

International Commission on Missing Persons. (2009). *Executive summary.*

Jeffreys, A., Allen, M., Hagelberg, E., et al. (1992). Identification of the skeletal remains of Josef Mengele by DNA analysis. *Forensic Science International,* 56:65-76.

Karen, D., McCarthy, J., & Mazal, H. (2004). The ruins of the gas chambers: A forensic investigation of crematoriums at Auschwitz and Auschwitz-Birkenau. *Holocaust and Genocide Studies,* 18:68-103.

Kissi, E. (2006). Genocide in Cambodia and Ethopia. In Gellately, R., & Kiernan, B., (Eds.), *The specter of genocide.* New York: Cambridge University Press.

Koff, C. (2004). *The bone woman: A forensic anthropologist's search for truth in the mass graves of Rwanda, Bosnia, Croatia, and Kosovo.* New York: Random House.

Komar, D., & Lathrop, S. (2008). The use of material culture to establish the ethnic identity of victims in genocide inves-tigations: A validation study from the American Southwest. *Journal of Forensic Science,* 53:1035-1039.

Leaning, J. (1999). Medicine and international humanitarian law. *British Medical Journal,* 319:393-398.

Lemkin, R. (1944). *Axis rule in occupied Europe.* New York: Carnegie Endowment for International Peace.

Lifton, R.J. (1986). *The Nazi doctors.* New York: Basic Books.

Lilenthal, G. (2007). *Regional Psychiatric Clinic of Hadamar. How healing becomes killing.* Houston: Holocaust Museum Houston, pp. 87-95.

Lipstadt, D. (1993). *Denying the holocaust: The growing assault on truth and memory.* New York: The Free Press.

Machel, G. (2001). *The impact of war on children.* London: Hurst & Co.

Manning, D. (2000). *Srebrenica investigation: Summary of forensic evidence—execution points and mass graves.* United Nations International Criminal Tribunal for the Former Yugoslavia.

Manning, D. (2003). Witness testimony in the trial of Milosevic (Case IT-02-54-T), September 23.

Mario, J. (2002) A review of Anglo-American forensic profes-sional Codes of Ethics with considerations for code design. *Forensic Science International,* 25:103-112.

Martin, C. (2002). Moral courage and resistance among doctors and nurses during the holocaust. *The Age of Genocide.* London: Blackwell Publishing.

Martin, C. (2007). The legacy of Nazi doctors and the Nuremberg Code. *Houston Medical Journal,* pp. 14-16.

McFarland-Icke, B.R. (1999). *Nurses in Nazi Germany: Moral choice in history.* Princeton: Princeton University Press.

Mejia, R. (2009). Digging Guatemala: Anthropologists look for clues to past political killings. *Scientific American.* Retrieved from www.scientificamerican.com/article.cfm? id+anthropologists-study-political-killings

Menneckee, M. (2009). Genocidal violence in the former Yugoslavia: Bosnia-Herzegovia and Kosovo. In Totten, S., & Parsons, W. (eds.), *A century of genocide.* New York: Routledge Publishing.

Mitscherlich, A., & Mielk, F. (1949). *Doctors of infamy.* New York: Henry Schuman, p. xxvi.

Mukamana, D., & Brysiewicz, P. (2008). The lived experience of genocide rape survivors in Rwanda. *Journal of Nursing Scholarship,* 5:379-384.

Neugebauer, W. (2007). Operation T-4. In U. Gehring-Munzel (Ed.), *How healing becomes killing.* Houston: Holocaust Museum, pp. 17-27.

Physicians for Human Rights. (2009). Perilous medicine: The legacy of oppression *and* conflict on health in Kosovo. Cambridge, MA: Physicians for Human Rights.

Posner, G.L., & Ware, J. (1986). *Mengele: The complete story.* New York: McGraw-Hill.

Proctor, R.N. (1988). *Racial hygiene: Medicine under the Nazis.* Cambridge: Harvard University Press.

Pross, C., & Gotz, A. (1991). *The value of the human being: Medicine in Germany 1918-1945.* Berlin: Arztekammer Berlin.

Rehn, E., & Sirleaf, E.J. (eds.). (2002). *Women, war, peace: The independent* experts' *assesssment on the impact of armed conflict on women and women's role in peace-building* (Vol. 1). New York: United Nations, pp. 1-155.

Roland, C.G. (1992). *Courage under siege-starvation, disease, and death in the Warsaw Ghetto.* New York: Oxford University Press.

Skinner, M., & Sterenberg, J. (2005). Turf wars: Authority and responsibility for the investigation of mass graves. *Forensic Science International,* 151:221-232.

Smith, M.J. (1995). *Dachau: The harrowing of hell.* Albany, NY: State University of New York Press.

Spitz, V. (2005). *Doctors from hell: The horrific account of Nazi experiments on humans.* Boulder CO: Sentient Press.

Steadman, D.W., & Haglund, W.D. (2005). The scope of anthropoloigcal contributions to human rights investiga-tions. *Journal of Forensic Science,* 50:23-40.

Steele, C. (2008). Archaeology and the forensic investigation of recent mass graves: Ethical issues for a new practice of archaeology. *Archaeologies: Journal of the World Archaeological Congress*, 4(3):414-428.

Swearingen, B.E. (1985). *The mystery of Hermann Goering's suicide.* New York: Harcourt Brace Jovanovich.

Schmitz, D., & Obrien, D. (2001). Testimony presented by Medecins Sans Frontieres during the French Parliamentary Hearings into the Srebrencia tragedy. Paris, France. Retrieved from www.doctorswithoutborders.org/ publications /article.

Taylor, T. (1992). *The anatomy of the Nuremberg trials.* New York: Little, Brown.

Totten, S., & Parsons, W. (2009). *A century of genocide: Critical essays and eyewitness accounts.* New York: Rutledge Publishing.

Trials of war criminals before the Nuremberg military tribunals under control council law No. 10. 10 vols. Washington, DC: U.S. Government Printing Office.

United Nations. (2009). Resolution 63/155 Intensification of Efforts to Eliminate All Forms of Violence Against Women. Adopted by the General Assembly on December 18, 2008. Genevea: United Nations, pp. 1-7.

United Nations. (2009). Resolution 63/156 Trafficking in Women and Girls. Adopted by the General Assembly on December 18, 2008. Genevea: United Nations, pp. 1-7.

Wagner, S. (2008). *To know where he lies.* San Francisco: University of California Press.

Wiesenthal, S. (1967). *The murderers among us.* New York: McGraw Hill.

Werth, N. (2006). The great terror in the Soviet Union, 1937-38. In Gellately, R., & Kiernan, B. (Eds.), *The Specter of Genocide.* New York: Cambridge University Press.

Werth, N. (2009). The great Ukranian famine of 1932-33. *Online Encyclopedia of Mass Violence*, pp. 1-13. Retrieved from www.massviolence.org/PdfVersion?id_article=166

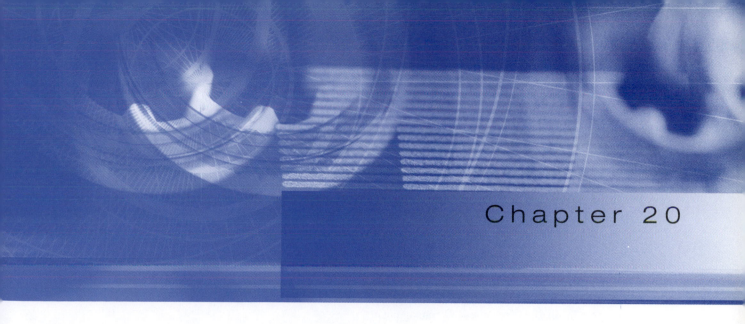

Chapter 20

DISASTER FORENSIC NURSING

Joyce Williams and David Williams

"Adapt or perish, now as ever, is nature's inexorable imperative."
H. G. Wells

Competencies

1. Understanding the subspecialties and roles of nurses in disasters.
2. Describing the laws, guidelines, and plans that dictate the federal emergency response to disasters.
3. Determining the appropriate steps to take to ensure a coordinated, appropriate emergency response.
4. Recognizing the various governmental, nongovernmental, and volunteer teams that respond to disasters.
5. Understanding the legal and ethical requirements for treating victims of disasters.

Key Terms

All hazard
Critical incident stress debriefing
Critical incident stress management
Disaster
Natural disaster
Technological disaster
Disaster Medical Assistance Team
Disaster Mortuary Operational
    Response Team
Emergency Management Assistance
    Compact
Emergency Medical Treatment and
    Labor Act
Emergency support function
Federal Emergency Management
    Agency
Hazard vulnerability analysis
Hospital incident command system
Homeland Security Presidential
    Directives
Incident command system

(key terms continued on page 392)

Key Terms (continued)

National Disaster Medical System
National Response Framework
Natural Disaster
Nongovernmental organizations
Occupational Safety and Health
    Administration
Post-traumatic stress disorder

Robert T. Stafford Act
Strategic National
    Stockpile
Technological disaster
Top Officials
Veterinary Medical
    Assistance Teams

INTRODUCTION

Hundreds of disasters occur around the world every day. A greater interest in disaster response and management among national and international agencies has occurred as a result of the devastating impact of disasters and need to rebuild communities affected by them. Many laws govern response capabilities and stress the need for personal safety. Health-care facilities must provide rapid and competent care to those affected directly by events. In addition, people may require mental health assistance to recover from the emotional consequences of a disaster.

Nurses, physicians, and other health-care workers are best prepared to provide care in a disaster. An excellent historical example, which illustrates the beginnings of disaster nursing, is the work of Florence Nightingale during the Crimean War. Nightingale was sent from London to Turkey to provide support for the British soldiers. Although soldiers were being wounded in battle, they were primarily being ravaged by epidemics of cholera and typhus due to unsanitary conditions. Nightingale instituted sanitation measures that decreased the mortality rate from 42.7% to 2.2% in just 6 months. Her efforts were instrumental in laying the foundation for sanitation guidelines, hospital design, and patient care. Additionally, her epidemiological outlook and statistical analysis methods established the foundation for modern evidence-based practice.

In this chapter, elements critical to disaster care are identified, and case studies provide insight into responses in various types of situations. Use of the "all hazard" approach demonstrates why and how reactions follow a conduit with options to mitigate the particular event. Governmental as well as nongovernmental organizations train, plan, and coordinate movements to respond to emergencies in collaboration with local authorities. No matter what the specific occurrence, data capture is of prime importance and provides the foundation for statistical analysis.

Best practices are derived from the evidence found in evaluations of current standards and making adjustments to improve care when indicated. This section demonstrates the basis for current actions and a future platform for leaders and providers to effectively respond when a disaster strikes.

KEY TERMS DEFINED

A **disaster** is an event that exceeds the resources immediately available. This is different from an emergency, which may cause an adverse effect but does not require extraordinary use of resources to bring conditions back to normal. The World Health Organization/Emergency and Humanitarian Action Department defines disasters as "any occurrence that causes damage, ecological disruption, loss of human life or deterioration of health and health services on a scale sufficient to warrant an extraordinary response from outside the affected community area." It also depends on perception: a fire that consumes an entire house would be a disaster for the family, but it would have little effect on the functioning of the community as a whole.

Disasters are classified as either *natural* or *technological*. **Natural disasters** are environmental events, such as volcanic eruptions, earthquakes, floods, cyclones, or more long-term epidemics, drought, or famine (catastrophic food shortage). **Technological disasters** are primarily caused by hardware failure and human error, resulting in toxic emissions, explosions, and transport accidents that may cause a chemical spill; insidious air, water, and soil pollution; or food contamination.

All hazard describes an incident, natural or human-caused, that warrants action to protect life, property, environment, and public health or safety and to minimize disruptions of government, social, or economic activities.

Critical incident stress debriefing (CISD) refers to Mitchell's model, a seven-phase, structured group discussion, usually provided 1 to 10 days after the crisis. It is designed to reduce acute symptoms, assess the need for follow-up, and if possible, provide a sense of post-crisis psychological closure for responders.

Critical incident stress management (CISM) is an integrated system of interventions designed to prevent and/or mitigate the adverse psychological reactions that often accompany emergency services, public safety, and disaster response functions.

The **Disaster Medical Assistance Team (DMAT)** is a volunteer group of medical and nonmedical individuals, usually from the same state or region of a state, who comprise a response team under the guidance of the National Disaster Medical System (NDMS) or under similar state or local auspices. DMATs usually include a mix of physicians, nurses, nurse practitioners, physician's assistants, pharmacists, emergency medical technicians, other allied health professionals, and support staff. Standard DMATs have 35 deployable personnel.

The **Disaster Mortuary Operational Response Team (DMORT)** is a volunteer group of medical and forensic personnel, usually from the same geographic region, who have formed a response team under the guidance of NDMS (or state or local auspices). DMORT personnel have specific training and skills in victim identification, mortuary services, forensic pathology, and anthropology methods. DMORTs usually include a mix of medical examiners, coroners, pathologists, forensic anthropologists, medical records technicians, fingerprint technicians, forensic odontologists, dental assistants, radiologists, funeral directors, mental health professionals, and support personnel. DMORTs are created for a particular mission on an "as needed" basis and typically deploy only with sufficient personnel and equipment specifically required for the current mission.

The **Emergency Management Assistance Compact (EMAC)** is the interstate mutual aid agreement that allows states to assist one another in responding to natural and human-caused disasters. In the aftermath of Hurricane Andrew in 1991, the Southern Governors' Association developed a simplified system for interstate assistance. This Southern Regional Emergency Management Assistance Compact, the precursor to EMAC, opened to other states around the country in 1995, and Congress ratified it into law as a national model in 1996. To date, nearly all states, the District of Columbia, and several U.S. territories have passed EMAC legislation.

The **Emergency Medical Treatment & Labor Act (EMTALA)** was enacted by Congress in 1986 to ensure public access to emergency services regardless of ability to pay. Additionally, section 1867 of the Social Security Act imposes specific obligations on Medicare-participating hospitals that offer emergency services to provide a medical screening examination (MSE) when a request is made for examination or treatment for an emergency medical condition (EMC), including active labor, regardless of an individual's ability to pay. Hospitals are then required to provide stabilizing treatment for patients with EMCs. Hospitals that do not have the capability to stabilize a patient should implement an appropriate transfer.

An **emergency support function (ESF)** is a specific area of response activity established to facilitate coordinated federal delivery of assistance required to save lives, protect property and health, and maintain public safety. These functions represent the types of federal assistance that the state likely will need most because of the overwhelming impact of a catastrophic event on local and state resources.

The **Federal Emergency Management Agency (FEMA)** has 3700 full time employees in Washington D.C. and regional and area offices across the country. FEMA also has nearly 4000 standby disaster assistance employees who are available for deployment after disasters. Often, FEMA works in partnership with other organizations that are part of the nation's emergency management system, such as state and local emergency management agencies, 27 federal agencies, and the American Red Cross.

A **hazard vulnerability analysis** identifies the disasters most likely to strike an organization or facility and estimates the potential impact of the disaster on the surrounding community. The goal of the analysis is to prioritize potential disasters that could affect a facility based on likelihood of occurrence and impact. The analysis can then be used as a starting point for emergency plans, enabling communities to use their resources most effectively.

The **hospital incident command system (HICS)** is an incident management system that assists hospitals in improving their emergency management planning, response, and recovery capabilities for unplanned and planned events. Use of the HICS will strengthen hospital disaster preparedness activities in conjunction with community response agencies.

Homeland Security Presidential Directives (HSPDs) are policies issued by the president of the United States on matters pertaining to homeland security. Several directives relate to disaster management:

- **HSPD-5 Management of Domestic Incidents.** Enhances the ability of the United States to manage domestic incidents by establishing a single, comprehensive national incident management system (NIMS).
- **HSPD-8 National Preparedness.** Aimed at strengthening the security and resilience of the United States through systematic preparation for the threats that pose the greatest risk to the security of the nation, including threatened or actual acts of terrorism, cyber attacks,

pandemics, catastrophic natural disasters, and other emergencies by requiring a national domestic all-hazards preparedness goal; establishing mechanisms for improved delivery of federal preparedness assistance to state and local governments; and outlining actions to improve the capabilities of federal, state, and local entities.

■ **HSPD-21 Public Health and Medical Preparedness**. Establishes a national strategy that will enable a level of public health and medical preparedness sufficient to address a range of possible disasters.

The **Incident Command System (ICS)** is the combination of facilities, equipment, personnel, procedures, and communications operating within a common organizational structure, designed to aid in the management of resources at emergency incidents. It is used for all types of emergencies and is applicable to small, as well as very large and complex, incidents.

National Disaster Medical System (NDMS) is a contingency system that comprises 150 disaster medical response units. The system provides for an evacuation plan and 100,000 voluntarily precommitted hospital beds throughout the United States. The federal government can activate the NDMS when a disaster overwhelms regional health-care resources and requires evacuation of patients to another region. Based on the Civilian Military Contingency Hospital System, NDMS is a cooperative effort of the Department of Health and Human Services, the Department of Defense, the Federal Emergency Management Agency, the Veterans Administration, state and local governments, and the private sector.

The **National Response Framework (NRF)** provides the template for governmental and nongovernmental organizations to work together to prevent, prepare for, respond to, and recover from domestic incidents.

Nongovernmental organizations (NGOs) are transnational organizations of private citizens that maintain a consultative status with the Economic and Social Council of the United Nations. NGOs may be professional associations, foundations, multinational businesses, or simply groups with a common interest in humanitarian assistance activities such as development and relief.

Occupational Safety and Health Administration (OSHA) specialists are personnel with specific training in occupational safety and health and in topics such as workplace assessment or occupational medicine. OSHA specialists and technicians help keep workplaces and workers safe. They promote occupational health and safety within organizations by developing safer, healthier, and more efficient ways of working. They analyze work environments and design programs to control, eliminate, and prevent disease or injury caused by chemical, physical, and biological agents or ergonomic factors. They may conduct inspections and enforce adherence to laws, regulations, or employer policies governing worker health and safety.

Post-traumatic stress disorder (PTSD) is a psychiatric disorder that can occur following the experience or witnessing of life-threatening events such as military combat, natural disasters, terrorist incidents, serious accidents, or violent personal assaults like rape. People who suffer from PTSD often relive the experience through nightmares and flashbacks, have difficulty sleeping, and feel detached or estranged. These symptoms can be severe and last long enough to significantly impair the person's daily life.

The **Strategic National Stockpile (SNS),** formerly the National Pharmaceutical Stockpile (NPS), is a national repository of antibiotics, chemical antidotes, antitoxins, life-support medications, IV administration and airway maintenance supplies, and medical and surgical items. The stockpile consists of two major components. The first is the 12-hour push package, and the second is the vendor-managed inventory (VMI). The SNS is designed to supplement and resupply state and local public health agencies in the event of a national emergency anywhere and at any time within the United States or its territories.

Robert T. Stafford Act, or The Robert T. Stafford Disaster Relief and Emergency Assistance Act, PL 100-707, signed into law November 23, 1988, amended the Disaster Relief Act of 1974, PL 93-288. This act constitutes the statutory authority for most federal disaster response activities, especially as they pertain to FEMA and FEMA programs.

Top Officials (TOPOFF) is a congressionally mandated, national, biennial exercise series designed to assess the nation's integrated crisis and consequence management capability against terrorist use of weapons of mass destruction (WMD). It examines national relationships among state, local, and federal jurisdictions in response to a challenging series of integrated, geographically dispersed terrorist WMD threats and acts.

Veterinary Medical Assistance Teams (VMATs) are volunteer teams of veterinarians, technicians, and support personnel, usually from the same region, that have organized a response team under the guidance of the American Veterinary Medical Association and the NDMS, and whose personnel have specific training in responding to animal casualties and animal disease outbreaks during a disaster. They help assess medical needs of animals, and conduct animal disease surveillance, hazard mitigation, biological and chemical terrorism surveillance, and animal decontamination. They usually include a mix of veterinarians, veterinary technicians, support personnel, microbiologists, epidemiologists, and veterinary pathologists.

DISASTERS

Disasters are occurring more frequently and are more devastating due to an overall increase in population numbers, the fact that populations are moving to more susceptible areas, and the fact that there is an increase in technology (which may be the source of the disaster). (See Box 20.1 for a list of disaster myths and realities.)

DISASTER NURSING

Disaster nursing, like disaster management itself, is an evolving field that can be divided into services for the living and those for the dead. It includes the subspecialties of:

- Medicolegal death investigator (identification of the dead)
- Researcher, investigator, epidemiologist (syndromic surveillance of infectious disease)
- First responder (emergency medical services)
- Direct care provider, generalist nurse, advanced practice nurse (trauma, critical care)

- Coordinator of care in hospital, nurse administrator
- On-site incident commander/director of care management
- Mental health counselor (CISD, PTSD, general care)
- Member of planning response team/member of community assessment team/member of decontamination team (citizens emergency response team, weapons of mass destruction (WMD) educator)
- Manager or coordinator of shelter (American Red Cross)
- Triage officer (DMAT)

Disaster nursing practice encompasses the four central concepts of nursing theory: person, environment, health, and nursing. Nurses who are trained and respond to disasters focus on key interventions as delineated in the basic and advanced disaster life support core principles. The primary focus of emergency response has changed from the traditional pillars of preparedness, planning, response, and mitigation to include prevention. Science has led to the emergence of both providing support during a disaster and educating individuals and populations on how to prepare for and avoid unnecessary injury.

The practice of nursing is regulated by the boards of nursing in accordance with the individual state nurse practice acts. These can vary between states, and knowledge of one's local practice act is critical to complying with the regulations set forth in it. Several states have established a voluntary corps to augment insufficient resources or to assist when a surge of personnel is needed.

Box 20.1   Disaster Myths and Realities

Myth: Dead bodies, left unburied, are a dangerous source of disease epidemics after disasters.
Reality: Disaster victims' bodies pose little or no threat to public health.
Myth: Burying victims quickly in mass graves gives survivors a sense of relief.
Reality: Survivors have a strong need to identify lost loved ones and grieve for them in customary ways.
Myth: Identifying large numbers of casualties is all but impossible. Mass graves are sometimes the only solution.
Reality: Even large numbers of bodies should be dealt with systematically, to facilitate their identification. Mass graves should always be avoided.
Myth: Any kind of international assistance is needed, and right away.
Reality: A hasty response that is not based on a needs evaluation can contribute to the chaos. It is better to wait until genuine needs have been assessed.
Myth: Foreign medical volunteers with any kind of medical background are needed following a disaster.

Reality: The local population almost always covers immediate life-saving needs. Only medical personnel with skills that are not available in the affected country are usually needed.
Myth: Natural disasters cause deaths at random.
Reality: Disasters cause more damage to vulnerable geographic areas, which are more likely to be inhabited by poor people. Especially in developing countries, disasters take a greater toll on the poor.
Myth: Locating disaster victims in temporary settlements is the best alternative.
Reality: It should be the last alternative. Funds may be better spent on building materials, tools, and other construction-related support in the affected area.
Myth: Things are back to normal within a few weeks.
Reality: The effects of a disaster last a long time. Countries deplete much of their financial and material resources in the immediate postimpact phase. Successful relief operations take account of the fact that donor interest tends to wane as needs and shortages grow more pressing.

Disaster Management

It is important to note that response to a disaster cannot be addressed simply by a change in the magnitude of the response. Hence, disasters generally cannot be managed adequately by merely mobilizing more personnel and materials. Additionally, disasters may extend beyond set jurisdictional boundaries and result in the need for collaboration across organizations or the creation of new organizations. A coordinated community response may not be able to quickly and effectively adapt to these changes (see below).

Formal emergency management in the United States began in the Truman administration and has evolved over the past half century. The names of the organizations have changed, and the primary focus has moved from preparedness against nuclear war to the all-hazards approach.

The Robert T. Stafford Disaster Relief and Emergency Assistance Act, PL 100-707, signed into law November 23, 1988, amended the Disaster Relief Act of 1974, PL 93-288. This Act constitutes the statutory authority for most federal disaster response activities, especially as they pertain to FEMA and FEMA programs (Box 20.2).

The Robert T. Stafford Disaster Relief and Emergency Assistance Act (The Stafford Act) is the federal law that specifies the statutory framework for a presidential declaration of an emergency or a major disaster. It provides the mechanism by which a governor or his or her representative may request federal assistance to either state or local authorities for disaster relief and recovery. It also stipulates that this assistance is to supplement the local and state resources and is not meant to furnish all of those resources alone.

Homeland Security Presidential Directive 5 (HSPD-5) establishes a "comprehensive approach to domestic incident management" and provides guidelines for a federal response that "will assist state and local authorities when their resources are overwhelmed, or when federal interests are involved." It identifies the secretary

---

Multilevel Response System

The U.S. response uses a coordinated multilevel system of plans, guidelines, and laws, which include the following:

- Federal
  - Robert T. Stafford Act
  - HSPD-5
  - HSPD-8
  - HPD-21
  - NRF
- State
  - State emergency response plan
  - Nurse practice act
- Local
  - Local emergency response plan
  - Laws
  - Ordinances

Box 20.2 Title I—Findings, Declarations, and Definitions

Sec. 101. Congressional Findings and Declarations (42 U.S.C. 5121)

(a) The Congress hereby finds and declares that
  1) because disasters often cause loss of life, human suffering, loss of income,
  2) and property loss and damage; and
  3) because disasters often disrupt the normal functioning of governments and communities, and adversely affect individuals and families with great severity; special measures, designed to assist the efforts of the affected States in expediting the rendering of aid, assistance, and emergency services, and the reconstruction and rehabilitation of devastated areas, are necessary.

(b) It is the intent of the Congress, by this Act, to provide an orderly and continuing means of assistance by the Federal Government to State and local governments in carrying out their responsibilities to alleviate the suffering and damage which result from such disasters by
  1) revising and broadening the scope of existing disaster relief programs;
  2) encouraging the development of comprehensive disaster preparedness and assistance plans, programs, capabilities, and organizations by the States and by local governments;
  3) achieving greater coordination and responsiveness of disaster preparedness and relief programs;
  4) encouraging individuals, States, and local governments to protect themselves by obtaining insurance coverage to supplement or replace governmental assistance;
  5) encouraging hazard mitigation measures to reduce losses from disasters, including development of land use and construction regulations; and
  6) providing Federal assistance programs for both public and private losses sustained in disasters

(**Source:** http://www.fema.gov/pdf/about/stafford_act.pdf)

of Homeland Security to be the principal official responsible for the coordination of federal operations within the United States and directs the secretary to coordinate the federal governmental resources that may be needed in response and recovery. It also "recognizes the role that the private and nongovernmental sectors plan in preventing, preparing for, responding to, and recovering from terrorist attacks, major disasters, and other emergencies."

Homeland Security Presidential Directive 8 (HSPD-8) mandates an all-hazards approach to response and notes that the "federal departments and agencies will work to achieve this goal by: (a) providing for effective, efficient, and timely delivery of federal preparedness assistance to state and local governments and (b) supporting efforts to ensure first responders are prepared to respond to major events, especially prevention of and response to threatened terrorist attacks." Also, "the primary mechanism for delivery of federal preparedness assistance will be awards to the states." It also delineates a mechanism for the training of first responders.

Homeland Security Presidential Directive 21 (HSPD-21) establishes a national strategy for public health and medical preparedness. This policy establishes a plan that enables provisions for public health and medical needs of the American people in the case of a catastrophic health event through continual and timely flow of information during such an event and rapid public health and medical response that marshals all available national capabilities and capacities in a rapid and coordinated manner. The four most critical components are bio-surveillance, countermeasure distribution, mass casualty care, and community resilience.

The National Response Framework (NRF) provides the template for governmental and nongovernmental response. It presents the guiding principles that enable all response partners to prepare for and provide a unified national response to disasters and emergencies. It establishes a comprehensive, national, all-hazards approach to domestic incident response. The National Response Framework became effective March 22, 2008.

The NRF defines the principles, roles, and structures that organize how we respond as a nation as it:

- Describes how communities, tribes, states, the federal government, private-sectors, and nongovernmental partners work together to coordinate national response
- Describes specific authorities and best practices for managing incidents
- Builds upon the National Incident Management System (NIMS), which provides a consistent template for managing incidents

The National Response Framework includes 15 emergency support functions and identifies who is responsible for them within the federal system. The emergency support functions have interlocking responsibilities of ESF 6–Mass Care; ESF 8–Health and Medical Services; and ESF 11–Food. The function under which mass casualty incidents (MCIs) are addressed is ESF 8. ESF 8 is the prime responsibility of the Department of Health and Human Services.

States have developed emergency response plans, laws, and regulatory agencies that mirror those of the federal government. These plans include specific details within the state and how the response will take place to minimize loss of life and community assets. Local jurisdictions are most affected by disasters, and their emergency plans are coordinated with the state plan.

Aviation Disaster Family Assistance Act of 1996

The National Transportation Safety Board (NTSB) has been investigating the nation's aviation incidents for nearly 30 years and has been to the scene of nearly 100,000 general and commercial airplane crashes. The Aviation Disaster Family Assistance Act of 1996 (PL 104-264, Title VII) was passed by Congress and signed by President Clinton on October 9, 1996. The act gave the NTSB the additional responsibility of aiding the families of aircraft accident victims. The new law is complemented by an earlier Presidential Executive Memorandum dated September 9, 1996, in which President Clinton designated the NTSB as the coordinator of federal services for families of major transportation disasters in the United States. This authority enables the NTSB to harness the collective resources of the federal government and direct aid to any area in which it is needed.

Prior to the passage of this act, the families of people killed or injured in a commercial aircraft accident had been primarily assisted in the aftermath of the accident by the individual airline. Additional support included local and state agencies, supported by volunteer organizations, but oftentimes the effort was uncoordinated and divisive.

The question of whether or not airlines are able to sufficiently manage family loss from an aviation disaster, or if services should be provided by an organized family assistance center trained to help families cope with the loss of a loved one is addressed in the following example.

Fragmented care became evident in the mid-1990s when the families' expectations were not met following an aviation crash because the perspective of the airlines was one of self-interest rather than interest in the families of the victims. Lack of coordination during such a mass fatality event left families waiting and wondering when and how identifications would be made on the deceased and who would inform them of the results. Additionally, discrepancies were demonstrated in the treatment of the families according to the ticket classes of passengers, with families of those paying for higher-priced tickets getting preferential treatment. Under the guidance of the NTSB, the issues and needs of families became an important aspect after an incident.

As a result of this incident, not only is investigation of the accident deemed important, but scientific identification of casualties and communication with the families of victims are important as well. Also, there is no longer a difference in treatment of the victims' families based on the price of the ticket that was purchased by the victim passenger. In addition, each airline is now expected to formulate a plan to effectively manage the needs of families after an accident.

While the airline continues to remain a major participant, the NTSB is now able to apply federal resources to augment local and state efforts and coordinate the overall family assistance support system. Issues, concerns, and needs of family members are significant, and interagency expectations have solidified, giving family members valid information with protection from secondary assaults and unwelcome intrusions by the media. These standards are a source of knowledge, and the core values of commitment, flexibility, communication, and sensitivity facilitate the complex needs of family members of those killed in accidents. Victim assistance programs are a vital asset to agencies responding to families and friends directly affected by the death of a loved one.

PERSONAL SAFETY OF RESPONDERS

Disasters by their nature can be dangerous to those who respond. These dangers may include natural hazards such as climatic and geologic or technologic hazards (primarily chemical and explosive) and hostile indigenous people. Personal safety of responders is a paramount responsibility of planners. Scene safety is demonstrated by a keen sense of awareness of potential and real risks. Surveys and assessments of affected areas are needed to determine the level of potential dangers to responders.

In the United States, OSHA is tasked with providing standards of safety for workers. Methods limiting environmental risks are engineering controls that physically prevent injury, such as confining access to a potentially contaminated area, and work practice controls that proscribe or prohibit actions, such as decontamination on leaving incident site or prohibiting eating within the morgue. Personnel, regardless of their role, must use the necessary personal protective equipment to avoid unnecessary health risk.

Hazards at Mass Casualty Events

Hazard levels vary by job title and hazard site. For example, the recovery of remains is more likely to expose one to hazardous materials than jobs that involve simply operating a computer. Therefore, safety measures for each of these jobs are different. The exposure control plan is pervasive and should be adhered to throughout the various phases of the operation—before, during, and after the event. Additionally, the Center for Disease Control and Prevention (CDC) provides standards for the safe handling of hazardous materials.

Scene Safety

The collapse of the World Trade Center (WTC) towers on September 11, 2001, created extraordinary forces that produced airborne particulate matter. In addition, fires burned within the rubble until mid-December 2001. More than 400 substances have been identified in airborne and settled samples of WTC dust. These agents, combined with the lack of availability of proper respirators and the minimal or nonuse of those available, exposed the nearly 11,000 personnel who worked at the site to widespread respiratory illnesses that can be directly related to this exposure. In fact, nearly one quarter of all conditions reported by local emergency departments may have been associated with the lack of proper personal protective equipment (PPE). In addition, there were injuries to the eyes as well as musculoskeletal conditions, including strains, sprains, lacerations, and contusions. These injuries continued at a constant rate for some weeks following the collapse, indicating that use of PPE was inadequate for some time following the first response. The CDC reported that less than 15% of the firefighters were using respiratory protection 2 weeks after the initial response, and less than half of the heavy equipment operators wore respirators 1 month after the attack. In his study, Izbicki found that the relative rate for "sarcoid-like granuloma" was 2.36 in the years 2 through 5 after WTC dust exposure.

Health Recommendations for Workers Who Handle Human Remains

Individuals in affected areas should exercise caution to avoid well-documented threats to health and safety, such as injury hazards from sharp debris and from unidentified structural damage to buildings, power lines, roads, and industrial facilities. Loss of sanitary infrastructure may result in exposure to raw sewage, a variety of soil and water organisms, and household and industrial chemicals. In addition, the loss of local drinking water treatment capacity and inability to maintain refrigeration for food and medical supplies may pose additional hazards. Disease(s) from human remains in floodwater are a minor part of the overall contamination. There are no additional practices or precautions for floodwater related to human remains, beyond what is normally required for safe food and drinking water, standard hygiene, and first aid for the general population.

There is no direct risk of contagion or infectious disease from being near human remains for people who are not directly involved in recovery or other efforts that require handling dead bodies. There is a risk of exposure to viruses or bacteria for workers who must handle human remains because remains may contain blood-borne viruses, such as hepatitis viruses and HIV, and bacteria that cause diarrheal diseases, such as shigella and salmonella. Recovery personnel or persons identifying remains or preparing the remains for burial or cremation should use the following precautions:

1. Protect the face from splashes of body fluids and fecal material.
2. Protect the hands from direct contact with body fluids, and also from cuts, puncture wounds, or other injuries that break the skin that might be caused by sharp environmental debris or bone fragments.
3. Maintain hand hygiene to prevent transmission of diarrheal and other diseases from fecal materials on your hands.
4. Give prompt care to any wounds sustained during work with human remains.
5. In addition to guarding physical safety, participate in available programs to provide psychological and emotional support for workers handling human remains.

Other Considerations

From the public health perspective of lowering the risk of possible infectious disease transmission, there is no requirement for mass burials or cremation. Response workers should assist local communities to identify a safe location for holding the deceased awaiting identification. This location should be shielded from public view if possible, and human remains should be protected from scavenging animals.

If available, use body bags to contain remains. Refrigeration can reduce the rate of decay and thereby maintain important forensic data. The sight and smell of decay are unpleasant, but they do not create a public health hazard.

THE SARS EPIDEMIC

The SARS epidemic can be traced to a series of atypical pneumonia infections in several cities in the Guangdong Province of China in November 2002. In February 2003, a physician who had been treating some of these patients in this area traveled to Hong Kong and stayed at a local hotel. Some of the individuals who stayed at this hotel acquired the infection and subsequently traveled to Vietnam, Singapore, and Toronto. In the end, the disease spread to 26 countries, with thousands infected, over 150 dead, and costs estimated between $11 billion and $18 billion.

Many of those contracting the disease were health-care workers. The outbreak was identified at the Prince of Wales Hospital in Hong Kong on Monday, March 10, 2003, when 11 health-care staff, 7 doctors, and 4 nurses went on sick leave simultaneously. The ward in which they worked was immediately closed to visitors. By the next day, the number of staff that had been taken ill had increased to 14. The hospital officials increased restrictions on ward 8A, the affected ward, and began to interview and give physical exams to those on sick leave. The 15 individuals who had a fever over 38°C (100.4°F), and another 8 who had chest x-rays that indicated signs of pneumonia, were then placed in an isolation ward. By Wednesday, the medical staff was divided into "dirty" and "clean" teams, with the "dirty" team caring for only those patients with atypical pneumonia and the "clean" team responsible for all other cases. There was no overlap between the teams. By Thursday, all nonemergency surgical procedures, same-day surgery, and cardiac outpatient clinics were cancelled, with patients diverted to other hospitals. There was increased training on droplet infection control for the staff, and the administration began to hold special meetings to make decisions regarding disease and infection control. On Friday there commenced daily press briefings to aid transparency in outbreak management and to provide background on the cases. The government was also investigating the cases of atypical pneumonia that had a tendency to affect hospital staff. The index case for the hospital epidemic was identified, and the decision was made to stop all clinical admissions to the medical department. By the next day, the World Health Organization (WHO) issued a travel advisory in response to the outbreak and named the disease severe acute respiratory syndrome (SARS). The coronavirus that was responsible for the outbreak was indentified at the University of

Hong Kong on March 22. The chief executive of hospital administration, who had visited the hospital eight times, was admitted to Queen Mary Hospital with suspected SARS on March 23. Between March 13 and 21, there were six mini-outbreaks in other health-care establishments.

Of the 1755 SARS infections in Hong Kong, 22%, or 386, were health-care workers, of whom 320 were infected while on duty. Factors leading to this high rate of infection were overwhelming caseloads, high viral loads, overcrowding and insufficient isolation facilities, and lack of experience or vigilance with regard to infection control procedures.

To prepare for the future, a committee was formed to review the details of the epidemic and make recommendations. These recommendations included strengthening the epidemiological capacity, providing a system for early detection, improving contingency planning, establishing clear command and control structures, providing mechanisms for an integrated response, improving surge capacity, and ensuring that communications are transparent and effective. The committee also wanted to ensure that a population-based framework be devised to coordinate services, use skills of health-care workers, involve private practitioners in providing services, and involve NGOs in providing care to those affected and those who are chronically ill. The committee was also concerned with the occupational health of the staff as well as the psychological impact of SARS on the patients and families of the patients, as well as the staff who cared for them. Of particular interest was the concern that there may be discrimination against former SARS patients.

The first case of SARS was recognized in Toronto in a woman who returned from Hong Kong on February 23, 2003. The virus was transmitted to other persons and resulted in a subsequent outbreak among 257 persons in hospitals in the greater Toronto area. In the period between April 15 and June 9, 2003, 74 cases of SARS were reported to Toronto Public Health. Of these, 29 (39%) occurred among health-care workers, 28 (38%) occurred as an exposure during hospitalization, and 17 (23%) occurred among hospital visitors. Therefore, 90% of the cases during this period were the direct result of hospital exposure.

In a study by Loeb et al, (2008), three patient activities were associated with a higher relative risk for infection: intubation, suctioning before intubation, and manipulating the oxygen mask. The use of PPE greatly reduced the risk to health-care providers. Consistent use of a gown reduced the attack rate from 42% to 15%; consistent use of gloves reduced attack rate from 40% to 18%; and the use of a N95 mask reduced attack rate from 56% to 13%.

In the words of a member of a Toronto hospital staff member:

> The word SARS instilled immense fear not just in the community, but within the walls of [the hospital] itself. With some 35 staff members contracting the disease, and one of our own dying from SARS, it was a threat that was all too real. But day after day our staff came to work, setting aside not only fears about their own safety and well-being, but an even greater dread about taking the disease home to their loved ones. Home, in many cases, provided little respite, as hospital staff became outcasts in the community. Shunned and isolated by family and friends alike, some reported seeing people cross the street to avoid even walking near their homes. Many staff felt—and were—truly alone. The sense of isolation was particularly acute for staff who contracted the disease. Their families could not visit them in hospital, and as soon as they were discharged they were sent into quarantine. Once home, Public Health and other officials visited them wearing protective gear, further frightening neighbors and friends. One of our staff members returned home only to learn that they were no longer welcome—their housemates had left our colleague's belongings outside. Media hysteria exacerbated the situation, creating what came to be called the "SARS pariah syndrome," making life outside the hospital difficult for health-care workers, patients, and their families. Despite the danger, our staff persevered, braving the crisis day by day.

Recommendations of the Ontario Expert Panel on SARS were more staff, more infection control practitioners, more epidemiologists, more community medicine practitioners, increasing awareness of health and safety issues in the health-care environment, balancing patient care with employee safety (a small number of employees refused to work based on perceived personal risk), enhancing the use of PPE, improving psychosocial education programs to help staff cope with psychological consequences of a similar health-care emergency, employing fewer part-time staff, reducing the risk of cross contamination due to working at multiple sites, and better deployment of human resources.

PSYCHOLOGICAL ISSUES BEFORE, DURING, AND AFTER A DISASTER

Critical incident stress management (CISM) is a technique that has been developed to help ordinary individuals who are exposed to extraordinary circumstances. These include counseling, medications, group therapy, and family therapy.

The psychiatric community does not universally embrace critical incident stress debriefing, yet from the recipient's point of view, the system seems to decrease traumatic stress over time (Box 20.3). Traumatic incident stress disorder or post-traumatic stress disorder (PTSD) has been recognized for over 150 years. During the Civil War it was called "soldier's heart," during World War I "shell shock," and during World War II, "battle fatigue."

When a person has been exposed to a traumatic event that threatens the physical integrity of self or others and the person's response involved intense fear, helplessness, or horror, this event may be persistently re-experienced in one or more of the following ways: recurrent distressing recollections or dreams, acting as if the event is recurring, or psychological stress when exposed to reminders of the event. These are called "flashbacks." Flashbacks may consist of images, sounds, smells, or feelings and are often triggered by ordinary occurrences, such as a door slamming or a car backfiring on the street. A person having a flashback may lose touch with reality and believe that the traumatic incident is happening all over again. Those with PTSD may avoid situations that remind them of the original incident, and anniversaries of the incident are often very difficult.

People with PTSD may startle easily, become emotionally numb (especially in relation to people with whom they used to be close), lose interest in things they used to enjoy, have trouble feeling affectionate, be irritable, become more aggressive, or even become violent. There may be persistent symptoms of increased arousal, including difficulty sleeping, irritability, difficulty concentrating, hypervigilance, and exaggerated startle reflex.

Not every traumatized person develops full-blown or even minor PTSD. Symptoms usually begin within 3 months of the incident, but occasionally emerge years afterward. They must last more than a month in order to be classified as PTSD. The course of the illness varies; some people recover within 6 months, while others have symptoms that last much longer. For a few, the condition becomes chronic.

Risk factors for developing PTSD include age, with school-aged victims being more susceptible at 62% versus 39% for adults. Location of the event is also a risk factor, with 79% of those from developing countries developing PTSD versus 27% in the United States and 46% in other developed countries. Lastly, the presence of mass violence increased impairment from 42% to 67%. Other factors

---

Box 20.3   Critical Incident Stress Debriefing: Implications for Best Practice

Critical incidents disrupt people's lives by creating strong emotional reactions, which may range from normal stress reactions to post-traumatic stress disorders. Critical incident stress debriefing (CISD) has been used since 1983 as a component of critical incident stress management. The processes are intended to help individuals manage their normal stress reactions to abnormal events. Although used extensively, research findings to date yield mixed results. Meta-analyses of research studies reviewed identify the methods, results, strengths, and weaknesses of the studies that can be used for evidence-based practice. Supportive methods describe decreased recovery time, fewer effects on family and work relationships, and allow for a return to normal precrisis functional levels. Many believe that CISD is not an isolated intervention, but rather is one that coexists with previous exposure, education, training, follow-up, and referral when necessary. The authors concluded that the data demonstrated a high degree of efficacy when CISD was implemented with a restrictive manual-driven protocol.

Nonsupportive studies include several extraneous variables that could explain how the risk of PTSD may be increased.

Some victims who received CISD also had physical injuries and therefore may have had greater emotional needs. Other victims may have misinterpreted the focus of CISD and assumed their reactions were pathological. It is also possible that the debriefing intervention led to an exacerbation of symptoms that were not countered with adequate emotional processing. There were limitations noted, however, that cited inconsistencies and variations in the application of CISD.

The conclusions point to a need for further research to evaluate the protocols and applications of CISD, explaining the intervention model, ensuring training of appropriate personnel, and providing assessment procedures to measure intervention effectiveness. Other important issues that remain to be examined include delineation of critical incidents; standardization of appropriate formats; additional measurement in specific populations; determining clearly defined time spans between the incident, debriefing, and follow-up evaluations; and specifying the number and type of health-care professionals and peer counselors involved. CISD remains a technique that is perceived to be clinically efficacious, while at the same time, research efforts continue to refine the techniques and measurement issues.

(From: Mitchell, M., Sakraida, T.J., & Kameg, K. (2003). Critical incident stress debriefing: Implication for best practice. *Disaster Management Response, 1*(2):46-51.)

include being female, having lower socioeconomic status, and the severity of the exposure.

All disasters should be considered a crime scene initially because of potential criminal prosecution or civil action. Some disasters are precipitated by individuals and constitute an obvious crime scene. An example of a criminal action is the Oklahoma City bombing where the perpetrator committed a crime and evidence was later needed for prosecution. An example for a civil matter is the instance of an airplane crash where victims' families may seek civil restitution for the loss of loved ones from the airline company. Evidence at a crime scene must be recognized, preserved, and collected for use in assigning responsibility for the incident. The Department of Justice (DOJ) trace evidence guidelines provide an excellent description of how this is best accomplished.

Field treatment of survivors is initiated by first responders assessing and performing triage to sort the acuity of those with injury. Secondary assessment of the injured is carried out upon arrival, with continuing assessments throughout the treatment phase at the receiving facility. Several methods are available that organize the system of determining acuity of injury for treatment. The goal is to render care and optimize survival, with only limited resources available in some cases. The severity of the disaster may require use of altered standards (discussed later) in order to render care and adapt to the extreme conditions.

Interruptions in infrastructure are possible that may compromise transportation of the injured and cause delays in the arrival at treatment sites of the most acutely injured. Many less-severely injured will present independently and require triage at the health-care facility (HCF) by the emergency room team member assigned. In the case of a large disaster, some HCFs will be overwhelmed by the walking wounded, necessitating transfer of those less acutely injured to alternate sites for treatment. In-house patients may be discharged early to make room for those arriving who require in-patient care.

In most disasters, a percentage of the injured do not survive. Some events are more lethal in nature, and in these cases many will be dead at the scene, while others will die later from their injuries. The recovery of the dead is an important step in identification and disposition of the remains. Forensic disaster nurses are trained to investigate and be part of the team that documents the preliminary findings and collaborates in the recovery of the dead. Large-scale events will require the assistance of recovery teams as determined by the medical examiner (ME) office or coroner protocols, with state or federal guidance.

Once the dead are recovered, the process of identification can begin. The individuals recovered are placed in either a temporary or permanent structure to allow appropriate procedures to be performed for the scientific identification process. This process consists of locating ante-mortem data and collecting postmortem information so that a comparison of information will provide a positive identification.

Identification of victims is accomplished using scientific methodology to distinguish unique characteristics of the victim and compare them with a known sample. The methodologies that provide medical certainty are fingerprints, DNA, dental identification, and medical devices. Nonscientific methods do not provide assurance of a positive identification (visual identification, tattoos, and personal effects are some methods employed). Forensic specialists work as a team to provide scientific determinations of identification to provide closure to families.

Case Study

Explosions in London Underground Transportation System

On the morning of July 7, 2005, at 8:50 a.m., four separate but connected explosions occurred in central London when terrorists detonated four bombs on the public transport system. Three explosions occurred within 1 minute in the Underground system at Edgeware Road, King's Cross, and Aldgate stations, and the fourth was detonated on a double-decker bus at Travistock Square approximately an hour later. Initial reports were confusing, indicating the source of the incident was a power surge. The incident was further exacerbated because the victims exited the underground trains from each end of the tunnel, so there were two evacuation sites

per individual incident. This was the largest mass casualty event in the United Kingdom since World War II.

At 9:23 a.m., a London-wide major incident was declared. The National Health Service placed hospitals that had accident and emergency services on alert, but did not alert some specialty hospitals, such as the Great Osmond Street Children's Hospital, which was closest to the Kings Cross and Travistock Square sites. Extrication of the injured was hampered by difficulties in accessing the scene, and lack of ambulance capacity hindered transportation of patients to health-care facilities because of the multiple active sites. Communications systems failed,

Case Study

leaving those at the receiving facilities in the position of not knowing when and how many patients they were to expect. Because the transportation system within the city had stopped, double-decker buses were used to transport the injured, which meant that without warning, as many as 50 or more injured would arrive at a medical facility.

Overall, 775 people were injured, 53 died at the scene, and 3 died subsequent to the incident. "Over triage," or assigning a noncritically injured victim to a higher priority level, is common in mass casualty events, especially when triage is done on-site. This increases the need for secondary triage and reprioritization of patients at entry into the health-care system and periodically throughout the incident to ensure that scarce resources are expended properly. Initial triage should also be used to ensure that the most critical patients are sent to the facility that is the most appropriate, not necessarily the closest. Higher-level trauma hospitals should receive the bulk of the most critical patients, while those victims with less severe injuries may be treated at a lower-level facility.

The first priority 1 and 2 patients arrived at the Royal London Hospital, London's primary trauma receiving hospital, at 10:05 a.m., and the resuscitation room capacity was reached within 15 minutes, with the first operation beginning at 10:45. In all, 17 patients needed operations, and these were done over 14 hours, with the maximum operating room surge of 4 patients per hour.

Morgue facilities were ready to receive deceased victims in 24 hours, and were fully functioning in 72 hours.

In the aftermath of the incident, it was felt that there was a lack of planning for care of survivors or traumatized relatives and friends of those affected by the bombing and that a point of contact for people who were worried about missing relatives or friends had not been set up in a timely manner.

There may be as many as 6000 people who were severely psychologically affected by the bombings, about half of them through direct experience.

References

Parish, C. (2005). The London bombings: How EDs and nurses responded to the terrorist attacks of July 7. *American Journal of Nursing, 105*(9):102-103.

Aylwin, C., et al. (2005). Reduction in critical mortality in urban mass casualty incidents: Analysis of triage, surge, and resource use after the London bombings on July 7, 2005. *Lancet 386*(12):2219-2225.

FAMILY ASSISTANCE CENTER

The family assistance center (FAC) is a private and comfortable location where individuals, families, and friends of the victims gather following a sudden extraordinary event. The importance of a well-chosen FAC cannot be stressed enough. It should be in a calm and quiet area in close proximity to the event site, but remote enough to diminish retraumatizing those impacted by the crisis. It is a site where families receive official, up-to-date information on the identification of the dead as well as coping strategies to mitigate the impact of the traumatic event on victims and to accelerate recovery processes. Forensic nurses meet with families to provide comfort and gather data to assist in the identification process. An informative questionnaire is completed by family members to document the unique characteristics of the deceased person. A DNA sample may be needed to compare to the sample retrieved from the human remains. Ante-mortem data are used by the mortuary personnel team to compare with the post-mortem data of the deceased.

Updates of the identification process and the release of positive identifications of individuals are provided to the families before any information is released to the media. Scheduling regular meetings during the day provides clear and accurate communication first to families and later to media. This demonstrates sensitivity to families who are already traumatized.

Support and counseling services are also a part of the FAC. Each family has stress placed on them from injury or the loss of a family member. Crisis intervention services take place the entire time families are present, during and long after the event has passed.

The National Association of Medical Examiners Mass Fatality Plan found at http://dmort.org/FilesforDownload/NAMEMFIplan.pdf speaks to the specifics of scene management responsibilities, morgue protocols, off-site examination center, family assistance center, logistic requirements, and an extensive appendix of forms and references to guide communities in the processes to be completed following an incident of large magnitude.

Case Study

HURRICANE KATRINA

Characteristics of the FAC contribute to the prospective outcomes during a mass fatality event. In 2005 Hurricane Katrina approached landfall with winds reaching 175 miles per hour and a tidal surge equivalent to a category 3. Because the storm was so large, highly destructive eye-wall winds and the strong northeastern quadrant of the storm pushed record storm surges onshore, smashing the entire Mississippi Gulf Coast and Louisiana after an initial landfall off the southern Florida peninsula 3 days earlier. Many families fled the widespread destruction and flooding, displacing nearly 1 million individuals. Nearly 80,000 to 90,000 people remained in the city of New Orleans, many of them taking refuge in the Superdome. The excess water from the storm flooded nearly 80% of the city, making life arduous for all. Most of the city's hospitals and other health-care resources were destroyed or inoperable.

During the post-assessment phase of the disaster, search and recovery efforts were complicated despite the plans in place to cope with and recover from an intense storm. The magnitude of this storm caused widespread loss of infrastructure, with communications lost throughout and among the communities. The needs of the population were exhaustive.

The Disaster Mortuary Operational Response Team was activated, with the family assistance center as a part of the response. Members reported to Jackson, Mississippi, on Friday, September 2, and Saturday, September 3, to begin the process of determining where and how to assist families in the aftermath. The first mission was an assessment of the situation compiled from reports received through the initial response team in the heart of the destruction along the coast of Louisiana and Mississippi. The FAC team continued planning and determining equipment needs, as well as finding a suitable place to locate the center. The group then split into two smaller groups to serve the residents in the states receiving the more significant damage. One group headed toward Gulf Port, Mississippi, and the second traveled to Baton Rouge, Louisiana.

The facilities of the FAC must be conducive to sensitive interaction between family members and staff. Ideally, privacy and security are paramount. This was no exception. The FAC was based at a hotel in Baton Rouge where staff could interact as necessary to obtain information needed on those missing or deceased. The rooms were arranged to facilitate multiple operations concurrently. Interagency collaboration was significant and no different from past events. Multiple communication lines were positioned for the FAC members as well as partnership agencies assisting in the mission.

Due to the widespread displacement of individuals and aggravating circumstances making recovery efforts challenging, it was necessary to develop an alternate way of communicating with family members. An 800 telephone number was established to allow families the opportunity to contact the FAC for information regarding their loved ones. They accepted these calls for those people who were missing, deceased, or unknown as to their whereabouts. 1-800 Find Family became the nationwide call-in number.

Calls were received at the center by the FAC members who spent time listening to callers and asking questions to complete the ante-mortem data information necessary and fill in the victim information profile (VIP). This was entered into a database for comparison to postmortem recovery information on human remains (Box 20.4).

To maintain sufficient services, the FAC established a larger bank of phones to receive calls. They secured as many as 100 additional phone lines and accessed additional volunteers to answer these lines to obtain preliminary information. The FAC members then returned calls to obtain the necessary VIP data.

Because children could not find their parents and parents could not find their children, the DOJ and the National Center for the Missing and Exploited Children collaborated in a reunification effort (Box 20.5). Several other state and federal agencies also worked together to assist in efforts to locate the missing.

Adapting to the circumstances of the event facilitates the direct outcome in the identification and location of the missing and deceased. Since Hurricane Katrina struck in September, there were 11,635 calls, with 9946 people found alive and 836 confirmed deceased.

Box 20.4   DMORT Victim Information Profile

Personal information data collection sheets are used by the FAC personnel when interfacing with family members. The antemortem information gathered on these forms is then used for comparison with postmortem findings on human remains. These forms may be downloaded at http://dmort.org/forms/index.html

Box 20.5   Technology Helps Reunite Children and Families

Chung and Shannon (2007) proposed the creation of a system to use advanced imaging and feature-extraction technology to expedite the reunification of children with their families. Children may become separated from family members or evacuated to relocation sites from schools or places hosting child activities. This data capture software will capture digital images including hair and eye color and transmit copies to a secure site where they are indexed and catalogued. Reunification is possible with the help of trained professionals who enter child's features into the system to compare images and identify the missing.

HOSPITAL INCIDENT COMMAND SYSTEM (HICS)

HICS Improves Integration and Communication

Management styles can be classified into hierarchical or collaborative styles. The hierarchical style uses a single person in charge with all others subordinate to that person. Communication flows from the person in charge to the subordinates and from subordinates back up the chain of command. The advantage of this style is both its efficiency and its concentration of responsibility with the person in charge. The disadvantages are there may be less input into the decision-making process and less agreement from the subordinates to the plan of action.

The collaborative style has one person in charge, but all the players collaborate together and are equal members of the group. The advantage is more agreement from the participants, but the decision-making process takes longer to complete and put into action. The shared responsibility for decisions may be a detriment as no one may be held responsible for the overall actions of the group. As disasters are in themselves chaotic and time is of critical importance with decisions being required rapidly, the hierarchical style is more appropriate.

The ICS provides a simple and adaptable management structure that is capable of being expanded or contracted to meet the needs of a specific situation. The hospital incident command system adapts the ICS to the hospital setting, and its use of the ICS nomenclature and terminology facilitates the communication and the sharing of resources between all agencies and health-care institutions involved.

HICS is the method of choice to define the management mechanism to provide optimal care using strained resources within the health-care system.

Adapting the Response to the Incident

Incidents vary in size, scope, and complexity; therefore, the response should be specific to that disaster. Disasters have commonalities governing the response, and the aspects universal to these events are widely used regardless of the type of disaster. However, the response must be "scalable, flexible, and adaptable" (NRF, p. 9-12).

In 2003 following the Bali bombing, Australian nurses cared for victims evacuated by air with ambulance transfer to the Royal Darwin Hospital in Australia's Northern Territory. Nearly 24 hours later, victims began arriving at the triage area, which allowed a generous amount of time to stock up and brief each other on burn formulas and analgesia. The patients proved to be unique in a number of ways, and the staff was required to adapt and set new priorities. Communication barriers were challenged, with victims representing several countries and cultures.

The core treatments consisted of:

- Airway management
- Breathing management
- Circulation
- Pain relief
- Temperature regulation
- Wound management
- Tetanus prophylaxis
- Psychological support

Local and Expanded Disaster Response

Incidents occur locally, with responses and resources brought in from the state, federal, and international components as needed. ICS is a proven method of providing a response to a disaster: it is tiered, scalable, flexible, and adaptable while maintaining a cohesive effort through unified command. This method allows all agencies to provide joint support through mutually developed objectives, yet each agency maintains its own authority and accountability.

Lessons learned in the clinical settings demonstrate that a large influx of patients can create chaos in unprepared and poorly administered events. Prior preparation to identify services, supplies, and personnel improves efficiency.

In the United States, the National Incident Management System (NIMS) is the methodology that is employed by governments and NGOs at all levels. Within the health-care system, ICS has been adapted to fit the specifics necessary to respond effectively.

CORE COMPETENCIES OF DISASTER NURSES

Training and competence improve process (knowledge, skills, and ability). Clinical skills are routinely used during patient care. Specific training in expanded functions is gained by accessing courses designed to reach beyond the normal day-to-day functions of health-care providers, such as ICS and academic course work designed to complement clinical practice. These competencies focus on critical elements and delineate a template consisting of key elements used in emergency conditions.

Core competencies for disaster nurses have been described by a variety of individuals and organizations. Some of these lists are extensive, whereas others are more abbreviated. Furthermore, some follow the core competencies of nursing in general, and others are more specifically attuned to the field of disaster management. There is no single authoritative source or approval body for emergency preparedness competencies, and as Slepski (2007) indicated, "the vision and resulting competency requirements are inconsistent across [health-care] groups."

It is our intention to clarify the concepts of core competencies, rather than add to the general confusion. To this end we propose the schema of organization, person, patient, and environment.

"Organization" reflects the legal basis for actions, how the system functions during the event, and information sharing. There must be a legal basis for all actions. These stem from the federal, the state, and the local governments, as well as other sources such as professional or international guidelines. To disregard this legal basis would expose the disaster nurse to potentially dire consequences. Justification or rationalization of actions taken that violate the law must not be contemplated. Information-sharing occurs before the event, through the duration of the event, and long after the event is over. Information includes the disaster plan and communication among all the participants in the preparedness phase, response phase, and recovery phase. It includes the written and the spoken information—that which is said in person or over a telecommunications system. Clarity is

essential, because decisions are made based on the information that is provided and actions are taken that are directed through communication. Unclear or misunderstood information can greatly hamper the response to a disaster.

Organization also reflects the system in which the individual works and how that individual fits into the system. This includes not only knowledge of the incident command system, but also how one's organization fits into the ICS. It also includes those principles and practices that the organization has in place to address the issues. An example of these may be staffing or logistical policies and procedures that are individualized to an institution.

"Person" considers the preparedness and safety of the individual, the mastery of skills typically accomplished within the normal workplace, and skills necessary for use in a disaster and professional development. As noted in the organization category, it is the responsibility of the individual to know what his or her part is within the entire response system. One also must be prepared physically and mentally for the rigors of the disaster scene. This may mean acquiring the proper clothing, PPE, and mental flexibility necessary to cope with a changing environment. Within this environment, one most likely will be called upon to perform his or her usual clinical duties, oftentimes in the face of scarce resources or large number of patients. In addition, individuals may be called upon to act in specialties with which they may be less familiar (pediatric, geriatric, trauma, orthopedics, etc.) in an environment that is totally foreign to them. These skills must be anticipated ahead of time and trained for so that their response is successful. This training will be in addition to the normal upkeep of clinical skills and will require the individual to take advantage of opportunities that he or she would not otherwise access. These may include basic disaster life support, FEMA's independent study courses, and Community Emergency Response Team (CERT) training.

"Patient" indicates the proper management of the individuals based upon the circumstances, with particular attention paid to those with special-needs. As noted earlier, the conditions may be austere and the equipment and supplies may be in short supply or nonexistent, but it is critical to maintain the highest level of care that may be afforded to the patients. In some cases, an altered standard of care may be instituted by the command authority, but even in these circumstances every effort must be made to provide the greatest amount of treatment to the largest number of victims. Special-needs individuals, including pregnant women, children, the elderly, and those with mental and physical limitations may present a particular challenge to treatment.

Lastly, the "environment" includes not only protection of the physical environment, but also the emotional and psychosocial health of the population. Those who may have lived through the event will have to rebuild their lives after the responders have gone and will have psychosocial and emotional issues that may require treatment far into the future. The overall plan must consider how to mitigate the effects of the environment on the responders and victims and how to care for their present and future needs.

ALTERED STANDARDS OF CARE

Do ethical considerations change in a mass disaster? The foundation of medical ethics is the Hippocratic Oath. Traditionally, health-care ethics have relied on the principles of respect, autonomy, beneficence, nonmalfeasance, and justice. The *Code of Ethics for Nurses* addresses these principles and the responsibilities derived from them and rely on humanist, feminist, and social ethics as well as the cultivation of virtues.

No emergency changes the basic standards of practice, code of ethics, competence, or values of a profession, but legal structures for health-care professionals may change if the emergency is in a state that allows for alterations under emergency powers. Faced with potentially hundreds, thousands, or even tens of thousands of victims, the decision-making process may shift to a utilitarian framework in which the clinical goal is the greatest good for the greatest number. This is contrary to the philosophy of "the most that can be done" and instead presents providers with what is sufficient, given the specific conditions at the time. It is important to note that there is a shift to what is best for the community and away from what is ideal for the patient.

It is hoped that the adoption of altered standards of care will take place within the ICS, using guidelines that have a basis for allocation that is fair and clinically sound. To this end, a number of organizations are addressing the challenges and working with communities, governmental officials, and health-care workers to provide protocols for a mass casualty response plan that will provide strategies for risk communication, modification of state laws, verification of credentials, and training of providers in the event of a disaster.

Prior training and practice removes limitations and concern during times of extreme stress. Rapid assessment and familiarity with situational awareness aids in the level of response, types of interventions, clinical protocols, standing orders, and other specifications useful in health and medical care regimens. The synthesis of core competencies and training overlap, which indicates the critical nature of additional training for adequate response to an emergency.

NATIONAL DISASTER MEDICAL SYSTEM

The National Disaster Medical System (NDMS) is a partnership that provides emergency medical services in a disaster, involving FEMA, the Department of Health and Human Services, the Department of Defense, the Veterans Administration (VA), as well as public and private hospitals across the country.

The purpose of the NDMS is to provide a nationwide medical response system that supplements state and local emergency resources during disasters or major emergencies. NDMS also provides backup medical support to the military/VA medical care systems during overseas conventional conflict. Circumstances for which NMDS may be activated include (1) a military contingency or overseas conventional armed conflict involving U.S. forces, (2) a presidential declaration of a disaster, or (3) a request for major medical assistance. The major responsibilities of the NDMS include medical response, patient evacuation, and definitive medical care. NDMS comprises the following specialty teams:

- Disaster Medical Assistance Team (DMAT)
- Disaster Mortuary Operational Response Teams (DMORT)
- Veterinary Medical Assistance Teams (VMATs)
- National Nurse Response Team (NNRT)
- National Pharmacy Response Teams (NPRTs)
- Disaster Portable Morgue Units (DPMU) Team

Disaster Medical Assistance Teams

Disaster Medical Assistance Teams (DMAT) are designed to be a rapid-response element to supplement local medical care until other federal or contract resources can be mobilized or the situation is resolved.

DMATs are the responsibility of the federal government, as prearranged sources of support. A DMAT consists of a volunteer group affiliated with NDMS consisting of approximately 35 individuals in each deployable unit. A "typical" DMAT may consist of 4 to 5 physicians, 10 to 15 nurses, 8 to 10 EMTs, and 8 to 10 administrative and logistics staff. Many teams also maintain a critical incident stress management subunit.

DMATs are categorized according to their ability to respond. DMATs are usually locally sponsored and community based but they maintain a Memorandum of Understanding (MOU) with the U.S. Public Health Service so they can be called upon for federal service when necessary. The normal length of deployment is 7 to 10 days.

DMAT Special Teams include pediatric, burn, orthopedics, urban search and rescue (USAR), and mental health teams. DMAT functions include triaging of victims at the disaster site, providing sophisticated medical care in austere conditions, and maintaining casualty clearing or staging locations just outside the disaster site. DMATs can also provide care at a reception area when the patient evacuation part of NDMS is activated. They can receive victims of the disaster in areas across the country that were unaffected and thus can handle a large quantity of injured.

When deployed, the DMAT functions under a Management Support Unit (MSU). The support that is provided is variable according to the magnitude of the event. Advance notice allows the opportunity to activate and predeploy units to augment current resources. DMATs are supplementary services and do not undertake the responsibility of planning that should occur by the local authorities and affiliated partners.

The response of DMATs has proven its worth for medical support for a number of events. Many of these include natural disasters such as hurricanes, earthquakes, and floods. They also provide support for major national events, including the Democratic and Republican conventions, the Centennial Olympic Games, and other gatherings of interest. Some of the most notable responses include the Oklahoma City bombing, the World Trade Center attack, major hurricanes such as Andrew, Wilma, Hugo, Floyd, Katrina, and Rita, as well as the California wildfires and numerous airplane crashes.

Burn nurses were used during the Pentagon terrorist incident in 2001 to complement the current resources available locally. Also in 2001, critical care nurses reinforced the local resources following the Texas floods in Houston, and in 2005 they provided care during the Katrina and Rita events. Overall, DMATs are used extensively as support for the local resources to receive, stabilize, and evacuate the injured and ill.

Disaster Mortuary Operational Response Teams

The Disaster Mortuary Operational Response Team (DMORT), is an outgrowth of an initiative that started in the early 1980s when a committee was formed within the National Funeral Directors Association (NFDA) to address the appropriate response of mass fatality incidents. Their concentration was in the mortuary field, but they soon realized that more than one discipline was needed to properly process the remains of victims. A multifaceted, nonprofit organization open to all forensic practitioners was thereby formed by the committee to support

the idea of a national-level response protocol for all related professions. The group purchased the first portable morgue unit in the country, and their equipment has subsequently supported DMORT missions across the United States and Guam.

DMORTs are multidisciplinary groups that work to support local authorities and provide technical assistance and personnel to recover, identify, and process deceased victims during disasters. A part of the Department of Homeland Security's National Disaster Medical System, DMORT may be activated under several legal authorities, including the National Response Framework, the Public Health Services Act, the Aviation Disaster Family Assistance Act, presidential mandate, and existing federal and state agreements.

Since the evolution of DMORTs, great comfort has been provided to families due to the teams' scientific ability to identify human remains of individuals in mass fatalities. Their mission is accomplished by using various experts, resources, and protocols to process the victims. The individual members of the team include forensic anthropologists, funeral directors, medical examiners, coroners, forensic pathologists, medical records technicians and transcribers, fingerprint specialists, forensic odontologists, dental assistants, x-ray technicians, mental health specialists, computer professionals, administrative support staff, and security and investigative personnel.

Forensic nurses serve within the DMORT by providing support to the various specialists on the team. In the morgue, they work side by side with pathologists, anthropologists, DNA analysts, and data management personnel. Their knowledge of the death investigation process, interaction with family members, and medical expertise make them ideal members of the team, and their role can extend to search and recovery efforts. Their responsibility extends to safety and health considerations of the team members and is also used on the Family Assistance Center team to console those whose family members have become victims of an event. Many have critical incident stress debriefing backgrounds and are accustomed to working under stressful situations. These nurses adapt to the situation at hand and are a great asset, maintaining flexibility in roles and providing assistance to each member of the team.

The success of DMORT response is evidenced by their ability to identify and provide closure to the families of victims of mass casualty events. Since their inception in 1992, DMORTs have responded to over 32 events in which more than 7600 victims were processed. Scientific rigor is achieved by employing current methodology and techniques, combined with a stringent peer review process. Several documents provide additional guidance to scientific rigor. They are the National Institute of Justice's *Mass Fatality Incidents: A Planning Guide for Human Identification*, the U.S. Army Soldier and Biological Chemical Command's *Guidelines for Mass Fatality Management During Terrorist Incidents Involving Chemical Agents,* and the National Transportation Safety Board protocol.

In January 2005, DMORT, the NTSB, the Department of Homeland Security (DHS), and FEMA created an interagency agreement describing the collaborative efforts with the National Disaster Medical System (NDMS) services on transportation incidents. This document is known as *DMORT Standard Operating Procedures for National Transportation Safety Board Activations*. It contains information needed to understand how DMORT operates in support of the local medicolegal authority in transportation accidents involving fatalities.

OTHER VOLUNTEER ORGANIZATIONS

Several national, state, local, and faith-based organizations respond to disaster sites. The Medical Reserve Corp, State Defense Forces, the American Red Cross, and Operation Blessing are examples of those that provide medical assistance. Many other organizations offer humanitarian relief in disaster areas, aid to refugees, food for the hungry, and assistance to the impoverished. The United Methodist Committee on Relief (UMCOR), Catholic Charities, and the Salvation Army each has a long tradition of aiding victims of disasters.

STATE DEFENSE FORCES

State defense forces, also known as state guards, state military reserves defense corps, or state militia, are military units under the exclusive jurisdiction of the state governor and are not entities of the federal government. Their potential missions include assisting civil authorities in the preservation of order and protection of life and property, assisting with domestic emergencies that may arise within the state, and protecting critical infrastructure. While their original missions were primarily those of a military police, there has been an increase in the medical component of the forces, and many of them have been activated through the Emergency Management Compact to assist in disasters beyond their own state borders.

The Medical Reserve Corps (MRC) was founded after President Bush's 2002 State of the Union Address in which he asked all Americans to volunteer in support of their country. MRCs are community based and prepare for and respond to emergencies and promote healthy living throughout the year. MRC units are not stand-alone or first-response entities. These volunteers provide personnel to support and supplement existing emergency and public health resources.

The Medical Reserve Corps responded during the 2005 hurricane season and furnished support for American Red Cross health services, mental health services, and shelter operations. MRC members also supported the U.S. Department of Health and Human Services response and recovery efforts by staffing special needs shelters, community health centers, and health clinics and by assisting health assessment teams in the Gulf Coast region.

DATA MANAGEMENT

Planning diminishes the nonfunctioning logistical aspects of an incident and serves to organize the complexities related to a disaster event. As demands increase in magnitude, it is essential to use forward thinking to respond effectively to operational processes. To have the ability to plan and operate during a disaster, high-quality and timely information is a necessity. Data management is a critical element of a decision-making process that can produce a successful outcome.

Data collection systems not only assist during a disaster but also in the aftermath. Maintaining accountability throughout the immediate impact and in the following months serves to demonstrate the characteristics of the displaced and the medical needs and interventions essential to properly care for affected individuals. Communication coordination is essential to categorize victims, coordinate and track the transportation of victims, manage emergency management resources, and allow hospitals to respond appropriately. The use of ICS alleviates additional chaos, streamlines efficiency, and coordinates effective integration within the community. Additionally, an Internet-based tracking system reduces the confusion during MCIs by tracking all victims receiving medical intervention.

Oklahoma completed a rapid needs assessment when Hurricane Katrina evacuees arrived in the state and found that many survivors experienced multiple emotional traumas, including witnessing grotesque scenes and dealing with the disruption of social systems. Many had preexisting psychopathologies predisposing them to PTSD. West Virginia also performed a needs assessment of evacuees and identified the following: 25% reported an acute illness and 46% had at least one chronic medical condition. A further breakdown determined that dental care, eyeglasses, dentures, and medical services (respectively) were the greatest needs. Georgia validated many of the aforementioned essentials, elaborating on medication demands for diseases and acute and chronic conditions. Issues can be effectively addressed only with the collection, analysis, and dissemination of data.

PREPARATION FOR PATIENT SURGE

The definition of "first responder" has expanded greatly since the terrorist attacks of 2001. No longer are police, fire, and emergency medical personnel the only first responders. Now those who work in public health and health-care facilities must be included in this definition. Not only must these diverse institutions function in their own field, but they also must constantly coordinate with each other to prevent duplication or omission of services.

All health-care facilities should have an emergency plan and exercise it periodically. Issues that must be addressed by the health-care facility include facility, staffing, supply, distribution of Strategic National Stockpile supplies, and laboratory and possibly evacuation needs.

Primary responsibility for hospital emergency preparedness varies widely, and there is no single discipline or professional group that can be identified as being responsible for preparedness. Also, many communities lack involvement of media outlets and volunteer organizations, and the hospitals have no community plans to respond to surge capacity with regard to pharmaceuticals, supplies, equipment, and isolation. Furthermore, most drills and exercises that are undertaken are short and include only staff on the day shift. Also, disease outbreak information is not collected by way of the Internet in one third of the states, which would cause serious delays in incident reporting.

Local government authorities have little direct control over private health-care assets and therefore have less leverage to promote health-care facility participation in partnership with the disaster response community. Particularly vulnerable are rural facilities that may have fewer connections with other facilities.

In the event of a surge, not only will the health-care facility need to increase bed capacity by 20% to 30%, but they will also need to staff and supply these beds as well. Systems must be in place for the accurate, rapid credentialing of those volunteer professionals who are needed to fill this staffing gap.

During Hurricane Katrina, the health-care facilities in New Orleans demonstrated their vulnerabilities. The hospital disaster plans did not include area-wide issues that developed, such as dependence on electrical power, water, security, and transportation. The facilities were often designed with important infrastructure of the hospital in the basement, which was vulnerable to flooding. There

was no coordination of evacuation of patients from the hospitals or a method for tracking them when they were evacuated. Plans did not include the potential for families of patients, families of staff, persons unaffiliated with the facility, and pets seeking refuge in what, in previous cases, had been a safe place.

Challenges to the ethical treatment of patients may include loss of essential services, loss of infrastructure, shortage of workers, size of affected population, and sudden increase of patients. The Joint Commission standards permit appropriate flexibility and effective response with a scalable approach to manage the variety, intensity, and the duration of disaster in six critical areas of emergency management: communication, resources and assets, safety and security, staff responsibilities, utilities management, and patient clinical and support activities (Box 20.6). Specifically, the most critical elements include ensuring worker and patient safety, maintaining airway and breathing, circulation and blood loss, and maintaining or establishing infection control. During times of surge, some less critical components of care will be delegated to family members.

Certain populations require nontraditional responses related to age, physical or mental limitations, and cultural and ethnic considerations. Knowledge and sensitivity to differences among individuals will expedite assessment and treatment throughout the event.

Professional organizations, academic institutions, and governmental agencies have reviewed past responses and lessons learned to revise and provide recommendations for the ethical treatment of those affected in a mass casualty incident. The local health officer is responsible for interagency collaboration within all communities to provide immediate, rapid, and accurate information necessary for appropriate treatment of victims.

PREPARATION AT HOME
AND ABROAD

The Federal Emergency Management Agency (FEMA) distributes and makes available publications and education for individuals and as training resources for groups. The motto found on the FEMA Web site is:

- Make a Plan
- Get a Kit
- Be Informed

FURTHER CONSIDERATIONS

Mass casualty incidents and large-scale disasters involving children are likely to overwhelm a regional disaster

The Joint Commission defines the specific actions of the organization and sets standards for health-care organizations. They are divided into six critical functions and standards:

- Communicating during emergency conditions
- Managing resources and assets during emergency conditions
- Managing safety and security during emergency conditions
- Defining and managing staff roles and responsibilities during emergency conditions
- Managing utilities during emergency conditions
- Managing clinical activities during emergency conditions

The standards are as follows:

Standard EC.4.13: The organization establishes emergency communications strategies.

Standard EC.4.14: The organization establishes strategies for managing resources and assets during emergencies.

Standard EC.4.15: The organization establishes strategies for managing safety and security during emergencies.

Standard EC.4.16: The organization defines and manages staff roles and responsibilities.

Standard EC.4.17: The organization establishes strategies for managing utilities during emergencies.

Standard EC.4.18: The organization establishes strategies for managing [patient] clinical and support activities during emergencies.

Standard EC.4.20: The organization regularly tests its emergency operation plan.

Standard IC.6.10: The hospital prepares to respond to an influx of infectious patients.

Standard HR.1.25: The hospital may assign disaster responsibilities to volunteer practitioners.

Standard HR.2.20: Staff and licensed independent practitioners describe or demonstrate their roles and responsibilities relative to safety.

Standard IM.2.30: Continuity of information is maintained.

response system. Children have unique vulnerabilities that require special considerations when developing pediatric response systems. The Institute of Medicine suggests that on a day-to-day basis the U.S. health-care system does not adequately provide emergency medical services for children. The variability, scale, and uncertainty of disasters call for a set of guiding principles rather than rigid protocols when developing pediatric response plans. The unique vulnerabilities of children can be categorized into the following: (1) terrorism prevention and preparedness, (2) all-hazards preparedness, (3) post-disaster disease and injury prevention, (4) nutrition and hydration, (5) equipment and supplies, (6) pharmacology, (7) mental health, (8) identification and reunification of displaced children, (9) day care and school, and (10) perinatology.

A complete and coordinated community response requires creation of integrated disaster plans. True readiness can be achieved only by testing and modifying these plans through integrated simulation drills and tabletop exercises. Hospital-wide drills are essential to educate all staff members as to their institutional plan and serve as the only substitute, at present, to firsthand experience.

IMPLICATIONS FOR NURSING

The fundamental concepts of nursing are relevant to disaster situations, such as caring, education, advocacy, treatment, and prevention. Primary, secondary, and tertiary prevention are the mainstays of mitigating adversity. It is recognized that nursing plays an essential role in the coordinated response to unexpected events and subsequent medical intervention.

The readiness of our health-care facilities to respond to terrorist acts or naturally occurring epidemics and disasters has been at the center of public attention since September 11, 2001. The many other tragic events that have occurred throughout the world since then further reinforce the need for all health-care facilities and medical personnel to increase their level of preparedness if they wish to optimize outcomes. Maximizing survival rates and minimizing disability during any MCI hinges on rapid, seamless, and coordinated response between first responders and first receivers.

Conclusions

Evidence-based practice integrates individual clinical expertise with the best available external clinical evidence from systemic research. Research in disaster practice presents a challenge for investigators because of the varied nature of disasters. Retrospective studies have benefited nursing practice by exploring lessons learned and incorporating them to improve the practices of caring for victims of unexpected events.

Research of unexpected events is framed by assumptions that answer the practice questions. The outcomes demonstrate the basis for current performance to improve care and respond effectively. Organizations that have well-thought-out all-hazards plans ready to respond to unexpected situations will have optimal outcomes with limited morbidity and mortality.

EVIDENCE-BASED PRACTICE

Reference Question: Was there a difference in care given between psychiatric nurses and forensic nurses after Hurricane Katrina?

Database(s) to Search: PubMed

Search Strategy: Use the MeSH term "cyclones" and use "OR" in a key word search of "Hurricane Katrina." Search the MeSH terms "forensic nursing" and "psychiatric nursing" individually. Use OR with the types of nursing, and then use AND with the set combining cyclones and Hurricane Katrina.

Selected References From Search:

1. Corrarino, J.E. (2008). Disaster-related mental health needs of women and children. *MCN: The American Journal of Maternal/Child Nursing, 33*(4):242-248.
2. Rhoads, J., Pearman, T., & Rick, S. (2008). PTSD: therapeutic interventions post-Katrina. *Critical Care Nursing Clinics of North America, 20*(1):73-81, vii.

Questions Used to Discern Evidence:

Read the two studies listed, and answer the following questions:

1. What are the differences between the two studies in the design, methods, and results?
2. What are the similarities between the two studies in the number of subjects, measures used, and interventions, if any?
3. What competencies do you need to acquire to work with survivors of disasters?

REVIEW QUESTIONS

1. What are some subspecialties of disaster nursing?
   A. Medicolegal death investigator
   B. First responder
   C. Mental health counselor
   D. All of the above

2. What are the five current pillars of emergency response?
   A. Prevention, preparedness, planning, response, and mitigation
   B. Triage, transport, evaluation, treatment, and counseling
   C. Staffing, training, planning, acting, and evaluating
   D. NDMS, ICS, FAC, FEMA, and DMORT

3. What federal law stipulates the statutory framework for presidential declaration of an emergency or major disaster?
   A. Stafford Act
   B. Comitatus Posse Act
   C. Family Assistance Act
   D. DMORT

4. What provides safety standards for workers and workplace safety standards in the United States?
   A. FDA
   B. OSHA
   C. EEOC
   D. Fair Labor Standards Act

5. What is the management mechanism of choice within the health-care system?
   A. Command and control
   B. Management by objectives
   C. Hospital incident command system (HICS)
   D. HIPAA

6. Describe the four determinations (methodologies) that provide medical certainty in the identification of individuals.
   A. DNA and fingerprints
   B. DNA and picture ID
   C. Dental comparison and medical devices
   D. Both A and C

REVIEW QUESTIONS—cont'd

7. The incident command system is used only for large-scale disasters.
- **A.** True
- **B.** False

8. Which initiative provides guiding principles for communities, states, and the federal government to work together during disasters?
- **A.** Homeland Security Presidential Directives
- **B.** FEMA
- **C.** National Disaster Medical System
- **D.** National Response Framework

9. Children are particularly vulnerable during disasters. Planning should include resources for their specific needs related to:
- **A.** Nutrition and hydration.
- **B.** Reunification with family.
- **C.** Equipment and supplies.
- **D.** All of the above.

10. Critical functions during emergency management, set by the Joint Commission, include:
- **A.** Establishing guidelines for implementing emergency drills.
- **B.** Providing triage, treatment, and psychological support for victims.
- **C.** Managing communication, safety, and staff roles.
- **D.** None of the above.

References

Agency for Healthcare Research and Quality (AHRQ). (2005). *Altered standards of care in mass casualty events: Bioterrorism and other public health emergencies.* AHRQ Publication No. 05-0043. Rockville, MD: AHRQ.

American Nurses Association. (1960). *Special Committee on Nursing in National Defense: The role of the nurse in disaster.* New York: American Nurses Association.

Auf der Heide, E. (1989). *Disaster response: Principles of preparation and response.* St. Louis: CV Mosby. Retrieved June 25, 2008, from http://orgmail2.coe-dmha.org/dr/flash.htm

Aylwin, C., Konig, T., Brennan, N., et al. (2006). Reduction in critical mortality in urban mass casualty incidents: Analysis of triage, surge, and resource use after the London bombings on July 7, 2005. Retrieved December 23, 2006, from www.thelancet.com

Bedfordshire & Luton Community Risk Register. Retrieved from http://www.luton.gov.uk/media%20library/pdf/chief%20executives/emergency%20planning/crr%20public%20version.pdf

Benson, M., Koenig, K.L., & Schultz, C.H. (1996). Disaster triage: START, then SAVE—A new method of dynamic triage for victims of a catastrophic earthquake. *Prehospital Disaster Medicine, 11*(2):117-124.

Bloch, Y.H., Schwartz, D., Pinkert, M., et al. (2007). Distribution of casualties in a mass-casualty incident with three local hospitals in the periphery of a densely populated area: Lessons learned from the medical management of a terrorist attack. *Prehospital Disaster Medicine, 22*(3):186-192.

Brandenburg, M., & Arneson, W. (2005). Pediatric disaster response in developed countries: Ten guiding principles. *American Journal Disaster Medicine, 2*(3):151-162.

Braun, B., Wineman, N., Finn, N., et al. (2006). Integrating hospitals into community emergency preparedness planning. *Annals of Internal Medicine, 144*(11):799-811.

Centers for Disease Control and Prevention. (2004). Personal protective equipment (PPE) in healthcare settings. Retrieved June 4, 2008, from http://www.cdc.gov/ncidod/dhqp/ppe.html

Centers for Disease Control and Prevention. Final Report, NLM Turoff, Hiltz, Department of Homeland Security, p. 17. Retrieved from http://emergency.cdc.gov/

Chung, S., & Shannon, M. (2007). Reuniting children with their families during disasters: A proposed plan for greater success. *American Journal Disaster Medicine, 2*(3):113-117.

Congressional Reports: S. Rpt. 109-322–Hurricane Katrina: A Nation Still Unprepared. Special Report of the Senate Committee on Homeland Security and Governmental Affairs. Retrieved June 14, 2008, from http://www.gpoaccess.gov/serialset/creports/katrinanation.html

Cox, E., & Briggs, S. (2004). New frontiers for critical care. *Critical Care Nurse, 24*(3):21.

Disaster Medical Assistance Team (DMAT). (2002). Retrieved from http://www.dmat.org/

Disaster Mortuary Operational Response Team. (2002). Retrieved from http://www.dmort.org/index.html

Disaster Nursing. (2006). Core Competencies Required for Disaster Nursing. Retrieved from http://www.coe-cnas.jp/english/group_education/core_competencies.html

Disaster Nursing Elective Course, N347/N395. (2007). Retrieved from http://www.utexas.edu/nursing/dp/html/courses/disaster.html

Disaster Victim Identification. (2002). Retrieved from http://www.interpol.int/Public/DisasterVictim/guide/chapitre6.asp

Dossey, B., Selanders, L., Beck, D., et al. (2005). Florence Nightingale today: Healing leadership global action. Silver Spring, MD: American Nurses Association.

Drabbek,T., & Hoetmer, G. (1991). *Emergency management: principles and practice for local government.* Washington, DC: International City Management Association.

Dunlop, A., Isakov, A., Compton, M., et al. (2006). Medical outreach following a remote disaster: Lessons learned from Hurricane Katrina. *Prehospital Disaster Medicine, 21*(6), 390-395.

Emergency Management Assistance Compact. (2008). Retrieved from http://www.emacweb.org

Emergency Nurses Association. (2008). Retrieved from http://www.ena.org/EmergencyPrepared/

Fagan, A., Moore, C., & Warren, H. (2005). Conceptual model of emergency management in the 21st century. Retrieved from http://www.dodccrp.org/events/10th_ICCRTS/CD/papers/147.pdf

Federal Emergency Management Agency (FEMA). (2008). Glossary. Retrieved from https://hseep.dhs.gov/pages/1001Gloss.aspx

Federal Emergency Management Agency (FEMA). (2008). National Response Framework. Retrieved January 25, 2008, from www.fema.gov

Federal Family Assistance Plan for Aviation Disasters. (2000). Retrieved from http://www.ntsb.gov/publictn/2000/SPC0001.pdf

Gray, B., & Hebert, K. (2006). *After Katrina: Hospitals in Hurricane Katrina.* Washington, DC: The Urban Institute. Retrieved from http://www.urban.org/UploadedPDF/411348_katrinahospitals.pdf

Hamilton, J. (2000). An internet-based bar code tracking system: Coordination of confusion at mass casualty incidents. *Prehospital Emergency Care, 4*(4):299-304.

Healthline Report. Retrieved from http://www.aacn.nche.edu/Education/pdf/INCMCECompetencies.pdf

Healthline Report. Retrieved from http://www.dhh.louisiana.gov/offices/publications/pubs-1/April%2012%202006.pdf

Herbert, R., Moline, J., Skloot, G., et al. (2006). The World Trade Center disaster and the health of workers: Five-year assessment of a unique medical screening program. *Environmental Health Perspective, 114*(12):1853-1858. Published online September 6, 2006. DOI: 10.1289/ehp.9592.

Hoard, M., & Tosatto, R. (2006). Medical Reserve Corps: Strengthening public health and improving preparedness. *Disaster Management & Resource, 3*(2):48-52.

Hsu, E. (2006). Healthcare worker competencies for disaster training. *BMC Medical Education, 6*:19.

International Nursing Coalition for Mass Casualty Education (INCMCE). (2003). Retrieved from http://www.aacn.nche.edu/Education/pdf/INCMCECompetencies.pdf

Izbicki, G., Chavko, R., Banauch, G., et al. (2007). World Trade Center "sarcoid-like" granulomatous pulmonary disease in New York City Fire Department rescue workers. *Chest, 131*(5):1414-1423. Epub March 30, 2007, http://chestjournal.org/cgi/content/abstract/131/5/1414

Jhung M., Shenab, N., Rohr-Allegrinni, C., et al. (2007). Chronic disease and disasters medication demands of Hurricane Katrina evacuees. *Journal of Health Care for the Poor and Underserved, 18*(2):369-381.

Joint Commission on Accreditation and of Healthcare Organizations. (2008). *Crosswalk: Current Standards & EPs to SII Standards and EPs.* Retrieved from http://www.jointcommission.org/Standards/Manuals/

Loeb, M. SARS Among Critical Care Nurses, Toronto. (2008). *Emerging Infectious Diseases, 10*(2):251-255.

Maryland Defense Force. (2008). Retrieved from http://www.mddefenseforce.org/units/medical.htm

Maryland Professional Volunteer Corps. Retrieved from http://www.mbon.org/main.php?v=norm&p=0&c=volunteer/index.html

Medical examiners, coroners, and biologic terrorism: A guidebook for surveillance and case management. (2004). *Morbidity and Mortality Weekly Report, 53*(RR-8). Retrieved from http://www.cdc.gov/mmwr/preview/mmwrhtml/rr5308a1.htm

Mitchell, M., Sakraida, T.J., Kameg, K. (2003). Critical incident stress debriefing: Implication for best practice. *Disaster Management and Response, 1*(2):46-51.

Moser Jr., R., Connelly, C., Baker, L., et al. (2006). Development of a state medical surge plan, part I: The procedures, processes, and lessons learned or confirmed. *Disaster Management and Response, 4*(1):19-24.

Moser Jr., R., Connelly, C., Baker, L., et al. (2006). Development of a state medical surge plan, part II: Components of a medical surge plan. *Disaster Management and Response, 4*(2):59-63.

NeSmith, E. (2006). Defining "disasters" with implications for nursing scholarship and practice. *Disaster Management & Response, 4*(3):80-87.

NIMS Training. (2008). Retrieved from http://www.fema.gov/emergency/nims/nims_training.shtm

Norris, F., Byrne, C., Diaz, E., et al. (2001). 50,000 victims speak: An empirical review of the empirical literature, 1981-2001. Washington, D.C.: National Center for PTSD and The Center for Mental Health Services.

O'Neill, P. (2007). The ABCs of disaster response. *Scandinavian Journal of Surgery, 94*(4):259-266.

Pan American Health Organization (PAHO). (2004). *Management of dead bodies in disaster situations.* Retrieved from http://www.paho.org/English/DeadBodiesBook.pdf

Pan American Health Organization. (2006). *Management of dead bodies after disasters: A field manual.* Retrieved from http://www.paho.org/english/dd/PED/DeadBodiesField-Manual.htm

Parish, C. (2005). The London bombings. *American Journal of Nursing, 105*(9). Retrieved from http://www.nursingcenter.com

Pattillo, M. (2003). Mass Casualty Disaster Nursing Course. *Nurse Educator, 28*(6):271-275.

Paturas, J. (2008). Joint Commission Emergency Management Standards revisited: Healthcare facility accreditation requirements for 2008. Retrieved from http://www.emforum.org/vforum/lc080326.htm

Persell, D. (2008). Toward a theory of Homeland Security nursing. *Journal of Homeland Security and Emergency Management, 5*(1), article 12. Retrieved from http://www.bepress.com/jhsem/vol5/iss1/12

Polivka, B. (2008). Public health nursing competencies for public health surge events. *Public Health Nursing*, 25(2):159-165.

Reiter, Y., Farfel, A., Lehavi, O., et al. (2007). Mass casualty incident management, triage, injury distribution of casualties and rate of arrival of casualties at the hospitals: Lessons from a suicide bomber attack in downtown Tel Aviv. Retrieved from Ridenour, M., Cummings, K., Sinclair, J., et al. (2007). Displacement of the underserved: Medical needs of Hurricane Katrina evacuees in West Virginia. *American Journal of Disaster Medicine*, 2(3):113-117.

Rodriguez, S., Tocco, J., Mallonmee, S., et al. (2007). Rapid needs assessment of Hurricane Katrina evacuees–Oklahoma, September 2005. *American Journal of Preventative Medicine*, 33(3):207-210.

Sanford, C., Jui, J., Miller, H., et al. (2006). Medical treatment at Louis Armstrong New Orleans International Airport after Hurricane Katrina: The experience of disaster medical assistance teams WA-1 and OR-2. Retrieved May 15, 2008, from Special Report of the Senate Committee on Homeland Security and Governmental Affairs, http://www.gpoaccess.gov/serialset/creports/pdf/sr109-322/ch24.pdf

Schultz, C. (2007). Improving hospital surge capacity: A new concept for emergency credentialing of volunteers. *Prehospital Disaster Medicine*, 22(3):186-192.

Slepski, L. (2007). Emergency preparedness and professional competency among health care providers during hurricanes Katrina and Rita: Pilot study results. *Journal of Emergency Nursing*, 5(4):99-110.

Suburban Emergency Management Project. (2005). Retrieved from http://www.semp.us/publications/biot_reader.php?BiotID=265

Texas Department of Health. Annex H (Health & Medical Services) to the State of Texas Emergency Management Plan. Retrieved from www.tdh.state.tx.us

University of Hyogo, Graduate School of Nursing. (2006). Core competencies required for disaster nursing. Retrieved from http://www.coe-cnas.jp/english/group_education/core_competencies_list.html

Virginia Defense Force. (2008). Retrieved from http://www.vdf.virginia.gov/pdf/National_Guard_Bureau_10-4.pdf

World Health Organization. (2004). Severe acute respiratory syndrome (SARS). Retrieved June 4, 2008, from http://www.who.int/csr/sars/en/

World Health Organization. (2007). The contribution of nursing and midwifery in emergencies. Retrieved from http://www.who.int/hac/events/2006/nursing_consultation_report_sept07.pdf

Wyand, C. (2006). A proposed model for military disaster nursing. Retrieved June 14, 2008 from http://www.nursingworld.org/MainMenuCategories/ANAMarketplace/ANAPeriodicals/OJIN/TableofContents/Volume112006/Number3/tpc31_416085.aspx

Recommended Resources

Air War College Gateway to the Internet. (2008). http://www.au.af.mil/au/awc/awcgate/awc-lesn.htm

All Hands Information Portal. http://www.all-hands.net/

American Journal of Disaster Medicine. http://www.disaster-medicinejournal.com/

Annals of Emergency Medicine. www.annemergmed.com

Auf der Heide, Erik. (2005). The importance of evidence-based disaster planning. Retrieved May 3, 2008, from http://www.atsdr.cdc.gov/emergency_response/importance_disaster_planning.pdf

Big Medicine. http://www.bigmedicine.ca/index.htm

Disasters. http://www.blackwellpublishing.com/journal.asp?ref=0361-3666&site=1

Emergency Management Institute. http://training.fema.gov/EMIWeb/grams/archives.asp

European Masters in Disaster Medicine. www.dismedmaster.com

The George Washington University Institute for Crisis, Disaster and Risk Management (ICDRM). www.gwu.edu/~icdrm

Health Actions in Crisis. www.who.int/entity/hac/about/structure/en/index.html

Health Resources and Services Administration (HRSA). http://www.hrsa.gov/

International Trauma Life Support (ITLS). http://itrauma.org

ISCRAM (Information Systems for Crisis Response and Management). http://iscram.org

Journal of Traumatic Stress. http://www.springerlink.com/content/104759/

Lessons Learned Information Sharing (LLIS). http://LLIS.gov

Medical Management of Radiological Casualties. (2003). http://www.afrri.usuhs.mil/outreach/pdf/2edmmrchandbook.pdf

Mental Health Web site. http://web4health.info

MMWR. (2004). Medical Examiners, Coroners, and Biologic Terrorism. A Guidebook for Surveillance and Case Management. Available at http://www.cdc.gov/mmwr/preview/mmwrhtml/rr5308a1.htm

National Association of County and City Health Officials. (2008). http://www.naccho.org/topics/emergency/pphr.cfm

National Center Forensic Science/National Institute of Justice. Mass Fatality Incidents: A Planning Guide for Human Identification. Available at http://ncfs.ucf.edu/massfatalityguide.

Pan-American Health Organization. (2005). Disaster myths and realities. *Perspectives in Health*, 10(1). Retrieved from http://www.paho.org/english/dd/pin/Number21_article01.htm

Pan-American Health Organization. www.paho.org.

Prehospital and Disaster Medicine. http://pdm.medicine.wisc.edu

Prevention Web: Building the resilience of nations and communities to disasters. (2008). Retrieved from http://www.preventionweb.net/

Radiation Event Medical Management (REMM). www.remm.nlm.gov

Ready.gov. www.ready.gov

Relief Web. www.reliefweb.int

Sigma Theta Tau International and the American Red Cross. (2008). Disaster preparedness and response for nurses. Retrieved from http://www2.nursingsociety.org/education/case_studies/cases/SP0004.html

Southern Medical Journal. http://www.sma.org/smj/

The Sphere Project. Humanitarian Charter and Minimum Standards in Disaster Response. (2008). Retrieved from www.sphereproject.org

Veenema, T. (2007). *Disaster nursing and emergency preparedness for chemical, biological, and radiological terrorism and other hazards*. New York: Springer Publishing.

WISER (Wireless Emergency Information System for Emergency Responders), a free download from the National

Library of Medicine and available for several handheld platforms as well as a pure online version (WebWISER). http://www.michigan.gov/documents/SalineHighSchool HC060906_163234_7.pdf

World Association for Disaster and Emergency Medicine. http://www.wadem.org

U.S. Army Soldier and Biological Chemical Command. *Guidelines for Mass Fatality Management During Terrorist Incidents Involving Chemical Agents*. Available at http://www.ecbc.army.mil/downloads/cwirp/ECBC_guid. . .'.

INDEX

"f" following a number indicates figure; "t" indicates table